INTERVENTIONAL

and

ENDOVASCULAR THERAPY

of the

NERVOUS SYSTEM

Springer
*New York
Berlin
Heidelberg
Barcelona
Hong Kong
London
Milan
Paris
Singapore
Tokyo*

PEARSE MORRIS, MD

INTERVENTIONAL

and

ENDOVASCULAR THERAPY

of the

NERVOUS SYSTEM

A Practical Guide

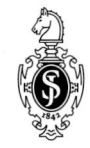

Springer

PEARSE MORRIS, MD
School of Medicine
Wake Forest University
Winston-Salem, NC 27157
USA
pmorris@rad-wfubmc.edu

LIBRARY OF CONGRESS CATALOGING-IN-PUBLICATION DATA
Morris, Pearse.
Interventional and endovascular therapy of the nervous system :
a practical guide / Pearse Morris.
p. ; cm.
Includes bibliographical references and index.
ISBN 0-387-95193-8 (h/c : alk. paper)
1. Cerebrovascular disease—Interventional radiology.
[DNLM: 1. Neuroradiography—methods. 2. Radiography,
Interventional—methods. WL141 M877i 2001] I. Title.
RC388.5 .M667 2001
616.8'106—dc21   00-068785

Printed on acid-free paper.

© 2002 SPRINGER-VERLAG NEW YORK, INC.

All rights reserved. This work may not be translated or copied in whole or in part without the written permission of the publisher (Springer-Verlag New York, Inc., 175 Fifth Avenue, New York, NY 10010, USA), except for brief excerpts in connection with reviews or scholarly analysis. Use in connection with any form of information storage and retrieval, electronic adaptation, computer software, or by similar or dissimilar methodology now known or hereafter developed is forbidden.

The use of general descriptive names, trade names, trademarks, etc., in this publication, even if the former are not especially identified, is not to be taken as a sign that such names, as understood by the Trade Marks and Merchandise Marks Act, may accordingly be used freely by anyone.

While the advice and information in this book are believed to be true and accurate at the date of going to press, neither the author nor the publisher can accept any legal responsibility for any errors or omissions that may be made. The publisher makes no warranty, express or implied, with respect to the material contained herein.

Production coordinated by Leslie Phillips; manufacturing supervised by Jeffrey Taub.
Text design by Steven Pisano.
Typeset by Matrix Publishing Services, Inc., York, PA.
Printed and bound by Maple-Vail Book Manufacturing Group, York, PA.
Printed in the United States of America.

9 8 7 6 5 4 3 2 1

ISBN 0-387-95193-8   SPIN 10790005

Springer-Verlag   New York Berlin Heidelberg
A member of BertelsmannSpringer Science+Business Media GmbH

*Dedicated with love to
Viki, Tristan, and Viveca*

"Forward"

YES, I KNOW that the proper spelling is "Foreword." But considering the subject matter of *Interventional and Endovascular Therapy of the Nervous System: A Practical Guide*, I believe the word "Forward" is actually more appropriate. Forward, because interventional neuroradiology looks boldly toward future concepts of pathophysiology, challenging long-held tenets of disease management. Forward, because neurointerventionalists are constantly moving into uncharted waters, offering new and exciting treatment options for a variety of difficult diseases.

Forward, because there is no turning back. With continual improvements in techniques and outcomes, neurointerventional procedures are likely to grow and prosper. Entrenched customs of practice that have dampened expansion of the field to date will ultimately succumb to the fundamental principle of medical ethics: We must all do what is best for our patients. As Dr. Morris points out in this book, there is a need for controlled trials to establish firmly the role of neurointerventional techniques in the noninvasive management of cerebrovascular diseases.

Turning to the text itself, I believe even physicians who do not personally perform neurointerventional procedures will still find it a valuable educational resource. Radiologists, neurosurgeons, and neurologists will all gain insight into treatment decisions for complicated patients when they better understand the neurointerventionalist's perspective.

In a remarkably succinct text, Dr. Morris has nevertheless managed to encompass the historical evolution of various treatment modalities, the state of the art of current treatment, and future avenues of development, imparting to the reader a comprehensive overview of the field. The current state of technology is thoroughly explained, as is the importance of pharmacological advances in the safe management of neurovascular diseases. Procedure-based discussions, technical table-side illustrations, and reviews of complications all enhance the value of this book to readers at many levels of training.

ALLEN D. ELSTER, MD
Director, Division of Radiologic Sciences; Professor and Chair, Department of Radiology, Wake Forest University School of Medicine, Winston-Salem, North Carolina

Preface

INTERVENTIONAL NEURORADIOLOGY is a wonderful field of work. The impact on people's lives of the techniques and procedures described in this book is often momentous. The nature of the diseases and the risks involved in treatment mean, however, that the costs of learning through mistakes can include great sorrows. This book is intended for students of interventional neuroradiology at various levels of achievement, with an emphasis on teaching where the dangers lie. It aims to provide the core body of knowledge necessary on which to start building a practical experience of one's own. It is intended to teach readers that safety and good patient outcome are the product of diligence not just during, but also before and after the procedure.

The range of neurovascular and other disorders that can be treated by endovascular methods is expanding. As the endovascular methods described herein become more accepted as an alternative to older treatment methods or become the standard of modern care, there will be a greater demand on radiology departments for such services. In an ideal world all practitioners of interventional neuroradiology would serve a two-year fellowship before beginning practice, and all patients in need of neuroendovascular treatment would be referred to a major university hospital. However, the reality is that practical considerations for emergency patients—and other circumstances for elective patients—demand otherwise.

Therefore, this book is written for radiologists or others placed in the position of having to perform neuroendovascular procedures based on a limited experience gained during a diagnostic neuroradiology or general vascular fellowship. It is also intended for neuroradiology fellows and residents rotating on the neurointerventional service during early training. The emphasis throughout is on patient safety and outcome, and learning from mistakes. An inconsequential complication or near-disaster is an infinitely more valuable experience than an elegant success; from the near-disaster one can learn a lesson that may save a future patient's life.

For the most part the basic techniques of interventional neuroradiology are easily learned. The difficulty comes in knowing when to use them, how to use them properly, and where the hidden spring of danger and complications lies. The heavy use of procedure discussions is intended to teach the reader practical case-based knowledge aimed at anticipation and avoidance of complications.

Acknowledgements

Most of the patients described in this book were taken care of at the Wake Forest University School of Medicine and at the University of Vermont Medical Center. This work, therefore, is primarily a reflection of the efforts of the faculty, staff, fellows, and residents of the Neuroradiology, Neurosurgery, Neurology, Anesthesiology, and Otolaryngology Departments of both hospitals, with whom it has been my great privilege to work. Particular thanks are due to colleagues Gary Alsofran MD, Jonathan Burdette MD, David Colonna MD, Stephen Copeland MD, David Durden MD, Allen Elster MD, Curtis Given MD, Steven Glazier MD, Frank Huang-Hellinger MD PhD, Jeffrey Mewborne MD, Michael Olympio MD, Dixon Moody MD, Bela Ratkovits MD, Patrick Reynolds MD, Stephen Tatter MD PhD, Charles Tegeler MD, Dan Williams MD, and John Wilson MD, who all contributed to this work in various ways. Especial acknowledgement is due to the nurses and technologists of the interventional neuroradiology service, and the nursing staff of the recovery units and intensive care units who work so unceasingly on behalf of these patients. The book is dedicated to my wife, Viki, and my family who selflessly, as always, made the time available for its writing. Finally, I thank Mr. Robert Albano of Springer-Verlag for his warm enthusiasm in editorial support of this project throughout.

Contents

"FORWARD," by Allen Elster, MD *vii*

PREFACE *ix*

1 *Platelets and Coagulation* 1
   Antiplatelet Therapy *1*
   Heparin Sodium *12*
   Hirudin/Lepirudin (Refludan) *14*
   Protamine Sulfate *14*
   Thrombolytic Agents *15*

2 *Room, Equipment, Basic Techniques* 21
   Rotational and 3D Angiography *23*
   Flush System *25*
   Catheters and Introducer Sheaths *27*
   Wires and Microwires *28*
   Microcatheters *28*
   Detachable Balloons *31*
   Nondetachable Balloons *34*
   Guglielmi Detachable Coils *34*
   Push Coils and Liquid Coils *37*
   Stents *38*
   Angioplasty Balloons *42*
   Liquid Embolic Agents *43*
   Polyvinal Alcohol *43*
   Gelfoam *44*
   Radiation Exposure and Monitoring *44*
   Catheterizing the Carotid Arteries *47*
   Advancing a Microcatheter *47*
   Closing the Arteriotomy Site *47*

3 *Aneurysms* 55
   Coil Embolization of Intracranial Aneurysms *55*
   Aneurysm Reconstruction with Balloons or Stents *67*
   Complications of Aneurysm Therapy *76*

        Thromboembolic Complications during Aneurysm Embolization *79*
        Arterial Sacrifice in the Treatment of Aneurysms *80*
        Arterial Sacrifice in the Treatment of Subarachnoid Aneurysms *88*

4   *Extracranial Carotid and Vertebral Angioplasty and Stenting* *95*
        The North American Symptomatic Carotid Endarterectomy Trial *97*
        Extracranial Vertebral Artery Angioplasty and Stenting *107*
        Suggested Medication Protocol for Extracranial Stenting *114*

5   *Intracranial Angioplasty and Stenting* *121*
        Clinical Efficacy of Intracranial Balloon Angioplasty *122*
        Risks of Intracranial Balloon Angioplasty *125*
        Intracranial Stent Deployment for Atherosclerotic Disease *134*
        Suggested Medication Protocol for Intracranial Stenting *135*

6   *Endovascular Treatment of Vasospasm* *139*
        Risk Factors for Vasospasm *140*
        Diagnosis of Vasospasm *141*
        Long-Term Histologic Effects of Vasospasm *141*
        Early Endovascular Intervention for Vasospasm *146*
        Papaverine versus Balloon Angioplasty *152*
        Papaverine *154*
        Side Effects and Risks of Papaverine *154*

7   *Dural Arteriovenous Malformations* *159*
        Risks of Dural Arteriovenous Malformationns Are Related to Impact on the
           Venous System *159*
        Clinical Presentation of Dural Arteriovenous Malformations *164*
        Carotid-Jugular Compression Protocol *165*
        Indications for Treatment *166*
        Endovascular Treatment of Dural AVMs *167*

8   *Carotid Cavernous Fistulas* *177*
        Early Treatments for Carotid Cavernous Fistulas *177*
        Endovascular Treatment of Carotid Cavernous Fistulas *178*
        Indications for Treatment *178*
        Materials and Methods *181*

9   *Balloon Test Occlusion and Postocclusion Patient Care* *193*
        Vertebral Artery Test Occlusion *193*
        Techniques of Internal Carotid Artery Test Occlusion *194*
        Complications of Balloon Test Occlusion *197*
        Patient Management Following Permanent Internal Carotid Artery Occlusion *198*

10 *Spine* *203*
        Vertebroplasty *203*
        Spine Arteriovenous Malformations *214*
        Spinal Tumor Embolization *224*

11 Tumor Embolization *229*

Preoperative Devascularization of Tumors *229*
Juvenile Nasal Angiofibroma, Glomus Tumors, and Other Vascular Head and Neck Tumors *237*
Chemotherapy *239*

12 Trauma and Hemorrhage *247*

Triage *247*
General Principles *247*
External Carotid Artery Injuries *252*
Post-Tonsillectomy Bleeding *254*
Postsurgical Vascular Injury *258*
Epistaxis *259*
Internal Carotid and Vertebral Artery Injuries *266*

13 Thrombolysis and Treatment of Acute Stroke *269*

Background *269*
Intraarterial Thrombolysis *270*
Technical and Procedural Considerations *273*
Emergency Angioplasty and Stent Placement *277*
Contraindications to Intraarterial Thrombolysis *279*

14 Venous Thrombotic Disease *281*

Indications for Endovascular Treatment *283*
Techniques *284*

15 Arteriovenous Malformations of the Brain *291*

Risk Factors Predictive of Hemorrhage *292*
Physiological Steal in the Vicinity of AVMs *292*
Normal Perfusion Pressure Breakthrough *293*
Microsurgical Treatment of Arteriovenous Malformations *293*
Radiotherapy for Arteriovenous Malformations of the Brain *294*
Embolization Therapy for Brain Arteriovenous Malformations *296*

INDEX *313*

INTERVENTIONAL

and

ENDOVASCULAR THERAPY

of the

NERVOUS SYSTEM

Chapter 1

Platelets and Coagulation

Antiplatelet Therapy

Platelets play an important role in normal hemostasis by direct effects at the site of vascular injury and by indirect effects through interaction with the hemostatic cascades of circulating blood (Fig. 1.1A–D). Under abnormal circumstances, such as those related to genesis factors of atherosclerosis or factors that prevail during neurointerventional procedures, platelet function plays an important role in the pathogenesis of occlusive and thrombotic complications. Arterial thrombus is frequently described as "white thrombus" composed of densely packed platelets and fibrin. This is in contrast to the loosely packed "red thrombus" of venous thrombosis which contains a greater proportion of erythrocytes. For safe neurointerventional work within the arteries, familiarity with the currently available antiplatelet and antithrombotic drugs is necessary.

The likelihood of arterial thrombosis under pathologic or procedural circumstances is influenced by factors summarized as Virchow's triad:

- Alterations in blood flow.
- The thrombogenicity of the endothelial surface.
- The thrombogenicity of circulating activated physiological and pathological hemostatic factors.

The role of platelets in hemostasis can be understood as taking place in two stages: adhesion, followed by activation/aggregation.[1] However, the processes of adhesion and aggregation have a complex interaction with the normal coagulation pathways of blood with numerous bioamplifying and biomodulatory feedback loops, which serve to maintain vessel integrity on the one hand, but prevent spontaneous thrombosis in the healthy state on the other (Figs. 1.1A,B).[2]

In many circumstances the initial platelet response is invoked at the time of exposure of subendothelial matrix or collagen through either intimal injury or pathogenic processes. Platelet adhesion and aggregation are mediated in large part by glycoprotein-receptors found on the surface of the platelet membrane. This initial step is not currently the focus of antiplatelet drugs in clinical use, but this may change in the future. Adhesion of the platelet membrane to collagen or the subendothelial matrix is mediated by specific binding between integrin and non-integrin glycoproteins on the platelet membrane with ligands such as collagen, fibronectin, laminin, von Willebrand factor, and thrombospondin (Fig. 1.1A). Among the most important sites recognized so far in this process are

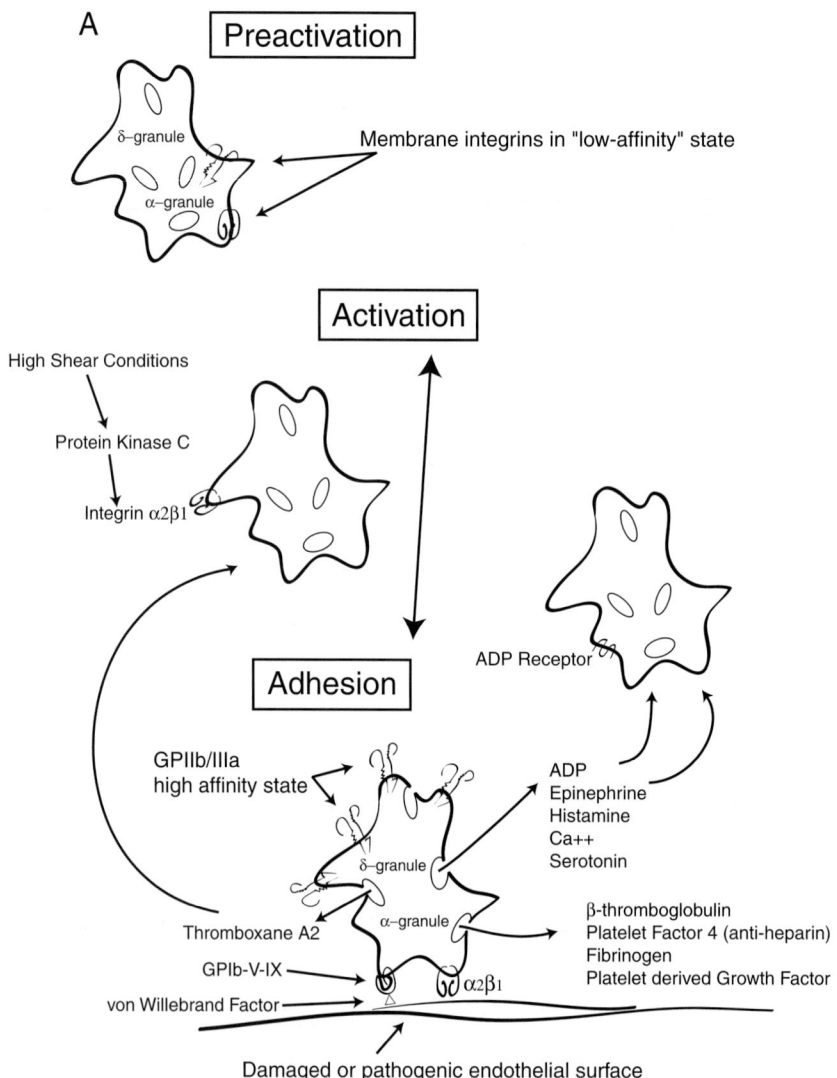

FIGURE 1.1A • The sequence of platelet activation and adhesion is a progressively self-amplifying process whereby release of α and δ granules from the activated platelet causes activation of adjacent platelets. An accompanying change in the affinity state of the glycoprotein receptors in the platelet membrane results in platelet binding with von Willebrand factor, facilitating platelet adhesion to the damaged or pathogenic endothelial surface.

the GPIb/IX receptor, the von Willebrand factor, and the membrane integrin α2β1.[3] Activation of the GPIb/IX receptor may be triggered by abnormal shear stress, as may prevail at the site of atherosclerotic disease. This occurs by a protein kinase C mediated pathway.[4] Moreover, there is evidence that stroke patients have a state of potentiated platelet aggregation in response to abnormal shear stress.[5] The GPIb/IX and integrin α2β1 adhesion sites on the platelet membrane are the focus of interest for potential future antiplatelet agents, including some snake venoms that exert a systemic hemorrhagic effect through a proteolytic action at these sites (Figs. 1.1C,D).[6–9] As the platelets adhere

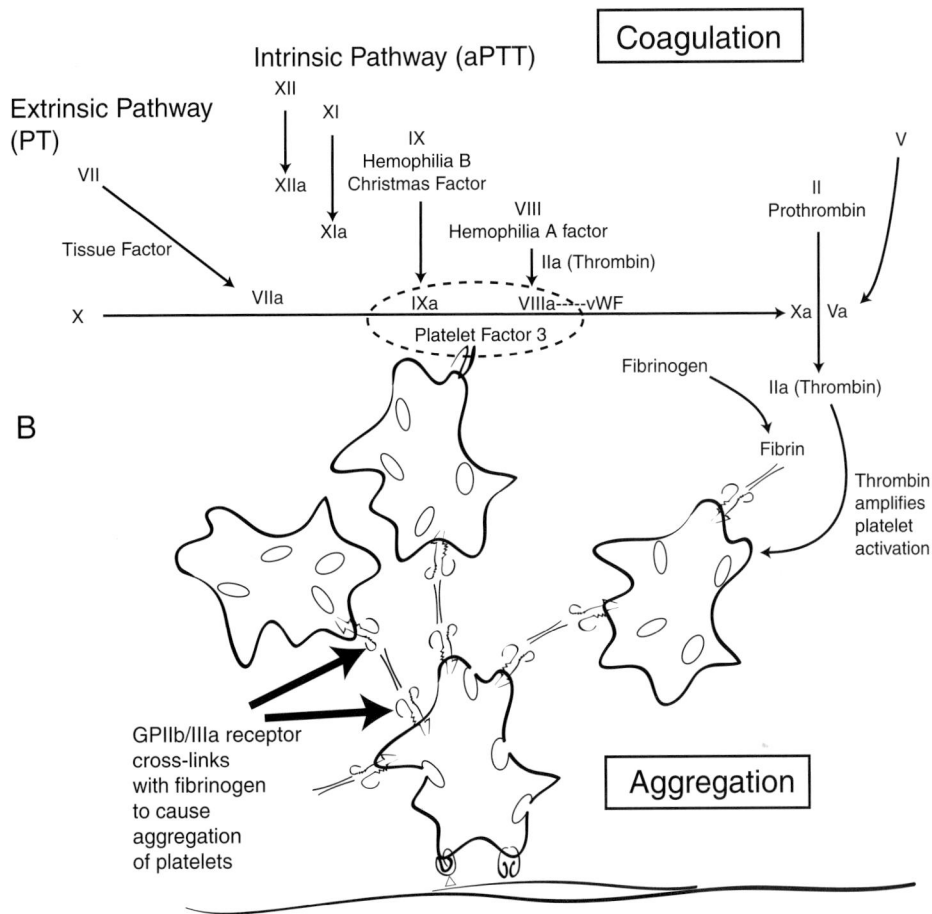

FIGURE 1.1B • A pivotal result of platelet activation is the change of the glycoprotein IIb/IIIa receptor to a state of high affinity for binding with fibrinogen. This step represents the final convergent focus of the coagulation cascade and platelet activation by which interaction "white" arterial thrombus is formed.

to collagen, there is "activation" of the platelet with alteration in shape and mobilization of intracellular calcium. Cytoplasmic α and δ granules merge with the outer membrane and release their contents into the plasma. These granular contents include adenosine diphosphate (ADP), thromboxane A2, norepinephrine, β-thromboglobulin, platelet factor 4 (PF4), serotonin, von Willebrand factor, and fibrinogen, acting to promote a cascade of excitatory events promoting further platelet activation and aggregation.

Activation of platelets can be stimulated by a variety of biochemical and mechanical routes, some of which are vulnerable to diverse pharmacological agents, but these various routes ultimately converge to a common final step. Among the most important of the surface glycoprotein receptors of platelets is an important integrin group composed of α (IIb) and β (IIIa) subunits with variable specific affinities for different ligands. An important result of the activation of platelets is a change in the GPIIb/IIIa receptor from a state of low affinity to one of high affinity for binding with fibrinogen. Platelet aggregation and platelet-stimulated thrombosis depend entirely upon this receptor because it is at this receptor that fibrin binds with the platelet membrane. There are approximately 50,000–80,000 such receptors per platelet, and activated

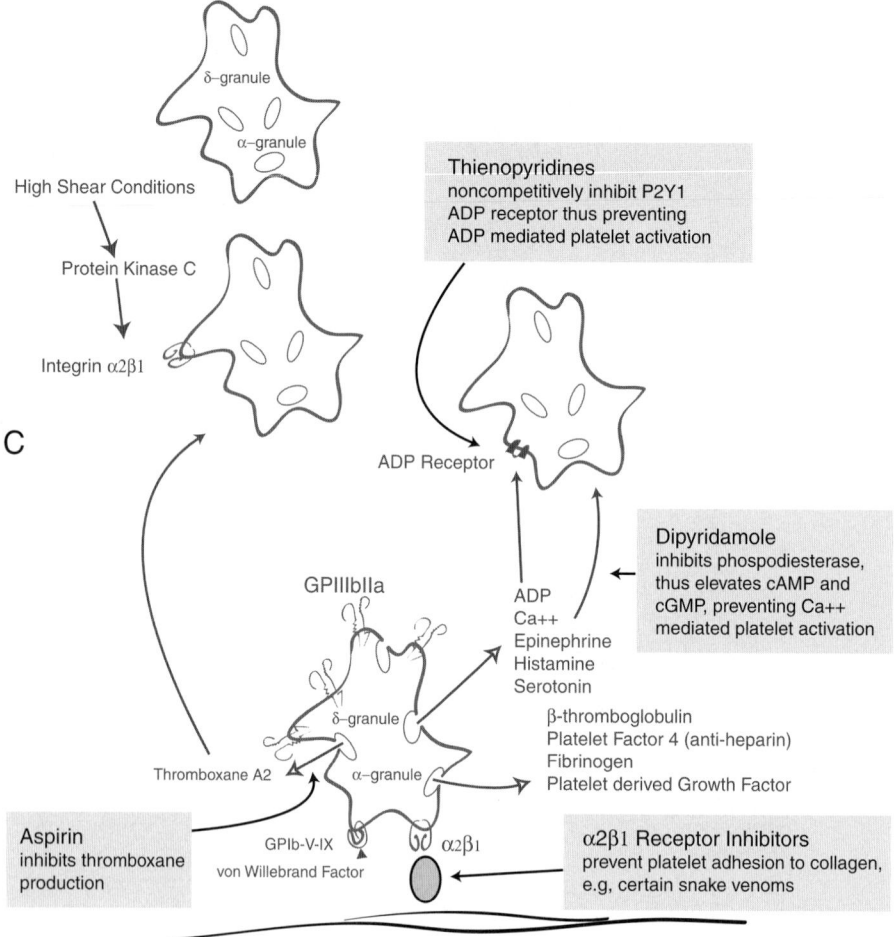

FIGURE 1.1C • The sites of action of the oral antiplatelet agents are illustrated using Figure 1.1A as a template. Their action is relatively early in the process compared with the GPIIb/IIIa inhibitors. Also illustrated is the potential site of action of future inhibitors of the $\alpha2\beta1$ surface receptor, similar in action to hemorrhagic toxins found in some snake venoms.[10] Such agents would have the potential of preventing platelet adhesion to endothelial surfaces.

platelets can bind >40,000 molecules of fibrinogen per cell. The final common pathway for platelet aggregation, regardless of cause, involves binding of fibrinogen to the activated glycoprotein IIb/IIIa receptor on the platelet membrane, making this a pivotal event in hemostasis and thrombosis (Fig. 1.1B). The ability of the glycoprotein IIb/IIIa inhibitor agents to suppress this final step in the process of platelet aggregation, described below, has had a significant impact on the clinical safety of percutaneous procedures.

The importance of the glycoprotein receptors of the platelet membrane is recognized in specific disease states. The role of the GPIIb/IIIa receptors was recognized from studies of Glanzmann's thrombasthenia, a hereditary condition with recurrent mucocutaneous bleeding related to diminution or absence of functional GPIIb/IIIa receptors.[10] Other rare platelet-related bleeding disorders, Bernard-Soulier syndrome, and platelet-type von Willebrand disease, are associated with abnormalities of the platelet GPIb-V-IX receptor.[11–13] The hemor-

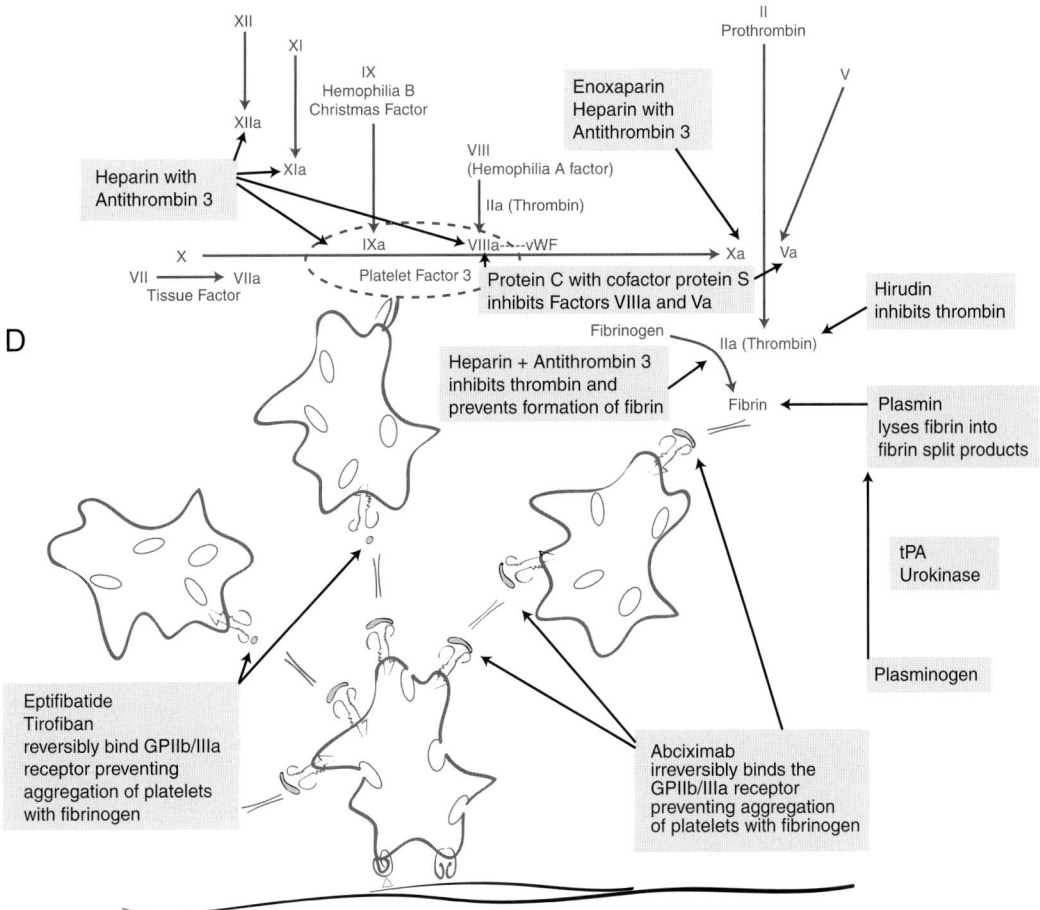

FIGURE 1.1D • The sites of action of the principal inhibitors of the coagulation cascade and thrombolytic agents are illustrated using Figure 1.1B as a template. Also illustrated are the GPIIb/IIIa inhibitor agents. Abciximab, a much larger molecule than eptifibatide or tirofiban, has a less specific action than its smaller counterparts. Binding by abciximab is noncompetitive and irreversible. Also illustrated is the site of action of Protein C and its cofactor Protein S, important inhibitors of spontaneous arterial or venous thrombosis.

rhagic effects of some snake venoms have been recognized to be due to the protease effects of the venom on the structure of the GPIb-IX receptor and on the adhesive von Willebrand factor.[6,9,14]

Aspirin

Prior to the advent of the thienopyridine derivatives, aspirin was the standard therapy recommended by the American Heart Association for patients with symptomatic atherosclerotic disease, with a 27% reduction in vascular mortality and morbidity in patients treated.[15] Aspirin inhibits platelet aggregation by irreversibly blocking the action of cyclooxygenase, an enzyme necessary for the production of thromboxane A_2. Thromboxane A_2 promotes thrombosis by causing vasoconstriction and promoting platelet activation (Fig. 1.1C).

Since it was first recognized in the 1950s that aspirin had a role in reducing the risk of myocardial infarction,[16] aspirin has been demonstrated in a larger number of trials at differing dose-levels to have a significant impact on reducing risk of stroke and myocardial infarction.[17,18] More recent studies have recommended doses of 50–325 mg daily, i.e., lower than those used previously, with evidence suggesting that the lower doses are equally effective. Aspirin is a relatively weak inhibitor of platelet function as it does not affect Thromboxane A_2 independent pathways of platelet aggregation.

Thienopyridine Derivatives

The thienopyridine agents, ticlopidine and clopidogrel, inhibit the $P2Y_1$ platelet-membrane receptor, which is responsible for ADP-mediated platelet aggregation (Fig. 1.1C). Ticlopidine and clopidogrel inhibit platelet aggregation through irreversible inhibition of the cytoskeletal effects of adenosine diphosphate (ADP) on the platelet membrane.[19–21] They have a synergistic effect with aspirin on efficacy of platelet inhibition. Compared with aspirin, the thienopyridines are generally tolerated well by most patients, except for cost concerns. The thienopyridine derivatives have fewer side-effects of gastrointestinal irritation but are more likely to cause skin rashes and diarrhea. They seem to be slightly more effective than aspirin alone in preventing major vascular events in the cranial and extracranial circulations.[22] For this reason the uncommon hematologic complications of neutropenia and thrombocytopenic purpura seem to be worthwhile risks in particular patients treated with these drugs. Clopidogrel is thought to be somewhat safer than ticlopidine.

Ticlopidine Hydrochloride (Ticlid)

Ticlopidine is a thienopyridine compound that causes inhibition of platelet aggregation and degranulation, producing a prolongation of bleeding time. It functions by inhibiting ADP-induced platelet-fibrinogen binding, thereby preventing the platelet-platelet aggregation that plays the initial role in hemostatic plug formation. The clinical efficacy of ticlopidine has been demonstrated in the TASS trial (Ticlopidine Aspirin Stroke Study)[23] in which ticlopidine 250 mg b.i.d. was more effective than aspirin 650 mg b.i.d. at preventing stroke in patients at risk (13.8% stroke rate with ticlopidine versus 18.1% with aspirin). In patients who have previously suffered a stroke, ticlopidine reduces the risk of subsequent stroke significantly, from 24% to 18%.[24] Ticlopidine with aspirin has been demonstrated to have a more powerful effect in preventing acute stent closure in the coronary arteries compared with oral anticoagulants with aspirin,[25] implying that thienopyridines have a synergistic effect with aspirin on platelet inhibition. This has been confirmed with ex vivo platelet aggregation studies comparing the effects of aspirin alone, ticlopidine alone, and a combination of the two in coronary stent patients.[26]

Ticlopidine has been found to have a number of life-threatening side-effects including neutropenia (2.4%), peaking in incidence 4–6 weeks after start of treatment,[27] and thrombotic thrombocytopenic purpura (1 in 2,000 to 10,000), peaking at 3–4 weeks after start of treatment.[28,29] Thrombotic thrombocytopenic purpura following ticlopidine therapy can have a 20% or higher mortality, but can be treated successfully with plasma exchanges.[30] During the first 3 months of treatment patients must be monitored every 2 weeks to detect hematologic side-effects, or for 2 weeks after discontinuation if treatment is stopped during the first 3 months. Less serious side-effects such as skin rashes or urticaria can be seen also, requiring cessation of therapy. The recommended dose is 250 mg b.i.d., with a minimum of 3 days of treatment in anticipation of elective percutaneous procedures.

Clopidogrel (Plavix)

Clopidogrel bisulfate is a thienopyridine derivative supplied as 75 mg tablets, and was developed as a safer alternative to ticlopidine. Clopidogrel exercises its effect on platelet aggregation by inhibiting ADP-mediated activation of the GPIIb/IIIa receptor. It works by irreversibly modifying the platelet ADP receptor; therefore its effect persists for the lifespan of the platelet. A steady-state effect of platelet inhibition is achieved after 5 days of a daily oral dose of 75 mg. For emergency procedures a loading dose of 300 mg orally has also been demonstrated to be effective in coronary patients.

Clopidogrel has been demonstrated to be at least as effective as aspirin in reducing rates of ischemic stroke, myocardial infarction, or vascular death in at-risk populations.[31] An animal study using unpolished nitinol stents demonstrated that clopidogrel was more potent than aspirin at preventing acute in-stent thrombosis in situations involving high shear.[32] It is speculated that under high shear conditions platelet aggregation is stimulated by a diacylglycerol-independent pathway of protein kinase C activation that is not affected by aspirin.[4] Clinically it has been shown that the combination of clopidogrel (300 mg loading dose and 75 mg daily for 4 weeks) with aspirin (325 mg daily) is as effective as ticlopidine (500 mg loading dose and 250 mg twice daily for 2 weeks) with aspirin at preventing stent thrombosis in the coronary arteries.[21,33]

The overall clinical toleration of clopidogrel by patients is similar to that of aspirin 325 mg daily. In the CAPRIE trial 6 out of 9,599 patients taking clopidogrel developed severe neutropenia, giving this drug a much safer profile than its chemical relative ticlopidine.[31] Thrombotic thrombocytopenic purpura has been identified in a small number of patients taking clopidogrel, usually within the first two weeks of treatment.[34] Milder but significant allergic-type reactions requiring withdrawal of the drug can be seen also. For long-term maintenance prophylaxis cost is an important factor; clopidogrel is considerably more expensive than aspirin.[20] For short-term treatment in preparation for and following a stenting procedure, this is a less important consideration.

Glycoprotein IIb/IIIa Inhibitors

Several powerful inhibitor agents that block the action of the GPIIb/IIIa receptor and thus prevent platelet aggregation are available for intravenous administration. Oral preparations are in development. The first of this group of drugs to be released in 1995 and the most extensively used since then is abciximab. Abciximab evolved from work involving isolation of a mouse monoclonal antibody against the GPIIb/IIIa receptor.[35] Development of eptifibatide derives from the recognition of naturally occurring GPIIb/IIIa inhibitors in snake venoms, particularly the protein barbourin from the southeastern pygmy rattlesnake *Sistrurus miliaris barbouri*.[36,37] Various related toxins have been discovered in the venoms of the Viperidae family, each toxin named for the genus of the particular snake from which it was purified.[9] These toxins have been named "disintegrins" because their effect is to blockade the arginine-glycine-aspartic acid RGD recognition site on the integrin family of membrane proteins (Fig. 1.1D). The integrin receptors play an important role in cytoadhesive homeostasis and cell-to-matrix binding phenomena, including those involved in blood clotting and platelet aggregation. The competitive effect of disintegrins at the RGD site has been therapeutically harnessed for the control of platelet function and is the focus of interest here. Other intriguing potential therapeutic effects of disintegrins include prevention of implantation of melanoma metastases and prevention of osteoporosis by virtue of interaction with the membrane receptors of osteoclasts.[38]

The efficacy and safety of the GPIIb/IIIa inhibitors have been studied in a number of large, international, double-blind, acronymous studies of patients undergoing percutaneous procedures for atherosclerotic coronary disease.

- The EPIC trial (Evaluation of 7E3 for the Prevention of Ischemic Complications)[39]
- The EPILOG trial (Evaluation in PTCA to Improve Long-Term Outcome with Abciximab GPIIb/IIIa Blockade)[40]
- The CAPTURE trial (c7E3 Fab Antiplatelet Therapy in Unstable Refractory Angina)[41]
- The EPISTENT trial (Evaluation in PTCA to Improve Long-term Outcome with Abciximab GPIIb/IIIa Blockade Study Group-Stent)[42]
- The RESTORE trial (Randomized Efficacy Study of Tirofiban for Outcomes and Restenosis)[43]
- The IMPACT-II trial (Integrilin to Minimize Platelet Aggregation and Coronary Thrombosis)[44]

These studies demonstrated in large numbers of patients that use of GPIIb/IIIa blockade agents during percutaneous coronary artery procedures has a significant and synergistic impact on patient outcome with 35% to 50% reduction in risk of death, myocardial infarction, and myocardial ischemia immediately following the procedure and at 30 days.[45,56] A randomized trial comparing coronary stenting in combination with abciximab and treatment with tissue plasminogen activator (alteplase) in acute myocardial infarction showed a significantly superior degree of myocardial salvage in the former group and a lower cumulative incidence of death, reinfarction, and stroke at 6 months (8.5% vs. 23.2%).[47] This particular study raises intriguing questions on whether the same results could be achieved in the cerebrovascular circulation with the same treatment methods.

Most patients in the large trials of GPIIb/IIIa blockade were treated simultaneously with aspirin. The EPIC trial used a higher dose regimen for heparin with a mean activated clotting time (ACT) of 401 seconds. The rates of adverse major bleeding in this trial (16.9%) were higher than those subsequently seen in the EPILOG trial (7.6%) when the ACT was maintained at 300–350 seconds. For most neurointerventional procedures involving abciximab or one of the other GPIIb/IIIa inhibitors, maintaining a procedural ACT of 200–300 seconds is probably therefore a reasonable balance of risks. The GPIIb/IIIa inhibitors have also been studied as the primary management of acute coronary syndrome in patients with unstable angina and non–Q wave infarctions[48–51] where results are more heterogeneous. Oral preparations of GPIIb/IIIa inhibitors are a focus of interest for the future.[52,53]

Abciximab (ReoPro)
Abciximab is the Fab fragment of a monoclonal antibody prepared from a process involving mammalian cell culture. It binds noncompetitively with the glycoprotein GPIIb/IIIa receptor of human platelets and inhibits platelet aggregation. It also affects the vitronectin ($\alpha V \beta 3$) receptor on platelets, endothelium, and smooth muscle cells (Fig. 1.1D). A typical loading dose in humans immediately blocks >80% of platelet receptors and virtually completely blocks all platelet aggregation. This effect begins to diminish quickly, but the degree of platelet inhibition can be kept at >80% by a continuous infusion of abciximab, generally for 12 hours following the procedure. The plasma half-life of free abciximab is approximately 10 to 30 minutes, but the effect of the drug on platelet aggregation takes 48 hours to wear off.[54] It has been speculated that the effect of abciximab on the vitronectin receptor might have a therapeutic role in preventing intimal hyperplasia and restenosis,[55] but this has not been clinically demonstrated.[56]

The role of abciximab and the other GPIIb/IIIa inhibitors in procedures involving balloon angioplasty and stenting of the cranial arteries appears likely to emulate that experienced with these agents in the coronary circulation. Anecdotally, they have been used very effectively in preventing fresh accumulation of thrombus during cases of intraarterial thrombolysis of the carotid and vertebrobasilar arteries. A powerful aspect of this adjunctive use of GPIIb/IIIa inhibitors in the emergency context of acute arterial thrombolysis is that part of the loading dose can be given systemically or intraarterially via the microcatheter directly into the point of thrombosis (Fig. 1.2). The adjunctive effect of abciximab during thrombolysis has been demonstrated in the coronary circulation, where an equivalent thrombolytic outcome can be achieved with half the control dose of alteplase (tPA) when used with abciximab, due to the direct thrombolytic effects of abciximab.[57,58]

Dose. Abciximab is supplied as a clear colorless fluid in 5 ml vials containing 2 mg/ml. The loading intravenous dose, 0.25 mg/kg for adults, is calculated by body weight and administered over the course of a minute or two. A 12-hour intravenous infusion at 0.125 μg/kg/min then follows. For those patients who will require abciximab or any of the intravenous GPIIb/IIIa inhibitors during a procedure, a second IV line is inserted before the case to facilitate infusion of this drug afterwards, separate from the site used for intravenous fluids and other drugs.

Precautions. Administration of abciximab provoked formation of human anti-chimeric antibodies in approximately 6% of subjects in the EPIC,

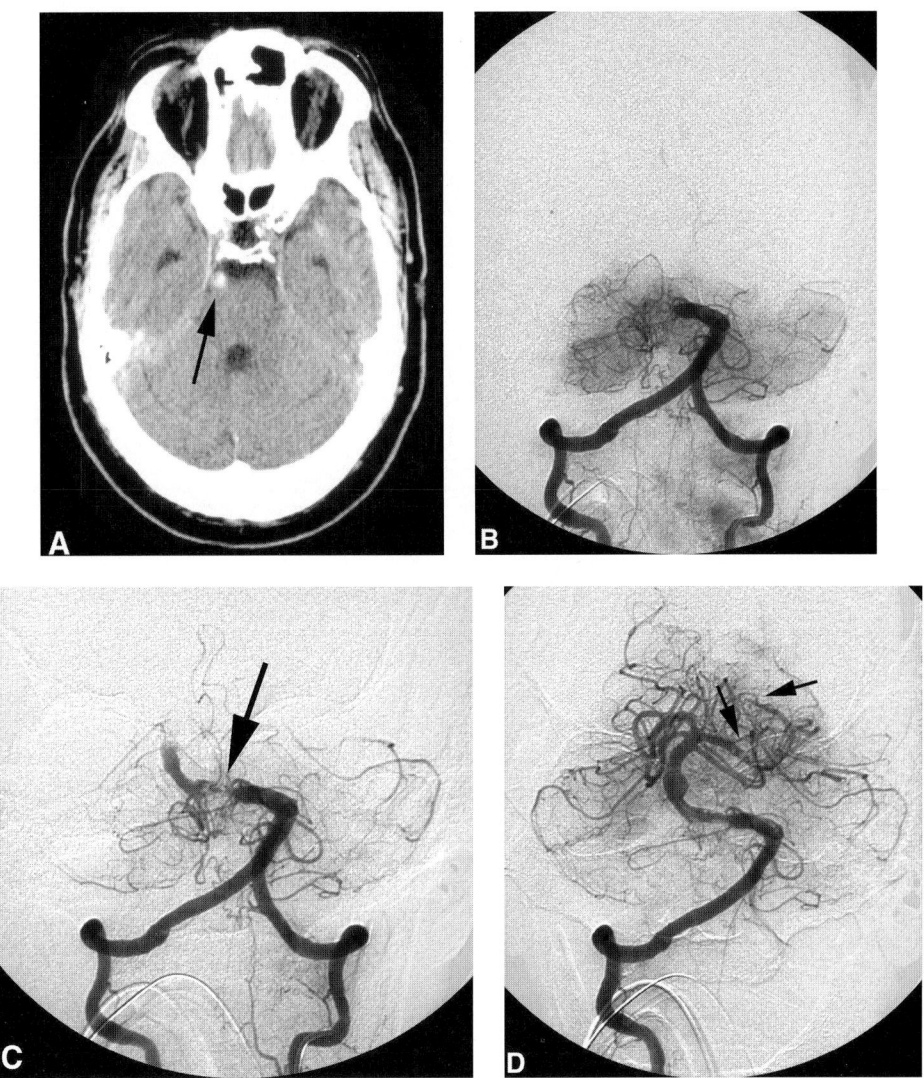

FIGURE 1.2 • A 60-year-old male presented abruptly with acute decline in brainstem function over the course of three hours. A noncontrast CT scan (arrow in image A) demonstrated density in the mid-basilar artery, suggesting thrombosis. After emergency intubation, a left vertebral artery injection (image B) demonstrated complete occlusion of the mid-basilar artery. Only the territories of the inferior cerebellar arteries are perfused. After 650,000 units of Urokinase (image C) only moderate progress at reopening the basilar artery has been achieved and an inciting severe stenosis of the basilar artery has been identified (arrow). Within a few minutes of this result the basilar artery had completely occluded anew and reverted to its pretreatment appearance. The 5F catheter system was exchanged for a 6F system and a 6F Envoy catheter (Cordis) was advanced in the right vertebral artery. A Traverse (Guidant) 0.014-inch wire was curved slightly at its tip and steered with a torque-device across the stenosis. A 3-mm Neptune (Bard) balloon catheter was advanced and inflated slowly for 10 sec at 6 atm. A bolus of abciximab was administered simultaneously followed by an infusion calculated by body weight. This resulted in immediate and sustained opening of the basilar artery (image D). Despite the presence of a small distal clot in the posterior cerebral arteries (arrows in D), the patient sustained only minimal acute brainstem injury from which he made a complete recovery.

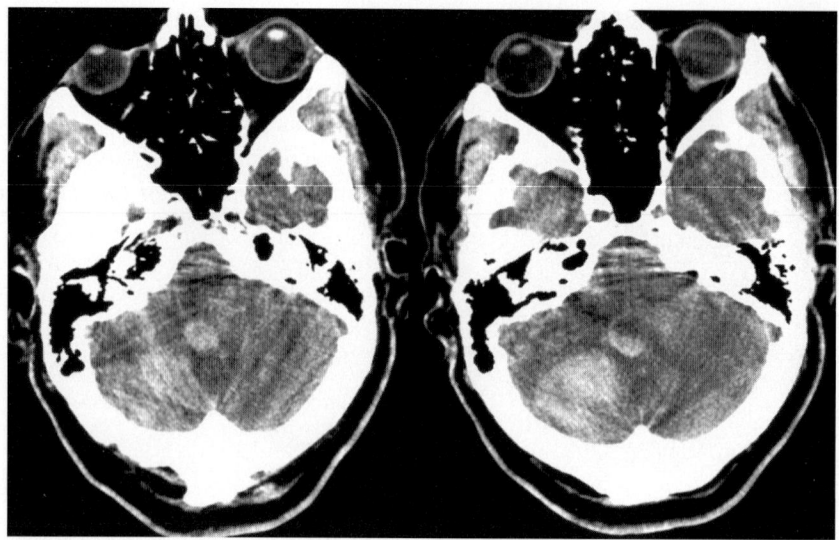

FIGURE 1.3 • A CT scan is shown of a severely hypertensive patient 2 days following a coronary stent procedure during which abciximab was administered. The patient's platelet count fell to <5,000 per µL within the first 24 hours and abciximab was discontinued. It was thought that the combination of severe hypertension, thrombocytopenia, and an embolic infarction of the cerebellar hemisphere resulted in a severe hemorrhage as shown, requiring surgical evacuation of hematoma. The patient sustained severe neurologic injury.

EPILOG, and CAPTURE trials. This suggests that prudent caution should be exercised when administering abciximab to patients with previous exposure to this drug, although all evidence suggests that readministration is safe.[45]

Abciximab is an extremely powerful drug. It is common to see petechial discoloration in the groin related to preprocedure shaving after this drug is used. Even minor trauma related to intubation of the patient before the procedure can cause some persistent oozing of mucosal sites afterwards. Petechiae or bruising can be easily induced by repetitive use of an automated blood pressure cuff during the procedure with use of abciximab. The possibility of spontaneous internal hemorrhage at sites of trauma, surgery, or infarction needs to be considered carefully in patients who might be candidates for this drug (Fig. 1.3). Therefore relative contraindications to abciximab in neurointerventional patients include:

- Active or recent (<6 weeks) internal bleeding, or recent surgery
- History of CVA within past 2 years. This is a relative contraindication, and the recommendation of a 2-year cautionary period probably represents an excessive concern for many patients with cerebrovascular disease. A prospective trial of abciximab in acute stroke demonstrated no significant increase in rates of intracranial hemorrhage compared with control patients (7% versus 5%), suggesting that this agent is safe to use in endovascular procedures, even in the setting of acute stroke.[59]
- Thrombocytopenia <100,000 platelets/µL
- Severe hypertension, systolic BPr >200 mm Hg
- Concurrent use of low-molecular-weight dextran. In the EPIC[39] trial a small number of patients were given abciximab and dextran during the same procedure and experienced a high rate of spontaneous internal bleeding.

A single-wall puncture of the femoral artery is recommended by the manufacturers when use of the GPIIb/IIIa inhibitors is anticipated, but in practice it is not absolutely essential. Following the procedure the femoral sheath should not be removed until the Activated Clotting Time has fallen below 200 seconds.

Thrombocytopenia with Abciximab. Abciximab and the other parenteral GPIIb/IIIa inhibitors can be associated with a precipitous drop in platelet count in a small number of patients (0.5% to 5.0%). This may be due to circulating antibodies[60] or to a paradoxical platelet activation and aggregation due to atypical interactions between the GPIIb/IIIa receptor and abciximab.[61] Thrombocytopenia is considered mild at 100,000–149,000 per μL, moderate at 50,000–99,000 per μL, and severe for levels lower.[62] Predictors of thrombocytopenia include age >65 years, weight <90 kg, and baseline platelet count <150,000.[63] A complete blood profile including platelet count is mandatory prior to the procedure as a baseline. Repeat platelet counts 2–4 hours following the procedure and on the following day are recommended to detect this side effect.

Management of GPIIb/IIIa-related thrombocytopenia involves excluding the possibility of pseudothrombocytopenia from platelet clumping in EDTA. A repeat sample in sodium citrate or a blood smear should be sent. If the platelet count falls below 100,000–120,000 per μL or falls by more than 25% of baseline, the abciximab infusion should be discontinued. If the count falls still lower, then heparin and antiplatelet agents should be suspended too, and platelet infusions are recommended for counts below 50,000 per μL.[64] A pooled analysis of the large GPIIb/IIIa-blockade trials indicated that thrombocytopenia was not significantly associated with eptifibatide or tirofiban.[65]

Eptifibatide (Integrilin)

Eptifibatide is a cyclic heptapeptide produced by a process of solution-phase peptide synthesis. In contrast to abciximab, binding by eptifibatide to the GPIIb/IIIa receptor is specific and reversible (Fig. 1.1D). After discontinuation of the drug, platelet function normalizes in 4 hours. The plasma half-life is approximately 2.5 hours, with approximately 50% of the clearance taking place in the kidneys. In patients with moderate renal impairment (serum creatinine 1–2 mg/dL) an adjustment of dose is not necessary. Because of the reversibility of the binding between eptifibatide and the GPIIb/IIIa receptor, some practitioners have favored this drug over abciximab with the view that potential complications of adverse bleeding might be more easily controlled. Additionally, surgery within 12 hours following discontinuation of an infusion of abciximab is associated with increased risks of hemorrhage, although the effects of abciximab can be counteracted by platelet infusions.[66]

Dose. Two dose schedules were studied in coronary patients. The PURSUIT study[50] used a loading dose of 180 μg/kg followed by a 2-μg/kg per minute infusion for 24 hours following a percutaneous procedure. The IMPACT II[44] study used lower doses, a bolus of 135 μg/kg followed by an infusion of 0.5–0.75 μg/kg per minute. Results with the higher dose of eptifibatide were more favorable without any dose-related increase in adverse hemorrhage. Eptifibatide is supplied as a clear, colorless solution for intravenous administration. The recommended dose for percutaneous procedures is a bolus of 180 μg/kg followed by a 2μg/kg per minute infusion for 24 hours. However, for patients with severe renal impairment, the lower dose regimen may be safer. In patients with compromise of flow or other difficulties requiring intensive management, the infusion of eptifibatide can be continued longer (up to 96 hours).

Tirofiban Hydrochloride (Aggrastat)

Tirofiban hydrochloride monohydrate is a nonpeptide tyrosine derivative delivered as a powder that is soluble in water. It is a reversible antagonist of fibrinogen binding with the GPIIb/IIIa receptor of platelets and provides a >90% inhibition of platelet aggregation after a 30-minute loading dose (Fig. 1.1D). Platelet function normalizes in approximately 4 hours following discontinuation. The plasma half-life is 2 hours. The major routes of excretion involve the kidney.

Studies of the efficacy of tirofiban in the coronary population[43,48,49] showed highly significant reduction in end points of myocardial ischemia, infarction, or death in patients treated with tirofiban and heparin compared with patients treated with heparin alone. Relative contraindications are similar to those for abciximab and eptifibatide.

The recommended intravenous dose of tirofiban is 0.4 μg/kg per minute for 30 minutes followed by an infusion of 0.1 μg/kg per minute for 12–24 hours following the procedure. There is some ex vivo evidence suggesting that the intensity of platelet inhibition following administration of tirofiban may be slightly less than that seen with eptifibatide and abciximab.[67]

Heparin Sodium

First discovered in 1916, heparin sodium is a preparation of covalently bonded glycosaminoglycan mucopolysaccharides[68] synthesized from bovine lung or porcine gut origins. Its molecular weight ranges from 5,000 to 30,000, explaining its variable pharmacokinetics and heterogeneity of antithrombotic effects. Higher-molecular-weight components are metabolized more quickly than low-molecular-weight components. In solution heparin acts as a strong acid. Heparin exerts its anticoagulant properties at a number of points in the coagulation process. In association with antithrombin III (heparin cofactor) it inhibits the conversion of prothrombin to thrombin and causes inactivation of activated Factor X.[69] By inactivating thrombin at higher concentrations, it prevents conversion of fibrinogen to fibrin. It also inhibits clotting factors IX, XI, and XII (Fig. 1.1D). The bioavailability and clearance of heparin is complex and varies according to the dose administered. Lower doses are cleared more quickly. Overall, heparin has a rapid α (distribution) phase of approximately 10 minutes, but for calculation of the effective half-life in vivo a period of 1.5 hours is usually accurate (range 0.5–2 hours).

A typical loading dose of heparin during neurointerventional procedures would be 60–100 units/kg, sufficient to raise the activated clotting time (ACT) close to 300 seconds.[70] However, many neurointerventionalists prefer to give even more heparin for some procedures, particularly those involving temporary arrest of flow with balloons or other devices. Hourly doses thereafter during a procedure are titrated to the decline of the ACT, typically in the range of 1000–2000 units for adult patients. Additionally, significant systemic doses of heparin can be given in the flush-systems.

A useful rule of thumb is that an arterial sheath should not be removed until the ACT has fallen below 200 seconds, or preferably under 180 seconds. An ACT machine in the neurointerventional room is an essential piece of equipment and provides a more accurate index of heparin function due to its linear dose-response, in contrast to the logarithmic response of the partial thromboplastin time.[71] The HemoTec (Medtronic HemoTec, Inc.) or Hemochron® (International Technidyne Corporation) devices use kaolin activators or diatomaceous earth, respectively, to stimulate coagulation in the tubed sample, and then time the movement of a plunger or a magnet through the sample as an indicator of clotting.[72] Checking the efficacy of loading and maintenance doses of heparin during each case is important for avoiding thromboembolic complications. Sometimes a dose of heparin might be administered incorrectly, or the intravenous line might fail for a number of reasons. Alternatively, postsurgical or infected patients can have variable degrees of resistance to heparin. In these circumstances proceeding with an interventional maneuver without confirming the ACT could have serious consequences. At the end of a case, confirming the reversal of the effect of heparin by protamine or by passage of time is important in avoiding arterial bleeding related to premature sheath removal.

After a case during which the ACT has been maintained at 200–300 seconds, an aPTT on return to the intensive care unit will be reported as high, typically >100–125 seconds. A target aPTT of 60–80 seconds is usually desirable for maintenance heparinization. However, when the heparin is completed suspended, the aPTT can fall precipitously from a very high level to a normal range in a short space of time; if this is not detected, thrombotic complications can occur quickly. Therefore, checking the aPTT every two hours initially after return to the ICU might be prudent in critical cases. Additionally, instead of suspending the heparin infusion temporarily while it descends to the desired therapeutic range, it may be safer to continue heparin at a lower dose so that the descent of the aPTT is more gradual and controlled.

Precautions

Heparin is a potent drug. Overdose or therapeutic doses of heparin can cause severe bleeding during or following neurointerventional procedures. Of particular concern is the combination of heparin with thrombolytic agents, which may be associated with increased risk of hemorrhagic transformation of cerebral infarction in patients undergoing intraarterial thrombolysis. Vigilance is necessary with monitoring of hematocrit and platelet counts in patients on maintenance heparin for early detection of retroperitoneal or pelvic/thigh hematomas. An unexplained falling hematocrit following a neurointerventional procedure is almost always an indication for an abdominal and pelvic CT examination, even in the absence of clinical findings.

Thrombocytopenia with Heparin

It is important routinely to monitor the complete blood count of patients on heparin, with particular emphasis on detecting a fall in hematocrit (internal bleeding) and a fall in the platelet count. Two mechanisms for thrombocytopenia with heparin have been identified. Type I (nonimmune) thrombocytopenia following administration of heparin can be seen in 15% to 30% of patients in a very mild self-limited form and recovers within 3–4 days after cessation of therapy. A more severe thrombocytopenia, Type II (immune) IgG-mediated thrombocytopenia (<100,000 platelets/μL), is less common but can cause systemic irreversible aggregation of platelets with thromboembolic sequelae. Even minimal heparin exposure such as that used to keep sheaths or intravenous lines clear is sufficient to induce this condition. This has been called the "white clot syndrome" and constitutes an emergency requiring immediate discontinuation of heparin. Patients may develop spontaneous venous or arterial occlusions anywhere in the body, myocardial infarctions, or pulmonary embolism. If unchecked this syndrome can lead to thromboembolic stroke, mesenteric infarction, renal infarction, gangrene of the extremities, and tissue necrosis. Patients test positive for heparin-dependent antiplatelet antibodies. After discontinuation of heparin, platelet counts recover after 3–20 days.[73,74] Chronic heparin use over 3–5 months can induce osteoporosis.[69]

Drug Interactions

Platelet inhibitors can have a synergistic effect on the risk of spontaneous hemorrhage when used in association with heparin, and caution should be exercised with this combination. When using GPIIb/IIIa inhibitors, an ACT in excess of 300 seconds can be associated with an increased risk of hemorrhage.[40,41]

Also of interest to neurointerventional procedures is the potential for an inhibitory action by systemically administered nitroglycerin on the anticoagulant effects of heparin. Close monitoring of the ACT during all procedures is important to detect this and other such unanticipated problems.

Low-Molecular-Weight Heparin and Heparinoids

Low-molecular-weight heparin preparations are fractionated components produced by enzymatic or chemical cleavage of parent compounds. They typically have molecular weights of 1–10 kd. Low-Molecular-Weight (LMW) heparins inhibit thrombin formation less than conventional heparin, have a greater affinity for inactivation of Factor Xa, and less interaction with platelets (Fig. 1.1D). Therefore, they are thought to have less risk of hemorrhagic complications than conventional heparin and a lower risk of heparin-induced thrombocytopenia.[75] Because of a lack of binding to endothelial cells and plasma proteins, they are considered to have a longer and more predictable half-life than standard heparin. Like heparin, they do not cross the placental barrier.[76] They are not completely neutralized by protamine sulfate.

Enoxaparin

Enoxaparin (Lovenox) is a preparation of low-molecular weight heparin supplied in prepackaged fixed doses, which can be self-administered subcutaneously at home by patients. Each milligram is the equivalent in inhibitory effects on Factor Xa of 1000 units of heparin (Fig. 1.1D). Daily or twice daily dosing with enoxaparin has been demonstrated to have a significant effect on reduction of thrombosis following orthopedic and abdominal surgery. The usual recommended dose for such patients is 30 mg B.I.D. or 40 mg daily subcutaneously, but higher doses are generally recommended for cerebrovascular patients switching from heparin or coumadin. Low-molecular-weight heparin can be a useful (but expensive) short-term alternative for particular patients for prevention of thromboembolic problems while awaiting or recuperating from a neurointerventional procedure. Precautions including those related to thrombocytopenia are similar to those mentioned for heparin sodium. Laboratory monitoring of the effects of subcutaneous low-molecular-weight heparin is difficult because the prothrombin time (PT) and activated partial thromboplastin time (aPTT) are relatively insensitive indicators of activity. As with any anticoagulant, the use of enoxaparin represents a contraindication to spinal procedures (such as lumbar puncture) that could lead to formation of epidural hematomas.

Hirudin/Lepirudin (Refludan)

For patients who develop heparin-related Type II immune-mediated thrombocytopenia, thrombotic complications are difficult to treat. These patients sometimes demonstrate cross-reactivity with low-molecular-weight heparin, too. An alternative agent which can be used in such situations is hirudin, or its recombinant form lepirudin, a direct thrombin inhibitor found in the salivary extracts of the medicinal leech, *Hirudo medicinalis*. It possesses a number of pharmacological advantages over heparin. Due to its small size it can access and directly inhibit clot-bound thrombin; it does not require the presence of antithrombin III for its effect; and it is not prone to deactivation by Platelet Factor 4 or other plasma proteins (Fig. 1.1D). Its effect can be monitored by following the activated partial thromboplastin time. The usual loading dose is 0.2–0.4 mg/kg followed by an infusion of 0.15 mg/kg per hour,[77,78] and the therapeutic effect is followed by the aPTT. The therapeutic window for this and similar agents is narrow, with at least a theoretical risk of overdosing. Clearance of lepirudin is markedly prolonged in patients with renal insufficiency. The efficacy of hirudin in the coronary circulation has been shown to be at least as effective as heparin in preventing myocardial infarction in patients with unstable angina or acute coronary syndrome without any greater risk of hemorrhagic complications.[79] In fact, hirudin or related agents may be even more effective than heparin in the first day or so following angioplasty at preventing thrombotic complications as shown in the OASIS-2 trial.[79–82]

Protamine Sulfate

Protamine is a preparation of low-molecular-weight fish proteins with strong basic properties. In the presence of acidic heparin, a stable salt is formed and the anticoagulant effect of heparin is neutralized. When administered alone or in excess of a neutralizing concentration of acidic heparin, protamine itself has weak anticoagulant properties due to interactions with platelets and fibrinogen. A useful rule of thumb for dosing is that 10 mg of protamine sulfate neutralizes 1000 units of circulating heparin. Therefore, taking the half-life of heparin as 1–1.5 hours, an estimate of the necessary dose of protamine can be calculated.

Rapid administration of protamine can be hazardous, and doses up to a maximum of 50 mg should be administered slowly over the course of 10 minutes. Administration should be performed only in locations with resuscitation equipment available. Rapid intravenous administration of protamine sulfate can induce hypotension, back pain, dyspnea, bradycardia, and flushing. Anaphylaxis and anaphylactoid reactions in association with protamine are a concern with the use of this drug, and patients should be observed carefully for signs of allergic reaction. Patients more likely to develop a hypersensitivity reactions include those who have developed immune response factors following previous exposure to protamine sulfate or to protamine in insulin preparations.

Thrombolytic Agents

Thrombolytic agents are activators of plasminogen that convert the inactive zymogen to plasmin in vivo. Plasminogen is a single-chain 92-kD glycoprotein that exists in two forms: glu-plasminogen and lys-plasminogen. Urokinase and t-PA catalyze the conversion of glu-plasminogen to lys-plasmin.

Urokinase

Urokinase is a thrombolytic serine protease derived by tissue culture from human neonatal kidney cells. The low-molecular-weight form is used for intraarterial thrombolysis and has a half-life of 12–13 minutes. It is supplied as a powder for reconstitution with 5 ml of sterile water per vial, yielding a concentration of 50,000 IU of urokinase per ml. Urokinase works on the endogenous fibrinolytic system by converting plasminogen to plasmin, which in turn causes degradation of fibrin and fibrinogen (Fig. 1.1D).

For intraarterial thrombolysis of acute stroke or direct infusion into thrombosed dural venous sinuses, urokinase can be administered without further dilution, for a total dose of 1.2 million units over the course of 1–2 hours. Doses as high as 2 million units have been used occasionally. Care should be exercised in the presence of circulating heparin, but doses on the lower end of the range for heparin are probably safe.[83]

Recombinant pro-UK is the 411 amino-acid zymogen precursor of urokinase derived from transfected murine SP2/0 hybridoma cells. It is activated at the surface of thrombus by plasmin associated with the fibrin mesh. Its thrombolytic effect is potentiated by the presence of heparin. The PROACT (Prolyse in Acute Cerebral Thromboembolism) study of recombinant pro-urokinase[84] used intraarterial doses of 6 mg and 9 mg delivered into the face of the thrombus and compared the effects with that of placebo and heparinization, respectively. Recanalization rates were significantly better and patient outcome was improved in the groups treated with rpro-UK. Increased hemorrhage rates were seen with rpro-UK and were influenced by the use of heparin.

Tissue-Type Plasminogen Activator t-PA

Tissue-type plasminogen activator is a 527 amino-acid serine protease glycoprotein with a half-life in humans of 3–8 minutes. Two forms of recombinant t-PA exist: a single chain (alteplase), and a two-chain form (duteplase). Trials of intravenous and intraarterial tPA for arterial thrombolysis are discussed in Chapter 13. Alteplase is synthesized using complementary human DNA from a human melanoma cell line inserted into a cell line of Chinese Hamster ovarian cells. It functions as a proteolytic enzyme (serine protease) converting plasminogen to plasmin (Fig. 1.1D). Intraarterial or intravenous alteplase is metabolized rapidly by the liver. Variability in biologic response to this agent in a number of trials may be related to the state of liver blood flow in each patient.[85] The half-life of alteplase is short, in the range of 2–5 minutes. Alternative forms of tPA such as TNK-tPA or reteplase have been devised with a longer half-life in the range of 16–18 minutes.[86] The question of doses for use during intraarterial thrombolysis of the intracranial vessels has not been clarified. Anecdotally successful doses at dissolving acute cerebral arterial thrombus range from 1 mg to 40 mg or more given over variable periods of time (0.5–2 hours).[87]

References

1. del Zoppo GJ (1998) The role of platelets in ischemic stroke. *Neurology* 51:S9–S14.
2. Becker RC, Bovill EG, Seghatchian MJ, Samama MM (1998) Pathobiology of thrombin in acute coronary syndromes. *Am Heart J* 136:S19–S31.
3. Becker RC (1999) Thrombosis and the role of the platelet. *Am J Cardiol* 83:3E–6E.
4. Kroll MH, Hellums JD, Guo Z, Durante W, Razdan K,

HARBOLICH JK, SCHAFER AI (1993) Protein kinase C is activated in platelets subjected to pathological shear stress. *J Biol Chem* 268:3520–3524.
5. KONSTANTOPOULOS K, GROTTA JC, SILLS C, WU KK, HELLUMS JD (1995) Shear-induced platelet aggregation in normal subjects and stroke patients. *Thrombosis & Haemostasis* 74:1329–1334.
6. KAMIGUTI AS, HAY CR, ZUZEL M (1996) Inhibition of collagen-induced platelet aggregation as the result of cleavage of alpha 2 beta 1–integrin by the snake venom metalloproteinase jararhagin. *Biochem J* 320:635–641.
7. DE LUCA M, WARD CM, OHMORI K, ANDREWS RK, BERNDT MC (1995) Jararhagin and jaracetin: novel snake venom inhibitors of the integrin collagen receptor, alpha 2 beta 1. *Biochem & Biophys Res Comm* 206:570–576.
8. KAWASAKI T, TANIUCHI Y, HISAMICHI N, FUJIMURA Y, SUZUKI M, TITANI K, SAKAI Y, KAKU S, SATOH N, TAKENAKA T (1995) Tokaracetin, a new platelet antagonist that binds to platelet glycoprotein Ib and inhibits von Willebrand factor-dependent shear-induced platelet aggregation. *Biochem J* 308:947–953.
9. KAMIGUTI AS, HAY CR, THEAKSTON RD, ZUZEL M (1996) Insights into the mechanism of haemorrhage caused by snake venom metalloproteinases. *Toxicon* 34:627–642.
10. VUCKOVIC SA (1996) Glanzmann's thrombasthenia revisited. *J Emergency Med* 14:299–303.
11. CLEMETSON KJ (1997) Platelet GPIb-V-IX complex. *Thrombosis* & Haemostasis 78:266–270.
12. KENNY D, MORATECK PA, GILL JC, MONTGOMERY RR (1999) The critical interaction of glycoprotein (GP) Ibeta with GPIX—a genetic cause of Bernard-Soulier syndrome. *Blood* 93:2968–2975.
13. BITHELL TC, PAREKH SJ, STRONG RR (1972) Platelet-function studies in the Bernard-Soulier syndrome. *Ann NY Acad Sci* 201:145–160.
14. KAMIGUTI AS, LAING GD, LOWE GM, ZUZEL M, WARRELL DA, THEAKSTON RD (1994) Biological properties of the venom of the Papuan black snake (Pseudechis papuanus): presence of a phospholipase A2 platelet inhibitor. *Toxicon* 32:915–925.
15. ANONYMOUS (1994) Collaborative overview of randomised trials of antiplatelet therapy—I: Prevention of death, myocardial infarction, and stroke by prolonged antiplatelet therapy in various categories of patients. Antiplatelet Trialists' Collaboration. *Br Med J* 308:81–106.
16. CRAVEN LL (1953) Experiences with aspirin (acetylsalicyclic acid) in the non-specific prophylaxis of coronary thrombosis. *Mississippi Valley Med J* 75:38–40.
17. ANONYMOUS (1978) A randomized trial of aspirin and sulfinpyrazone in threatened stroke. The Canadian Cooperative Study Group. *N Eng J Med* 299:53–59.
18. PATRANO C (1994) Aspirin as an antiplatelet drug. *N Eng J Med* 330:1287–1294.
19. SCHAFER AI (1996) Antiplatelet therapy. *Am J Med* 101:199–209.
20. GORELICK PB, BORN GV, D'AGOSTINO RB, HANLEY DF JR, MOYE L, PEPINE CJ (1999) Therapeutic benefit. Aspirin revisited in light of the introduction of clopidogrel. *Stroke* 30:1716–1721.
21. QUINN MJ, FITZGERALD DJ (1999) Ticlopidine and clopidogrel. *Circulation* 100:1667–1672.
22. HANKY GJ, LUDLOW CLM, DUNBABIN DW (2000) Thienopyridines or aspirin to prevent stroke and other serious vascular events in patients at high risk of vascular disease? A systematic review of the evidence from randomized trials. *Stroke* 31:1779–1784.
23. HARBISON JW (1992) Ticlopidine versus aspirin for the prevention of recurrent stroke. Analysis of patients with minor stroke from the Ticlopidine Aspirin Stroke Study. *Stroke* 23:1723–1727.
24. GENT M, BLAKELY JA, EASTON JD, ELLIS DJ, HACHINSKI VC, HARBISON JW, PANAK E, ROBERTS RS, SICURELLA J, TURPIE AG (1989) The Canadian American Ticlopidine Study (CATS) in thromboembolic stroke. *Lancet* 1:1215–1220.
25. URBAN P, MACAYA C, RUPPRECHT HJ, KIEMENEIJ F, EMANUELSSON H, FONTANELLI A, PIEPER M, WESSELING T, SAGNARD L (1998) Randomized evaluation of anticoagulation versus antiplatelet therapy after coronary stent implantation in high-risk patients: the multicenter aspirin and ticlopidine trial after intracoronary stenting (MATTIS). *Circulation* 98:2126–2132.
26. RUPPRECHT HJ, DARIUS H, BORKOWSKI U, VOIGTLANDER T, NOWAK B, GENTH S, MEYER J (1998) Comparison of antiplatelet effects of aspirin, ticlopidine, or their combination after stent implantation. *Circulation* 97:1046–1052.
27. SZTO GY, LINNEMEIER TJ, BALL MW (1999) Fatal neutropenia and thrombocytopenia associated with ticlopidine after stenting. *Am J Cardiol* 83:138–139.
28. JAMAR S, VANDERHEYDEN M, JANSSENS L, HERMANS L, JAMAR R, VERSTREKEN G (1998) Thrombotic thrombocytopenic purpura: a rare but potentially life-threatening complication following ticlopidine administration. *Acta Cardiologica* 53:285–286.
29. STEINHUBL SR, TAN WA, FOODY JM, TOPOL EJ (1999) Incidence and clinical course of thrombotic thrombocytopenic purpura due to ticlopidine following coronary stenting. EPISTENT Investigators. Evaluation of Platelet IIb/IIIa Inhibitor for Stenting. *JAMA* 281:806–810.
30. CHEN DK, KIM JS, SUTTON DM (1999) Thrombotic thrombocytopenic purpura associated with ticlopidine use: a report of 3 cases and review of the literature. *Arch Intern Med* 159:311–314.
31. ANONYMOUS (1996) A randomised, blinded, trial of clopidogrel versus aspirin in patients at risk of ischaemic events (CAPRIE). CAPRIE Steering Committee. *Lancet* 348:1329–1339.
32. MAKKAR RR, EIGLER NL, KAUL S, FRIMERMAN A, NAKAMURA M, SHAH PK, FORRESTER JS, HERBERT JM, LITVACK F (1998) Effects of clopidogrel, aspirin and combined therapy in a

porcine ex vivo model of high-shear induced stent thrombosis. *Europ Heart J* 19:1538–1546.
33. Moussa I, Oetgen M, Roubin G, Colombo A, Wang X, Iyer S, Maida R, Collins M, Kreps E, Moses JW (1999) Effectiveness of clopidogrel and aspirin versus ticlopidine and aspirin in preventing stent thrombosis after coronary stent implantation. *Circulation* 99:2364–2366.
34. Bennett CL, Connors JM, Carwile JM, Moake JL, Bell WR, Tarantolo SR, McCarthy LJ, Sarode R, Hatfield AJ, Feldman MD, Davidson CJ, Tsai HM (2000) Thrombotic thrombocytopenic purpura associated with clopidogrel. *N Engl J Med* 342:1773–1777.
35. Coller BS (1985) A new murine monoclonal antibody reports an activation-dependent change in the conformation and/or microenvironment of the platelet glycoprotein IIb/IIIa complex. *J Clin Invest* 76:101–108.
36. Scarborough RM, Rose JW, Naughton MA, Phillips DR, Nannizzi L, Arfsten A, Campbell AM, Charo IF (1993) Characterization of the integrin specificities of disintegrins isolated from American pit viper venoms. *J Biol Chem* 268:1058–1065.
37. Scarborough RM, Rose JW, Hsu MA, Phillips DR, Fried VA, Campbel AM, Nannizzi L, Charo IF (1991) Barbourin. A GPIIb/IIIa specific integrin antagonist from the venom of *Sistrurus m. barbouri*. *J Biol Chem* 266:9359–9362.
38. Gould RJ, Polokoff MA, Friedman PA, Huang TF, Holt JC, Cook JL, Niewiarowski S (1990) Disintegrins: A family of integrin inhibitory proteins from viper venoms. *Proc Soc Exper Biol Med* 195:168–171.
39. Anonymous (1994) Use of a monoclonal antibody directed against the platelet glycoprotein IIb/IIIa receptor in high-risk coronary angioplasty. The EPIC Investigation. *N Engl J Med* 330:956–961.
40. Anonymous (1997) Platelet glycoprotein IIb/IIIa receptor blockade and low-dose heparin during percutaneous coronary revascularization. The EPILOG Investigators. *N Engl J Med* 336:1689–1696.
41. Anonymous (1997) Randomised placebo-controlled trial of abciximab before and during coronary intervention in refractory unstable angina: the CAPTURE Study. *Lancet* 349:1429–1435.
42. Anonymous (1998) Randomised placebo-controlled and balloon-angioplasty-controlled trial to assess safety of coronary stenting with use of platelet glycoprotein-IIb/IIIa blockade. The EPISTENT Investigators. Evaluation of Platelet IIb/IIIa Inhibitor for Stenting. *Lancet* 352:87–92.
43. Anonymous (1997) Effects of platelet glycoprotein IIb/IIIa blockade with tirofiban on adverse cardiac events in patients with unstable angina or acute myocardial infarction undergoing coronary angioplasty. The RESTORE Investigators. Randomized Efficacy Study of Tirofiban for Outcomes and REstenosis. *Circulation* 96:1445–1453.
44. Anonymous (1997) Randomised placebo-controlled trial of effect of eptifibatide on complications of percutaneous coronary intervention: IMPACT-II. Integrilin to Minimise Platelet Aggregation and Coronary Thrombosis-II. *Lancet* 349:1422–1428.
45. Tcheng JE (1999) Differences among the parenteral platelet glycoprotein IIb/IIIa inhibitors and implications for treatment. *Am J Cardiol* 83:7E–11E.
46. Giri S, Mitchel JF, Hirst JA, McKay RG, Azar RR, Mennett R, Waters DD, Kiernan FJ (2000) Synergy between intracoronary stenting and Abciximab in improving angiographic and clinical outcomes of primary angioplasty in acute myocardial infarction. *Am J Cardiol* 86:269–274.
47. Schömig A, Kastrati A, Dirschinger J, Mehilli J, Schricke U, Pache J, Martinoff S, Neuman FJ, Schwaiger M (2000) Coronary stenting plus platelet glycoprotein IIb/IIIa blockade compared with tissue plasminogen activator in acute myocardial infarction. *N Engl J Med* 343:385–391.
48. Anonymous (1998) A comparison of aspirin plus tirofiban with aspirin plus heparin for unstable angina. Platelet Receptor Inhibition in Ischemic Syndrome Management (PRISM) Study Investigators. *N Engl J Med* 338:1498–1505.
49. Anonymous (1998) Inhibition of the platelet glycoprotein IIb/IIIa receptor with tirofiban in unstable angina and non-Q-wave myocardial infarction. Platelet Receptor Inhibition in Ischemic Syndrome Management in Patients Limited by Unstable Signs and Symptoms (PRISM-PLUS) Study Investigators. *N Engl J Med* 338:1488–1497.
50. Anonymous (1998) Inhibition of platelet glycoprotein IIb/IIIa with eptifibatide in patients with acute coronary syndromes. The PURSUIT Trial Investigators. Platelet Glycoprotein IIb/IIIa in Unstable Angina: Receptor Suppression Using Integrilin Therapy. *N Engl J Med* 339:436–443.
51. Anonymous (1998) International, randomized, controlled trial of lamifiban (a platelet glycoprotein IIb/IIIa inhibitor), heparin, or both in unstable angina. The PARAGON Investigators. Platelet IIb/IIIa Antagonism for the Reduction of Acute coronary syndrome events in a Global Organization Network. *Circulation* 97:2386–2395.
52. Kereiakes DJ, Kleiman NS, Ferguson JJ, Masud AR, Broderick TM, Abbottsmith CW, Runyon JP, Anderson LC, Anders RJ, Dreiling RJ, Hantsbarger GL, Bryzinski B, Topol EJ (1998) Pharmacodynamic efficacy, clinical safety, and outcomes after prolonged platelet Glycoprotein IIb/IIIa receptor blockade with oral xemilofiban: results of a multi center, placebo-controlled, randomized trial. *Circulation* 98:1268–1278.
53. Cannon CP, McCabe CH, Borzak S, Henry TD, Tischler MD, Mueller HS, Feldman R, Palmeri ST, Ault K, Hamilton SA, Rothman JM, Novotny WF, Braunwald E (1998) Randomized trial of an oral platelet glycoprotein IIb/IIIa antagonist, sibrafiban, in patients after an acute coronary syndrome: results of the TIMI 12 trial. Thrombolysis in Myocardial Infarction. *Circulation* 97:340–349.
54. Kleiman NS (1999) Pharmacokinetics and Pharmacodynamics of Glycoprotein IIb/IIIa inhibitors. *Am Heart J* 138:S263–S275.

55. COLLER BS (1999) Potential non-glycoprotein IIb/IIIa effects of abciximab. *Am Heart J* 138:S1–S5.
56. ANONYMOUS (1999) Acute platelet inhibition with abciximab does not reduce in-stent restenosis (ERASER study). The ERASER Investigators. *Circulation* 100:799–806.
57. ANTMAN EM, GIUGLIANO RP, GIBSON CM, MCCABE CH, COUSSEMENT P, KLEIMAN NS, VAHANIAN A, ADGEY AA, MENOWN I, RUPPRECHT HJ, VAN DER WIEKEN R, DUCAS J, SCHERER J, ANDERSON K, VAN DE WERF F, BRAUNWALD E (1999) Abciximab facilitates the rate and extent of thrombolysis: results of the thrombolysis in myocardial infarction (TIMI) 14 trial. The TIMI 14 Investigators. *Circulation* 99:2720–2732.
58. AMBROSE JA, HAWKEY M, BADIMON JJ, COPPOLA J, GEAGEA JP, RENTROP P, DOMIGUEZ A, DUVVURI S, ELMQUIST T, ARIAS J, DOSS R, DANGAS G (2000) In vivo demonstration of an antithrombin effect of abciximab. *Am J Cardiol* 86:150–152.
59. THE ABCIXIMAB IN ISCHEMIC STROKE INVESTIGATORS (2000) Abciximab in Acute Ischemic Stroke. A randomized, double-blind, placebo-controlled, dose-escalation study. *Stroke* 31:601–609.
60. BEDNAR B, COOK JJ, HOLAHAN MA, CUNNINGHAM ME, JUMES PA, BEDNAR RA, HARTMAN GD, GOULD RJ (1999) Fibrinogen receptor antagonist-induced thrombocytopenia in chimpanzee and rhesus monkey associated with preexisting drug-dependent antibodies to platelet glycoprotein IIb/IIIa. *Blood* 94:587–599.
61. PETER K, STRAUB A, KOHLER B, VOLKMANN M, SCHWARZ M, KUBLER W, BODE C (1999) Platelet activation as a potential mechanism of GP IIb/IIIa inhibitor-induced thrombocytopenia. *Am J Cardiol* 84:519–524.
62. MADAN M, BERKOWITZ SD (1999) Understanding thrombocytopenia and antigenicity with Glycoprotein IIb/IIIa inhibitors. *Am Heart J* 138:S317–S326.
63. KEREIAKES DJ, BERKOWITZ SD, LINCOFF AM, TCHENG JE, WOLSKI K, ACHENBACH R, MELSHEIMER R, ANDERSON K, CALIFF RM, TOPOL EJ (2000) Clinical correlates and course of thrombocytopenia during percutaneous coronary intervention in the era of abciximab platelet glycoprotein IIb/IIIa blockade. *Am Heart J* 140:74–80.
64. JUBELIRER SJ, KOENIG BA, BATES MC (1999) Acute profound thrombocytopenia following C7E3 Fab (Abciximab) therapy: case reports, review of the literature and implications for therapy. *Am J Hematol* 61:205–208.
65. DASGUPTA H, BLANKENSHIP JC, WOOD GC, FREY CM, DEMKO SL, MENAPACE FJ (2000) Thrombocytopenia complicating treatment with intravenous glycoprotein IIb/IIIa receptor inhibitors: a pooled analysis. *Am Heart J* 140:206–211.
66. DYKE CM (1999) Safety of Glycoprotein IIb/IIIa inhibitors: A Heart Surgeon's perspective. *Am Heart J* 138:S307–S316.
67. KEREIAKES DJ, BRODERICK TM, ROTH EM, WHANG D, SHIMSHAK T, RUNYON JP, HATTEMER C, SCHNEIDER J, LACOCK P, MUELLER M, ABBOTTSMITH CW (1999) Time course, magnitude, and consistency of platelet inhibition by abciximab, tirofiban, or eptifibatide in patients with unstable angina pectoris undergoing percutaneous coronary intervention. *Am J Cardiol* 84:391–395.
68. MCLEAN J (1916) The thromboplastic action of cephalin. *Am J Physiol* 41:250–257.
69. HIRSH J, RASCHKE R, WARKENTIN TE, DALEN JE, DEYKIN D, POLLER L (1995) Heparin: mechanism of action, pharmacokinetics, dosing considerations, monitoring, efficacy and safety. *Chest* 108(suppl):258S–275S.
70. QURESHI AI, LUFT AR, SHARMA M, GUTERMAN LR, HOPKINS LN (2000) Prevention and treatment of thromboembolic and ischemic complications associated with endovascular procedures: Part II—Clinical aspects and recommendations. *Neurosurgery* 46:1360–1376.
71. QURESHI AI, LUFT AR, SHARMA M, GUTERMAN LR, HOPKINS LN (2000) Prevention and treatment of thromboembolic and ischemic complications associated with endovascular procedures: Part I—Pathophysiological and pharmacological features. *Neurosurgery* 46:1344–1359.
72. BOWERS J, FERGUSON JJ (1994) The use of activated clotting times to monitor heparin therapy during and after interventional procedures. *Clin Cardiol* 17:357–361.
73. WARKENTIN TE (1997) Heparin-induced thrombocytopenia. Pathogenesis, frequency, avoidance and management. *Drug Safety* 17:325–341.
74. KING DJ, KELTON JG (1984) Heparin associated thrombocytopenia. *Ann Intern Med* 100:535–540.
75. ADAMS HP, LEIRA EC (1997) Acute therapeutic intervention. Antithrombotic and antiplatelet-aggregating drugs. *Neurosurgery Clinic of North America* 8:207–217.
76. HIRSH J, FUSTER V (1994) Guide to Anticoagulant Therapy Part 1: Heparin. *Circulation* 89:1449–1468.
77. BRIEGER DB, MAK KH, KOTTKE-MARCHANT K, TOPOL EJ (1998) Heparin-induced thrombocytopenia. *J Am Coll Cardiol* 31:1449–1459.
78. ORTEL TL, CHONG BH (1998) New treatment options for heparin-induced thrombocytopenia. *Sem Hematol* 35:26–34.
79. ANONYMOUS (1996) A comparison of recombinant hirudin with heparin for the treatment of acute coronary syndromes. The Global Use of Strategies to Open Occluded Coronary Arteries (GUSTO) IIb investigators. *N Engl J Med* 335:775–782.
80. WHITE HD, AYLWARD PE, FREY MJ, ADGEY AA, NAIR R, HILLIS WS, SHALEV Y, BROWN MA, FRENCH JK, COLLINS R, MARAGANORE J, ADELMAN B (1997) Randomized, double-blind comparison of hirulog versus heparin in patients receiving streptokinase and aspirin for acute myocardial infarction (HERO). Hirulog Early Reperfusion/Occlusion (HERO) Trial Investigators. *Circulation* 96:2155–2161.
81. SERRUYS PW, HERRMAN JP, SIMON R, RUTSCH W, BODE C, LAARMAN GJ, VAN DIJK R, VAN DEN BOS AA, UMANS VA, FOX KA (1995) A comparison of hirudin with heparin in the prevention of restenosis after coronary angioplasty. Helvetica Investigators. *N Engl J Med* 333:757–763.

82. Antman EM (1996) Hirudin in acute myocardial infarction. Thrombolysis and Thrombin Inhibition in Myocardial Infarction (TIMI) 9B trial. *Circulation* 94:911–921.
83. Tennant SN, Dixon J, Venable TC, Page HL Jr, Roach A, Kaiser AB, Frederiksen R, Tacogue L, Kaplan P, Babu NS (1984) Intracoronary thrombolysis in patients with acute myocardial infarction: comparison of the efficacy of urokinase with streptokinase. *Circulation* 69:756–760.
84. del Zoppo GJ, Higashida RT, Furlan AJ, Pessin MS, Rowley HA, Gent M (1998) PROACT: a phase II randomized trial of recombinant pro-urokinase by direct arterial delivery in acute middle cerebral artery stroke. PROACT Investigators. Prolyse in Acute Cerebral Thromboembolism. *Stroke* 29:4–11.
85. van Griensven JM, Koster RW, Burggraaf J, Huisman LG, Kluft C, Kroon R, Schoemaker RC, Cohen AF (1998) Effects of liver blood flow on the pharmacokinetics of tissue-type plasminogen activator (alteplase) during thrombolysis in patients with acute myocardial infarction. *Clin Pharmacol Ther* 63:39–47.
86. Cannon CP, McCabe CH, Gibson CM, Ghali M, Sequeira RF, McKendall GR, Breed J, Modi NB, Fox NL, Tracy RP, Love TW, Braunwald E (1997) TNK-tissue plasminogen activator in acute myocardial infarction. Results of the Thrombolysis in Myocardial Infarction (TIMI) 10A dose-ranging trial. *Circulation* 95:351–356.
87. Qureshi AI, Suri FK, Shatla AA, Ringer AJ, Fessler RD, Ali Z, Guterman LR, Hopkins LN (2000) Intraarterial recombinant tissue plasminogen activator for ischemic stroke: an accelerating dosing regimen. *Neurosurgery* 47:473–479.

Chapter 2

Room, Equipment, Basic Techniques

THE MOST IMPORTANT RESOURCE of the neurointerventional service is the staff, the technologists, nurses, and anesthesia teams. With encouragement, respectful communication, and teaching, most personnel are capable of making important contributions to patient safety, case management, materials use, etc., through suggestions or observations that may not always be apparent to a single operator. The motivation for such behavior can be cultivated by working toward creating an environment in which individuals realize that their work has personal meaning and is therefore important. Pride in one's work will translate into an attention to detail, an interest in the case in progress, a willingness to participate with suggestions, and a sense of vigilance necessary for the nature of this work. Similarly, an outlook of inclusion toward the nursing staff and anesthesia team in the case will extract from them a greater level of collaboration redounding to the ultimate advantage of the patient.

However, when the number of technologists and nurses is large or the team changes from day to day, then the system must be self-perpetuating so as to resist the unfortunate regression of standards that can plague most human group endeavors. The task of monitoring and maintaining standards must be performed by the leader of the team. If not, then the lowest common denominator established by some other individual or by group consensus will prevail. Therefore, there must be an insistence on the same standards of work and vigilance for all cases, diagnostic or interventional, performed in the room. For instance, letting a poorly draped patient or badly prepared flush-line go by once because the case in hand is "only" a diagnostic case will assure that the same problem will come up again later. Mistakes must be corrected the first time and every time thereafter.

Keeping the room neat and tidy at all times is important. For instance, before each case relevant films are hung on the light box and reviewed. Films from previous cases are tidied away. After the room has been cleaned, mops and buckets are stowed away and not simply placed against the wall; extraneous equipment, wheelchairs, and so forth are parked neatly or put away. Fluid splashes on TV monitors and other equipment are cleaned scrupulously. Apart from obvious hygienic and regulatory concerns, there are important psychological reasons for these scruples. A high standard of neatness in the room creates an atmosphere of vigilance in which personnel become more aware of their own

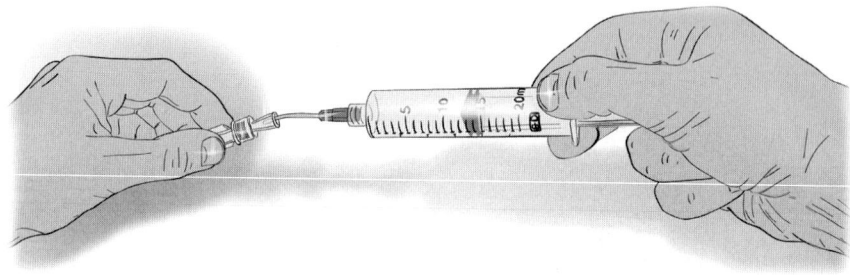

FIGURE 2.1 • Habitual irrigation of microcatheter hubs with a shaped intravenous cannula and a syringe of heparinized saline flush is imperative. It clears sites of potential clot formation and raises a clean meniscus to eliminate adherent bubbles of air that might otherwise be injected. Fellows must be instructed from the beginning that standards of blood spillage that might be reasonable for peripheral vascular work are not acceptable for neurointerventional procedures. A blood-free work area assures that one's perception will be sensitive to any inadvertent back-leakage through a loose valve.

behavior and become more attentive to the details of their work. The human mind needs order. Focusing on the drip chambers of the flush systems is easier to do, for instance, across a neatly draped table than in a situation of disarray and chaos. The collective effect on patient safety of such a carefully maintained working environment is difficult to quantify, but it would take only a small number of avoided complications to realize the value of working with a collaborative team, rather than with a group of hourly employees. Occasions arise, for instance, on which you may have overlooked a drug allergy and been reminded by the nurse. A malfunctioning flush-line detected by a technologist while your attention was elsewhere might prevent a thromboembolic complication only once every few years, but when it happens it is of pivotal importance to that particular patient.

Fellows must be trained from the beginning that standards of table cleanliness adequate for peripheral vascular cases are not acceptable for neurointerventional work. Gloves must be kept clean and bloodless. Syringes and Tuohy-Borst adapters must be bloodless inside and out (Figs. 2.1–2.2). This is to avoid any clot formation on the table, but also to enhance one's sensitivity to any inadvertent back bleeding that might occur via a poorly closed valve. Gowns must be tied at the back to avoid contamination of a colleague's hands during the close-quarters work of a long case. The rub of the matter from the point of view of managing human nature is insisting on these standards for all cases, diagnostic and interventional, at all times. Otherwise the standard requiring the least effort will ultimately prevail.

A contrast can be drawn between the methodical, self-monitoring philosophy of airlines with reference to safety in commercial flying and the way in which medicine is practiced. Changes in airline-safety regulations came about through the recognition that most airline accidents happened because of human error rather than mechanical failure. A change in pilot training to address failures in communication and improve teamwork has resulted in significant improvements in the safety statistics of commercial airlines.[1] A change of this nature may be relevant to some aspects of medicine, particularly to complex procedures such as those involving interventional neuroradiology. Procedures of this nature require the cooperation of many individuals of diverse skills, not just a single-handed pilot. An environment in which a methodical, critical philosophy is upheld will encourage all members to speak out on potential errors, make suggestions, or be on the qui vive for potential problems.

Fellows involved with or rotating on the neurointerventional service must learn at an early stage that complications during the procedure represent

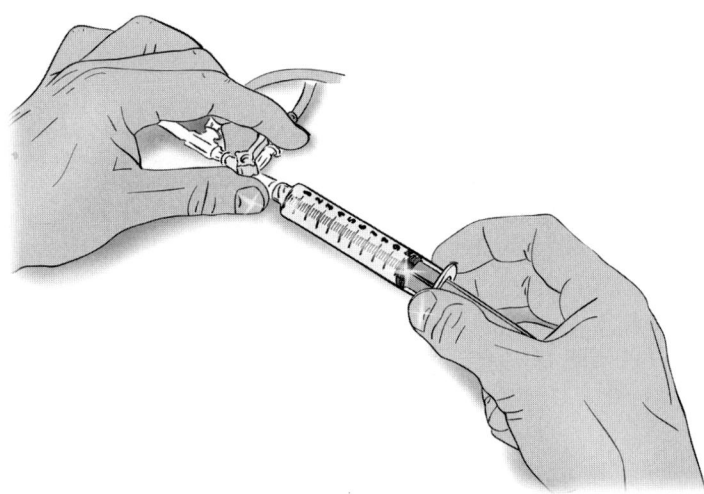

FIGURE 2.2 • All devices on the tabletop should be clean and blood-free inside and out. Luer-lock syringes can accumulate blood on the inside of the lock. This is most easily cleared by rotating the filled syringe 90° partially off the loading port and flushing forward approximately 1 cc. Bubbles should be avoided by filling the contrast syringe slowly and eliminated from the syringe by rolling it back and forth until the bubbles ascend to the tip where they are expelled. Catheter injections are always made pointing the syringe down toward the table as a final protection against inadvertent bubbles in the syringe.

only a proportion of undesirable events that can occur. Adequate patient evaluation, consent documentation, and discussion prior to the procedure are extremely important. Most particularly, fellows need to learn that continued patient surveillance after the procedure is imperative for good procedural outcome.

A procedure is never considered complete until the patient is delivered to the recovery room or ICU and the report is given to the nurse there. Quite apart from the obvious benefits of direct communication with the nursing staff and continuity of patient care, this simple rule helps to prevent ill-will on the part of the anesthesia team, who are invariably left with the task of patient transportation if the radiology team disappears when the arterial site is sealed. A synopsis of the patient's care and status is given to the ICU nurse with particular emphasis on aspects of care peculiar to that patient. Contact should always be made with the primary treatment service or referring surgeon after the procedure too.

Most postprocedure complications can be either avoided or mitigated by vigilant patient monitoring. Fellows must learn that responsibility for particular post-procedure precautions, heparinization regimens, mobilization schedules, arterial care, etc., rests with the neurointerventional team and not necessarily with the primary treatment service.

Treating neurointerventional procedures as just an elaborate angiogram that ends when the patient rolls out the door of the suite is a recipe for poor patient outcome. Daily or twice-daily patient rounds to the ICU and patient floors are the only way of maintaining vigilance for post-procedural problems.

Rotational and 3D Angiography

Rotational angiography in 2D or 3D mode is available on most new neurointerventional rooms. At the cost of increased radiation exposure and a prolonged injection of contrast, a better understanding of extracranial and intracranial lesions can be obtained. Planning of surgical and particularly neurointerventional procedures can be improved con-

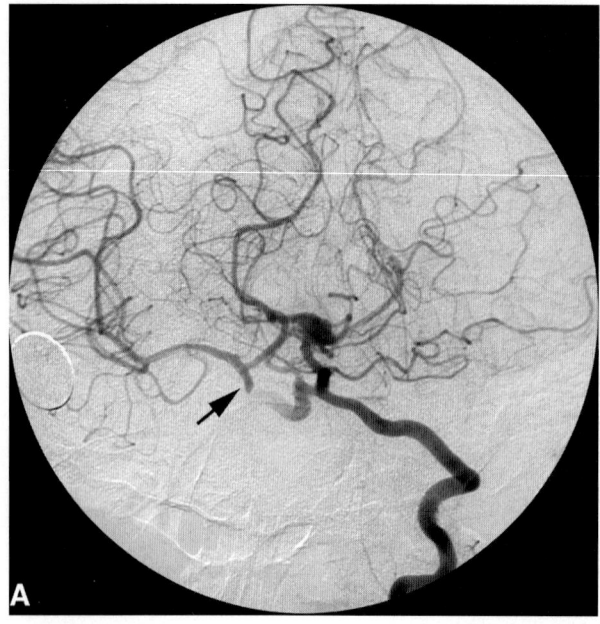 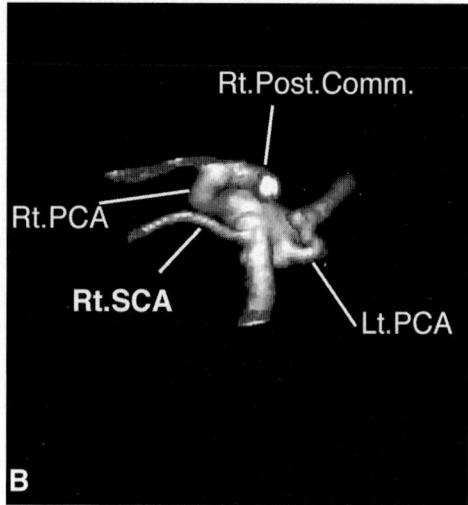

FIGURE 2.3 • A left vertebral artery injection (A) in a 46-year-old female patient fills the supraclinoid right internal carotid artery (arrow) via the right posterior communicating artery because of a previous carotid occlusion on that side. A complex dysplastic aneurysm of the basilar artery tip was difficult to interrogate adequately despite multiple conventional images in many planes. The configuration of the aneurysm was more clearly demonstrated by 3D angiography (B) showing the involvement of the origin of both posterior cerebral arteries (PCA) and the left superior cerebellar artery (SCA) with the dysplastic aneurysm.

siderably in certain patients as a result. This is particularly true for complex intracranial aneurysms.[2] By virtue of the increased numbers of views obtained in a rotational angiographic run, a better understanding of complex stenoses and dissections can be achieved too, compared with a limited number of DSA images (Figs. 2.3–2.5, 3.4, 3.17). Rotational angiography increases the sensitivity of digital subtraction angiography to the severity of carotid stenosis present in patients with suspected atherosclerotic disease.[3]

Different subtraction protocols are available from various manufacturers of angiographic suites. Some use a set of zero images without contrast which are then subtracted from a second run done with contrast. Some manufacturers acquire a single run with contrast and extract the vessels from the data by thresholding of pixel densities.

Patient motion is a hindrance during rotational angiography. It is useful to cover the patient's eyes with a cloth so that the swinging C-arm cannot be seen during the run and is less likely to cause alarm. Additionally, motion can be reduced by adequately warning the patient in advance of the prolonged sensation of injection, particularly felt in the eye during carotid injections and in the neck during vertebral artery injections. Respiratory motion can be eliminated in most cooperative patients by hyperventilating the patient for 9–10 breaths in advance of the run and then having them hold their breath in inspiration. For patients with slower circulation times or proximal stenoses, a delay in filming of 2–6 seconds after the contrast injection starts can reduce the likelihood of the initial images being acquired without contrast in the vessels. Rates of 3 ml/s for a duration of 6 seconds are typically satisfactory in the vertebral artery and internal carotid artery, 4 ml/s in the common carotid artery.

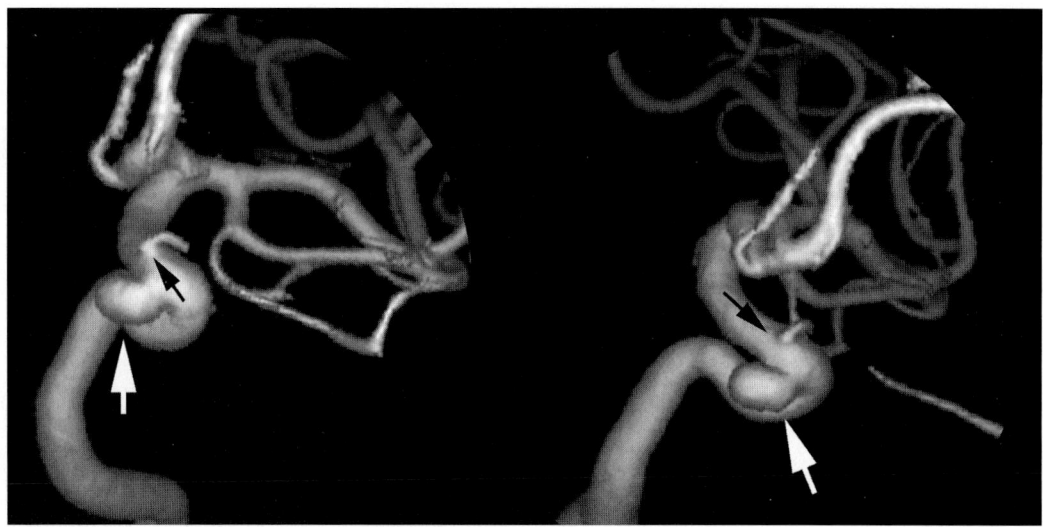

FIGURE 2.4 • An aneurysm (white arrows) of questionable provenance on planar views is well seen on these 3D images lying proximal to the ophthalmic artery (black arrows). The aneurysm almost certainly lies too proximally to involve the intradural carotid cave and therefore is best understood as cavernous in location. Being asymptomatic, it does not require treatment.

Flush System

There are two types of flush system for keeping coaxial catheters cleared with heparinized flush during angiography cases: mechanical pumps and pressurized drips.

A mechanical pump can be set at a fixed volume of infusion per unit time. However, with alarms sounding and needing to be reset, and the ever present possibility of mechanical failure, electronic pumps tend to be seen as troublesome and unreliable by most neurointerventionalists.

A pressurized bag is preferred by most with the rate of flow regulated by a simple flow-valve at the tabletop. Generally, liter bags of saline containing 1,000–5,000 units of heparin are used. The heparin is injected using a small needle (21G), and excess air is extracted from the bag. This is very important so as to prevent embolization of pressurized air into the flush system if the bag runs low or if the patient is being transported with a catheter or sheath still in place at the end of the procedure. There are two drip chamber options available. The first has a large drip configuration (15 drops/ml) and has the advantage of being easy to prime and easy to clear of bubbles along the line. However, fluid regulation is more difficult with this system, and the rate of flow is a little more difficult to gauge by eye because the drops are more infrequent than with the microdrip alternative. The second type of drip chamber appears identical except that the drops of saline are smaller (60 drops/ml). This allows a finer adjustment of the rate of flow, very important for children and other patients needing close monitoring of fluid status. The disadvantage of this system is that when the flow valve is inadvertently opened up fully, the rate of flow through such a small-bore opening generates turbulence in the drip chamber, causing bubbles to travel into the flush-line (Figures 2.6, 2.7).

Studies of clinically detectable complications following cerebral angiography have been superseded by the greater sensitivity of diffusion-weighted MRI (DWI) to embolic complications. Studies of clinically silent embolic complications of diagnostic and interventional cerebral angiographic procedures using diffusion-weighted MRI discovered that embolic complications may be seen in 0% to 23% of patients.[4,5] This risk is lower when systemic he-

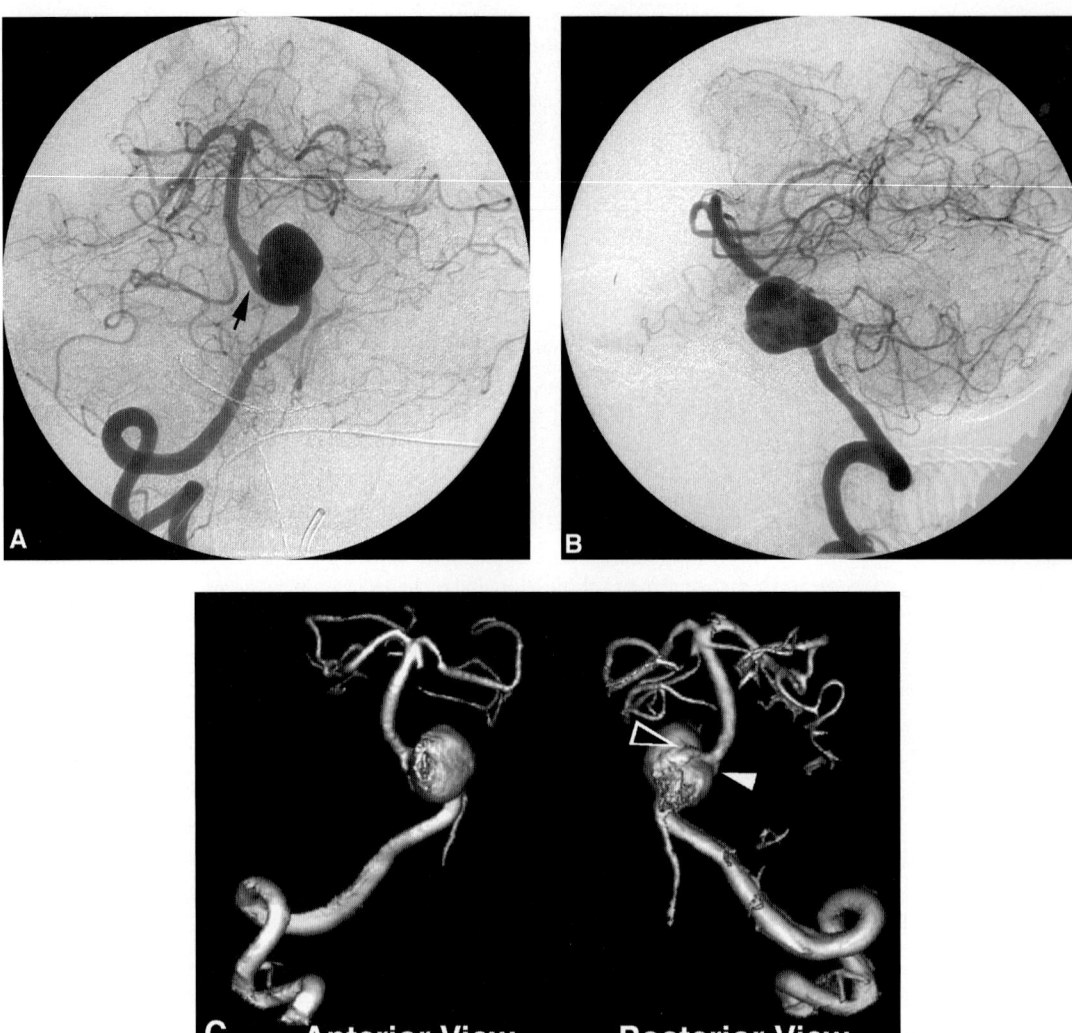

FIGURE 2.5 • A 68-year-old female presented with extensive subarachnoid hemorrhage of the posterior fossa related to a large aneurysm of the vertebrobasilar junction. Its location and configuration are very suggestive of the presence of an underlying fenestration, but this is difficult to confirm on the planar views (A, B). A glimpse of one limb of the fenestration is seen on the Caldwell view (arrow in A). The 3D images confirm the presence of the fenestration (arrowheads in C) and the involvement of both limbs of the fenestration proximally with the aneurysm, an inauspicious situation for surgical or endovascular treatment. Bridging the right vertebral artery to the left limb of the fenestration with an endovascular stent followed by coil embolization would probably represent the best hopes of securing an aneurysm such as this.

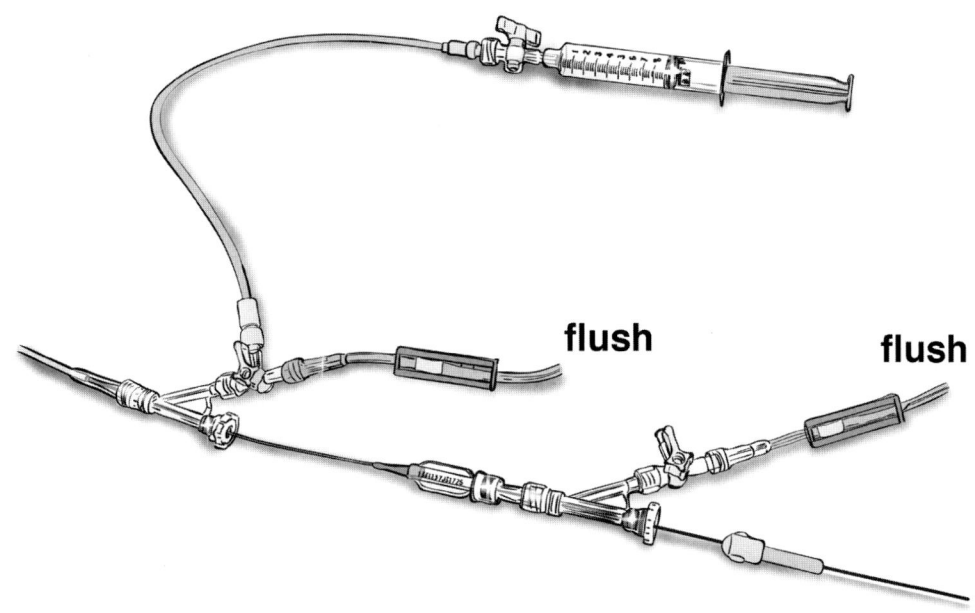

FIGURE 2.6 • An illustration of the basic coaxial set-up for all neurointerventional procedures. A high-pressure 12-in side-arm of pliable tubing is an option not used universally, but allows syringe attachment or injector hook-ups without disturbing a tenuously seated catheter. Pressurized saline flush at 300 mm Hg is regulated at tabletop by the color-coded lines.

parinization is used and is higher when technical difficulties are encountered with catheter manipulation and vessel selection. It is known from the use of intraprocedural transcranial Doppler monitoring that 50–100 microembolic signals can be detected during the course of a diagnostic cerebral angiogram.[6–8] The microembolic signals observed with Doppler are assumed to be mostly benign bubbles that pass through the cerebral microvasculature without causing injury. However, this is not known for sure, and in the absence of such proof one must assume that standards of tableside technique should at all times be as meticulous as possible.

Catheters and Introducer Sheaths

Most of the modern large-bore catheters are braided in construction. This represents a great improvement on the catheters of a few years ago when kinking, breakage, and lack of steerability were major problems. Many long sheaths are now on the market, allowing the option of accessing the carotid or vertebral arteries with a larger introducer lumen while minimizing the size of the arteriotomy site. These are most useful for stenting procedures.

Length of devices can be problematic, and for unusual or difficult cases it is worthwhile spending 10 minutes in advance doing some homework or trials outside the body to assure that a case will not be confounded by incompatible devices. The lengths of interest to neurointerventional work for introducer devices are 70-cm, 90-cm, 100-cm, and 110-cm. In most adult patients, a 7 Fr 70-cm sheath will extend from the common femoral artery to the mid-proximal common carotid artery. This is useful for test-occlusions where one intends using a 100-cm 5 Fr occlusion balloon. A 90-cm sheath or catheter will reach the internal carotid artery or distal vertebral artery in most patients; occasionally a 100-cm catheter is necessary when arteries are very tortuous.

An extremely useful device to keep in stock is a cerebral catheter longer than the standard 100 cm, e.g., a 110-cm 5 Fr Davis catheter or a 125-cm Vitek

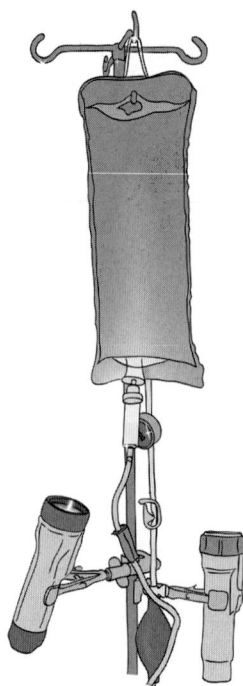

FIGURE 2.7 • Clamps from a chemistry laboratory contrive inexpensively to focus light on the drip chambers of the flush-lines, crucial at times of low light conditions for monitoring the rate of flow.

(Cook) cerebral catheter. The extra length of these catheters can be pivotal in selecting major vessels during cases in which exchange-length wires must be inserted or where the diagnostic catheter is first advanced to act as a coaxial guide for a following introducer device.

When a few centimeters of length are of critical importance in coaxial device management, the Tuohy-Borst valve can be removed from the introducer and replaced with a simple flap-valve flushed through a side-arm available in 4–6 Fr and 7–9 Fr sizes (Maxxim/Argon). This will gain you about 5 cm extra in length for the device being inserted.

WIRES AND MICROWIRES

Neurointerventional microwires are generally of 0.014–0.016-in caliber and with convergence of technology tend to be very similar in performance from one company to another (Figs. 2.8–2.10). Similarly, the 0.010-in wires for directing smaller microcatheters are very comparable in performance. Ultralight wires, e.g., the Mizzen wires (Target, Fremont, CA), can be used inside a nominally flow directed microcatheter to add body to the microcatheter or even steer it at the tip. Most of the newer wires have hydrophilic coating and must be kept wet in saline while not in use. Some of the older wires still have a particular niche to fill during interventional cases. For example, a Dasher-14® wire can be used through a 10-series catheter for very precise intracranial manipulation or steering into an aneurysm. Occasionally the Stubbie®, a very stiff steel wire, can be useful in extracranial situations of extreme tortuosity where the microcatheter is unsupported and other wires are too deformable.

For intracranial stenting and balloon angioplasty, the 300-cm 0.014-in microwires currently in use in the field of cardiology are extremely variable in performance. Some of the stiffer wires are completely unsuitable for intracranial use. Even with the softer and mid-range wires, e.g., ACS Hi-Torque Traverse®, the ACS Hi-Torque Balance® (Guidant, Santa Clara, CA), or the Choice PT® (Boston Scientific, Maple Grove, MN), extreme care is necessary intracranially to avoid perforation of distal small vessels or intimal tears on tight corners.

MICROCATHETERS

There are two types of microcatheters: wire-directed of 0.010–0.016-in caliber, and flow-directed, usually close to 0.010 in. The distinction between them is more blurred than before with the possibility of wire-manipulation of the flow-directed microcatheters and the advent of extremely floppy-tipped braided microcatheters.

Flow-directed microcatheters are used for delivering flow-sensitive coils to an AVM, liquid material to an AVM, or smaller PVA particles. They are usually so floppy that they have to be mounted on a stylet or wire to allow them to be advanced within the introducer catheter. Care should be taken during preparation of the flow-directed microcatheters to avoid any kind of proximal microcatheter perforation with the stylet. This can translate during subsequent em-

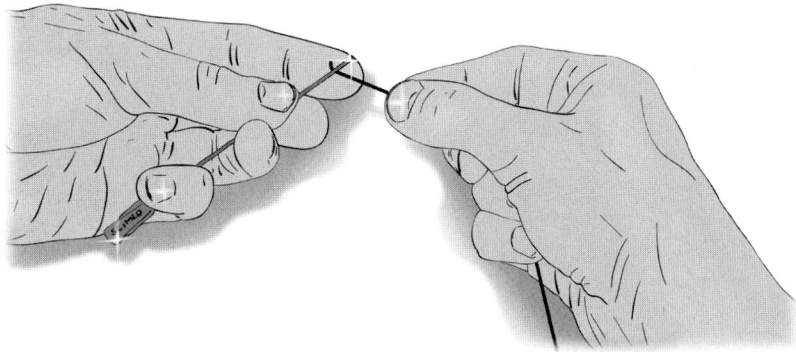

FIGURE 2.8 • Most modern wires are hydrophilically coated. Therefore any shaping or use of the wire requires wetting it with saline in advance. Wires vary in the degree of force necessary to induce a distal curve. Wires of 0.010-in caliber are generally very susceptible to being over curved and should be stroked very gently. When the wire is too curved to advance into the microcatheter hub, the provided introducer device (illustrated) can be backloaded at the end of the wire and advanced up to straighten the curve during introduction.

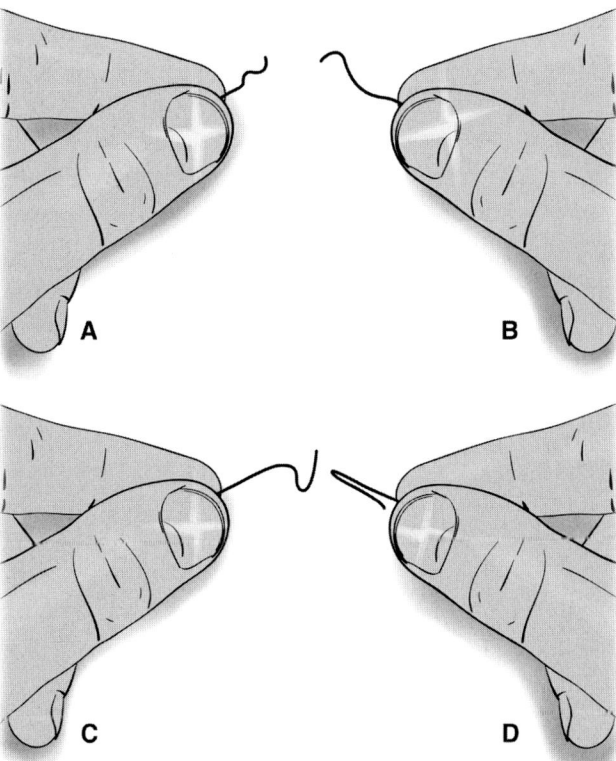

FIGURE 2.9 • Examples of the types of curves necessary for difficult intracranial navigation, with particular emphasis on the anterior cerebral artery. With all carotid and vertebral artery navigations, a J curve on the wire after it emerges from the microcatheter will help to reduce the risk of a traumatic dissection.

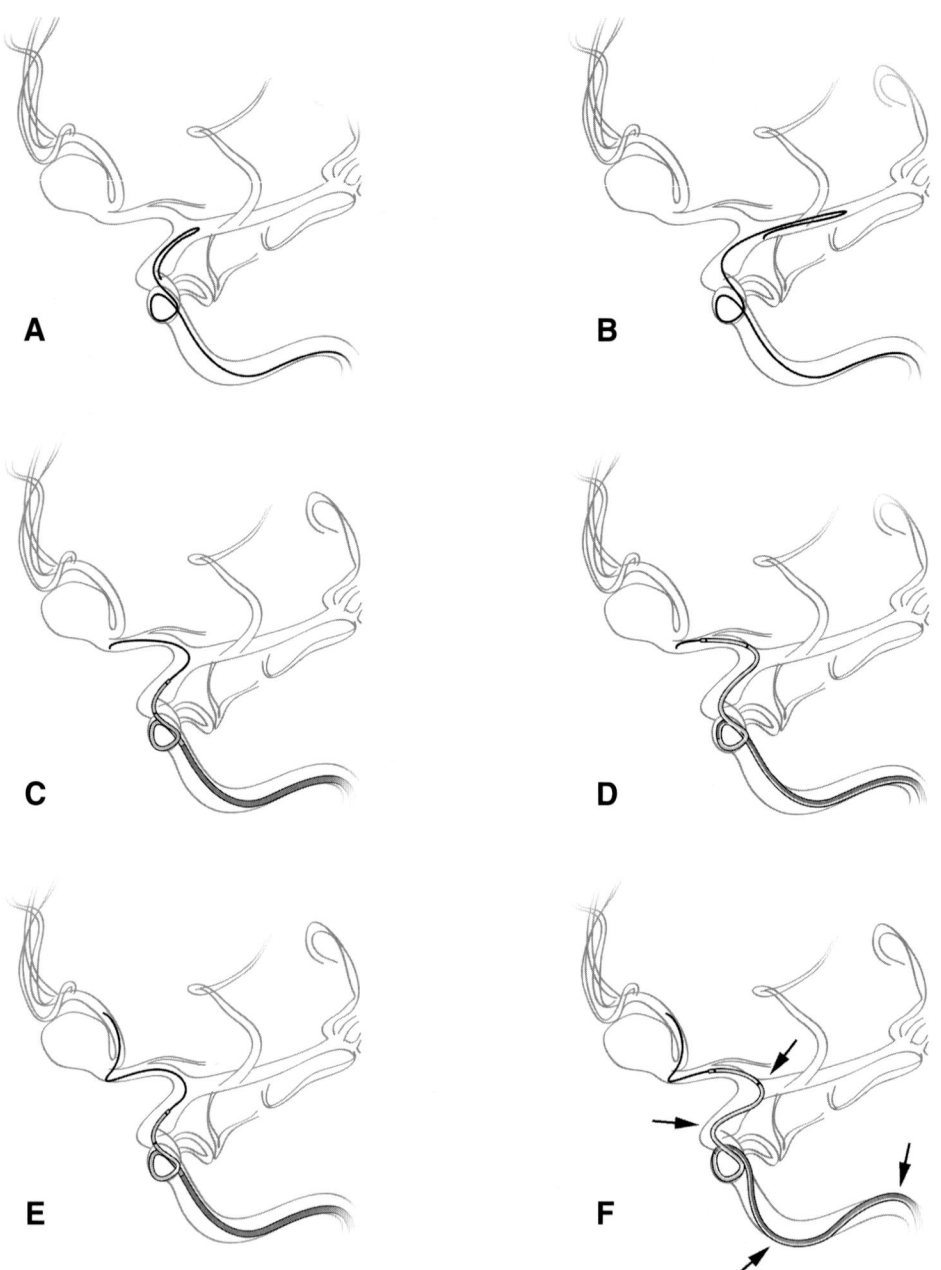

FIGURE 2.10 • The dragging loop method for anterior cerebral artery navigation described by Graves et al.[35] is analogous to using a Simmons curve in the aortic arch for selecting a difficult carotid artery. In this set of illustrations the loop has been advanced into the middle cerebral artery (A, B) and dragged back into the A1 segment (C). In illustration D the microcatheter is represented as having been advanced only proximally in the A1 segment. One needs to be extremely careful about accumulation of catheter tension in making difficult curves (arrows in F). When this happens, the microcatheter can suddenly release its tension by harpooning forward and perforating an aneurysm or arterial wall. When difficulties are encountered, the wire can sometimes be navigated more safely past the danger point (E). After the microcatheter has been advanced, the tension at the curves in the microcatheter should be eased at the proximal curves by retracting the microcatheter before selecting the aneurysm with the wire.

bolization into a proximal release of embolic material into the brain with disastrous consequences.

Wire-directed microcatheters vary a great deal in distal maneuverability. They are generally braided, which makes them more difficult to steam-shape than nonbraided products, but this also makes them less vulnerable to kinking or rupture. Hydrophilic coating allows them to gain more distal access than nonhydrophilic microcatheters, but at the cost of greater instability. Microcatheters for delivery of aneurysm coils have two markers at the distal end to allow alignment of the detachment zone with the microcatheter tip.

Detachable Balloons

Two types of detachable balloons are available:

1. Latex balloons (Nycomed, France) have some advantages in size and profile compared with silicone balloons. They have a gold marker within, allowing them to be more easily seen while deflated. Their coefficient of friction with the vessel wall is better, and they have less propensity to slip forward after detachment. They are not approved for use by the Federal Drug Administration (FDA) and cannot be used in patients with known allergies to latex material. They tend to deflate spontaneously in the days to weeks following insertion, by which time surrounding thrombosis and fibrosis have become established (Figs. 2.11–2.13).
2. Silicone DSB Balloons (Target, Fremont, CA) are approved for use by the FDA. The closure valves are color-coded for three levels of resistance to detachment. They are larger in profile than equivalently sized latex balloons, and therefore require a larger introducer catheter. They are inflated with isotonic contrast, Visipaque 320 (iodixanol) with osmolality 290 mOsm/kg. Under normal circumstances they do not deflate over time, unlike latex balloons, and do not incite a strong surrounding inflammatory reaction in adjacent tissue. They tend to be slippery inside the vessel and have a propensity for forward movement under the hydrostatic pressure of forward flow (Fig. 2.14).

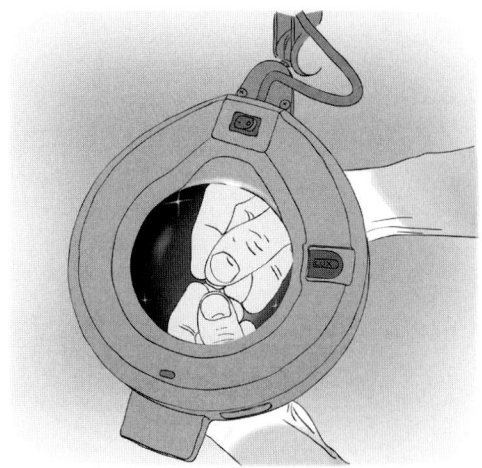

FIGURE 2.11 • A stand-mounted illuminated magnifying glass is a very useful piece of laboratory equipment for mounting contrary balloons or other intricate devices.

Histopathological evaluation of the differences between the two types of balloons in experimental aneurysms in laboratory animals confirm anecdotally observed differences between the two types of balloons.[9] More exuberant fibroblastic reaction and endothelialization over the surface of experimental aneurysms were seen with latex balloons compared with silicone balloons in dogs. Silicone balloons were less likely to incite a fibroblastic and inflammatory response in surrounding tissue than latex, resulting in greater mobility of the silicone balloon. In fact, during 2 months of follow-up after balloon placement in the dog aneurysms, greater mortality was seen in the silicone group due to spontaneous aneurysmal rupture thought to be related to trauma against the dome of the aneurysm by the mobile silicone balloon. These observations on the lack of thrombogenicity of silicone versus latex suggest that latex balloons may be more effective and stable when complete arterial closure is required. Silicone balloons, on the other hand, might be safer when preservation of flow in the adjacent artery is needed, e.g., balloon treatment of a carotid-cavernous fistula, because a silicone balloon might be less likely to generate surface thrombus that could be shorn off by the bypassing bloodstream.

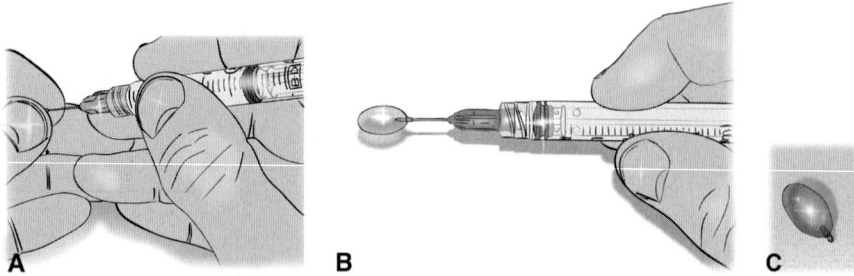

FIGURE 2.12 • Latex balloons have a long valve, which must be penetrated fully with a blunt inflation needle or stubbie provided in the package (A). After they are inflated with contrast, bubbles of air within are fished out by directing the tip of the stubbie directly at the bubbles and partially deflating (B). They are then detached from the stubbie and observed for competence of the valve over a period of a few minutes before mounting them on a microcatheter. Placing them on a dry towel over a period of a few minutes will allow one to detect any leakage from the balloon (C). A rapidly deflating balloon within the body due to a faulty or torn valve could be a cause of disaster.

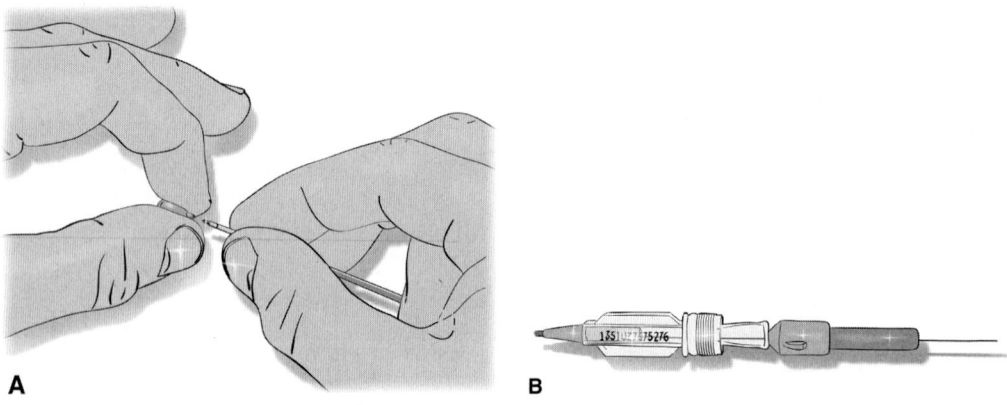

FIGURE 2.13 • Latex balloons can be mounted on a coaxial 2F/3F Red/Black delivery system (Nycomed) or on an extended-tip microcatheter (Target). An extended-tip microcatheter has a longer segment of catheter (5 or 20 mm) than standard microcatheters distal to the platinum marker to facilitate ease of balloon mounting. The Nycomed system is supplied with a stiffening stylet already in place. Usually it is better not to remove this stylet until the balloon is mounted because the stylet is very difficult to insert back into the microcatheter. An extended-tip microcatheter, on the other hand, must be backloaded with the stiff end of a standard microwire until a millimeter of wire protrudes from the tip (A). The position of the wire within the microcatheter can be stabilized at the hub by using the torque device as a brake (B). A commonly used method for preparing a latex balloon is to mount the contrast-filled balloon onto the microcatheter and to allow it to deflate in that position, thus eliminating air from the lumen of the microcatheter.

The Nycomed system requires that the red inner microcatheter be supported externally by the black outer sleeve so as to give it enough body to be advanced into the Tuohy-Borst valve. This involves advancing the outer black sleeve close to but not touching the balloon. Obviously this involves the potential for pushing the balloon off the red catheter if not done carefully. Once the combined system is securely in the introducer catheter, the assistant at the lower end of the table advances the red inner microcatheter (holding the balloon) farther up the catheter. It is important to secure the position of the red and black components with reference to one another from this point to avoid the possibility of pushing the balloon off the central red microcatheter with an independently moving outer black sleeve.

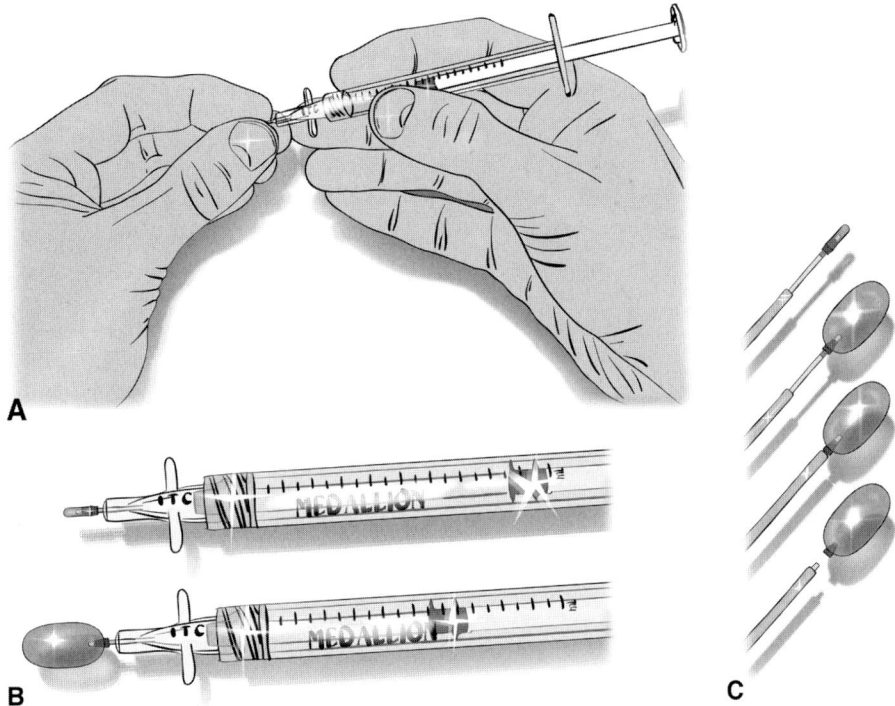

FIGURE 2.14 • Silicone detachable balloons (DSB, Target) can be prepared in a fashion similar to latex balloons (A, B) as described in Figs. 2.12, 2.13. Near isotonic nonionic contrast is necessary for silicone balloons. A detaching microcatheter system involving an outer sleeve (Target) is one of the options available for mounting and detaching (C), although other microcatheters can be used. Manufacturer recommendations may be followed according to one's preference. If one so wishes, the uninflated balloon can be mounted on a coaxial microcatheter system stiffened with a venting mandrel. The mandrel is flushed gently with isotonic contrast as it is withdrawn, filling the balloon and microcatheter lumen and eliminating air. The valve system on the DSB is larger than an equivalently sized latex balloon, and the manufacturers provide a wall chart detailing the 6Fr–8.3Fr introducer systems necessary for each of the various balloon sizes. The valves are color-coded into three groups according to the degree of friction or grip that the valve exercises on the mounting device.

These histological observations by Miyachi et al. in dogs[9] are in concordance with clinical observations of a tendency for silicone balloons to be mobile immediately after placement or even on a delayed basis. Latex balloons, on the other hand, have a definite tendency to undergo spontaneous deflation within a matter of days to weeks. When this happens, acute complications such as recanalization of vessels or occluded fistulas can occur. In both instances—early deflation on the part of latex balloons and migration on the part of silicone balloons—an argument can be made for supporting the key therapeutic balloon deposition with what might appear initially to be a superfluous number of balloons. Some authors argue that two balloons are adequate for arterial sacrifice, others prefer to place up to four. Latex balloons are not immune from the risks of sudden antegrade migration, and either type of balloon when used as a singleton carries a risk of sudden motion due to hemodynamic pressure.[10,11] With both types of balloons one has to be extremely vigilant during the time that the first balloon placed in an artery is exposed to the full hemodynamic pressure before a second supporting balloon is deployed. Measures to prevent migration include placing a simultaneous lower "shepherd-balloon" for control of flow. If motion of

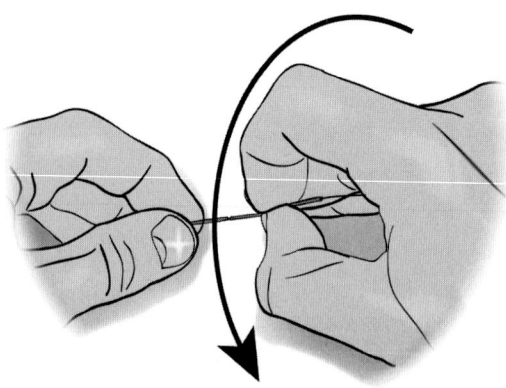

FIGURE 2.15 • Guglielmi detachable coils (GDC®) are supplied in a plastic sleeve necessary for stiffness while introducing them into the microcatheter. To avoid slipping of the coil within the sleeve, the sleeve is crimped tightly at its proximal end. To facilitate ease of movement of the coil, the crimping is loosened by twisting counterclockwise with the right hand.

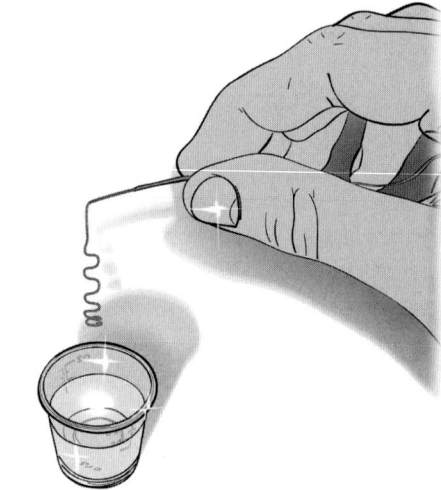

FIGURE 2.16 • Most authorities recommend extruding the coil from its sleeve and dipping it in heparinized saline before starting the insertion process.

the topmost balloon is seen, the introducer catheter can be jammed roughly into the carotid artery to staunch flow and induce spasm while the second balloon is in preparation. External compression of the carotid artery might also be useful.

NONDETACHABLE BALLOONS

Various nondetachable compliant balloons are available for temporary vessel occlusion. Larger vessels such as the proximal internal carotid artery or common carotid artery can be occluded with a 5 Fr or 7 Fr double-lumen balloon catheter (e.g., Cook, Meditech). Smaller compliant balloons suitable for small-vessel occlusion or for intracranial vasospasm angioplasty include wire-directed balloon systems:

- Sentry balloon (Target)
- Commodore (Cordis)
- Equinox balloon (MTI)

A nonwire-directed balloon, the Endeavor (Target), is a soft-compliant balloon catheter with a single lumen used to inflate the balloon. Although this would seem to limit its performance and versatility, this balloon was the only balloon available for a number of years for the purposes of intracranial vasospasm angioplasty or aneurysm reconstructive techniques. Therefore, a considerable experience with this balloon has reflected favorably on its safety. Its stability and steerability can be improved by inserting a shaped 0.010-inch wire within its lumen extending up to the balloon and by using a Tuohy-Borst valve to inflate around the wire.

GUGLIELMI DETACHABLE COILS

The Guglielmi Detachable Coil (GDC) is manufactured from a tightly wound platinum wire measuring from 0.0015 in (in the GDC 10 ultrasoft category) to 0.003 in (in the GDC 18 series). A primary helix is wound to a 0.010-in (Tracker 10) or 0.016-in (Tracker 18) caliber, and then wound in turn to a secondary helix measuring 2mm to 20mm in diameter with varying lengths. When the coil is in a satisfactory position within an aneurysm, a 9V current is passed through the coil, causing an electrolytic detachment from the stainless steel pusher-wire (Figs. 2.15–2.19).

More complex configurations of the GDC have had a significant impact on the versatility of this device for aneurysm embolization. The 2D coil has an initial turn of smaller diameter on the first loop. This encourages a pathway within the aneurysm for this

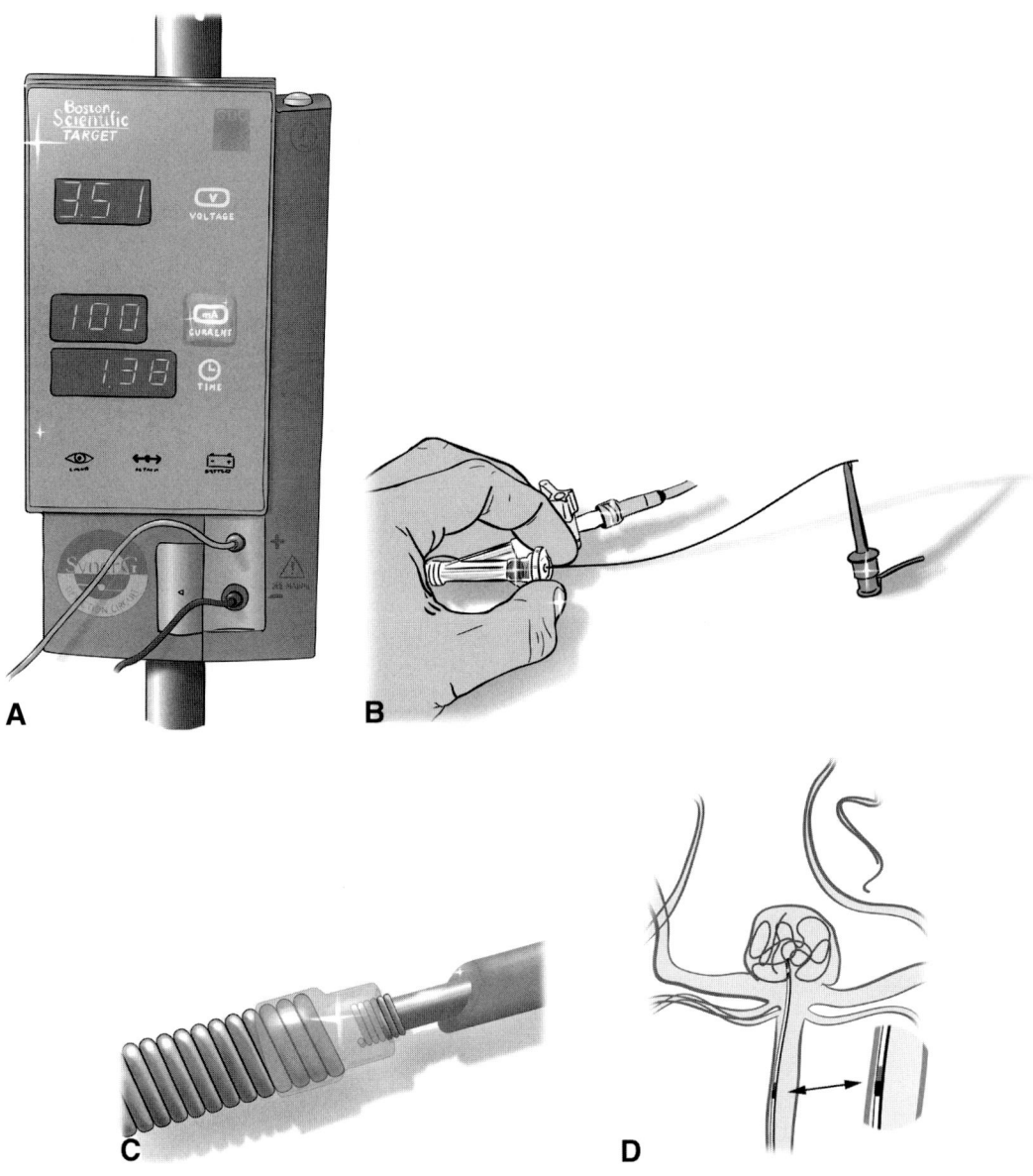

FIGURE 2.17 • The newest iteration of electrical detachment mechanism GDC4 (Boston Scientific, Target) is similar to and compatible with previous equipment but involves a greater range of current selections up to 2 mA and more internal circuitry for detection of current shorting (A). To avoid short-circuiting the detachment current into a wet towel, the red electrode is stood on its end as demonstrated (B). Only the proximal 3 cm of wire can be used for detachment, because of an insulating layer on the remainder of the wire (B). The newest generation of detachment mechanism (C) uses an insulation device at the junction of the pusher wire and coil to accelerate detachment by preventing dissipation of the current throughout the coil. Coils are advanced until the moderately opaque marker on the coil pusher is just beyond the proximal platinum marker of the double-marker introducer catheter (D). The pusher wire used to advance the coil is of stainless steel and therefore not seen well on fluoroscopic images, in contrast to the coil or the markers.

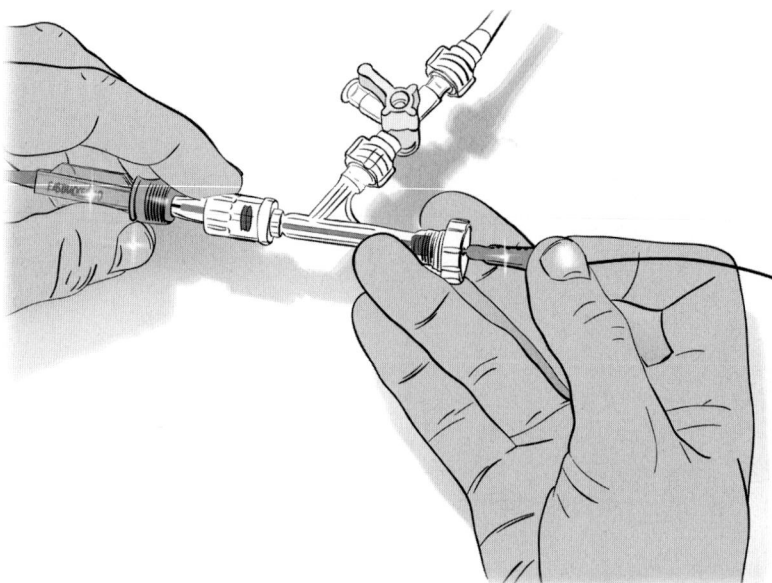

FIGURE 2.18 • Sometimes the pusher wire of a coil can kink during a difficult advancement. In situations other than an intracranial aneurysm, resistance can be overcome by straightening the pusher with an introducer rod. Greater push can be imparted to the coil in small increments in the manner illustrated without kinking the wire.

first loop that will curve back into the body of the aneurysm, as opposed to emerging from the outflow zone into the parent vessel. This helps the following loops of coil to follow suit and stay confined within the aneurysm. The 3D coil has a complex configuration composed of omega-like curves. When fully deployed, it tends to form an almost spherical over- all shape and can serve as a basket for successful placement of other coils within. Some potential disadvantages of 3D coils can be seen, however. By virtue of defining the overall scope of subsequent intraaneurysmal coil deployment during a case, any corner pocket of aneurysm excluded by the initial 3D coil(s) can be subsequently very difficult to access

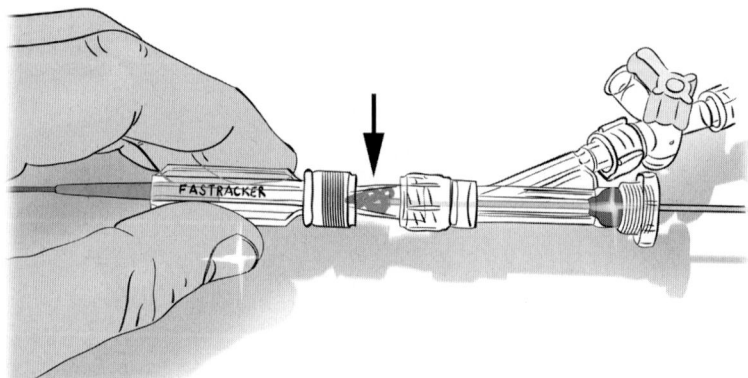

FIGURE 2.19 • During the initial coil advancement in the microcatheter, if the sleeve is not adequately pushed into the hub of the microcatheter it can bunch up on itself as illustrated. If this happens, do not pull back on the coil because it may tangle on itself and become damaged. Loosen the skein of coil in one piece from the hub before retracting it gently into the plastic introducer.

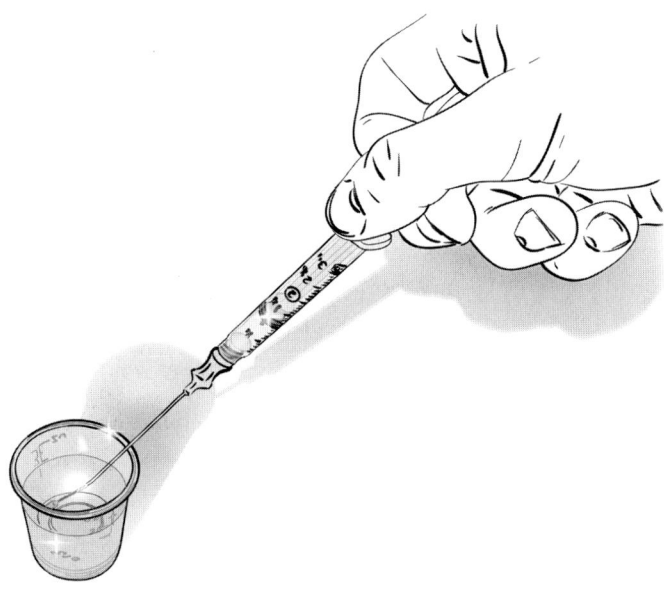

FIGURE 2.20 • Liquid coils are provided in a launching tube from which they are injected into the microcatheter using saline. To eliminate air from the tubing, suction of saline into the tube is performed as demonstrated. To help prevent inadvertent loss of the flimsy coil, a stopper at the end of the launching tube is supplied. It does not have to be removed while the coil is being prepared, but obviously it is discarded before the coil is launched into the microcatheter.

(Fig. 3.12). If the 3D coil seems to exclude an important lobe or part of the neck of the aneurysm, it might be worthwhile considering use of a reconstructive balloon technique to achieve more complete aneurysm filling. This will most often have to be used from an early stage in the procedure to achieve coil stability in the pocket in question.

Stretch-resistant (SR) coils have a 9.0 polypropylene thread through the primary helix. This gives greater strength to the coil if it needs to be withdrawn from the aneurysm. Soft coils without this SR feature have a vulnerability to being stretched or broken during withdrawal. Therefore, they are usually best used only in short lengths if no SR coils are available, and only where one is confident that problems with insertion of the coil will not be encountered.

Push Coils and Liquid Coils

A large variety of fibered thrombogenic coils is available from numerous vendors in 0.010, 0.016, and 0.035-in caliber. Fibered 0.016-in coils that can be electrolytically detached from a stainless steel pusher are also available and are very useful for high-flow or otherwise tenuous situations where coil loss is feared. Different vendors have various loading mechanisms for their coils. In general the holding device supplied with the coil must be held tightly in line with the hub of the microcatheter to allow initiation of the coil into the shaft. From there, the coil can be advanced with a push of saline if the situation is safe. More commonly, precise deposition of the coil is required and a coil-pusher is used to advance the coil. The coil-pusher looks like a wire but has a flatter tip of gold or other radiographically dense material.

Liquid Coils® (Target, Fremont, CA) are ultralight 0.008 or 0.016-in platinum coils which are advanced by an injection of saline or contrast within the microcatheter. They are most commonly used for AVM embolization to slow down flow and are easily manipulated and cut during surgical resection of the AVM (Fig. 2.20).

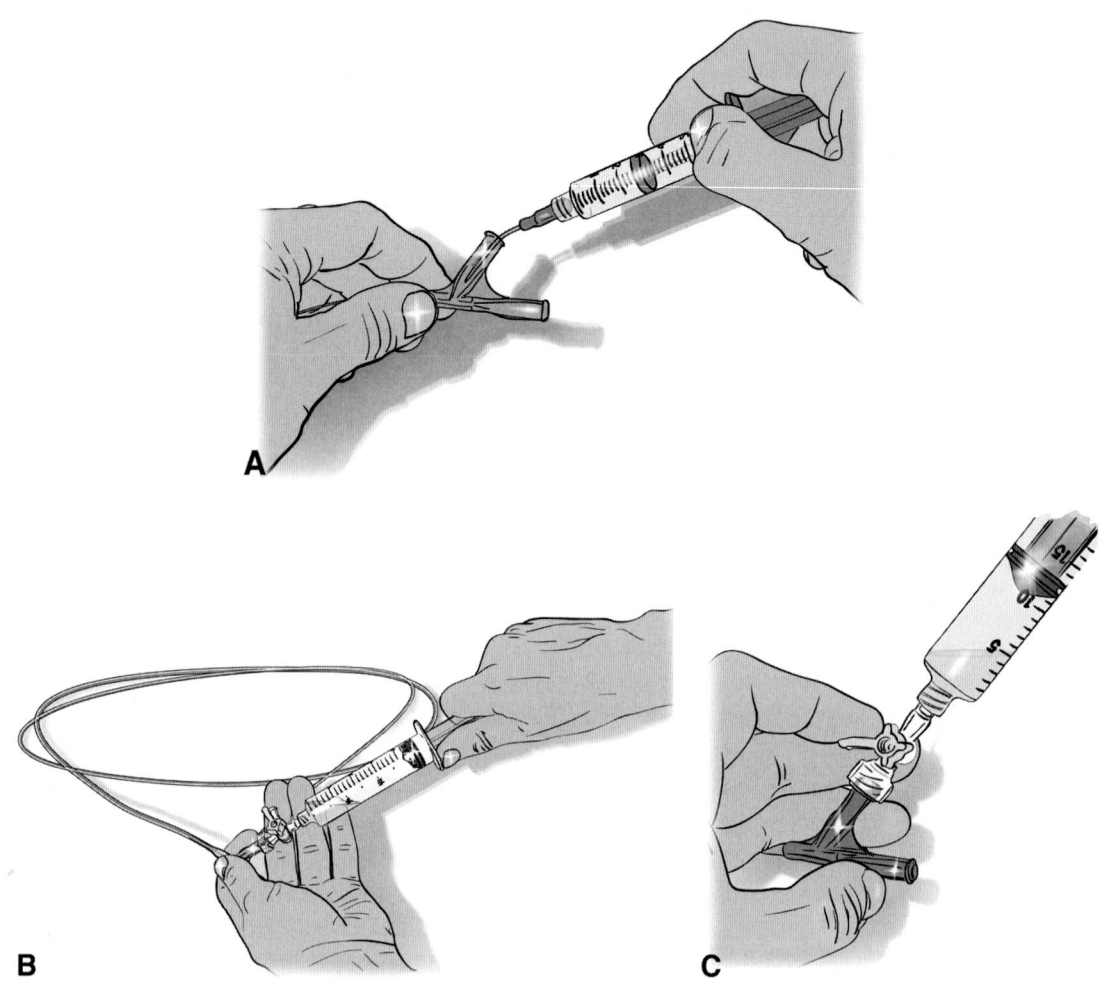

FIGURE 2.21 • Balloon-mounted coronary stents are prepared in a manner similar to coronary angioplasty balloons. The central lumen for the wire is flushed with saline. The balloon lumen is primed with contrast to eliminate air. This process can be accelerated a little by filling the side-arm with contrast (A) and then applying suction with a 20-ml syringe containing 2–4 ml of contrast (B). When suction has been applied a few times, the stopcock can be flicked into closed position to maintain the vacuum within the balloon-lumen (C).

Stents

Vascular stents are deployed either by balloon expansion of a collapsed stainless steel stent, or release of a self-expanding nitinol or steel stent from a constraining sheath. Coronary stents cover the size ranges up to 4-mm diameter. With maximal dilatation of a coronary balloon-expandable stent, diameters up to 4.3 mm can be covered. Larger stents cover the range between 6 mm and 10 mm. Between 4 mm and 6 mm stent options are more limited, although the Palmaz balloon-expandable stent or Magic Schneider self-expanding stents can cover this size range. Self-expanding stents are preferred in exposed locations where minor trauma or deformity of the surrounding tissues might be expected in the course of normal patient activity. Balloon-expandable stents may be at risk for being deformed and crushed in exposed locations of the neck (Figs. 2.21–2.27).

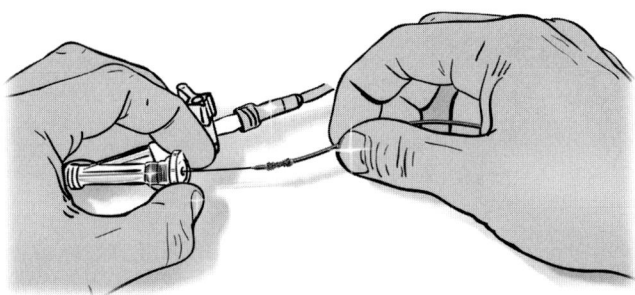

FIGURE 2.22 • For intracranial angioplasties and stent placements, stability of the wire in the distal intracranial circulation is crucial. In this illustration, there is probably excessive play in the configuration of the wire-catheter combination. The left hand must keep control of the wire until the balloon catheter reaches the valve. The assistant must give tension sufficient to keep the catheter straight thereafter, but not cause retraction of the wire at the same time. With excessive slack in the catheter as illustrated here, advancing the catheter with the right hand will cause the distal intracranial wire to advance considerably.

Balloon-expandable stents are manufactured in two general designs. A "slotted tube" stent such as the Palmaz stent or the NIR stent tends to be more rigid and tends to remain relatively straight after deployment. This can be advantageous in certain circumstances. On the other hand, a stent composed of discrete jointed sections, such as the S670 stent (Medtronic AVE) or MultiLink Tristar stent (Guidant) may be more flexible during delivery and may conform better to a curved vessel after deployment. This may confer advantages or disadvantages, depending on the circumstances.

Some manufacturers have attempted to improve the delivery and expansion characteristics of their stents by altering the distal shape of the balloon to a stepped configuration or by partially wrapping the ends of the collapsed stent in the folds of the balloon. These designs are aimed at preventing a

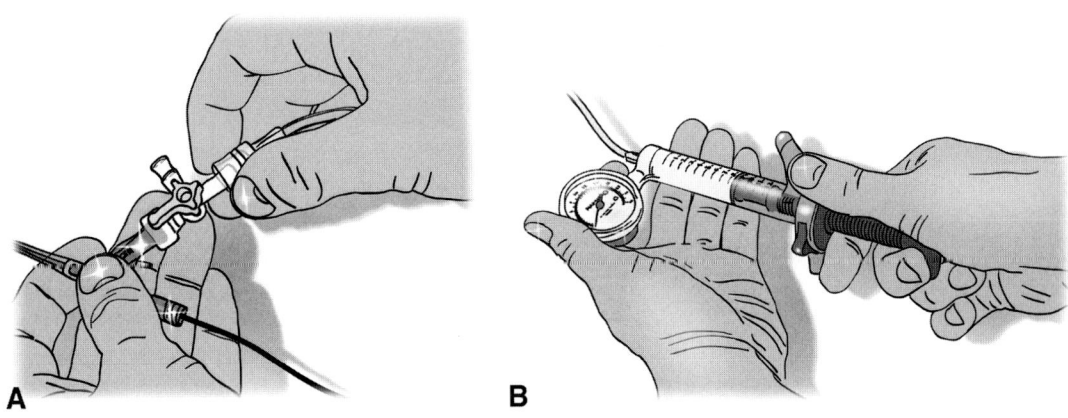

A   B

FIGURE 2.23 • Using an inflation handle or manometer is important for controlling the rate and degree of inflation of the balloon, particularly for intracranial devices. The primed manometer and primed catheter can be joined as illustrated with the stopcock still sealed (A). When air has been eliminated from the stopcock by cranking the manometer forward, it can be opened to the manometer. A very slow rate of inflation is recommended for delicate intracranial vessels (B) (see Chapter 5). Fractions of a revolution are used as the balloon nears full expansion with long pauses between increments.

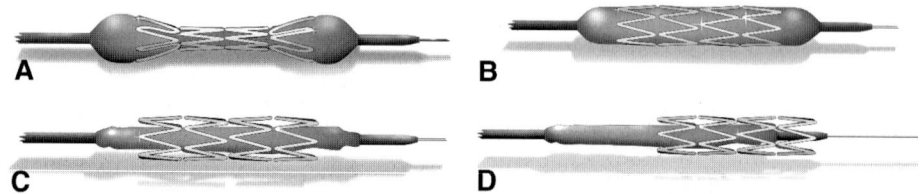

FIGURE 2.24 • Some balloon-mounted microstents have a tendency to "dog-bone" as they inflate (A, B). This is a theoretical concern for vessel damage or rupture, and admonishes against oversizing stents during intracranial use. Package inserts provided with the stents indicate nominal pressures for required diameters. Additional pressure within prescribed limits can allow an additional 0.1–0.3 mm of diameter of stent deployment, but one must stay below the rupture pressure of the balloon in use. When the balloon is deflated, the folds of the balloon are always a little more bulky than during the insertion. One must watch the stent carefully during retraction of the balloon to avoid any traction on the stent (C, D). On rare occasions when the stent is still adherent to the folds of the balloon, separation can be effected by twisting the balloon catheter within the stent or by advancing the wire to alter the tension of the catheter within the stent.

"dog-bone" appearance of the stent as it expands, which occurs when the early expression of balloon pressure is manifest only in the noncovered balloon.

Extracranial Use of Coronary Stents

Many of the currently available coronary stents are suitable for use in smaller extracranial vessels in the 2.5-mm to 4.5-mm diameter range. The designs are essentially divided into those consisting in a laser-cut metal tube or, alternatively, a series of short segments linked together by bridging struts. The advantage of the former "slotted tube" design is greater stiffness and integrity, which may be useful if straightening a segment of vessel is required or for overcoming the elastic recoil of a

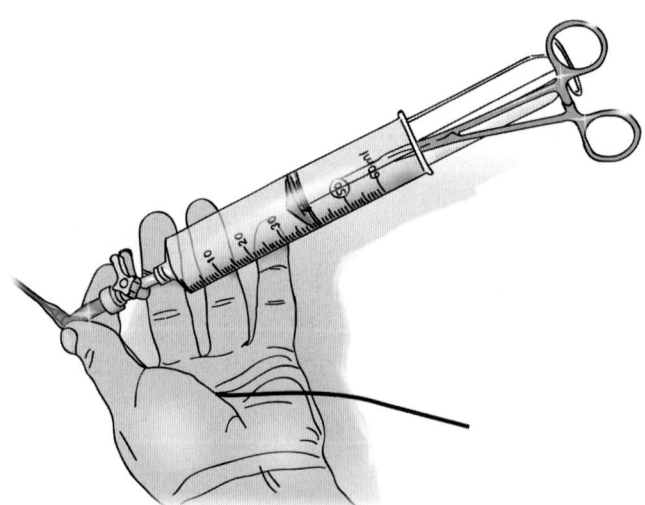

FIGURE 2.25 • Stent balloons and angioplasty balloons need to be as fully deflated as possible before retracting the balloon within the stent. Greatest suction can be applied with a 50–60 ml syringe, the plunger of which can be locked in the vacuumed state by applying a clamp as illustrated.

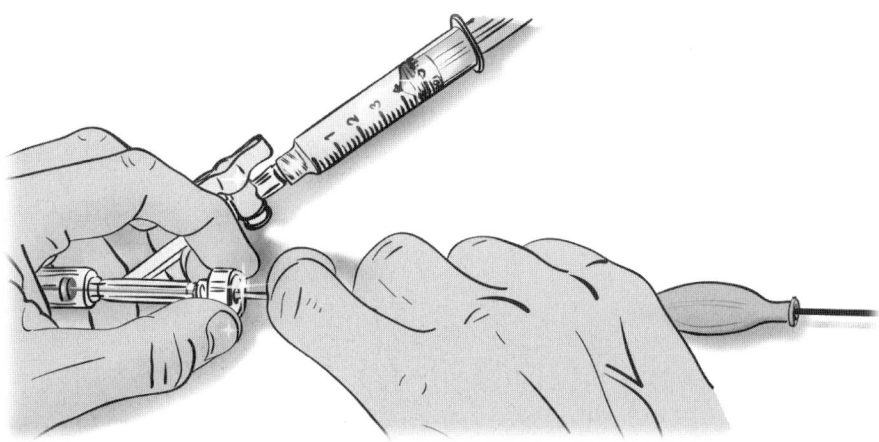

FIGURE 2.26 • Larger self-expanding stents such as the Wall stent (Schneider) or SMART stent (Cordis) are deployed by similar means. The right hand secures the central lumen which stabilizes the stent, while the left hand retracts the Tuohy-Borst adapter attached to the other sleeve, this action exposing the stent and allowing it to deploy. As one retracts the sleeve with the left hand, it is common to see the whole stent device move with reference to the target site. This is undesirable and will require as much straightening of the delivery catheter as possible in order to reduce movement. In some cases play in the catheter is inevitable. Therefore it is always desirable to aim for deployment a little on the distal or upper side of the site because it is easier and safer to retract than advance the delivery device with a partially released stent.

vessel ostium. The general comparative advantages of the segmented design of the stent are greater flexibility during delivery and greater conformity to the native tortuous anatomy of the vessels.

- Nir with SOX (balloon-expandable) (Boston Scientific/Medinol) 2.5–4 mm. This design features a folding of the balloon over the proximal and distal ends of the "slotted-tube" stent to prevent intimal trauma from the tines of the stent and to assure an even expansion of the stent.
- Nir on Ranger (balloon-expandable) (Boston Scientific/Medinol) 2.5–4 mm. This is an excellent stent for the straight segments of vertebral arteries with good radial strength resistant to arterial recoil. The Nir Royal stent is a similar stainless steel stent with gold electroplating for increased fluoroscopic visibility.
- Magic Wall Stent (self-expanding stainless steel) (Boston Scientific/Schneider) 3.0–5.0 mm.
- Radius (self-expanding nitinol) (Boston Scientific) 3.0–4.0 mm.

Intracranial Use of Coronary Stents

- S670 (Medtronic/AVE) (balloon-expandable) 3.0–4.0 mm diameter. The AVE stents formerly marketed as GFX and GFX2 are segmented stainless steel stents with remarkable capacity for distal navigation. Shorter stents obviously track more easily than longer stents. In difficult distal anatomy placing two short stents to cover a stenotic lesion or dissection might be a necessary fall-back stratagem when a single longer stent will not advance.[12,13]
- S660 (Medtronic /AVE) (balloon-expandable) 2.5-mm diameter is an even smaller segmented stent capable of distal small-vessel navigation.
- ACS Multi-Link TriStar or ACS Multi-Link Duet (Guidant).[13,14] The Multi-Link Tristar design features a step-like graduation in the contour of the mounting balloon to prevent any dog-bone configuration at the proximal and distal ends during stent expansion. It is available in standard over-the-wire ("OTW" marked on the package) configuration and rapid exchange monorail ("RX").

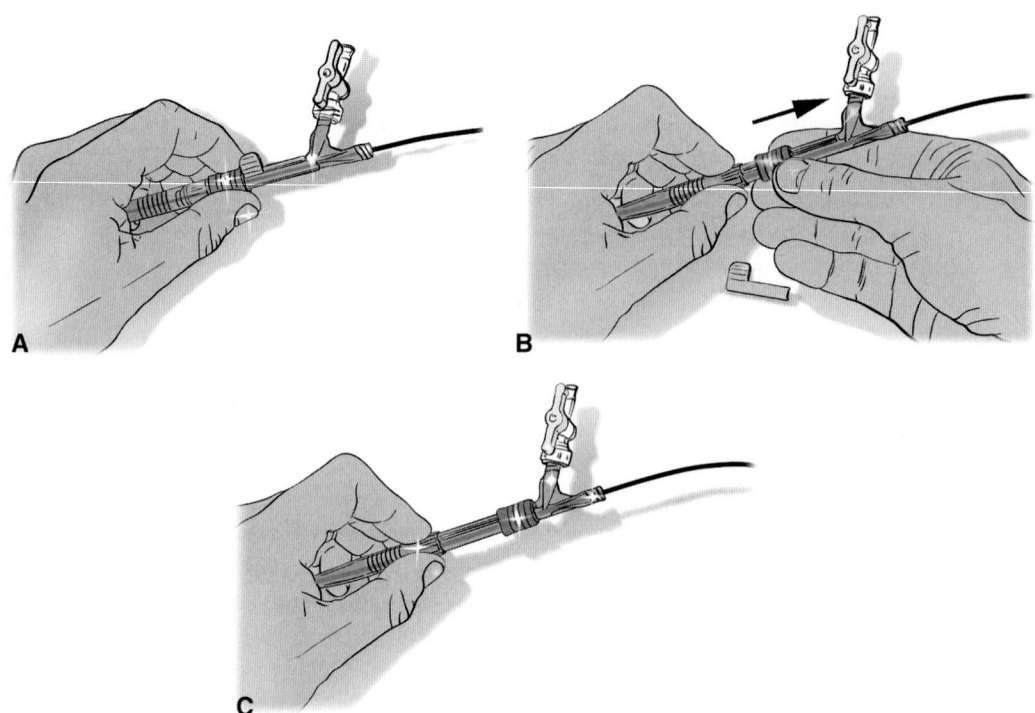

FIGURE 2.27 • The Radius self-expanding stent is deployed by a mechanism somewhat similar to that of larger self-expanding stents. After the stent catheter is in position (A), a protective spacer is removed (B). In contrast to the larger stent systems described in Fig. 2.26, the left hand stabilizes the catheter while the right hand retracts the sheath into the deployed position (C).

Coronary wires (length 300 cm diameter 0.014 in) recommended to the reader as suitable for various neurointerventional uses include:

- ACS Hi-Torque Traverse and Floppy II wires are the softest of the Guidant range. They have excellent performance for distal access. Hydrophilically coated wires such as the Choice and Choice PT range of wires (Boston Scientific) are preferred by some interventionalists because their manufacturing specifications are similar to those of dedicated intracranial wires. Some interventional cardiologists believe that hydrophilic wires are more likely to induce intimal dissections. With all wires it is important to be wary of any motion or jabbing of the wire-tip during exchange procedures so as to avoid the risks of intracranial perforation.
- Wires of intermediate stiffness such as the ACS Hi-Torque Balance (Guidant) and ACS Hi-Torque Balance Middle Weight (Guidant) can occasionally be helpful in gaining intracranial access when softer wires have failed.
- The most stiff of the 0.014-in wires such as the ACS Hi-Torque All Star or Iron Man wires (Guidant) or the 0.018-in V-18 wire (Boston Scientific/Meditech) are generally not suitable for any kind of intracranial use. However, they might be very useful on occasion in the proximal carotid or vertebral arteries where tortuous anatomy requires extra support.

ANGIOPLASTY BALLOONS

Many of the coronary angioplasty balloons lend themselves easily to use in the cranial circulation. The industry standard for coronary guide-wires is 0.014-in caliber, and most of the available balloons will fit through a 6 Fr introducer catheter. Interventional cardiologists sometimes like to use devices with a "monorail" design, in which the lumen for the guide-wire extends over a small section only of the angioplasty balloon or stent catheter. Other than for very proximal easily accessed lesions, this design is unsuitable for cranial use because the monorail design is not as suitable for advancing the wire through a difficult segment of vessel.

Coronary angioplasty balloons suitable for neurointerventional use include virtually all of the available coronary angioplasty balloons, although monorail balloon systems are sometimes a little more difficult to track distally through tortuous anatomy:

- Ranger (Boston Scientific). The Ranger angioplasty balloon is a standard that gives excellent performance. Shorter lengths obviously track better for more distal tortuous access. There are minor differences in balloon compliance in the various balloons of the Ranger set of products.
- Quantum Ranger. This balloon has a compliance profile intermediate between that of the Ranger and the NC (Non-Compliant) Ranger. It is a good balloon for performing post-deployment stent expansion.
- NC Ranger. This balloon is useful for severe difficulties with stent expansion due to lesion calcification or recoil.
- Big NC Ranger. This is a useful balloon with diameter up to 5 mm. It is very useful as an initial angioplasty balloon for carotid bifurcations.
- Photon (Guidant). This product has a lubricious hydrophilic coating which gives excellent distal trackability through tortuous anatomy.

The low profile of the coronary balloons makes them all excellent for crossing a tight stenosis with minimal trauma and performing an initial angioplasty over a 0.014-in wire.

Liquid Embolic Agents

Use of liquid embolic agents (acrylate glues and alcohol) is generally associated with embolization of brain arteriovenous malformations and are discussed in Chapter 15. Several newer liquid embolic agents are in development and are likely to reach the stage of clinical trials in the near future.

Polyvinyl Alcohol

Polyvinyl alcohol particles (PVA) are supplied in size ranges from 45 μm to 1000 μm. PVA particles in the size range of 50–150 μm induce a very effective devascularization with tumor necrosis, as is seen with gelfoam particles in the same size range.[15] However, the risks of collateral damage to adjacent tissue are considerable, in many instances prompting caution. Skull-base tumors frequently share arterial supply with important adjacent structures such as cranial nerves. To avoid injury to the vasa nervorum, PVA particles in the size range of 150–250 μm are usually preferred as a staple for preoperative tumor devascularization. Larger particles are used if there is arteriovenous shunting in the target tumor or if there are suspected collateral channels to dangerous anastomoses.

Polyvinyl alcohol particles induce devascularization by clumping along the endothelium of the vessel wall.[16,17] They provoke an inflammatory reaction in surrounding tissues with histopathological evidence of foreign-body giant cell reaction, mural angionecrosis, and necrotizing vasculitis. Less noxious, however, than other embolic agents such as acrylate or pure alcohol, PVA embolization in AVMs is characterized by a higher likelihood of recanalization within days to weeks.[18,19]

When using PVA particles, clearly marked sets of 1 ml syringes and towels are recommended to prevent any inadvertent dissemination of particles to other devices or wires that might be used later in the case in vulnerable territories (Fig. 2.28). PVA is injected in light suspension of contrast monitored fluoroscopically. Reflux into critical vessels or collateral communication through dangerous anastomoses are the paramount concerns during embolization. The mixing of PVA particles with contrast is generally based on experience. As a rule of thumb, clumping of particles in the hub of the catheter suggests that the concentration of particles is too high. The larger the size of particle, the less PVA one should add to the contrast. Additionally,

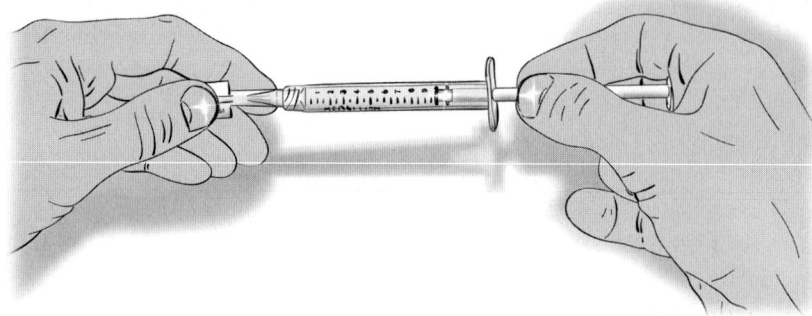

FIGURE 2.28 • With PVA or Gelfoam injections, clumping of the particles in the microcatheter can require additional force to push them clear. This could result in sudden decompression and change in resistance which would cause reflux of particles if the force on the plunger were excessive. To prevent this from happening, holding the syringe as illustrated with the right hand will assure that a sudden surge of the plunger will be braked by the thumb and forefinger on the stem.

it is worthwhile to use high-density contrast for particle injection. Most modern DSA machines provide excellent images with 200–240 strength nonionic contrast. However, for the PVA injections by hand, a separate bottle of 300 or 320 nonionic contrast can be used to enhance visualization.

Gelfoam

Gelfoam is a water-insoluble embolic agent prepared from pork-skin gelatin granules and is supplied in powder or sponge form. It is capable of holding up to 45 times its weight in blood within its interstices, accounting for its hemostatic qualities. It is resorbed by the body within 2–6 weeks without much sclerosing effect.

Gelfoam sponge is usually cut by scissors or scalpel into little pledgets or torpedoes, and injected into vessels where ultimate recanalization is acceptable or desirable, e.g., post-traumatic bleeding or epistaxis. The strips are cut as small as possible and rolled with dry gloves. The microcatheter is flushed with saline. At the last instant the dry Gelfoam torpedo is tapped into the Luer-lock tip of a 1 ml syringe containing contrast and launched into the proximal shaft of the microcatheter before it has time to swell excessively. It can be advanced from there with a firm push of saline or contrast. A sudden change in resistance with release of contrast from the microcatheter tip indicates delivery of the Gelfoam from the microcatheter tip. Because a certain degree of force is necessary to inject the gelfoam through the microcatheter, injection technique is important (Fig. 2.28). This technique should be used only in situations where a margin of error for reflux of the gelfoam exists. Therefore, injecting Gelfoam close to the origin of the external carotid artery is not a good idea because of ease of reflux into the internal carotid artery.

Gelfoam powder with particle dimensions of 40–60 μm has a powerful ischemic and necrotizing effect on pathologic and normal tissue due to its penetration of distal arterioles. It should be used only in situations where no risk to collateral vessels prevails and where a therapeutic effect more aggressive than simple presurgical devascularization is required.

Radiation Exposure and Monitoring

Monitoring and minimizing radiation use in the angiography suite is important for the welfare of patients and operating personnel. Modern fluoroscopic units are limited by law to maintaining exposures at tabletop (i.e., skin) of 10 roentgens per minute, with provision for higher-dose fluoroscopy to 20 roentgens per minute on demand for dense

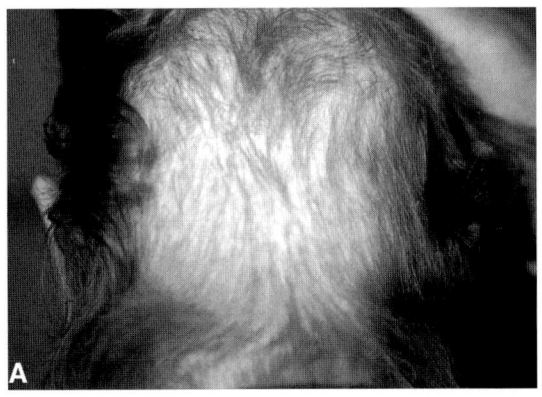
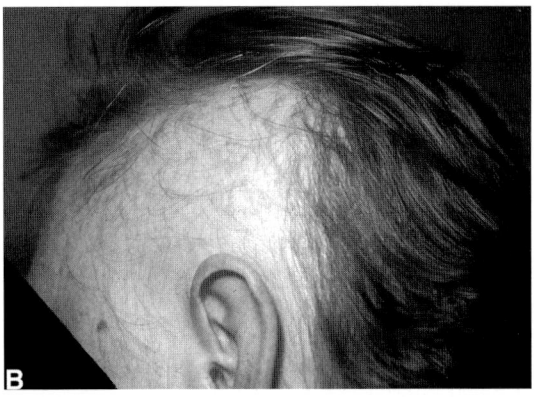

FIGURE 2.29 • Posterior (A) and oblique views (B) of a patient with sharply defined radiation burns to the head corresponding with the portals used during a prolonged neurointerventional procedure. This elderly patient was understanding of the complication due to her greater concern for her neurovascular problem. However, one should never be complacent about the risks involved either to patients or operating personnel. In the excitement of dealing with novel devices or challenging neurovascular problems, one should always have an eye for the cumulative radiation dose involved. Skin breakdown, scarring, and exposure of underlying bone structures have been reported following prolonged peripheral interventional procedures. Such things are best avoided completely in neurovascular work. Sometimes, for example with elective pediatric or other cases, it is a good idea to start the procedure with a firm decision concerning a cut-off time for fluoroscopy. At that time the procedure will be discontinued, to be resumed another day.

body parts. Exposures to the patient are reduced by interposition of filters or an air-gap between the X-ray tube and the patient's skin. Exposures are driven up by interposition of screens or an air-gap between the patient and the image intensifier. The biggest determinant of radiation exposure, however, is time on the pedal. As neurointerventional procedures have become more complex, newer devices have made new procedures possible, but at the cost of increased use of fluoroscopic exposure. This has significant implications for the health of everybody in the room (Fig. 2.29).

Radiation Effects: Deterministic and Stochastic

The deleterious effects of radiation exposure are categorized into deterministic and stochastic effects. Deterministic effects of radiation are those affecting a large number of cells in the field with immediate or imminent biologic response, e.g., skin erythema or retrolenticular opacities. In healthy tissue there is a capacity to resist and repair the effects of radiation, and therefore a threshold level of exposure can be established below which deterministic effects are not likely to be seen. Above this threshold level the severity of the biologic effect rises rapidly with increasing dose, and deterministic effects are therefore considered to be directly dose related in severity. Stochastic effects of radiation are less predictable and can occur at any level of exposure, e.g., radiation-related neoplasm. Stochastic effects are more likely to occur with higher exposures, but the severity of the effect is not proportional to dose. Stochastic responses are considered to be monoclonal in character or affecting a single cell at the outset. Therefore stochastic effects are seen later than deterministic effects.

Both of these effects are of major concern during long neurointerventional cases, and with more such intricate and tedious cases being performed each year, it is likely that radiation exposure will become an even greater concern from a patient-care and a regulatory point of view. The organ of greatest concern during neurointerventional procedures is the skin and its appendages (Table 2.1).

TABLE 2.1
SKIN EFFECTS FROM SINGLE DOSE IRRADIATION[20]

Effect	Threshold (Gy)	Onset	Peak
Temporary epilation	3	3 wk	
Permanent epilation	7	3 wk	
Transient erythema	2	hours	24 hrs
Erythema	6	10 d	2 wk
Dry desquamation	10	4 wk	5 wk
Moist desquamation	15	4 wk	5 wk
Late erythema	15	6–10 wk	
Ulceration	20	>6 wk	
Necrosis	18	>10 wk	
Atrophy	11	>14 wk	
Teleangiectasia	12	>52 wk	
Invasive fibrosis	10		

Temporary epilation following long neurointerventional procedures is probably more common than is reported in the medical literature and most neurointerventionalists have seen at least a few cases, many with prolonged erythema.[21] Depending on the dose of exposure, the epilation may be transient or permanent. With doses of 3–5 Gy epilation may be noticed by the patient 3 weeks after the procedure with gradual improvement after another 5 weeks. With higher doses—over 7 Gy—permanent epilation can be seen.[20] Rapidly growing cells are more sensitive to radiation; therefore scalp hair is more sensitive than eyebrow hair, for instance. Early transient erythema at skin doses in excess of 2 Gy can be seen due to release of histamine-like agents and proteolytic enzymes. This transient effect fades after 24 hours. More prolonged erythema with possible pigmentation can be seen with dose thresholds of 2–8 Gy after a single exposure.

More severe skin effects are rarely seen. Ulceration and necrosis under otherwise normal circumstances with responsible management of fluoroscopy times should not occur following neurointerventional procedures on the head. However, such effects can be seen and be very difficult to manage in patients who have the following risk factors:

- Previous fluoroscopic procedures within a few weeks
- Diabetes mellitus
- Connective tissue diseases, e.g., scleroderma, systemic lupus erythematosus, mixed connective tissue disease[22–24]
- Rash from any current illness or from previous radiation dose
- Ataxia teleangiectasia[25]
- Rapidly growing tissue, e.g., childhood

Estimates of patient exposures during cerebral diagnostic angiographic and neurointerventional procedures vary between an H_E value of 3.6 mSv and 43 mSv, with skin entrance doses as high as 6.6 Gy, translating into an estimated risk of subsequent radiation-induced neoplasm of 0.3% or less.[26–29]

Radiation Risk to Interventional Personnel

There is a great variation in degree of radiation awareness from one department to another. Use of a lead screen can reduce operator radiation exposure by a factor of 3,[30] but such screens are not consistently used in all suites. Similarly, use of a thyroid collar alone can reduce one's calculated effective dose (H_E) in half,[31] but thyroid collars are frequently neglected. Direct exposure of one's hand in the primary beam must be avoided at all times.

As a shorthand rule, exposures to operating personnel can be considered to be somewhere between 0.01 to 0.001 that of the patient.[28,29] Peripheral angiographers and interventional cardiologists in a busy department with 120–200 interventional cases per year receive an H_E dose of approximately 3.6–10 mSv per year, or 86 μSv per case.[28,32] Interventional neuroradiologists, on the other hand, probably receive less scatter radiation from the head per unit time by virtue of the relatively smaller body part involved and the presumed longer distance down the table, but fluoroscopy times are longer, compensating for this difference. Niklason et al.[31] estimated that the risk to the interventional radiologist represented approximately the equivalent of one fatal cancer per 10,000 careers.

The radiation-related risks to patients and operating personnel of current practice in interventional neuroradiology are not known, and estimates quoted in the literature are based on deduction. Long-term effects of the current pattern of use of radiation will not be evident for another 10–20 years. In the interim minimizing use of radiation exposure whenever possible is in the best interests of all involved.

Catheterizing the Carotid Arteries

Sometimes, redundant or tortuous vessels can be extremely difficult to catheterize with large introducer catheters or sheaths (Figs. 2.30, 2.31). If a stiff wire such as an Amplatz or stiff-shaft Terumo wire is necessary, it is probably safer to place the tip of the wire as far distally as possible in the external carotid artery before exchanging for a larger device. Often it is better to advance the large introducer over a 5 Fr long catheter (110–125 cm) to avoid the exchange maneuver. Most bad cerebral emboli during peripheral or subclavian angiography happen during exchange-wire maneuvers in the arch. One should be extremely cautious about using exchange wires in the carotid arteries or in the ascending aorta, and then only when the patient is already heparinized and preferably has antiplatelet medications active.

Advancing a Microcatheter

An over-the-wire (OTW) microcatheter is usually fairly atraumatic to the endothelium of an artery. However, if there is a dissection flap or tear in the surface, an advancing microcatheter has the ability to create a false lumen and extend the dissection. Therefore, it is safer to advance an OTW microcatheter with a J-curved microwire. The wire is invariably softer and will distort more easily in a flap or other obstruction, prompting one to be careful. Even in a heparinized patient, it is alarmingly easy to form clot in a stagnant microcatheter. Therefore, while advancing the microcatheter over the wire, it is preferable to continue flushing the microcatheter either with a standard 300 mm Hg flush-line, or with a 1 ml syringe attached to a Tuohy-Borst valve. When the inner lumen of the microcatheter and the microwire are of the same size, the fit is too snug to allow flushing to occur with the pressurized line. In this instance, the 1 ml syringe is more effective. When the wire is removed, the flush-line can then be attached.

Closing the Arteriotomy Site

Various devices are available for internal closure of the arteriotomy site or for external compression after sheath removal. External clamps are useful for cooperative patients in whom the arterial puncture site is known precisely. However, the compression pad is small, and where the site is uncertain or when the patient is moving around, the compression clamp is ineffective. Furthermore, the clamp is difficult to use once the patient is placed on a soft mattress. A pneumatically inflated and calibrated pad held in place by a firm belt constitutes the Femostop® device (Radi Medical Systems AB, Sweden). The pneumatic ball is transparent, allowing monitoring of the site. For situations where a hematoma has already developed and precise localization of the artery has become difficult, the Femostop is an excellent bail-out device well tolerated by patients even at high pressures. Its use does not require that the patient be on a firm surface, and it can be used on a soft mattress or ICU bed. Excessive prolonged use beyond a few hours can cause skin desquamation or superficial necrosis.

Internal closure devices for arterial closure include those using a suture (Closer® 6 Fr, or ProStarXL® 8 Fr, or 10 Fr from Perclose Inc., Menlo Park, CA) (Fig. 2.32), a coagulant plug of collagen (Vasoseal®, Datascope, Montvale, NJ) (Fig. 2.33), or

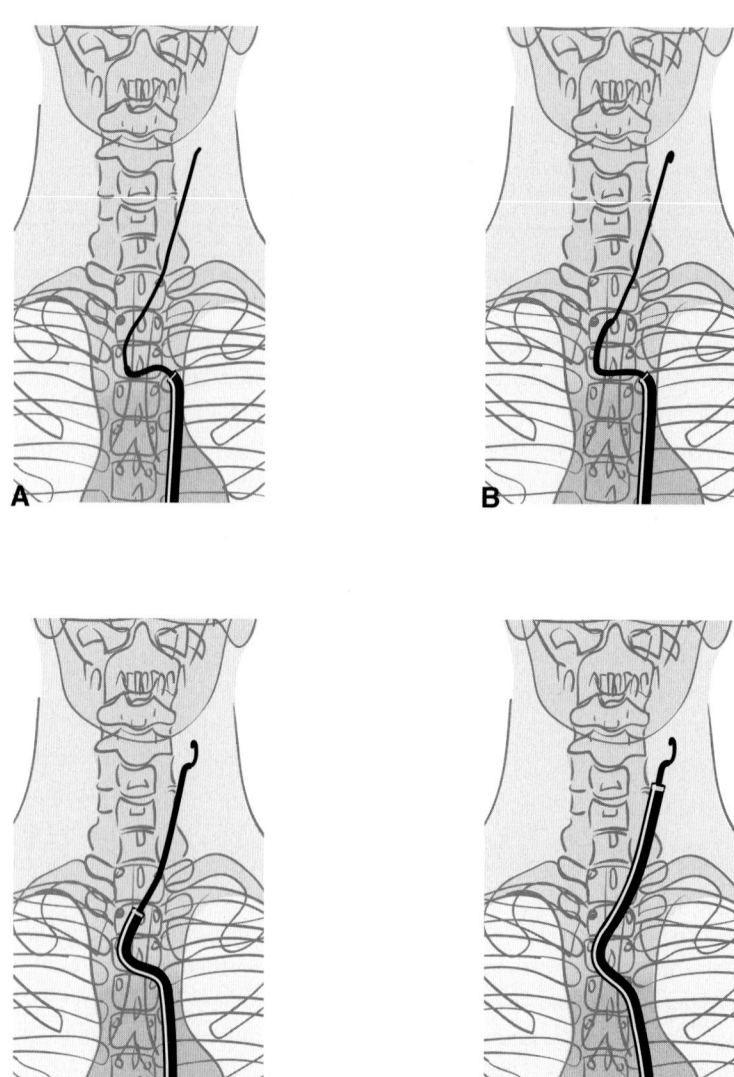

FIGURE 2.30 • The carotid arteries can sometimes be very difficult to select with a large introducer catheter or sheath for PTA/stent procedures. In this set of illustrations a long cerebral catheter (110–125 cm) is used to select the common carotid artery using a standard wire. With the catheter advanced as much as possible into the common carotid artery, the larger outer device can sometimes then be advanced. Using a stiffer, nonstandard wire (e.g., Amplatz) will sometimes be necessary to accomplish this maneuver. However, advancing an outer sheath or catheter that does not match the caliber of the inner catheter exactly can be problematic. It can cause a dissection or can scrape plaque from the inner vessel wall.

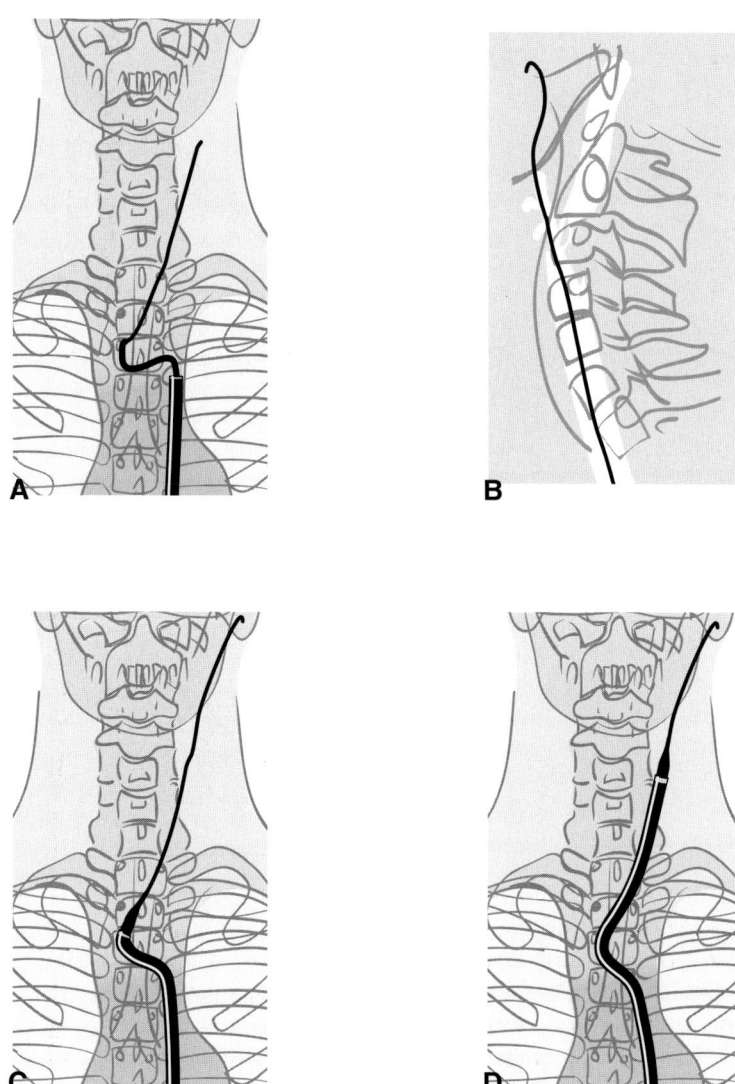

FIGURE 2.31 • An alternative method for selecting difficult carotid arteries is to use a long inner catheter to select the external carotid artery on the side in question and to place a stiff exchange length wire in the distal circulation (B). The catheter can then be exchanged for an inner dilator matching the introducer device. This will assure minimal wall trauma due to the smooth transition from dilator to shaft as the device is advanced into the common carotid artery. As described in the text, exchanges in the carotid or vertebral arteries should only be done after heparinization and antiplatelet agents have been administered.

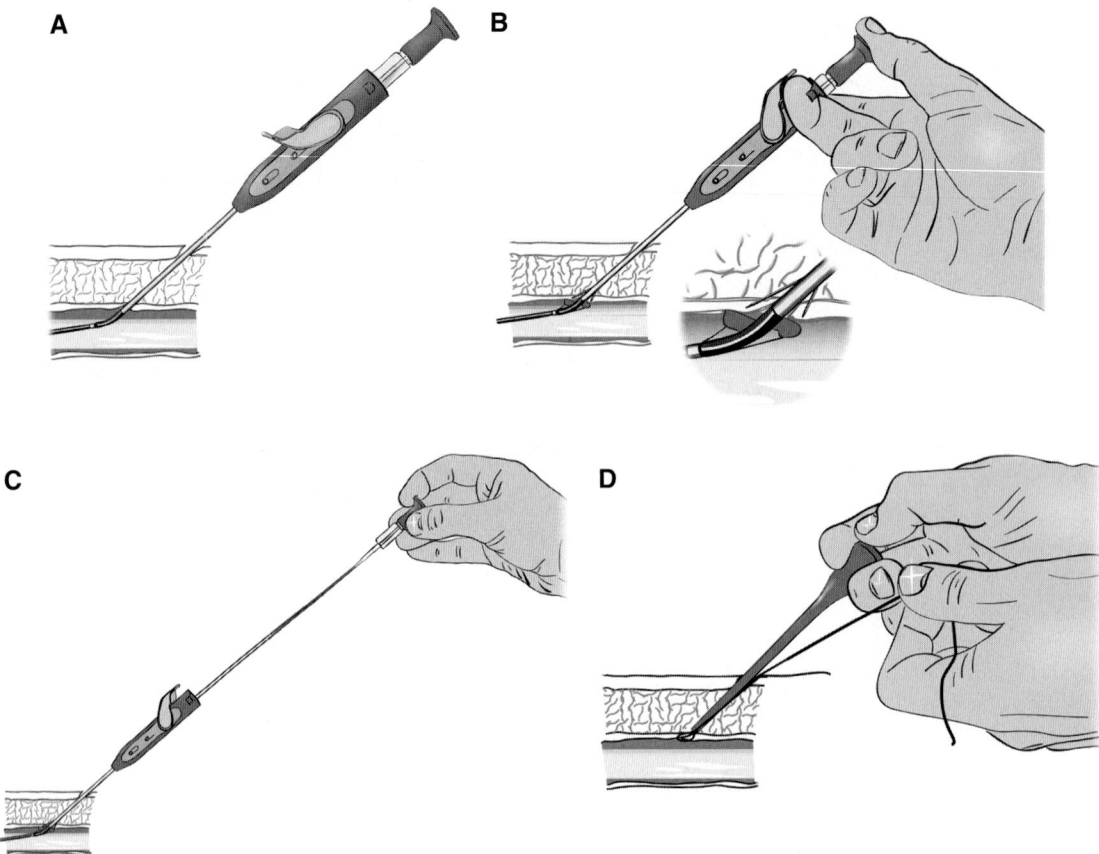

FIGURE 2.32 • The Perclose® arteriotomy closure device is inserted into the artery at the beginning or end of the case over a 0.035-in wire until blood spurts from the transparent side-arm (A). The feet are then deployed within the lumen with the external lever, and retracted against the inner wall of the artery (B). In that position the needles are plunged into the feet where they engage toggles on the suture threads. The needles are then withdrawn (C), which pulls the suture thread through the arteriotomy walls forming the basis for the grip of the threads on the arterial wall. An improved clinch knot (as used for fly-fishing) is formed by hand or with the provided knot-forming device. The knot is then pulled into the artery as the shaft of the device is retracted from the artery and cinched into place with the provided pusher device (D). The suture is then cut as close as possible to the arterial wall.

The Perclose 6F device can be deployed at the beginning of the case, and after deployment of the sutures, access to the artery with a wire can be regained through the device. The arteriotomy can then be expanded to 10F or greater and sutured with the same single thread at the end of the case, usually with very reliable results. For long cases, it is probably prudent to wrap the sutures in a sterile gauze and administer an antibiotic at the time of ligation.

With all of the suture-closure devices, complications and difficulties are possible, and manufacturers' warnings about the learning curve should be heeded.

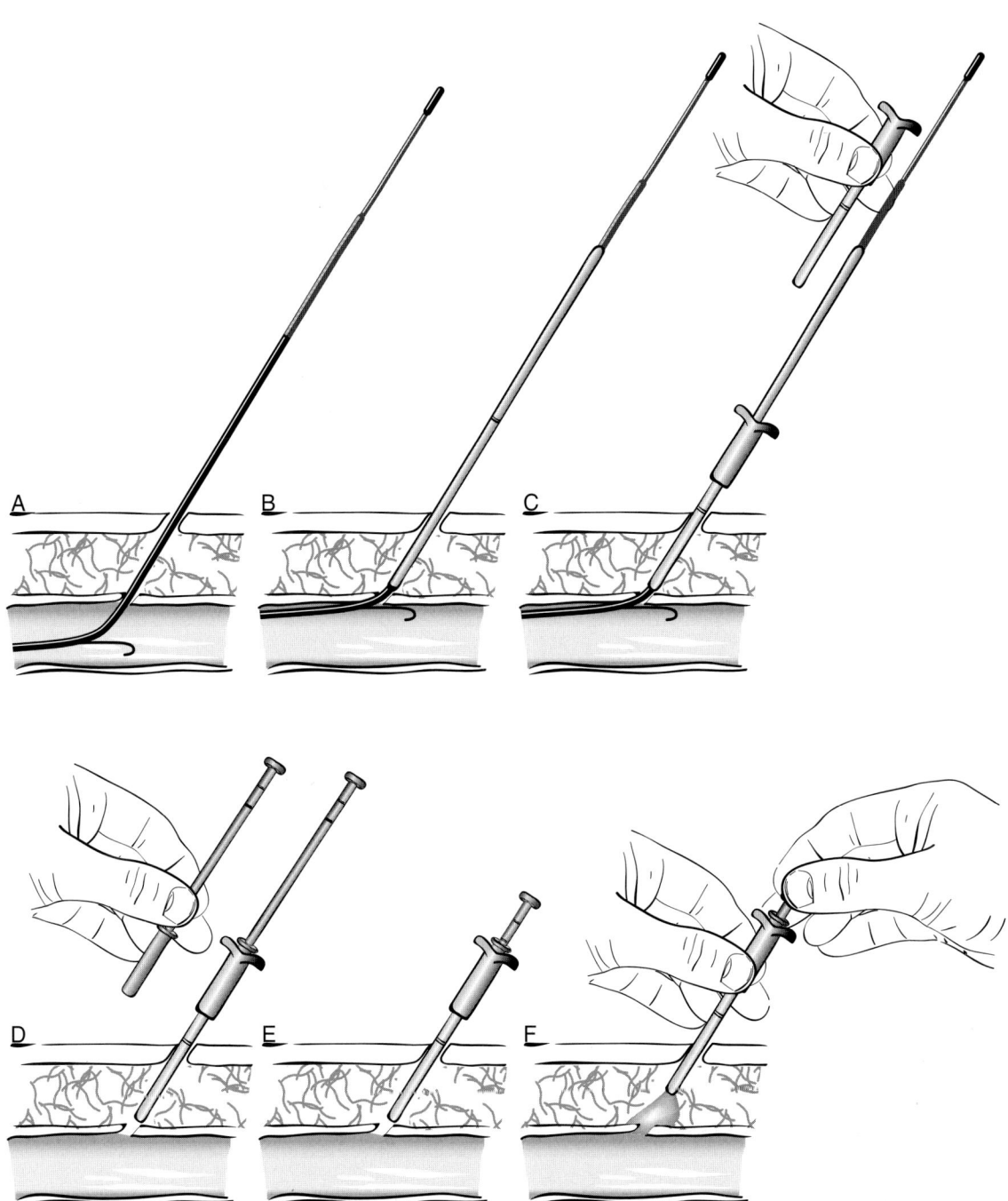

FIGURE 2.33 • The Vasoseal device involves initially defining the depth of the artery with a short hydrophilic minicatheter placed over a standard wire. A retractable wire-hook is deployed (A) and retracted against the arterial wall. A rod is advanced snugly against the outer wall of the artery, over which in turn an introducer tube is advanced against the arterial wall (C). While an assistant compresses the artery upstream, the wire-hook is withdrawn and all components are removed except the introducer tube. Through the latter (D) a plug of collagen is injected to a depth defined by markers on the plunger (E). The collagen is then extruded by retracting the tube along the plunger, which is being stabilized by the right hand.

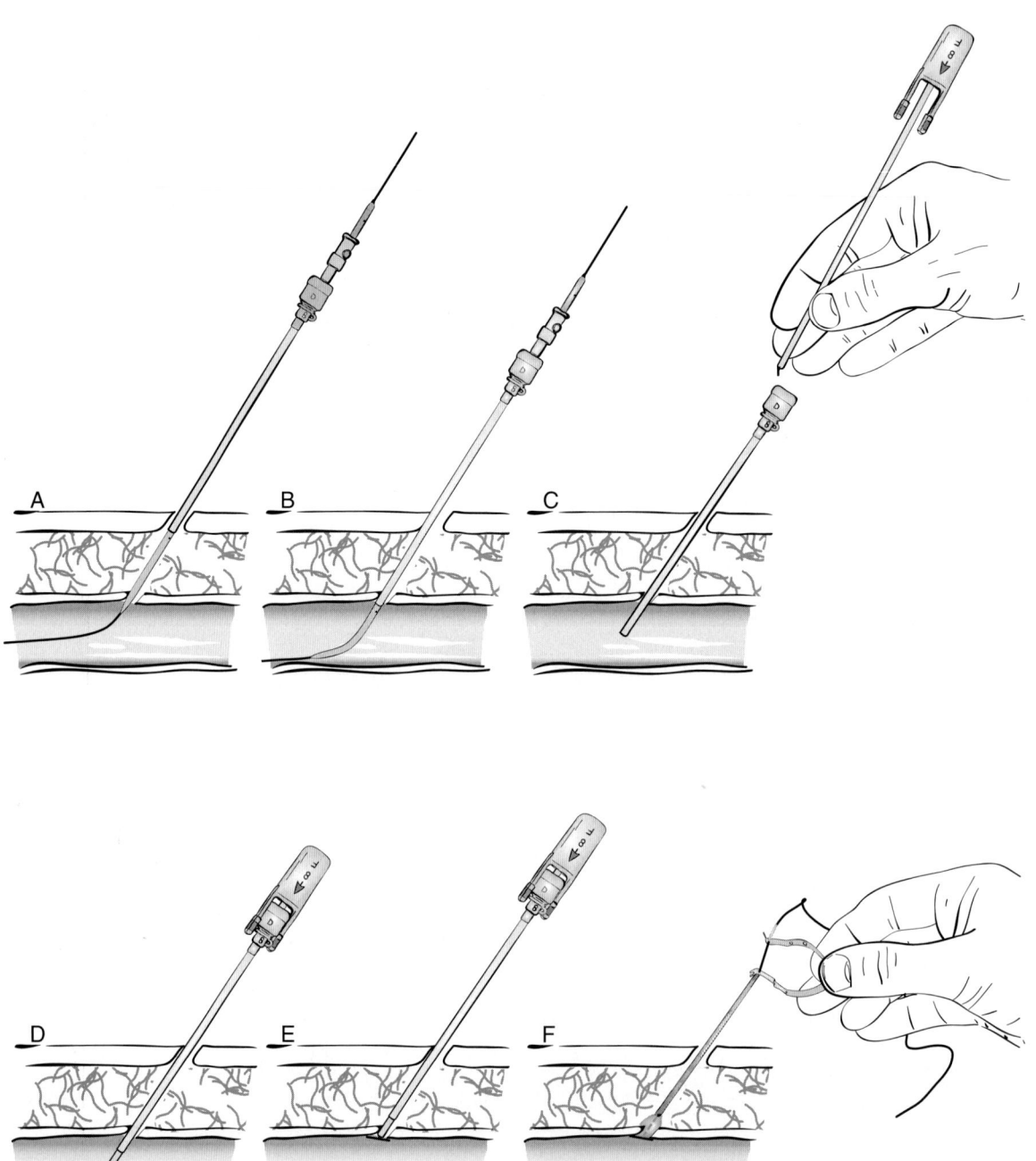

FIGURE 2.34 • The Angioseal device involves placing an 8Fr equivalent sheath in the artery over a wire at the end of the case (A). Holes distally and proximally in the central dilator allow blood to escape when the device is sufficiently advanced (B). While an assistant compresses the artery proximally to prevent bleeding, the inner dilator is exchanged without moving the position of the outer sheath (C), and an 8Fr component is inserted and rotated (D), causing the foot of polyglycolic acid to deploy. This is retracted against the inner wall of the artery (E) and tension is applied along the suture by means of a counterpoised metal spring and pusher (F). After hemostasis is achieved, the pusher is removed and the suture is cut.

a seal of polyglycolic acid (Angioseal®, Sherwood Davis & Gleck, St. Louis, MO) (Fig. 2.34). Potential serious complications are possible with all of these devices, and a learning curve is observed. However, for larger sheaths with anticoagulation and antiplatelet drugs active, they are an extremely valuable tool. A single-wall puncture is recommended when use of these agents is contemplated. Prior to the availability of these devices it was common to maintain a femoral arterial sheath in place in the neurointensive care unit for periods up to days while the patient was heparinized following a neurointerventional procedure. However, this strategy is fraught with a high risk of complications. Whether they are perfused with heparinized saline or not, over 70% of femoral arterial sheaths form clots overnight[33] with the potential for ischemic or septic complications. Use of internal closure devices has achieved general acceptance in the field of interventional cardiology where early mobilization and discharge of the patient from the hospital is a desirable consequence of their use. In the field of interventional neuroradiology early mobilization of the patient following the procedure is not as prevalent a goal as in cardiology, but these devices probably have a significant impact on reduction in rates of arteriotomy-related complications, pseudoaneurysms, and hematomas.[34]

References

1. HELMREICH R. Quoted by Stolberg SG. "Breaking down medicine's culture of silence." *New York Times* (1999) 4, 1–18.
2. TU RK, COHEN WA, MARAVILLA KR, BUSH WH, PATEL NH, ESKRIDGE J, WINN HR (1996) Digital subtraction rotational angiography for aneurysms of the intracranial anterior circulation: injection method and optimization. *AJNR* 17:1127–1136.
3. ELGERSMA OEH, BUIJS PC, WÜST AFJ, VAN DER GRAAF Y, EIKELBOOM BC, MALI WPTM (1999) Maximum internal carotid arterial stenosis: assessment with rotational angiography versus conventional intraarterial digital subtraction angiography. *Radiology* 213:777–783.
4. BENDSZUS M, KOLTZENBURG M, BURGER R, WARMUTH-METZ M, HOFMANN E, SOLYMOSI L (1999) Silent embolism in diagnostic cerebral angiography and neurointerventional procedures: a prospective study. *Lancet* 354:1594–1597.
5. BRITT PM, HEISERMAN JE, SNIDER RM, SHILL HA, BIRD CR, WALLACE RC (2000) Incidence of postangiographic abnormalities revealed by diffusion-weighted MR imaging. *AJNR* 21:55–59.
6. GERRATY RP, BOWSER DN, INFELD B, MITCHELL PJ, DAVIS SM (1996) Microemboli during carotid angiography. Association with stroke risk factors or subsequent magnetic resonance imaging changes. *Stroke* 27:1543–1547.
7. DAGIRMANIJIAN A, DAVIS DA, ROTHFUS WE, DEEB ZL, GOLDBERG AL (1993) Silent cerebral microemboli occurring during carotid angiography: frequency as determined with Doppler sonography. *AJR* 161:1037–1040.
8. MARKUS H, LOH A, ISRAEL D, BUCKENHAM T, CLIFTON A, BROWN NM (1993) Microscopic air embolism during cerebral angiography and strategies for its avoidance. *Lancet* 341:784–787.
9. MIYACHI S, NEGORO M, HANDA T, TERASHIMA K, KEINO H, SUGITA K (1992) Histopathological study of balloon embolization: silicone versus latex. *Neurosurgery* 30:483–489.
10. LANGFORD KH, VITEK JJ, ZEIGER E (1983) Migration of detachable mini-balloon from the ICA causing occlusion of the MCA. Case report. *J Neurosurg* 58:430–434.
11. AYMARD A, HODES JE, RUFENACHT D, MERLAND JJ (1992) Endovascular treatment of a giant fusiform aneurysm of the entire basilar artery. *AJNR* 13:1143–1146.
12. MORRIS PP, MARTIN EM, REGAN J, BRADEN G (1999) Intracranial deployment of coronary stents for symptomatic atherosclerotic disease. *AJNR* 20:1688–1694.
13. RASMUSSEN PA, PERL J, BARR JD, MARKARIAN GZ, KATZAN I, SILA C, KRIEGER D, FURLAN A, MASARYK TJ (2000) Stent-assisted angioplasty of intracranial vertebrobasilar atherosclerosis: an initial experience. *J Neurosurg* 92:771–778.
14. GOMEZ CR, MISRA VK, LIU MW, WADLINGTON VR, TERRY JB, TULYAPRONCHOTE R, CAMPBELL MS (2000) Elective stenting of symptomatic basilar artery stenosis. *Stroke* 31:95–99.
15. WAKHLOO AK, JUENGLING FD, VAN VELTHOVEN V, SCHUMACHER M, HENNIG J, SCHWECHHEIMER K (1993) Extended preoperative polyvinyl alcohol microembolization of intracranial meningiomas: assessment of two embolization techniques. *AJNR* 14:571–582.
16. DAVIDSON GS, TERBRUGGE KG (1995) Histologic long-term follow-up after embolization with polyvinyl alcohol particles. *AJNR* 16(suppl):843–846.
17. QUISLING RJ, MICKLE JP, BALLLINGER WB (1984) Histopathologic analysis of intraarterial polyvinyl alcohol microemboli in rat cerebral cortex. *AJNR* 5:101–104.
18. GERMANO IM, DAVIS RL, WILSON CB (1992) Histopathological follow-up study of 66 cerebral arteriovenous malformations after therapeutic embolization with polyvinyl alcohol. *J Neurosurg* 76:607–614.
19. WHITE RI, STRANDBERG JV, GROSS GS (1977) Therapeutic embolization with long-term occluding agents and their effects on embolized tissues. *Radiology* 125:677–687.
20. WAGNER LK, EIFER PJ, GEISE RA (1994) Potential biological

effects following high X-ray dose interventional procedures. *J Vasc Intervent Radiol* 5:71–84.
21. CARSTENS GJ, HOROWITZ MB, PURDY PD, PANDYA AG (1996) Radiation dermatitis after spinal arteriovenous malformation embolization: case report. *Neuroradiology* 38(suppl)1:S160–S164.
22. VARGA J, HAUSTEIN UF, CREECH RH, DWYER JP, JIMENEZ SA (1991) Exaggerated radiation-induced fibrosis in patients with systemic sclerosis. *JAMA* 265:3292–3295.
23. MAYR NA, RIGGS CE, SAAG KG, WEN BC, PENNINGTON EC, HUSSEY DH (1997) Mixed connective tissue disease and radiation toxicity: a case report. *Cancer* 79:612–618.
24. ROSS JG, HUSSEY DH, MAYR NA, DAVIS CS (1993) Acute and late reactions to radiation therapy in patients with collagen vascular diseases. *Cancer* 71:3744–3752.
25. WAGNER LR, MCNEESE MD, MARX MV, SIEGEL EL (1999) Severe skin reactions from interventional fluoroscopy: case report and review of the literature. *Radiology* 213:773–776.
26. MARSHALL NW, NOBLE J, FAULKNER K (1995) Patient and staff dosimetry in neuroradiological procedures. *Br J Radiol* 68:495–501.
27. HUDA W, PETERS KR (1994) Radiation induced temporary epilation after a neuroradiologically guided embolization procedure. *Radiology* 193:642–644.
28. BERTHELSEN B, CEDERBLAD A (1991) Radiation doses to patients and personnel involved in endovascular surgery of the head and neck. *Acta Radiologica* 32:492–497.
29. BERGERON P, CARRIER R, ROY D (1994) Radiation doses in patients in neurointerventional procedures. *AJNR* 15:1809–1812.
30. VANO E, GONZALEZ L, GUIBELALDE E, FERNANDEZ JM, TEN JI (1998) Radiation exposure to medical staff in interventional and cardiac radiology. *Br J Radiol* 71:954–960.
31. NIKLASON LT, MARX MV, CHAN HP (1993) Interventional radiologists: occupational radiation doses and risks. *Radiology* 187:729–733.
32. GUSTAFSSON M, LUNDERQUIST A (1981) Personnel exposure to radiation at some angiographic procedures. *Radiology* 140:807–811.
33. KOENIGSBERG RA, WYSOKI M, WEISS J, FARO SH, TSAI FY (1999) Risk of clot formation in femoral arterial sheaths maintained overnight for neuroangiographic procedures. *AJNR* 20:297–299.
34. MORRIS PP, BRADEN G (1999) Neurointerventional experience with an arteriotomy suture device. *AJNR* 20:1706–1709.
35. GRAVES VB (1998) Advancing loop technique for endovascular access to the anterior cerebral artery. *AJNR* 19:778–780.

Chapter 3

Aneurysms

Coil Embolization of Intracranial Aneurysms

A pioneering paper on neurosurgical use of balloons in 1980 by Mullan et al.[1] contains one of the very first descriptions of successful carotid balloon angioplasty. The same paper also describes transvenous embolization of a carotid cavernous fistula, and balloon-occlusion of an exsanguinating carotid artery. It also reports in detail a procedure for coil obliteration of an inoperable carotid aneurysm using phosphate bronze coils. The bronze coils were inserted through the aneurysm wall after direct exposure of the aneurysm at craniotomy. Intravascular balloons were used to prevent prolapse of the coils into the carotid artery and were removed at the end of the procedure. The patient had a successful recovery. This single brief paper therefore pointed the direction for a number of innovations that would be developed over the following decades. The strategy of using balloons to keep coils within an aneurysm would later be developed into the balloon reconstructive technique for endovascular aneurysm coil therapy.

The Guglielmi Detachable Coil (GDC) was introduced in 1990[2,3] and has become an important tool in the treatment of intracranial aneurysms (Figs. 3.1–3.6). Surgical clipping by craniotomy has been the standard method for aneurysm control for decades. Surgical clipping of unruptured aneurysms involves a mortality risk of 0% to 8% and a morbidity risk of 0% to 30%, depending on the size and location of the aneurysm and on the experience of the treating institution.[4,5] The outcome from clipping a ruptured aneurysm is dependent in part on the same factors, but to a greater extent is dependent upon the consequences of the rupture, including occurrence of rebleeding, age of the patient, clinical grade of the patient at the time of surgery, and occurrence of vasospasm. Because it is the established mode of treatment, the risks and outcomes of surgical clipping of intracranial aneurysms set the standard by which the performance of endovascular techniques can be judged, preferably within the context of randomized trials.

Trials Comparing Surgical Clipping and Coil Embolization

A prospective randomized trial by Vanninen et al.[6] from Finland comparing endovascular treatment of ruptured aneurysms with surgical clipping confirms the efficacy and safety profile of coil em-

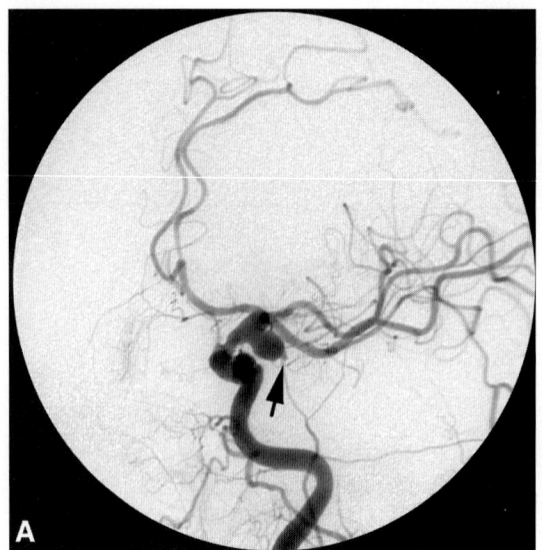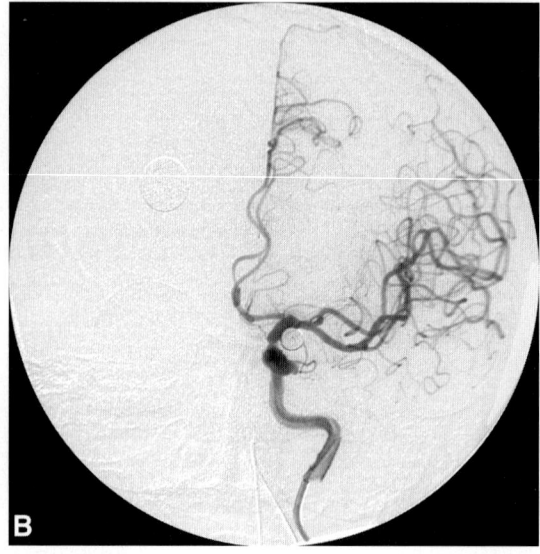

FIGURE 3.1 • *Aneurysm Occlusion with Preservation of the Parent Artery.*
An 85-year-old female presented with Grade III subarachnoid hemorrhage related to a ruptured aneurysm of the left posterior communicating artery. An apical teat or site of presumed rupture is easily seen on the pretreatment image (arrow in A). The neck was relatively broad, and a 2D 9-mm coil could not be stabilized within the aneurysm. Balloon assistance could not be used easily because of severe atherosclerotic disease in the cervical carotid artery limiting the size of introducer catheter that could be placed. An 8-mm 2D coil was then used to form the initial basket or framework for the coiling procedure (posttreatment, B). The apical teat was excluded from the circulation early in the procedure.

bolization of ruptured aneurysms. Mortality related to the technique of coiling was comparable to or less than that seen in the surgical group, while there was no difference in short-term clinical outcome between the two treatment methods. Angiographic outcome in the anterior circulation was better in the surgical group, while endovascular treatment fared better in the posterior circulation. This group of patients ($n = 111$) was screened into the study from a larger group ($n = 321$) of consecutive admissions. Criteria for admission to the study based on the width of the neck of the aneurysm have since been superceded by progression in coil design and by development of balloon-assisted and stent-assisted techniques for dealing with wide-necked aneurysms.[7,8] This implies that the results seen by Vanninen et al. could be generalized to a greater proportion of the total population of patients with ruptured aneurysms.

A different single-institution study from Belgium in which endovascular coiling was considered as the first treatment option for a group of 103 patients was reported by Raftopoulos et al.[9] Within this series, totaling 132 aneurysms, 64 aneurysms were assigned prospectively to endovascular treatment. Treatment failures and some patients with procedural complications from within the endovascular group were subsequently treated by surgical clipping, as were all those initially thought unsuitable for coiling. Final outcomes in this study indicated that thromboembolic complications and perforations (9.4%) or treatment failures in the endovascular treatment group influenced the comparison of coiling versus surgery substantially in favor of the latter. Within the surgically treated group, 93.9% of patients had good or favorable outcomes, while 86.7% of endovascular patients were so classified. Nevertheless, the authors concluded that because coil embolization offers a less

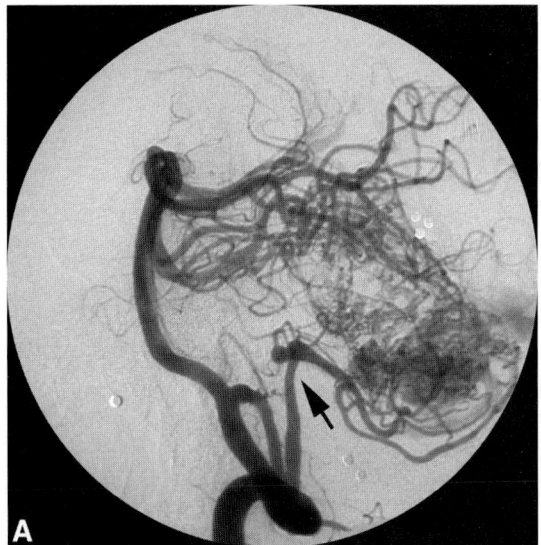 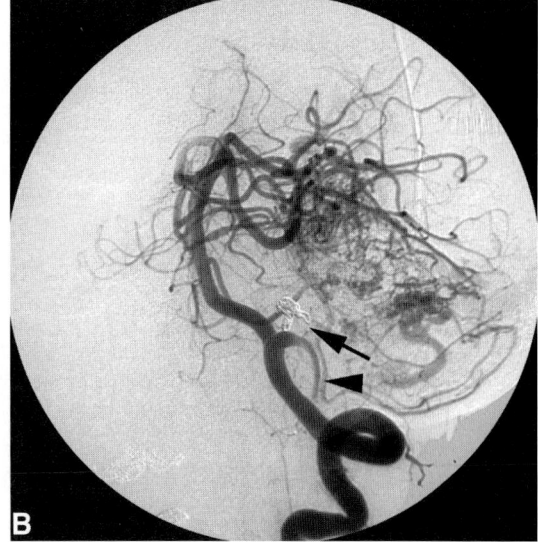

FIGURE 3.2 • *Aneurysm Occlusion with Sacrifice of the Parent Artery.*
A 52-year-old female presented with subarachnoid hemorrhage from a cerebellar arteriovenous malformation feeding principally from a dysplastic enlarged left posterior inferior cerebellar artery. An aneurysm most likely representing the site of hemorrhage (arrow in A) is evident at the choroidal point of the posterior inferior cerebellar artery proximal to the AVM. A small hemispheric branch arises from the aneurysm.

In this case an attempt was made to coil the aneurysm and preserve flow in the distal posterior inferior cerebellar artery, so as to facilitate subsequent embolization. However, at the apex of the loop of the artery, the turn into the aneurysm was sharp and abrupt. This would have required considerable catheter tension to overcome. With so small an aneurysm there is little safety margin for intraaneurysmal catheter motion, meaning that the risk of rupturing the aneurysm was thought to be too high. Therefore, the aneurysm was occluded with its parent vessel using GDCs (arrows in B). The patient recovered from the hemorrhage without evidence of a clinical deficit related to the occlusion procedure. In most instances, if absolutely necessary, the posterior inferior cerebellar artery can be occluded with impunity provided that the proximal lateral and posterior brainstem perforators proximal to the choroidal point are preserved. In this case the posterior inferior cerebellar artery fills slowly (arrowhead) to the point of occlusion.

invasive but effective treatment option, it should be offered as the first choice of treatment, after due consideration by a neurovascular team.

A retrospective analysis of outcomes following surgery versus embolization of unruptured aneurysms using data from 60 university medical centers was published by Johnston et al.[10] in 1999. Allowing for factors such as age, sex, race, mode of admission to hospital, and year of treatment, endovascular coil embolization resulted in fewer adverse outcomes than surgery for unruptured cerebral aneurysms. Rates of in-hospital mortality, adverse outcomes defined by subsequent discharge to rehabilitation institutions or nursing homes, length of stay, and cost of treatment were all substantially greater for surgical patients compared with endovascular coiling.

Several studies that examined uncontrolled series of patients have been published, demonstrating the safety and efficacy of embolization of cerebral aneurysms. These are for the most part operator dependent and contain various selection biases in the patient populations studied. However, the results are congruent from multiple centers in demonstrating that coiling represents a realistic alternative form of treatment for intracranial aneu-

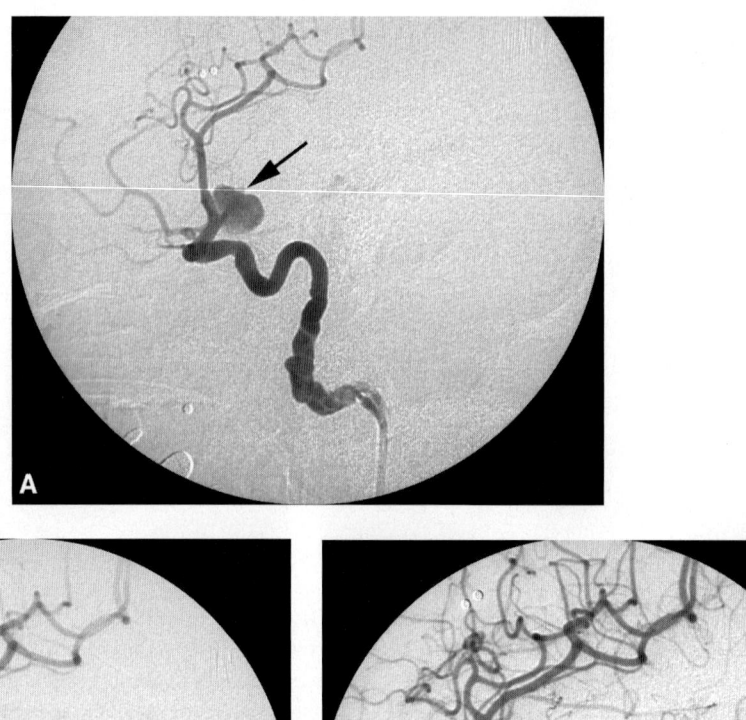
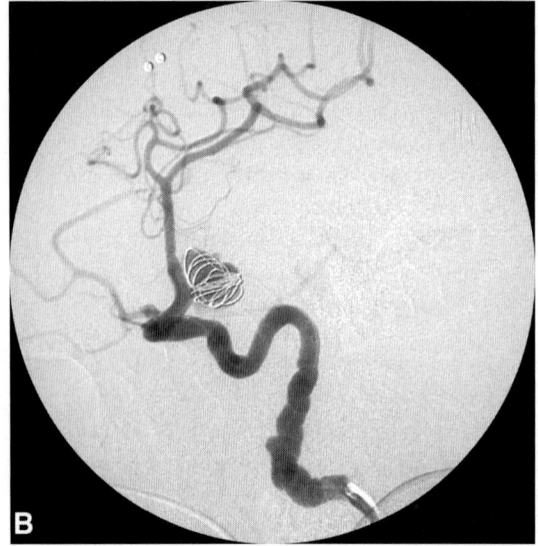
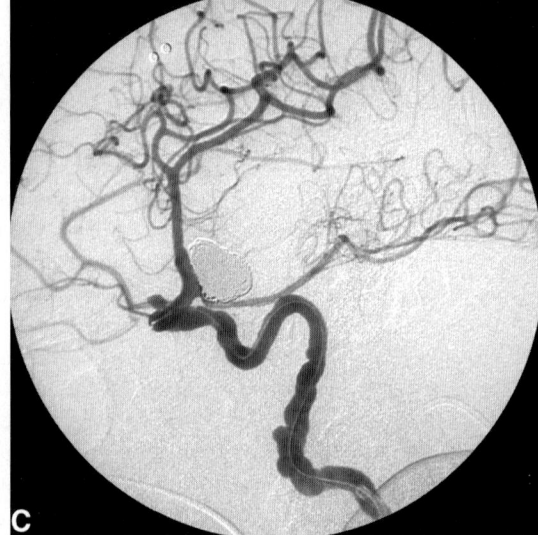

FIGURE 3.3 • *Avoid Any Procedural Trauma to the Site of Rupture during Catheter Manipulation or Coil Extrusion.*
A 74-year-old female who presented with a ruptured aneurysm of the left posterior communicating artery demonstrated a prominent jet effect of the aneurysmal inflow which strikes the rupture point on the aneurysm (arrow in A). Changes of fibromuscular dysplasia and a smaller more proximal carotid-ophthalmic aneurysm are also evident. Coil stabilization was performed using an Endeavor (Target) balloon placed parallel to the microcatheter through a single 7F introducer catheter (Cordis). An 8 × 30 mm 2D coil was placed initially (image B taken after first coil; C, final image after 11 coils). It is important to anticipate in an anatomic situation such as this that the microcatheter and extruding coil have a remarkable tendency to follow the line of the inflow jet into the apical rupture point. This could result in rebleeding from the aneurysm. Steam-shaping the microcatheter might reduce this risk, but one should be extremely careful about the course taken by the first coil. When the first or any coil detaches within the aneurysm, any tension in the microcatheter at that time might cause the microcatheter tip, now no longer constrained by the coil, to surge forward within the aneurysm. If there is tension within the microcatheter, pull back on it until the loop closest to the tip begins to move slightly.

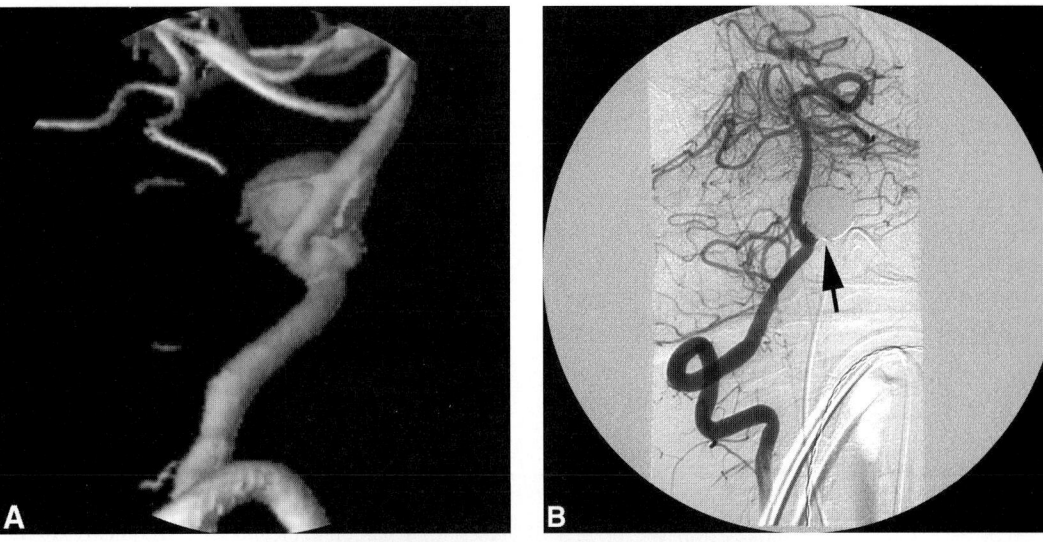
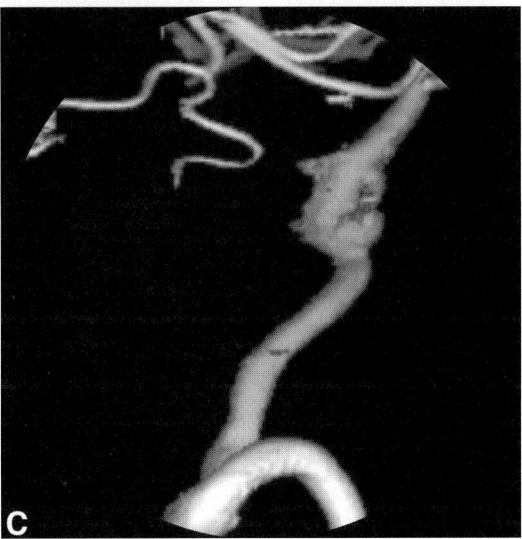

FIGURE 3.4 • *Coil Embolization of a Vertebrobasilar Junction Aneurysm.*
A 3D image (A) of an unruptured aneurysm arising from a fenestration of the vertebrobasilar junction affords the opportunity of understanding the anatomy of the aneurysm before undertaking the case. Rotating the image in 3D mode helps enormously in selecting the optimal angle of projection that will best allow a profile view of the aneurysm. With this projection the parent artery can be monitored easily during the progress of the case until complete packing of the aneurysm is attained (B). A 3D image after the procedure (C) shows that the residual neck of the aneurysm seen on the planar images is really an integral part of the native vessel fenestration.

rysms. For instance, in a series of 21 ruptured and unruptured basilar artery aneurysms 90% to 100% occlusion was achieved in 90% of patients,[11] but retreatment following aneurysm regrowth can still be required in 14% of patients. In the Food and Drug Administration multicenter clinical trial in the United States involving 150 patients with ruptured or unruptured basilar tip aneurysms considered unsuitable for surgery, near complete occlusion of the aneurysm was seen in 75% of patients with a periprocedural mortality rate of 2.7%[12] (Figs. 3.7, 3.8). In their 6-year experience with GDC treatment of 45 ruptured or unruptured basilar tip aneurysms, Bavinzski et al.[13] reported that 87% of aneurysms could be occluded by 90% to 100%. Only one patient demonstrated rebleeding.

In a series of 208 patients with intracranial aneurysms (150 presenting with subarachnoid hemorrhage), complete aneurysm occlusion was achieved in 81% of cases, while technique-related mortality rates of 2% and morbidity of 4% were seen.[14] Delayed rebleeding was seen in only one patient who had declined retreatment for a known neck remnant. In a follow-up multicenter series of 166 patients (187 aneurysms) from France,[15] aneurysm recurrence rates of 14% were seen, not all of which required retreatment.

The paraclinoid (Fig. 3.9) and carotid-ophthalmic area (Fig. 3.10) represent particular challenges for surgical clipping. Coil embolization has been demonstrated to be an effective and safe method of treatment in this anatomic location.[16,17] In a prospective study of 26 patients with ruptured and unruptured aneurysms of the paraclinoid internal carotid artery, rates of aneurysm occlusion with coils close to 75% to 85% were seen in the ophthalmic and superior hypophyseal regions when the neck of the aneurysm was small.[17] One patient had a permanent neurologic deficit from the procedure, and no delayed bleeding was seen.

Disadvantages of Coil Embolization

Patients treated by endovascular coiling are more likely than patients treated surgically to demonstrate a residual neck of aneurysm on follow-up angiogra-

FIGURE 3.5 • *Coil Embolization of a Large Ruptured Posterior Communicating Aneurysm with a Combination of Balloon-Reconstructive Technique and 3D Coils.*
A 75-year-old female presented with Grade IV subarachnoid hemorrhage related to a 20-mm aneurysm of the right posterior communicating artery (A, skewed lateral view). Although the ratio between the height of the dome and the mouth of the aneurysm appears favorable, the 3D view (B) shows that the aneurysm neck is wide to a degree that the native vessel would be incorporated into the sweep of the radius of the aneurysm. In other words, unconstrained coils placed in the aneurysm conforming to the wall of the aneurysm would almost certainly encroach on the carotid lumen.

A 16-mm 3D coil was deployed within the aneurysm (C) using a balloon at the mouth of the aneurysm to ballotte the coil loops back toward the aneurysm as they emerged. After detachment, the 16-mm 3D coil appeared to have been too small for the aneurysm in that the coil did not have good apposition against the circumference of the aneurysm on many aspects. Subsequently, an 18-mm 3D coil was deployed within the first 16-mm 3D coil, forming an excellent framework for complete packing of the aneurysm (D).

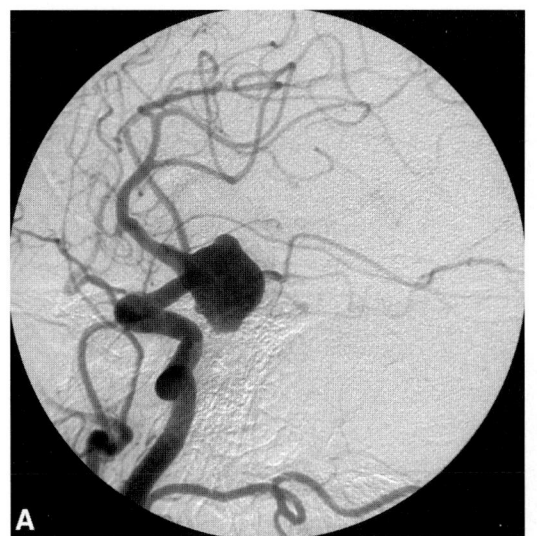
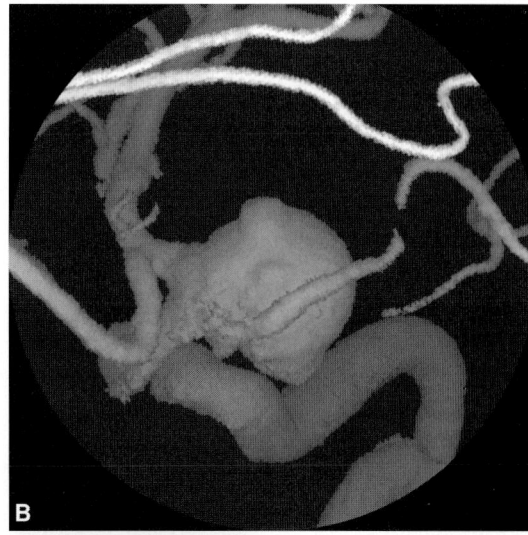
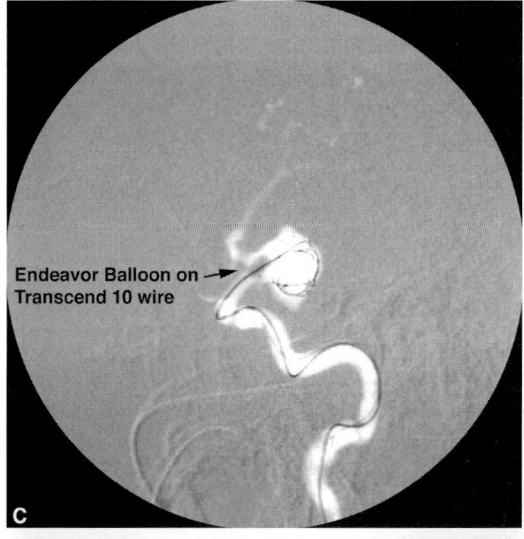
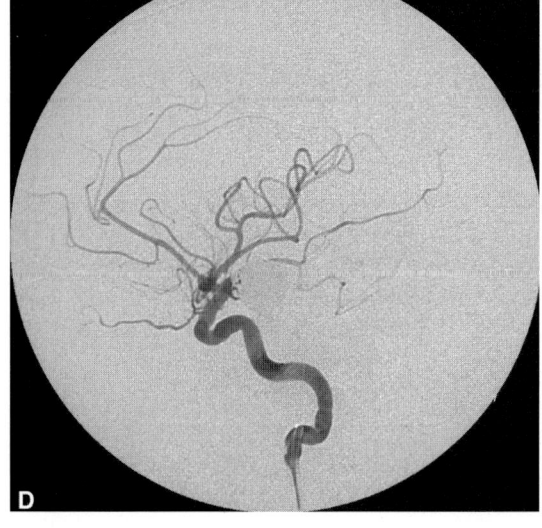

ANEURYSMS 61

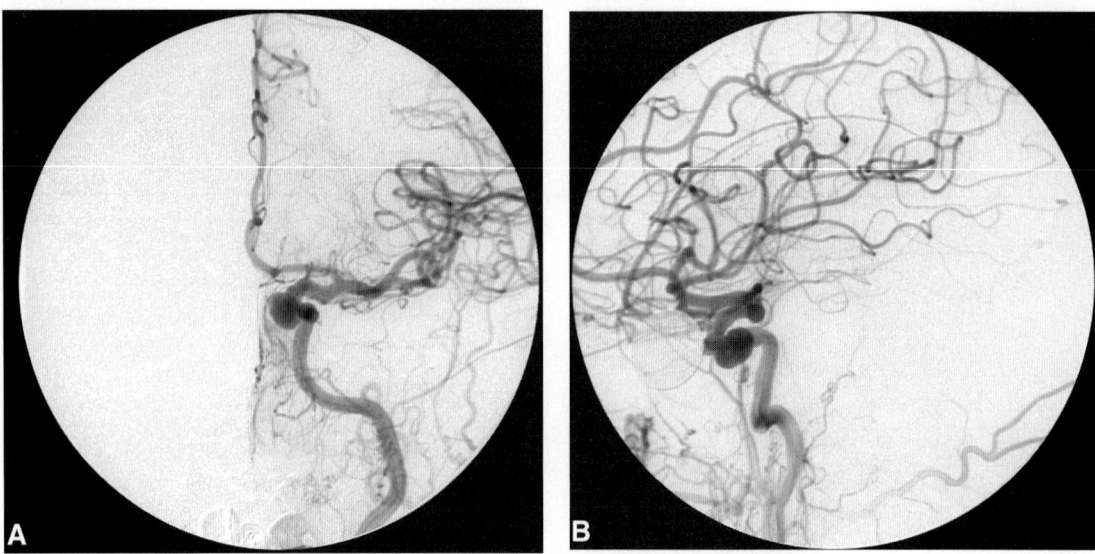

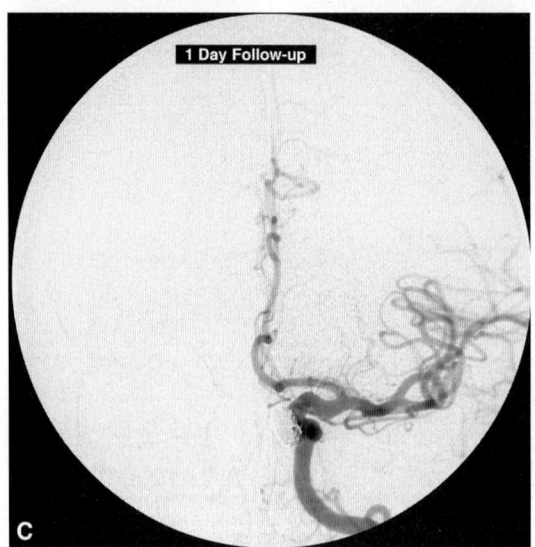

FIGURE 3.6 • *Coil Embolization of a Cavernous Carotid Aneurysm.*
A symptomatic cavernous aneurysm of the left internal carotid artery presenting with headache represents an uncommon combination of low technical risk with a favorable anatomic configuration (A, pretreatment, Caldwell projection; B, pretreatment lateral projection; C, posttreatment, Caldwell projection). While the risks of arterial injury and thromboembolic complications apply in this case as always, the risk of aneurysm perforation by the wire or microcatheter is virtually nonexistent. This is an example of a good first case for a fellow or other neophyte. The aneurysm is difficult to project in profile on the lateral view distinct from the parent artery. Therefore, the Caldwell projection is very useful in examining and treating aneurysms of this region as it allows an "over-and-under" view of the supraclinoid and cavernous segments of the internal carotid artery.

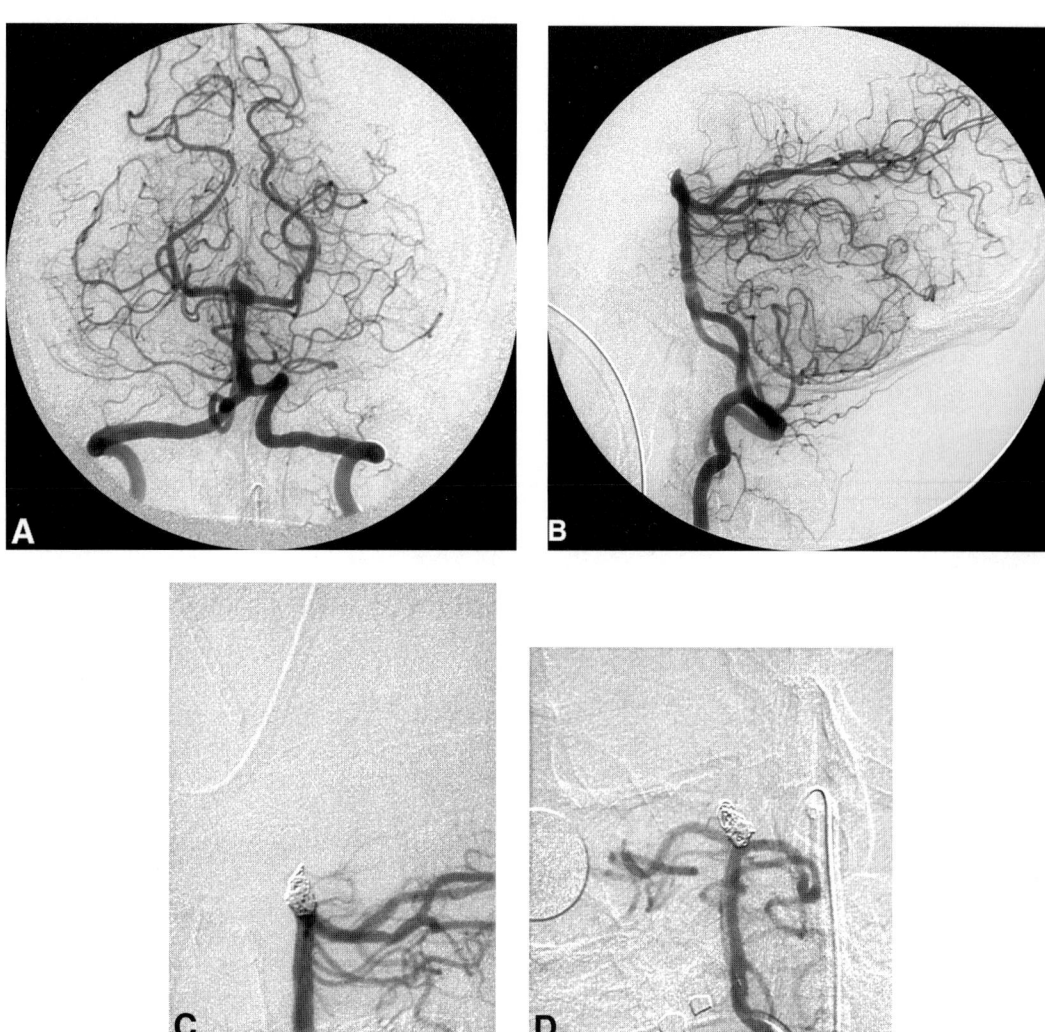

FIGURE 3.7 • *Basilar-Tip Aneurysm Embolization with Balloon-Assistance I.*
A 41-year-old male patient with deteriorating nephropathy (serum creatinine 4.1 mg/dL) presented with a Grade IV subarachnoid hemorrhage related to a 5-mm aneurysm of the basilar tip (A, B). Coil embolization of the aneurysm was performed using a parallel balloon in the basilar artery to stabilize the coils within the wide-mouth aneurysm. Following embolization, all of the thalamoperforators are intact (C, lateral image postembolization). However, on the Water's view (D, posttreatment) there is overlap of the coil nidus and the artery, and the possibility that the coils encroach on the lumen of the basilar bifurcation must be considered. The patient was treated with peritoneal dialysis after the procedure. Heparin was continued for 3 days after the procedure with no complications suggesting compromise of the vessel.

The configuration of this aneurysm is innately unfavorable for aneurysm coiling because it is wider at its base than at the apex. One must be extremely cautious during basilar aneurysm embolizations to avoid thalamoperforator compromise, because this is such a devastating injury to the patient. In this patient the repeated inflation of the balloon over the aneurysm mouth with a stable pattern was the most reliable assurance during the procedure that the parent vessel was not being compromised. After each coil insertion a DSA run was performed to evaluate the perforators before detachment of the coil.

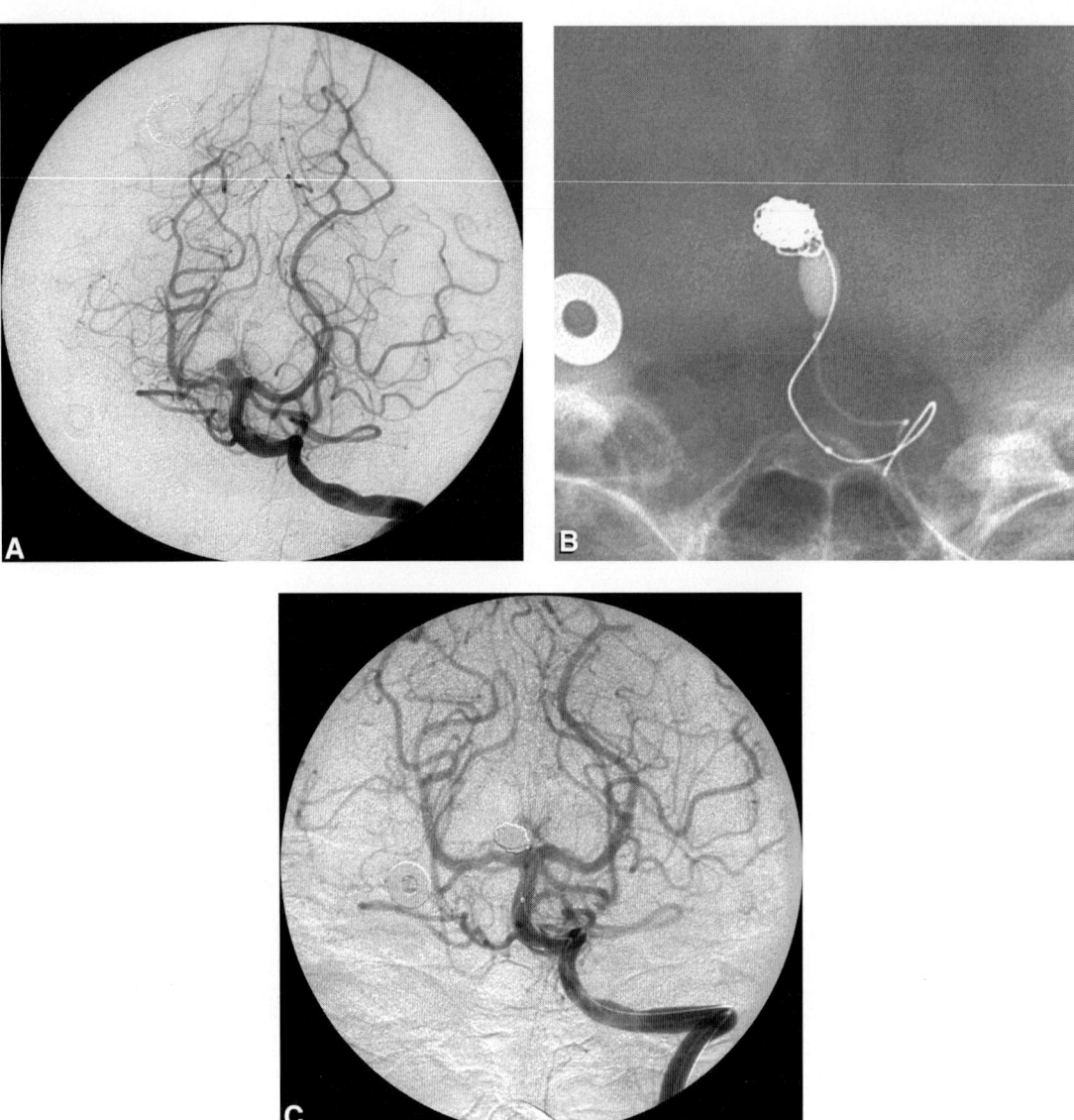

FIGURE 3.8 • *Basilar-Tip Aneurysm Embolization with Balloon-Assistance II.*
A 45-year-old female presented with Grade IV subarachnoid hemorrhage from an eccentric aneurysm of the basilar tip with a wide mouth (A, Towne's view prior to treatment). An intraprocedural image in mid-coil extrusion (B) demonstrates an Endeavor balloon inflated in the basilar artery, preventing the coils in the neck from slipping back into the artery. The balloon also pins the microcatheter down and discourages it from moving back when resistance is encountered. One can get a much tighter and complete packing in this manner (C, Towne's view postembolization), compared to coiling without balloon assistance.

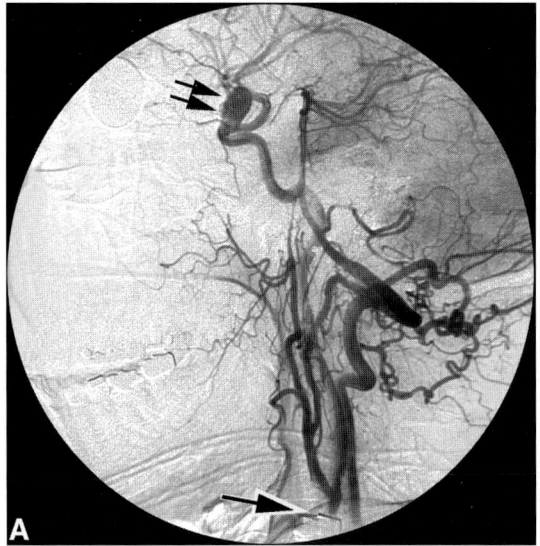 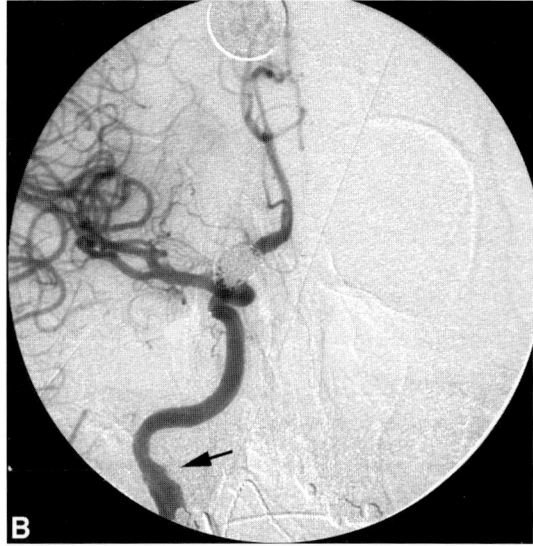

FIGURE 3.9 • A 60-year-old female patient presented with headaches. She was known to have an aneurysm of the right carotid-ophthalmic region for which a Selverstone clamp had been placed on her right common carotid artery 20 years previously. A right vertebral artery injection (A, lateral view) shows prompt reconstitution of the right internal carotid artery via the right external carotid artery (single arrow) and opacification of a large intradural aneurysm (double arrow).

The patient opted for coil embolization of the aneurysm. This was performed via a cervical puncture using a standard 4 Fr sheath. A small dissection of the internal carotid artery (B, arrow) was induced at the tip of the sheath, but with antiplatelet medication and heparinization for 3 days after the procedure no complications were evident.

Lessons learned: The cervical puncture in this case was performed in the operating room after surgical exposure of the internal carotid artery. This precluded use of the fluoroscopy unit to monitor the luminal position of the wire during sheath advancement. Unless one has specifically noted the relative lengths of wires, dilators, sheaths, etc., in a situation such as this, one can be left not knowing for sure how much wire one has advanced into the vessel at the time of sheath insertion. Too little wire risks arterial injury, possibly a factor in this patient; too much risks injury to the aneurysm higher up.

phy.[6,18] Moreover, the center of the aneurysm in circumstances of loose coil-packing or a wide neck does not thrombose immediately and continues to communicate with the parent vessel in many patients for some period of time. It is recognized that the immediate angiographic appearance of a coiled aneurysm overestimates the extent of complete exclusion of the aneurysm from the circulation.[19] Gradually, however, organized thrombus, capillaries, fibrous connective tissue, and inflammatory cells invade the aneurysm centripetally. Several postmortem studies of patients with coiled aneurysms have been published showing a variable tissue response over time to the presence of coils within an aneurysm.[20–24] The process of complete aneurysm resolution following coil therapy requires deposition of vascular, fibrous connective tissue leading to fibroblastic invasion and collagen formation across the neck of the aneurysm. This can then serve as a base for endothelialization of the interface between the aneurysm and the lumen of the parent vessel. It is probable that this process is slower in intracranial aneurysms than, for instance, in experimental animal models, due to the relatively avascular nature of the containing aneurysm wall and the

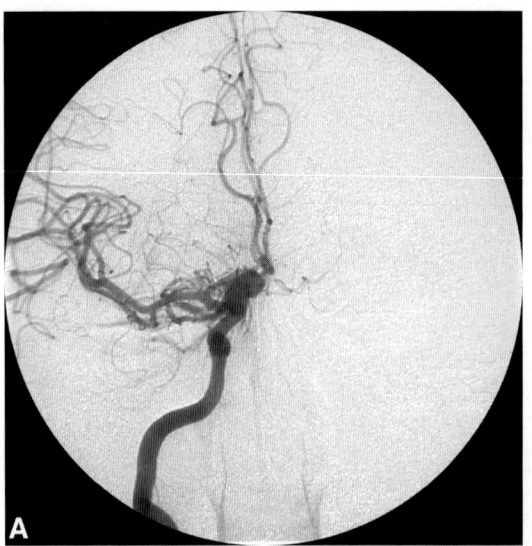
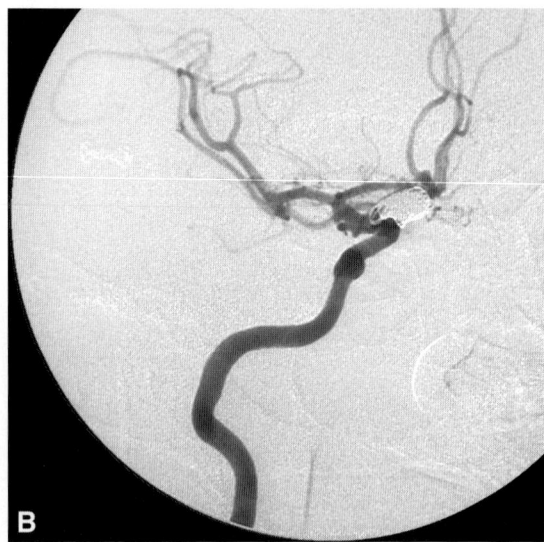
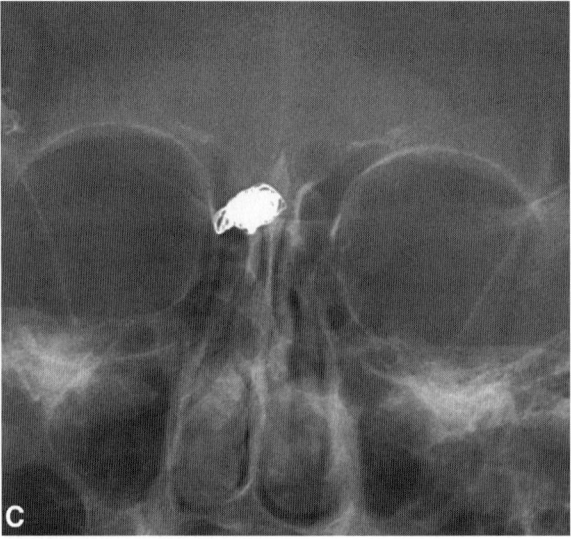

FIGURE 3.10 • *Balloon-Assisted Coil Embolization III.*
A 56-year-old female was referred for craniotomy and clipping of this 12-mm unruptured carotid-ophthalmic aneurysm (A), but it proved difficult to access surgically at craniotomy. The aneurysm was relatively wide-based and was coiled using an Endeavor balloon for coil stabilization. A satisfactory postembolization result was obtained (B). The nonsubtracted image (C) of the coils shows the contour of the coil nidus created by the intraluminal balloon. A relatively dense packing was obtained, which prevented any compaction of the coils on subsequent follow-up. Loose coils on the right side of the aneurysm at the merging of the neck and parent vessel were difficult to pack further and have remained stable at 1-year follow-up.

surrounding avascular subarachnoid space.[24] Based on postmortem studies and on animal studies, this process of complete isolation of coiled intracranial aneurysms probably requires some weeks.[25,26]

In contrast to aneurysm clipping, in which there is immediate apposition of intimal surfaces, the delayed process by which sealing of the aneurysm occurs following coil therapy is a concern for the risk of acute rebleeding. However, in published series this seems to be an uncommon event, and it is hypothesized that even loose coil-packing within an aneurysm can strengthen the wall of the aneurysm by reducing the surface tension on the aneurysm wall.[23]

The dangers related to the persistence of residual aneurysm after endovascular coiling involve aneurysm regrowth and late rupture. Persistence of an aneurysm neck following clipping occurs in approximately 4% of surgical patients[27] and is known to carry a small risk of delayed rupture and of aneurysm regrowth.[28–30] Even patients with unruptured cerebral aneurysms who undergo successful clipping are at higher risk of delayed subarachnoid hemorrhage than the general population due to bleeding from persistent or de novo aneurysms.[31] It has therefore been extrapolated that the higher incidence of residual aneurysm neck in coil patients might lead to an unfavorably high rate of rehemorrhage. This does not appear to be a prominent risk so far, however, and the evidence suggests that endovascular coils protect against rebleeding satisfactorily.[32–35] In the short term (<6 months) rebleeding is seen in less than 1% of patients[14] despite the presence of a residuum in up to 19% of cases. Long-term follow-up on patients treated with coil embolization shows a stable occluded appearance in over 85% of aneurysms regardless of size, with a 0.8% risk of rebleeding in the first year, 0.6% in the second year, and 2.4% risk in the third year of follow-up, as reported by Byrne et al.[36] Similar results with a 0.9% risk of delayed rebleeding were reported on a series of 112 patients presenting with ruptured posterior circulation aneurysms by Lempert et al.[37]

The question becomes whether the small risk of late rebleeding following coil embolization[34] is acceptable compared with the initial risks related to surgical craniotomy. For instance, persistent cognitive and neuropsychological impairments have been identified in 8.7% to 10.6% of patients undergoing craniotomy for unruptured aneurysm treatment,[38] in addition to a 3.8% rate of surgery-related mortality and 15.7% to 17.5% rates of neurologic morbidity in long-term outcome. It is not known at this time whether the short-term significant benefits of minimally invasive coil embolization compared with surgery justify any longer-term increased relative risk of rebleeding and aneurysm regrowth.

Aneurysm Reconstruction with Balloons or Stents

Considerable advances have been made in the ability to use coils for endovascular treatment of intracranial aneurysms in situations that would have appeared unsuitable a short time ago. Newer designs for coils including the 3D and 2D configurations have had a significant impact on the ease of attaining a desirable extrusion of the initial coil (Figs. 3.11, 3.12). Attention to the neck of the aneurysm as the critical focus concerning success of the procedure and likelihood of aneurysm recurrence has stimulated the development of techniques for tighter packing of the aneurysm using adjunctive devices, particularly temporary balloons or permanently placed stents. Alternative devices such as baffles, coils shaped like flowers or umbrellas to straddle the aneurysm neck, intraaneurysmal sacs to be packed with coils, or asymmetrically constructed stent-like devices are also in progress.

Balloon Reconstructive Technique

The most commonly used reconstruction technique for coil stabilization within intracranial aneurysms is the balloon reconstructive technique popularized by several authors.[7,8] This technique involves placing a nondetachable balloon parallel to the microcatheter and inflating the balloon across the mouth of the aneurysm as the coil is being placed in the aneurysm (Figs. 3.8, 3.10, 3.13, 3.14). The balloon is deflated prior to detachment of the coil, and the coil is observed carefully for signs of instability prior to detachment. Several compliant

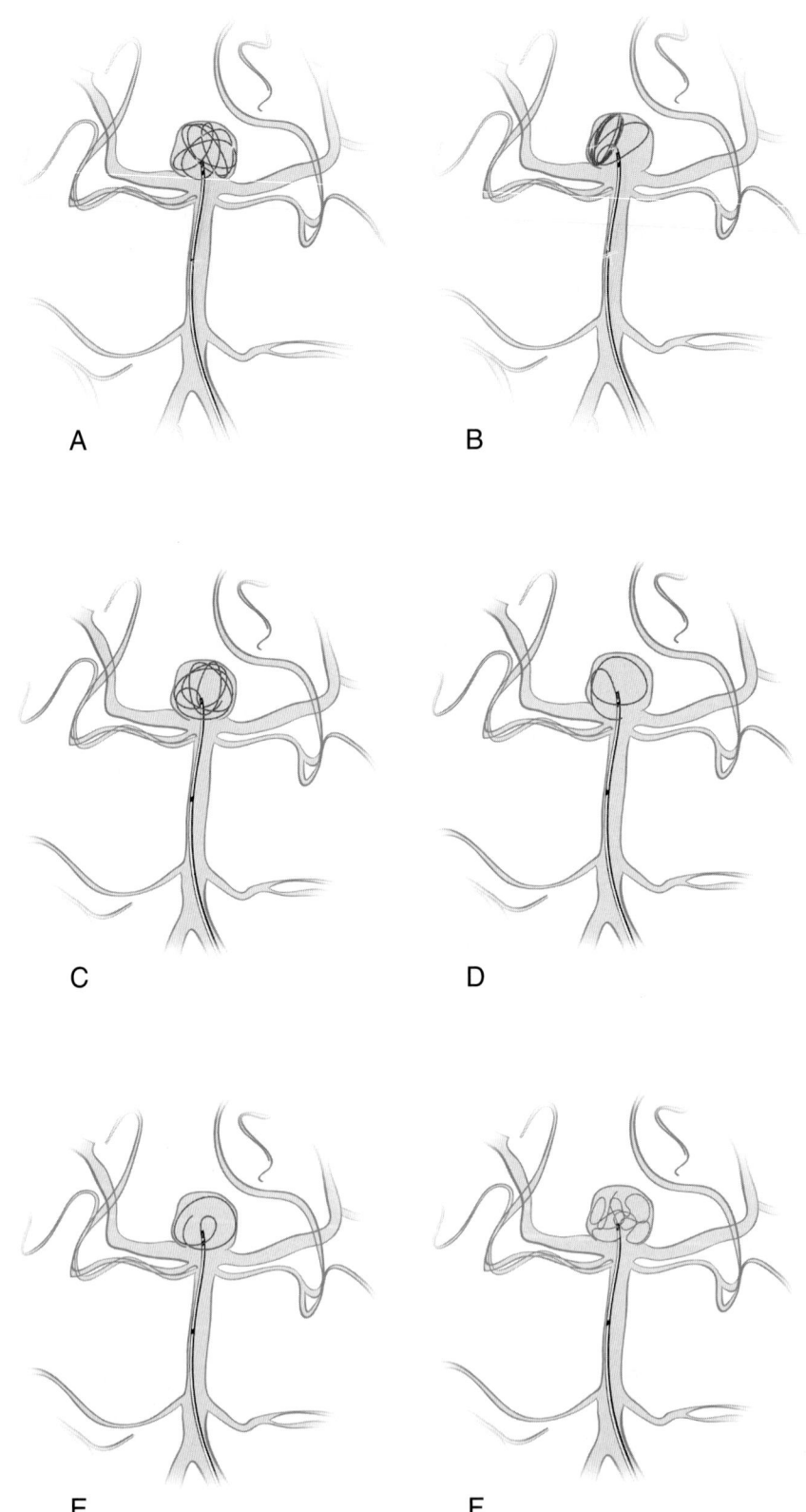

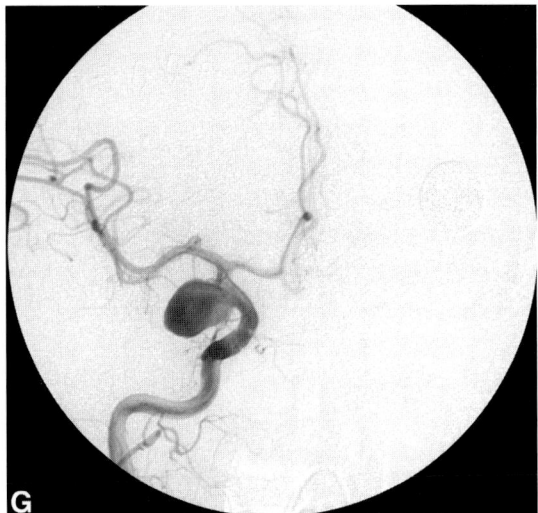
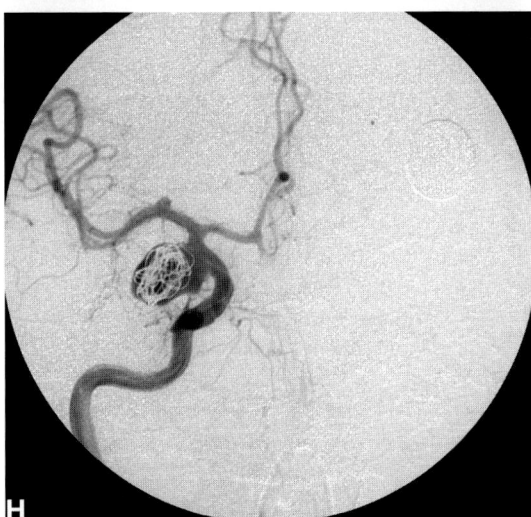
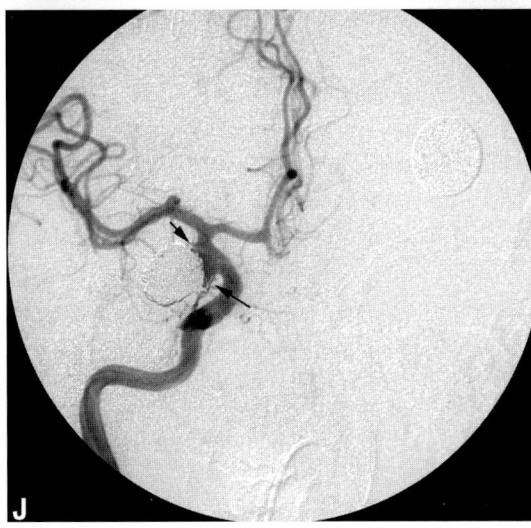

FIGURE 3.11 • *Aneurysm Packing and the Importance of the First Coil.*
An illustration of various difficulties that can be encountered during the early stages of aneurysm embolization. The first coils placed within the aneurysm usually have a disproportionate bearing on the safety and adequacy of the ultimate outcome. Ideally a framework or "basket" of coil(s) is established early in the case, encompassing the volume of aneurysm lumen that will be subsequently targeted for tighter packing.

In a favorable aneurysm (A, C) with shoulders defining a relatively narrow neck, a standard coil of diameter close to that of the aneurysm is deployed. It is important that there be a little tension between the coil and the aneurysm wall so that the coil will cease tumbling and will stabilize itself as it emerges to form a three-dimensional framework. A coil that is too small will emerge in a two-dimensional flattened helix within the aneurysm (B). The coil configuration depicted in B suggests that the coil is undersized for the diameter of the aneurysm. The resulting deployment within the aneurysm is therefore ineffective at forming an initial mesh. Furthermore, because the coils are too small for the aneurysm, they are likely to be unstable and prone to motion.

When the neck of the aneurysm is too wide (D), a coil appropriately sized for the aneurysm diameter will unfortunately prolapse into the parent vessel. This can sometimes be avoided by using a 2D coil (E) where the tighter curvature of the initial coil loop stays within the aneurysm and encourages the subsequent larger loops to follow suit. A 3D coil (F) has still greater internal integrity of shape and size and will often sit in a stable position where a 2D coil fails.

An example of timid undersizing of the first coils in a large aneurysm of the right posterior communicating artery is shown in images G, H, J. The initial oblique image (G) shows the aneurysm to be wide-based with little by way of shoulders with which to constrain the coils within the aneurysm. After the first coil has been placed, a prominent area of the neck of the aneurysm is excluded from the basket or framework of the coil mesh (H). The final image (J) shows how it is difficult to recover procedurally from the constraints defined by the initial coil. A wide neck of the aneurysm with upper and lower "dog-ears" persists. A larger sized 3D coil and/or balloon assistance would represent a better standard of technique now. In the future placement of a stent or other device across the aneurysm mouth will probably become routine.

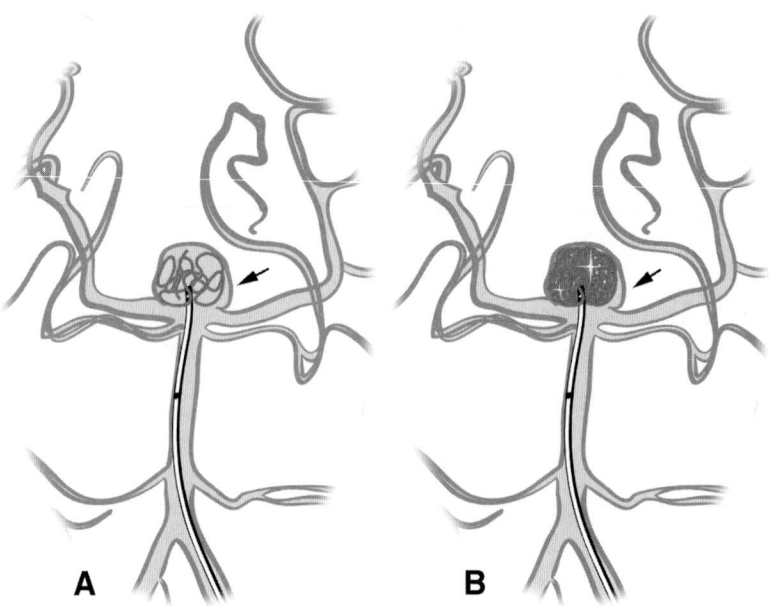

FIGURE 3.12 • *Use of 3D Coils for Initial Framing of the Aneurysm.*
The utility of 3D coils for forming an initial framework of coils within an aneurysm can occasionally work to one's disadvantage. So effective are 3D coils at confining the scope of deposition of subsequent coils that pockets of aneurysm excluded from the initial framework can be very difficult to access later in the case (arrow in B). An alternative problem with 3D coils is the possibility that the microcatheter tip will be restricted to a peripheral pocket of the aneurysm, and coil deposition within the center of the aneurysm can thus become difficult. When one anticipates such problems early in the case, it is worth spending a deal of time working to achieve a more favorable initial framing. Options include moving the microcatheter slightly during coil extrusion to achieve a different configuration within the aneurysm, using a larger 3D coil with the already opened coil (3D coils are very expensive!) deployed later within, or following the suboptimal 3D coil framework with a larger diameter 2D coil in the hope of reaching the excluded pocket.

balloons are suitable for this purpose: Endeavor (Target), Sentry (Target), Commodore (Cordis), and Equinox (MTI). Noncompliant balloons also have been used in certain locations, but are generally not recommended. The key technical points for the balloon reconstructive technique are:

- The need to minimize the occlusion time with the balloon. Therefore, the coil can be advanced all the way up to the aneurysm or partially into the aneurysm before inflating the balloon.
- The balloon must be deflated prior to detaching the coil so that any instability of the coil can be detected and adjustments made accordingly.
- The risk of thromboembolic complications is

probably higher with this technique so an adjustment upwards of the ACT and level of heparinization is recommended.
- Two catheters, 5 Fr and 6 Fr, can be used for the procedure requiring bilateral femoral arterial sheaths. Alternatively, a single 7 Fr catheter can accept both devices. A single-valve Tuohy-Borst adapter will usually suffice (Fig. 3.15), although a double-limbed Tuohy-Borst adapter is available (Microvena).
- With small aneurysms, care is necessary to avoid dislodging or pushing the microcatheter with the balloon at the time of inflation. This could result in loss of catheter position or even aneurysm perforation. A technique that can help to diminish this risk

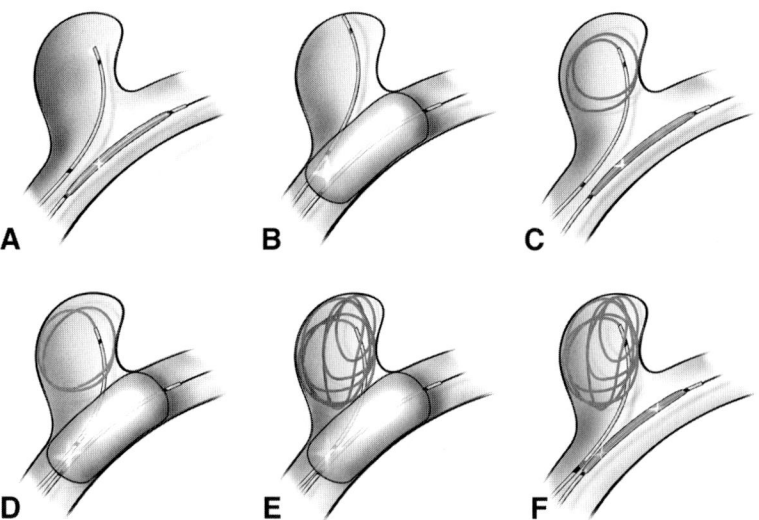

FIGURE 3.13 • *Balloon-Assisted Coil Embolization IV.*
In this series of illustrations the principles of using an intraarterial balloon parallel to the microcatheter are demonstrated. Obviously, it is desirable to minimize the occlusion time of the artery with the balloon. Therefore, it is usual to load the coil all the way to the tip of the microcatheter before inflating the balloon. The coil can then be advanced. The balloon is deflated and the coil is observed for stability prior to detachment. At the end of the case a theoretical risk exists of pulling some of the coils from the aneurysm with the withdrawing microcatheter. Therefore, it is probably prudent to inflate the balloon alongside the aneurysm to stabilize the coils as one extracts the microcatheter.

In practice, some difficulties can be commonly encountered with this technique. Often the hemodynamic thrust in the vessel can cause balloon motion within the artery as it is inflated, even with wire-directed balloons. Of particular concern is the possibility of transmitting this motion to the parallel microcatheter with the risk of impacting the tip against a fragile aneurysm dome. The same problem can be seen during balloon inflation when the balloon deflects the catheter shaft (B). The safety of this procedure can sometimes be improved by protecting the microcatheter tip with a loop or two of coil before inflating the balloon (C).

is to extrude a loop or two of coil from the catheter into the aneurysm before inflating the balloon. This will help to stabilize the microcatheter due to the buffeting effect of the softer coils (Fig. 3.13).

Double Microcatheter Technique for Wide-Necked Aneurysms

An alternative technique for achieving a stable intraaneurysmal nidus of coils has been described by Baxter et al.[39] and involves catheterizing the aneurysm with two parallel microcatheters. Simultaneous extrusion of two coils into the aneurysm can allow the coils to function as a brace against one another and prevent prolapse into the parent artery. However, the balloon reconstruction maneuver has been so successful that the double microcatheter is not commonly needed and has not achieved significant currency.

Aneurysm Reconstruction Using Stents

Use of intracranial stents for aneurysm reconstruction holds great promise for success, particularly in the proximal larger vessels of the Circle of Willis in cases of unruptured aneurysms (Fig. 3.16).[40–42] Stent placement involves greater risk of thromboembolic complications, and therefore premed-

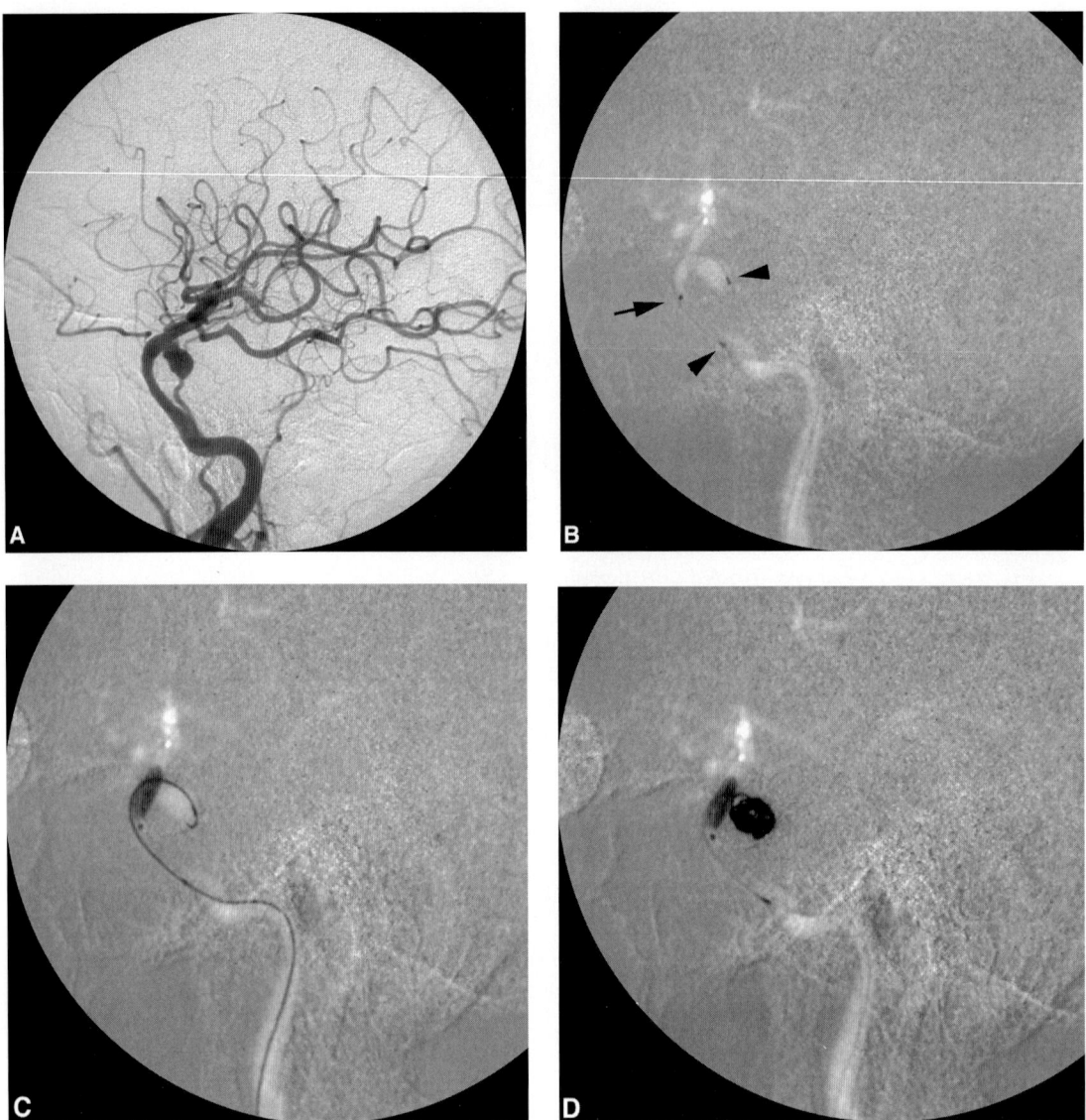

FIGURE 3.14 • *Balloon-Assisted Coil Embolization V.*
A lateral view of the left internal carotid artery (A) in a 70-year-old female who presented with mass-effect and cranial nerve deficits shows the opacified nonthrombosed portion of a larger aneurysm. Splaying of the carotid siphon is evident. In an aneurysm like this it is probably important to achieve a dense packing of the coils so as to reduce the likelihood of compaction of a loose coil mesh into the surrounding laminar thrombus. A road-map image (B) shows the double-marker (arrowheads) microcatheter in the dome of the aneurysm and a marker for the uninflated Endeavor balloon (arrow). After the first coil is advanced up to or partially into the aneurysm, the balloon is inflated (C). After the coil is extruded, the balloon is deflated. If the coil is stable, it is detached, and the process repeated (D).

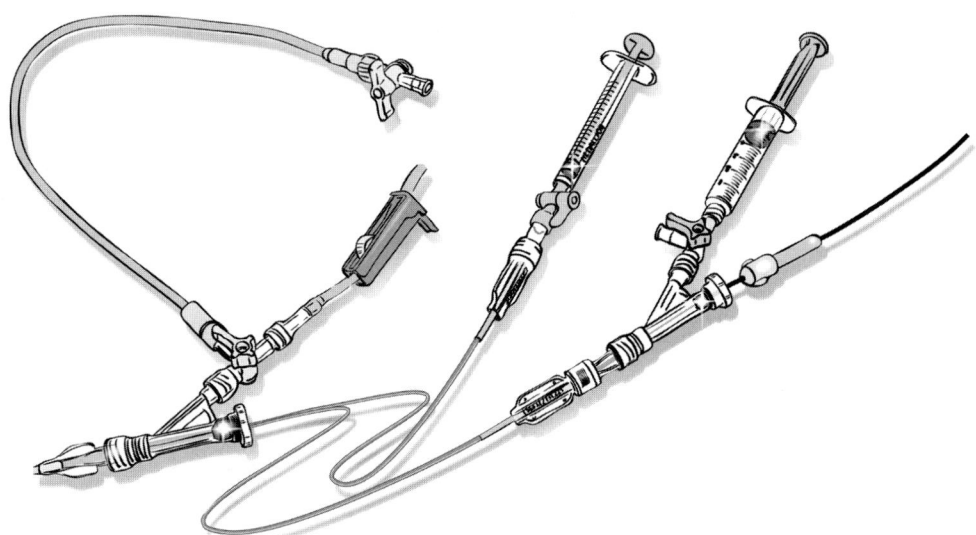

FIGURE 3.15 • *Parallel Balloon and Microcatheter for Balloon-Assisted Aneurysm Embolization.*
Balloon-assisted coil embolization can be performed with two introducer catheters or, as illustrated, through a single Tuohy-Borst adapter and a 7Fr catheter. In this diagram an Endeavor balloon can be inflated by a 1-ml syringe. For greater stability a 0.010-in wire can be placed within the balloon shaft and inflation accomplished by using another Tuohy-Borst adapter. The newer wire-directed balloons described in the text will probably prove more versatile for this purpose, and can also be used in the manner illustrated. A double-adapter is also available for parallel use of devices via a single introducer catheter.

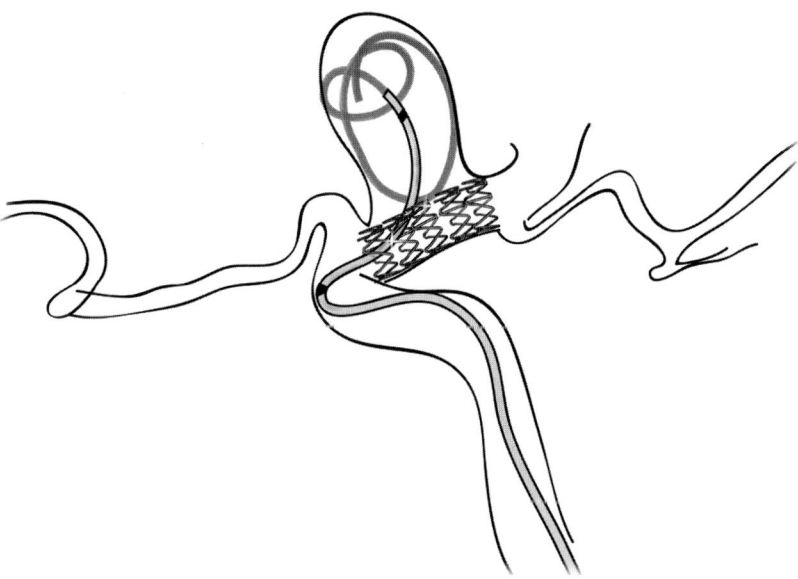

FIGURE 3.16 • *Stent-Assisted Coil Embolization.*
If they can be navigated to the intracranial sites of aneurysm formation, stents offer the potential of allowing greater packing of aneurysms and of aneurysm embolization in previously unfavorable locations. Although the diagram shows that this stent conveniently skirts the ophthalmic and posterior communicating arteries, such diligence is not always possible, and perhaps not necessary. Experience with stenting for atherosclerotic disease so far suggests that side-branch "jailing" by stents is not problematic.

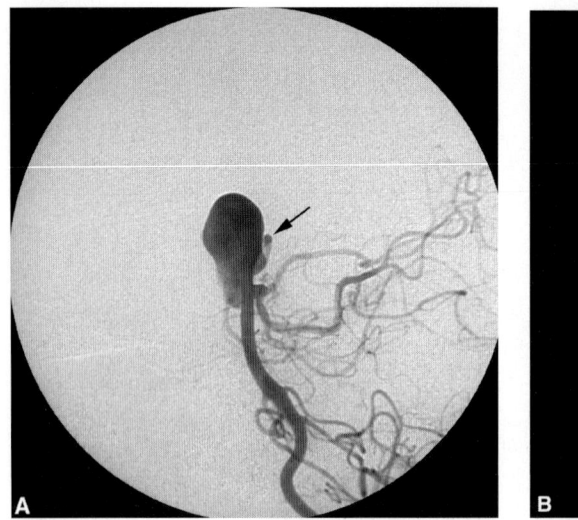
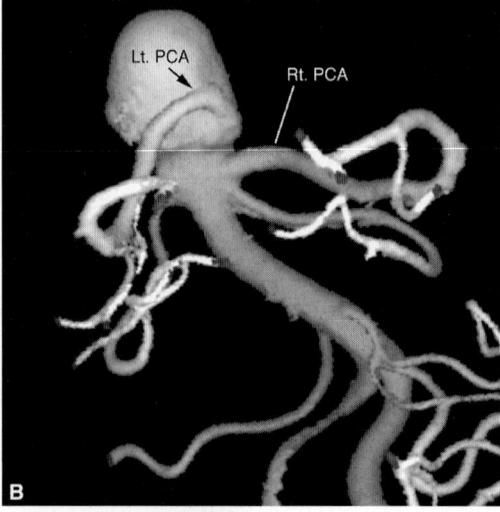
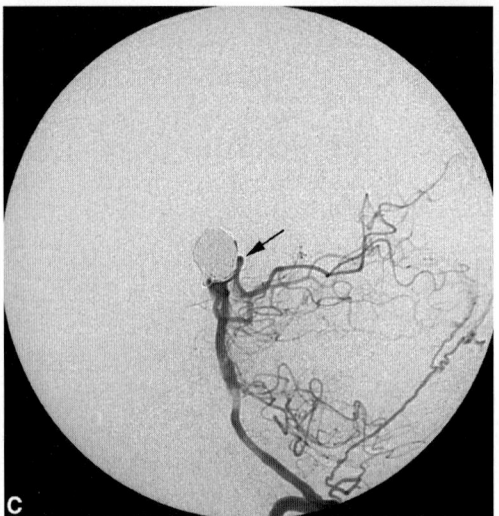

FIGURE 3.17 • *Stent-Assisted Coil Embolization of a Basilar Artery Aneurysm.*
A 71-year-old female presenting with worsening headache was found to have a large aneurysm of the basilar artery. The lateral view (A) demonstrates that the left posterior cerebral artery (arrow) is looped behind the aneurysm, and that the anterior wall of the aneurysm extends proximally along the anterior wall of the basilar artery below the level of the superior cerebellar arteries. A 3D view (B) from a posterior vantage shows the left posterior cerebral artery arising from the posterior right aspect of the aneurysm. The left posterior communicating artery was diminutive, precluding any consideration of sacrificing the left posterior cerebral artery proximally during a coiling procedure. A reasonable result was obtained from the initial embolization (C, lateral view) with preservation of the left posterior cerebral artery (arrow in image C) and filling of the major portion of the dome with coils.

However, 3 months later with return of severe headache, a follow-up angiogram (D) demonstrated an alarming degree of regrowth of the neck of the aneurysm anteriorly (arrowhead). Balloon reconstructive technique was unsuccessful at stabilizing a 3D coil within the aneurysm. A 4 × 12 mm S670 stent (AVE) advanced easily up to the aneurysm over a Fasdasher 14 wire (Target), but the stent delivery catheter was too stiff to make a turn into either posterior cerebral artery to a degree that would allow the stent to de-

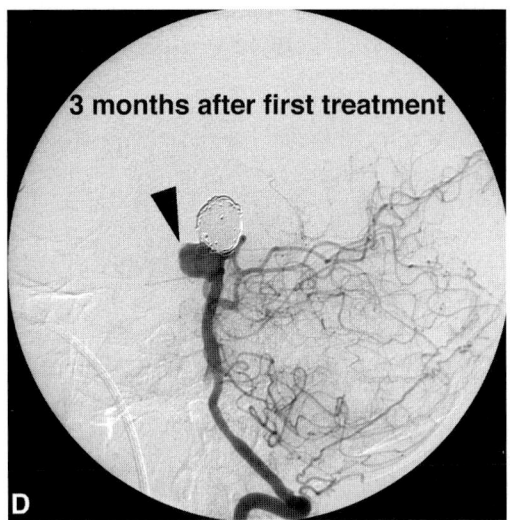
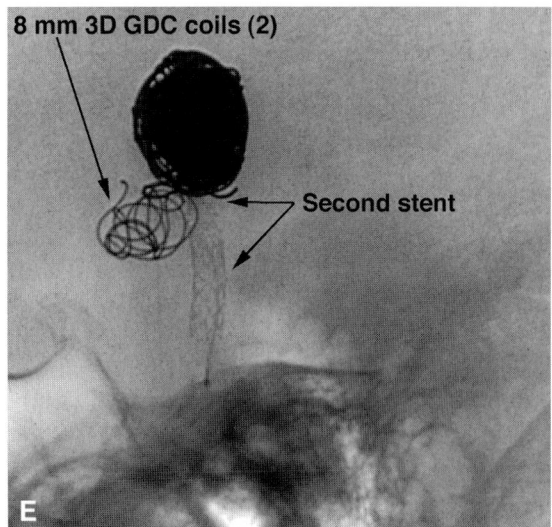
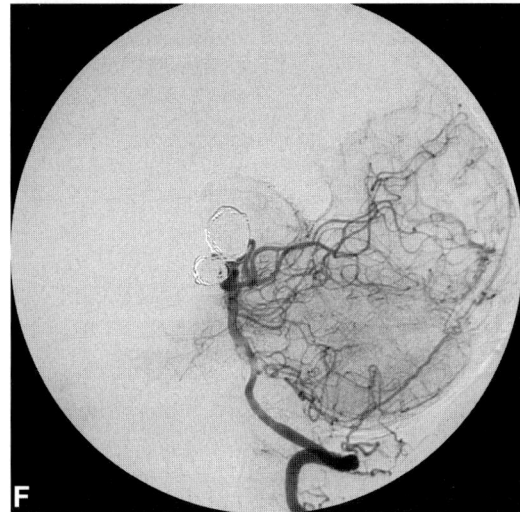

ploy adequately across the neck of the aneurysm. The stent was finally deployed in a compromise position so that it partially overhung the neck of the aneurysm, but even here with balloon assistance, coil stability could not be achieved. The procedure was abandoned after many hours.

The patient returned 2 weeks later with critical exacerbation of headache, and a repeat embolization was attempted. Premedication with clopidogrel and aspirin, and procedural platelet suppression with eptifibatide were used as during the first procedure. On this occasion a 3.5 × 9 mm S670 stent (AVE) was used, but encountered the same difficulties. The delivery system for the stent was too stiff to advance sufficiently into the posterior cerebral artery. After some prolonged attempts, it was noticed that the stent had moved distally on the balloon by approximately 2 mm. This would normally be a very dangerous event, but was used to advantage in this patient because it allowed the second stent to be deployed more distally within the first stent (E). Coiling of the resurgent dome of the aneurysm could then be performed (F). She was discharged on coumadin and clopidogrel. At last follow-up the patient continues to suffer from severe, but improved, headaches, and the residual components of the aneurysm appear stable without further growth.

ication and intraprocedural antiplatelet medication is desirable if not imperative for such cases. The use of antiplatelet agents involves greater risk in the setting of recent rupture of an aneurysm or ventriculostomy placement.

Technical considerations for coil placement within the aneurysm involve deciding whether to place the microcatheter in the aneurysm *parallel* to the stent, i.e., outside the stent, or alternatively *through* the struts of the stent (Fig. 3.17). Placing the microcatheter parallel to the stent catheter carries some advantages in that the microcatheter will be somewhat pinned against the arterial wall and thus held in a stable position during coil delivery. Furthermore, this approach will avoid the difficulty of having to advance the microcatheter tip through the apertures of the stents, a task that can sometimes be very difficult. However, expanding the stent parallel to the microcatheter can kink or deform the microcatheter and prevent the coils from advancing within the microcatheter. It may be necessary to extract the microcatheter in such an instance and advance through the struts of the stent.[43]

COMPLICATIONS OF ANEURYSM THERAPY
Aneurysmal Rupture during Coil Embolization

Among the most severe complications that can occur during coil embolization of a ruptured intracranial aneurysm is perforation of the aneurysmal dome by a coil, wire, or microcatheter (Figs. 3.18, 3.19). This has a published incidence of 2% to 5%.[44,45] Although this has the potential to be a catastrophic event with sudden elevation of intracranial pressure and compromise of cerebral perfusion, many intraprocedural perforations can be handled without major neurologic consequences.

First, the effects of the hemorrhage can be mitigated if a ventriculostomy is placed in advance. This should be considered in every patient with a ruptured intracranial aneurysm prior to coiling, even if the ventricles are just mildly enlarged. The possibility of hydrocephalus developing in an anesthetized patient during the course of a long proce-

FIGURE 3.18 • *Complication of Aneurysm Embolization: Intraprocedural Aneurysmal Rupture.* A 50-year-old female presented with Grade IV subarachnoid hemorrhage and had a ventriculostomy placed. However, during a diagnostic angiogram her condition deteriorated and pooling of extravasated contrast could be seen at the C1–2 level near the aneurysm of the left vertebral artery (A, arrow). It was unclear at first whether the aneurysm (B, arrowhead) arose along the course of the posterior inferior cerebellar artery arising from the C2 level of the vertebral artery (B, arrow). However, a selective injection in the C2 branch did not show the aneurysm (C). In retrospect, a small inflowing branch (C, arrow) was seen on one image from this run. The aneurysm was catheterized from the intradural vertebral artery, and embolization with soft GDC coils without heparinization was attempted.

However, the third coil clearly perforated the contour of the aneurysm. It was not pulled back but rather was deployed in the aneurysm (D, arrowhead). This failed to stop the extravasation (D, arrow), and balloon occlusion of the vertebral artery was then performed above the C2 origin of the posterior inferior cerebellar artery (E, arrowhead marks the upper of two balloons). Interestingly, the basilar artery opacified despite the inflated balloons, due to the fact that the posterior inferior cerebellar artery origin had a duplicated origin, allowing the C2 posterior inferior cerebellar artery to continue perfusing the basilar artery. The aneurysm with coils within (small double-arrows) no longer opacifies.

Lessons learned: In retrospect, given that extravasation was seen on the diagnostic angiogram, it might have been simply safer to perform arterial closure of the vertebral artery using balloons or coils adjacent to the aneurysm. The unusual anatomy of this patient required interrogation, however, in order to understand the origin of the aneurysm.

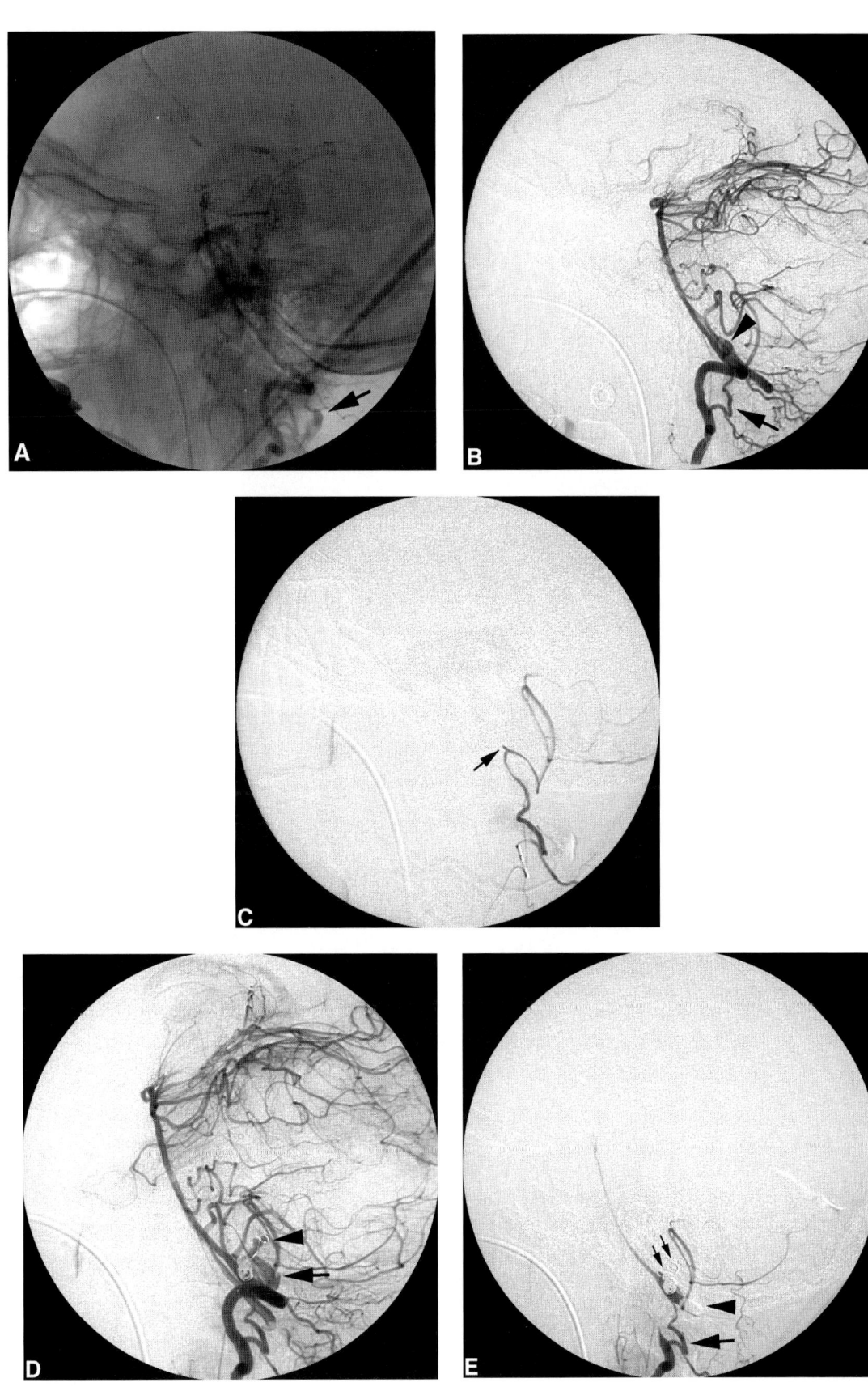

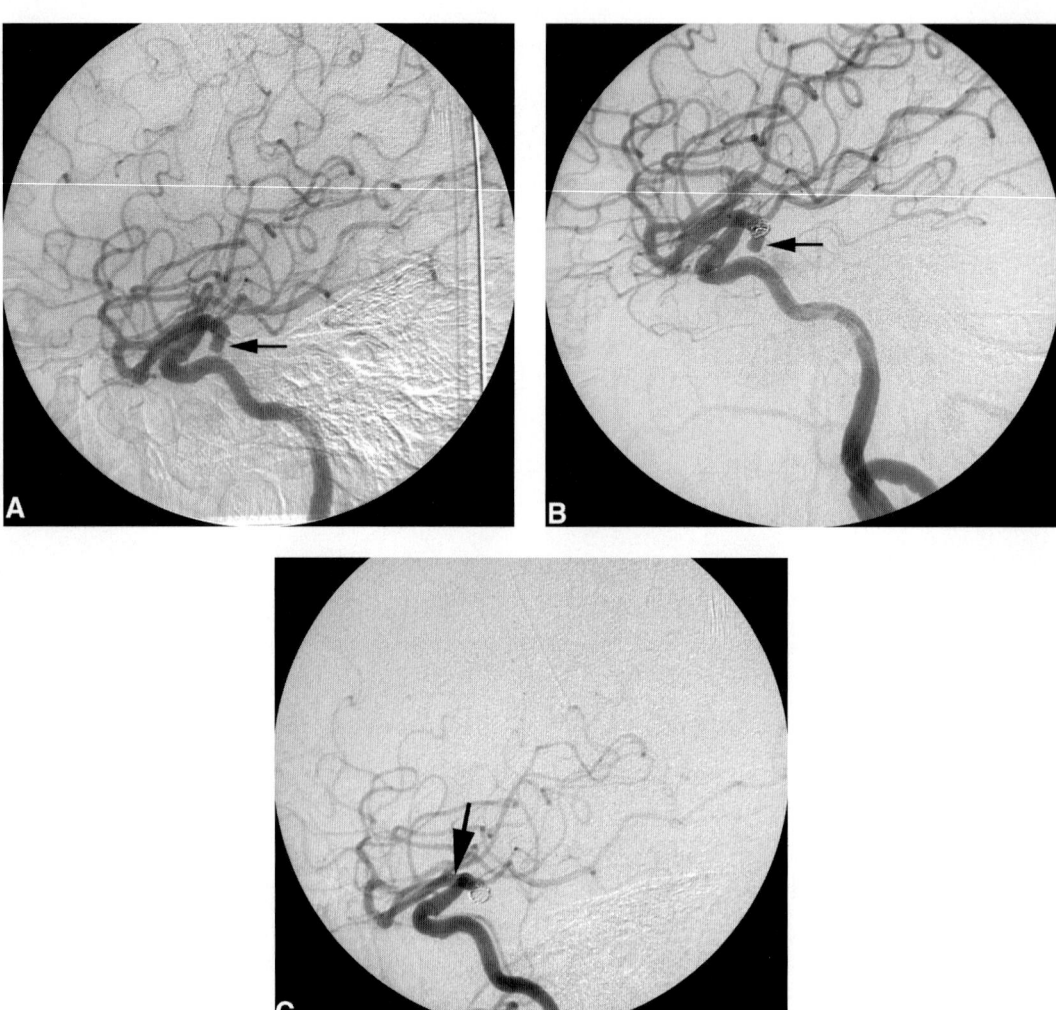

FIGURE 3.19 • *Avoidance of Trauma and Manipulation of Rupture Points Is Important to Reduce Risk of Procedural Rupture.*
A 62-year-old female presented with a Grade II subarachnoid hemorrhage from a posterior communicating artery aneurysm. Pointing inferiorly from the aneurysm is a large apical teat (A, lateral view, pretreatment, arrow) almost as big as the aneurysm itself. This apical teat represents the site of vulnerability of the aneurysm from the point of view of rupture during the procedure and it is better to avoid any trauma to this area if it can be avoided. An image after the first coil (B) and a final postembolization image (C) show that after dense packing of the aneurysm body itself, the apical teat is now excluded from the circulation. The teat was not entered during the procedure by the wire, microcatheter, or coils.

This patient had extremely tortuous cervical vessels, and balloon assistance could not be used. The final coil gave resistance in the last centimeter and could neither be advanced nor retracted. It was eventually detached at the mouth of the aneurysm, where it prolapsed distally into the middle cerebral artery at a length of approximately 7 mm (arrow in C). The patient was heparinized for 3 days afterwards and then discharged fully recovered on aspirin. No change in the patient's fully recovered clinical status or in the aneurysm has occurred since.

Lessons learned here include an affirmation of the need to choose *short* coils toward the end of a case when one cannot be certain of how much space remains within the aneurysm.

dure is a serious danger and cannot be monitored well under general anesthesia. A ventriculostomy will protect against the danger of sudden hydrocephalus and will also provide a safety valve for the intracranial pressure in the event of aneurysmal perforation. If there is not a ventriculostomy present at the time of perforation, one should be placed as a matter of emergency in the angiography suite after these primary control measures have been taken:

- Reverse the heparinization. Protamine sulfate must be immediately available in the room from the beginning of all coil procedures involving ruptured aneurysms.
- If there is a balloon present across the neck of the aneurysm for reconstruction purposes, inflate the balloon to tamponade the aneurysm.
- Do not extract the coil that has transgressed the aneurysmal wall. Finish the delivery of the coil at the perforation site in the hope that it might seal the perforation. There is concern that the coil partially within and outside the aneurysm wall in this manner could act as a "wick" to perpetuate flow across the perforation, but most experience suggests that extruding the coil rather than withdrawing it represents the better course.
- If the microcatheter ruptures the aneurysm wall, extruding a coil to help seal the perforation as one retracts the microcatheter is probably a worthwhile maneuver.

The risk of aneurysm perforation seems to be greater with small aneurysms rather than large, and most perforations occur at the time of deposition of the first coil.[18,44] The reasons for this are threefold.

- First, smaller aneurysms have less room for maneuvering with the microwire and microcatheter on initial approach to the aneurysm. A small degree of relaxation of proximal tension in the microcatheter, particularly at the time of removal of the microwire, will allow the microcatheter to move forward, risking a perforation of the aneurysm.
- Second, a small mismatch in coil size and aneurysm size in smaller aneurysms translates into a greater differential of surface tension compared with a similar degree of mismatch in a larger aneurysm.
- Third, smaller coils relative to their diameter have more memory in their shape than larger coils, implying that the relative tension imparted to the wall of the aneurysm may be greater in smaller aneurysms. Availability of newer soft and ultrasoft coils will improve performance in this regard.

THROMBOEMBOLIC COMPLICATIONS DURING ANEURYSM EMBOLIZATION

Thromboembolic complications are an ever-present concern during coil embolization of aneurysms (Figs. 3.20, 3.21). Many operators consider that the risk of emboli is so high without heparinization that even with ruptured aneurysms they heparinize the patient from the very beginning of the procedure. Others wait until the first coils have been placed in a ruptured aneurysm before starting the heparin or administer the heparin by increments. Even with heparinization, significant thromboembolic complications can be seen in 5% to 8% of patients[9,46] undergoing this procedure. Some groups have shown that with increasing experience and close monitoring of anticoagulation, these figures can be reduced to near zero.[47] Generally, these complications respond very well to intraarterial thrombolytic therapy or mechanical clot fragmentation with balloons or wires, because the thrombus is fresh. However, organized resistant thrombus might be seen in previously treated aneurysms that are undergoing a repacking of the residual or recurrent aneurysm.

Intravenous aspirin, where available, is used routinely during coil procedures to reduce this risk. Premedication of elective patient with oral clopidogrel and aspirin is probably also prudent. For emergency thrombolysis in unruptured aneurysms, use of parenteral GPIIb/IIIa inhibitors is probably also worth remembering. The difficult cases are the situations of thromboembolic complications in the setting of a ruptured aneurysm. In these situations the decision of how aggressively to use fibrinolytic drugs to dissolve the clot versus the risk of provoking a rebleed from the aneurysm needs to be considered. The first-pass hepatic metabolism of tPA suggests that delivering this agent if possible distal to the ruptured aneurysm may substantially reduce the risk of rebleeding in the aneurysm because so little of the tPA will recirculate into the systemic circulation. Alternatively, depending on what point has been reached with the procedure and how bad the thromboembolic complication appears, one may consider securing the aneurysm still further with more coils, while temporizing with more heparin and elevation of the mean arterial blood pressure, before diverting one's attention to the clot.

Postembolization TCD monitoring of patients with large aneurysms or wide-necked aneurysms with a large coil-artery interface has confirmed the intuitive suspicion that such patients are at higher risk for delayed thromboembolic complications. Klötzsch et al.[48] observed that 31% of their postembolization patients had high rates of microemboli detectable by TCD, particularly with wide-necked aneurysms. The frequency of these observations correlated with the likelihood of an adverse clinical ischemic deficit. The heparin protocol used at the time of this particular study has since been superseded by heavier use of heparin (ACT >300 s) during and after the procedure at most centers. Many centers now continue heparinization for a period of time following a coil-embolization procedure. In cases of extreme danger from clot formation in a loosely packed aneurysm, coumadin therapy is sometimes necessary. Additionally, antiplatelet agents are now favored by most operators, particularly for elective unruptured cases, and are extremely important in posttreatment management of aneurysms with undesirable coil prolapse (Figs. 3.22, 3.23).

Arterial Sacrifice in the Treatment of Aneurysms

Although pioneering neurointerventional incursions into the field of intracranial aneurysm therapy involved permanent deployment of detachable balloons within the aneurysm, first described by Serbinenko,[49] these techniques have generally been outmoded by other technological innovations. Bal-

FIGURE 3.20 • *Complication of Aneurysm Embolization: Intraprocedural Compromise of Flow.* A 52-year-old female with a strong family history of ruptured aneurysms was found to have bilateral middle cerebral artery aneurysm, the aneurysm on the left (A, B) being complex and multilobulated. Generally, aneurysms of the middle cerebral artery are inauspicious from the viewpoint of coil embolization. It is common for such aneurysms to involve divisions or branches of the middle cerebral artery. In this instance, the referring neurosurgeon was apprehensive about clipping such a complex aneurysm. A 3D image suggested that coil embolization (B, view from posterior position) might be feasible, and this was the patient's preference.

Embolization of the larger dome was uneventful. However, a digital run after the third coil placed in the smaller dome showed compromise and slow filling of an angular branch of the middle cerebral artery (C, arterial and parenchymal phases). The coil was removed and the patient's blood pressure elevated. Flow improved significantly in the vessel and the patient awoke from anesthesia neurologically intact. She was maintained in the ICU on heparin and pressor agents after the procedure, but became dysphasic whenever her systolic blood pressure dropped below 150 mm Hg.

Finally, after 5 days she was weaned from the pressor agents. A follow-up angiogram on day 6 showed good flow in the previously compromised vessel (D, arrowhead). During compression of the femoral artery the patient developed a vagal response with hypotension and bradycardia. Until she was resuscitated with atropine and intravenous fluids, she was again densely aphasic and paretic. Fortunately, the patient made an excellent recovery from that point, and a follow-up angiogram at 1 year showed complete occlusion of both aneurysms of the middle cerebral artery (E).

Lessons learned from this case included an affirmation of the dangers of middle cerebral artery aneurysms during coiling and of the need to perform digital runs of the vessel before each coil detachment in critical situations to detect problems such as this one early. The postprocedure management of the patient was equally pivotal to her successful outcome.

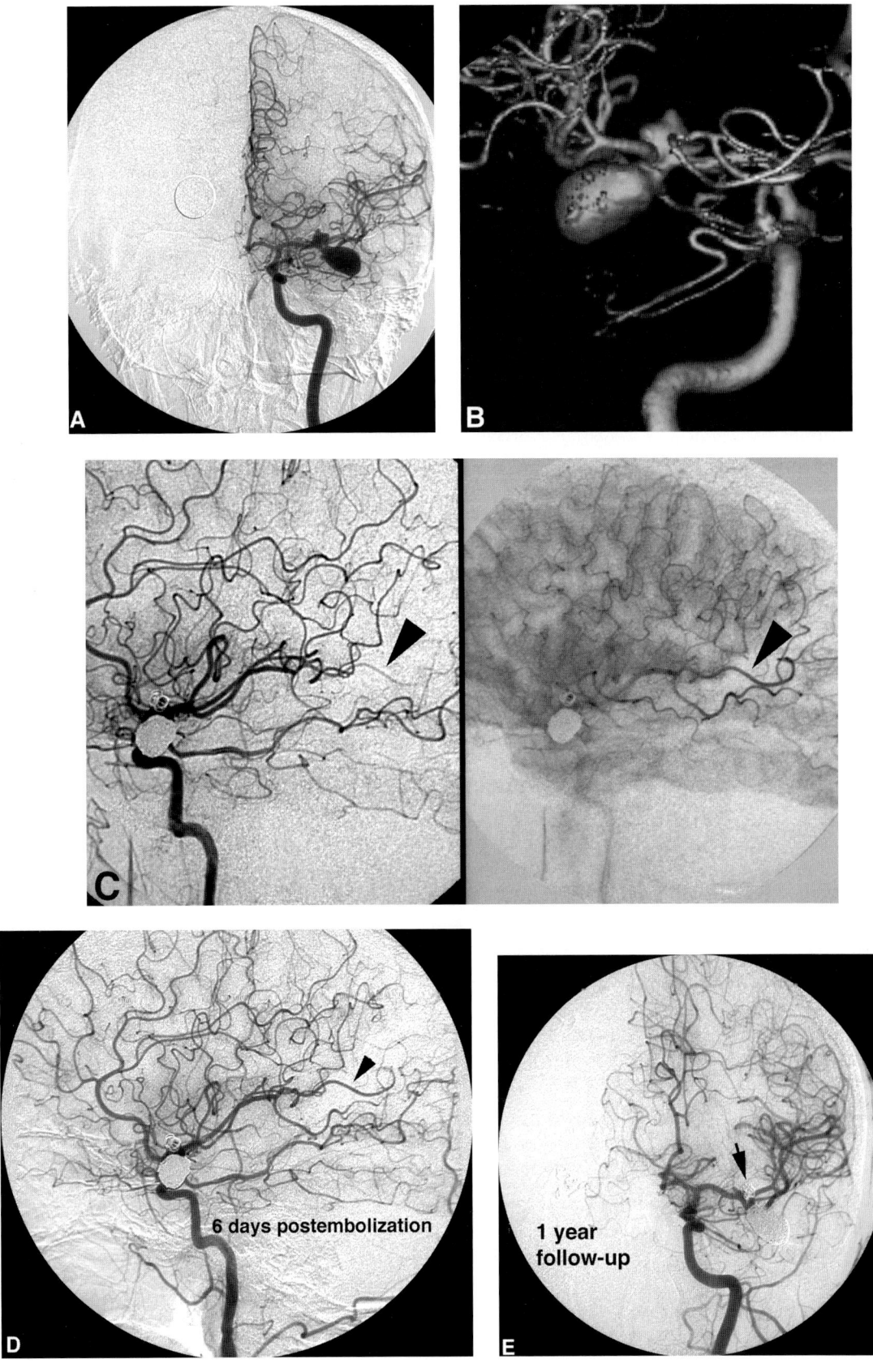

loons continue to have a role in the permanent closure of the carotid or vertebral arteries in situations where alternative treatments that might preserve flow within the artery either are not available or involve excessive risk (Fig. 3.24).

Proximal arterial ligation or clamping is accepted as an alternative treatment for inoperable intracranial aneurysms in the anterior and posterior circulations.[50,51] Proximal arterial ligation permits a change in the hemodynamic patterns of flow adjacent to an aneurysm with the hope that at least partial thrombosis will occur and that the risk of rupture will be attenuated. More recently, endovascular closure of arteries has become accepted as a preferable method for inducing this desired alteration in the pattern of flow in the circle of Willis. The reasons for this are:

- The procedure can be performed with an awake patient, and the effects of arterial sacrifice can be assessed by conducting a test occlusion first.
- A second catheter can be placed in an alternative artery during the test occlusion to evaluate angiographically the effects of the planned closure.
- The size of the distal arterial stump between the site of arterial closure and next point of inflow from the collateral circulation can be minimized, and with it the risk of delayed thromboembolic complications (Fig. 8.7).

Arterial sacrifice can be performed safely using intravascular coils or balloons depending on the anatomic limitations of the location and the preferences of the operator. Indications for use of this technique involve primarily symptomatic aneurysms of the cavernous internal carotid artery. Symptomatic dissections, pseudoaneurysms, or inoperable intracranial aneurysms may also be treated in this way, by either occluding flow proximally or "trapping" the lesion with balloons or coils placed distally and proximally. Deposition of coils within a flowing artery involves theoretical risks that the initial coils or the forming thrombus could be swept forward by flow during the time that it takes to arrest flow completely. Graves et al.[52] have described a technique using proximal arrest of flow with a balloon catheter while coils are being in-

FIGURE 3.21 • *Complications of Aneurysm Embolization: Acute Postprocedure Embolus.*
A 67-year-old female was referred for embolization of an unruptured 8-mm left carotid-ophthalmic aneurysm. A satisfactory dense packing of the wide-mouth aneurysm was obtained (A) using balloon stabilization. An unusual fenestration of the left middle cerebral artery is also noted.

The patient was placed on heparin in the ICU but her aPTT drifted into the normal range close to midnight following the procedure. She became abruptly paretic on the right side of her body and dysphasic. An emergency angiogram showed no discernible emboli or branch occlusions. Her heparin status was corrected and she was given a loading bolus of eptifibatide, followed by a 24-hour infusion. Her blood pressure was elevated using pressor drips and fluid boluses. Over the next 24 hours her neurological status fluctuated between near normal on one extreme to almost complete aphasia and right-sided paresis on the other. An MRI DWI scan (B) showed a small focal infarction in the left frontal area from a presumed embolus from the aneurysm. Contrast-enhanced T1-weighted images (C, arrows) showed pooling of contrast in an area more extensive than that demonstrated on the DWI. This, in association with her clinical fluctuation, suggests that a more extensive area of penumbra or "at-risk" tissue was present and was saved from infarction by the prompt handling of her complication. The patient made an uneventful complete recovery and was discharged on aspirin and clopidogrel. Many complications can be mitigated or prevented from worsening by prompt intervention in the ICU. It is important for interventional neuroradiologists to be involved with patient care following all cases.

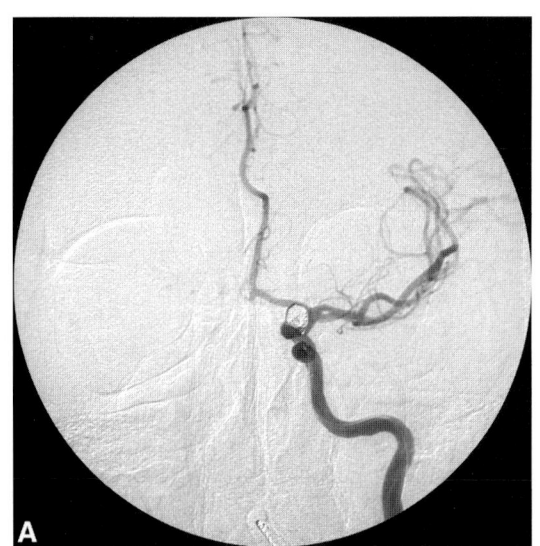
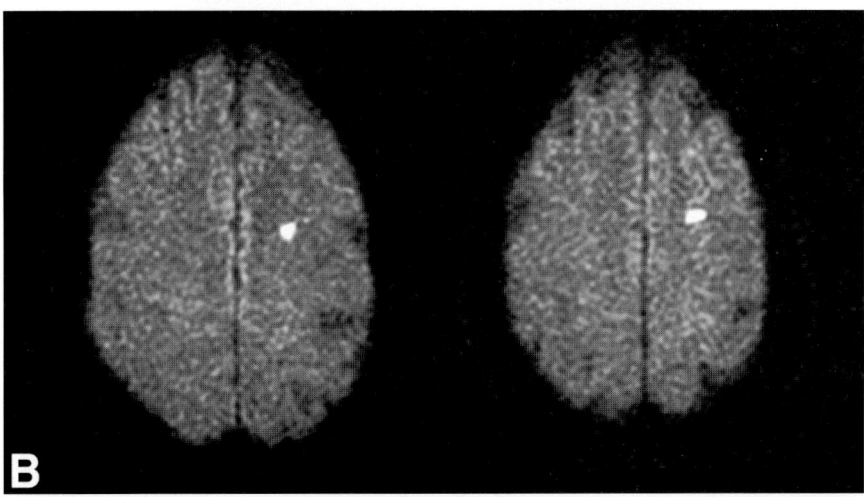
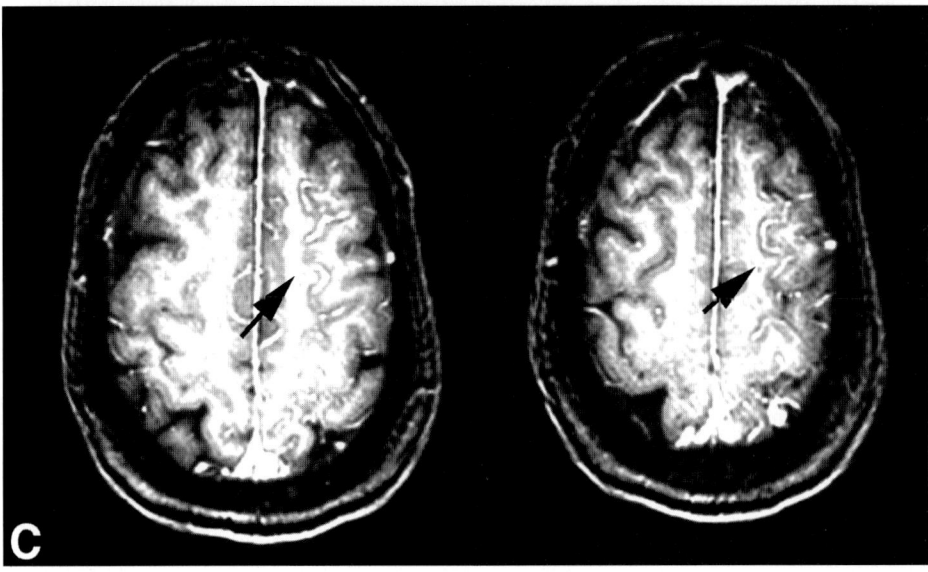

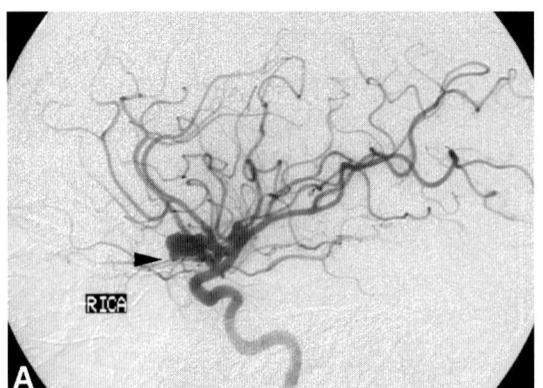
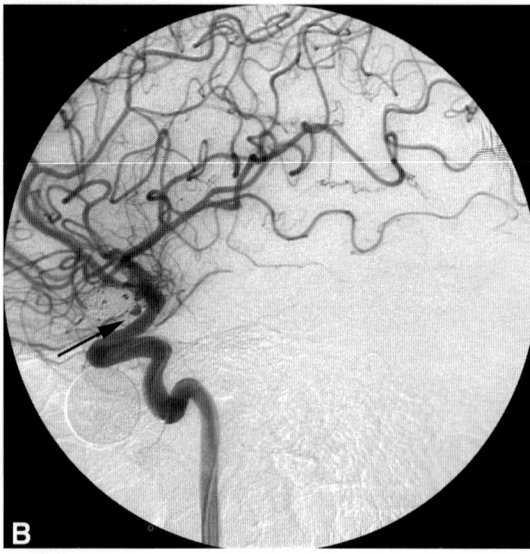

FIGURE 3.22 • *Intraprocedural Crisis Due to Coil Stretching.*
A 35-year-old female presenting with Grade II subarachnoid hemorrhage from a multilobed anterior communicating aneurysm was referred for embolization. The point of hemorrhage was thought most likely to be an anterior inferior teat (A, lateral view, arrowhead). This teat was sealed off early in the case by coils placed in the dome of the aneurysm. However, a second more posterior lobule, which appeared to be covered by coils, continued to opacify late in the case (B, lateral view, arrow), and a specific attempt was made to focus soft coils into that area near the neck to seal the second lobule. This was difficult, and in the course of placing an 8-cm soft coil in the posterior aspect of the already fairly well packed aneurysm, difficulty with coil manipulation was encountered. The coil would neither advance nor withdraw, and in trying to manipulate it, it became evident that the coil was damaged and stretched. The coil was then purposefully stretched into the descending aorta with the reasoning that a wire so small (<0.003 in) would pose very little embolic potential and would become endothelialized.

Three days later the aneurysm was stable and the residual pocket of aneurysm posteriorly seemed to be shrinking (C). However, a head CT showed that hemodynamic shear stress on the stretched coil had carried the coil up into the middle cerebral artery where it was looped at the bifurcation (D) and then returned back down the internal carotid artery. The appearance of the coil is deceptively large on the soft-tissue CT windows. On bone windows the wire (having been stretched, it is now no longer a coil) was hardly discernible. The patient was asymptomatic at this time and was discharged on aspirin. After 2 years of angiographic follow-up, the aneurysm and the looped coil remain stable and asymptomatic.

Lessons learned: The choice of an 8-cm soft coil in this situation was an error. Soft coils are prone to stretching with any difficulties encountered during manipulation. The newer, soft, stretch-resistant (SR) coils are designed to help avoid such problems. However, one should always choose short coils when one is near the end of an aneurysm packing, precisely to avoid this problem. Second, the decision to stretch the coil deliberately into the aorta was probably not the very best choice in view of the manner in which blood flow subsequently carried the coil into the middle cerebral artery. A more stable position might have been achieved by looping the stretched coil into the distal ipsilateral external carotid artery.

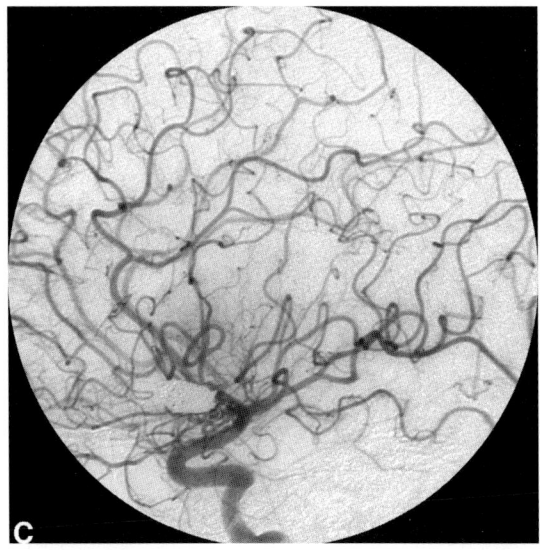 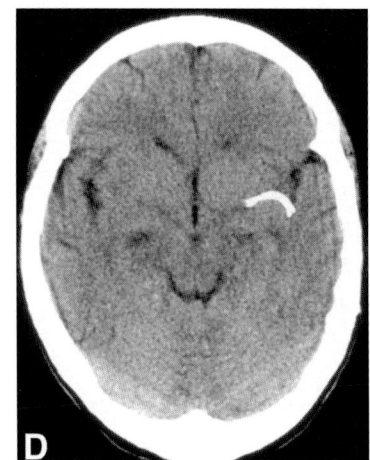

serted via a coaxial microcatheter, and have achieved excellent results. In their opinion, the technique is easier and safer than use of intravascular balloons. If double-lumen balloon catheters of a size capable of admitting a coaxial microcatheter are not available, this technique can be performed using a parallel system of balloon and microcatheter.

Patients who cannot tolerate test occlusion of the internal carotid-artery will need to have an external-internal carotid artery bypass procedure first. Therefore, in the angiographic evaluation of all giant or large intracranial aneurysms or symptomatic cavernous aneurysms, it is important to obtain good images of the ipsilateral external carotid artery to facilitate surgical planning of the bypass route.

Arterial Sacrifice in the Treatment of Cavernous Aneurysms

Aneurysms of the cavernous segment of the internal carotid artery are common. Most are small and asymptomatic. They do not require treatment. Large asymptomatic cavernous aneurysms are best left alone too. Cavernous aneurysms that become symptomatic usually present with mass-effect: headache, ophthalmoplegia, and ptosis. Occasionally, they may be the source for presenting cerebral emboli. Spontaneous rupture of cavernous aneurysms generally results in a direct carotid cavernous fistula. Rarely the rupture may extend into the subdural or subarachnoid space.

Large series of cavernous internal carotid-artery aneurysms treated by balloon occlusion report mortality rates of 0% to 2% and morbidity rates of <6.7%, significantly less than those reported for open surgical treatment of equivalent lesions.[53–55] Complete closure of the cavernous aneurysm is achieved in 90% to 100% of cases, with either improvement of clinical symptoms or imaging evidence suggesting substantial shrinkage of the aneurysms.[56,57] If possible it is desirable to place the first balloon above the aneurysm to trap it. This will reduce the likelihood of migration of thromboembolic clot from the aneurysm to the intracranial circulation. Where mass-effect and paracavernous cranial nerve dysfunction are the main presenting symptoms, endovascular therapy can result in reversal of the deficit in 80% of patients.[58]

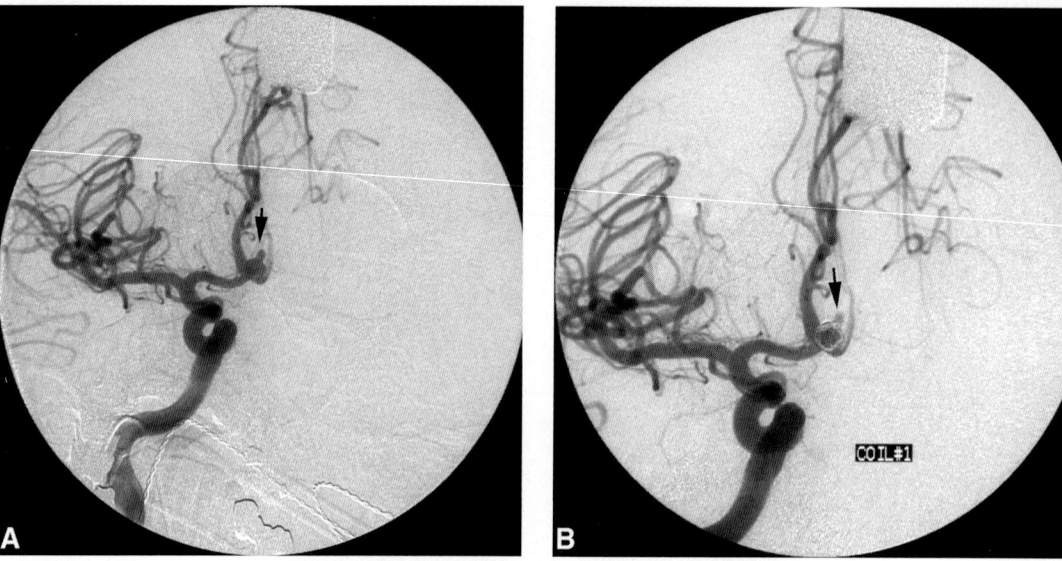
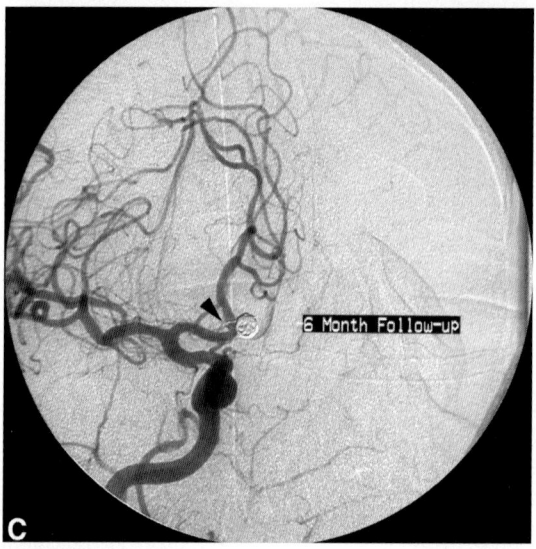

FIGURE 3.23 • *Undesirable Prolapsed Coil Loops Are Often More Safely Managed Medically Than by Hazardous Extraction Procedures.*
A 61-year-old male made an uneventful recovery following coil embolization of a Grade II ruptured aneurysm of the anterior communicating artery. A rupture point (A, arrow) on the aneurysm was avoided during the embolization and was sealed early from the circulation (B). An errant loop of coil was underestimated in size early in the case and later prolapsed farther into the parent artery. However, no further coil prolapse was seen and the patient was managed with aspirin after 3 days of heparinization. The 6-month follow-up angiogram (C), by which time the prolapsed loop is almost certainly endothelialized, is stable, and the patient continues to be asymptomatic.

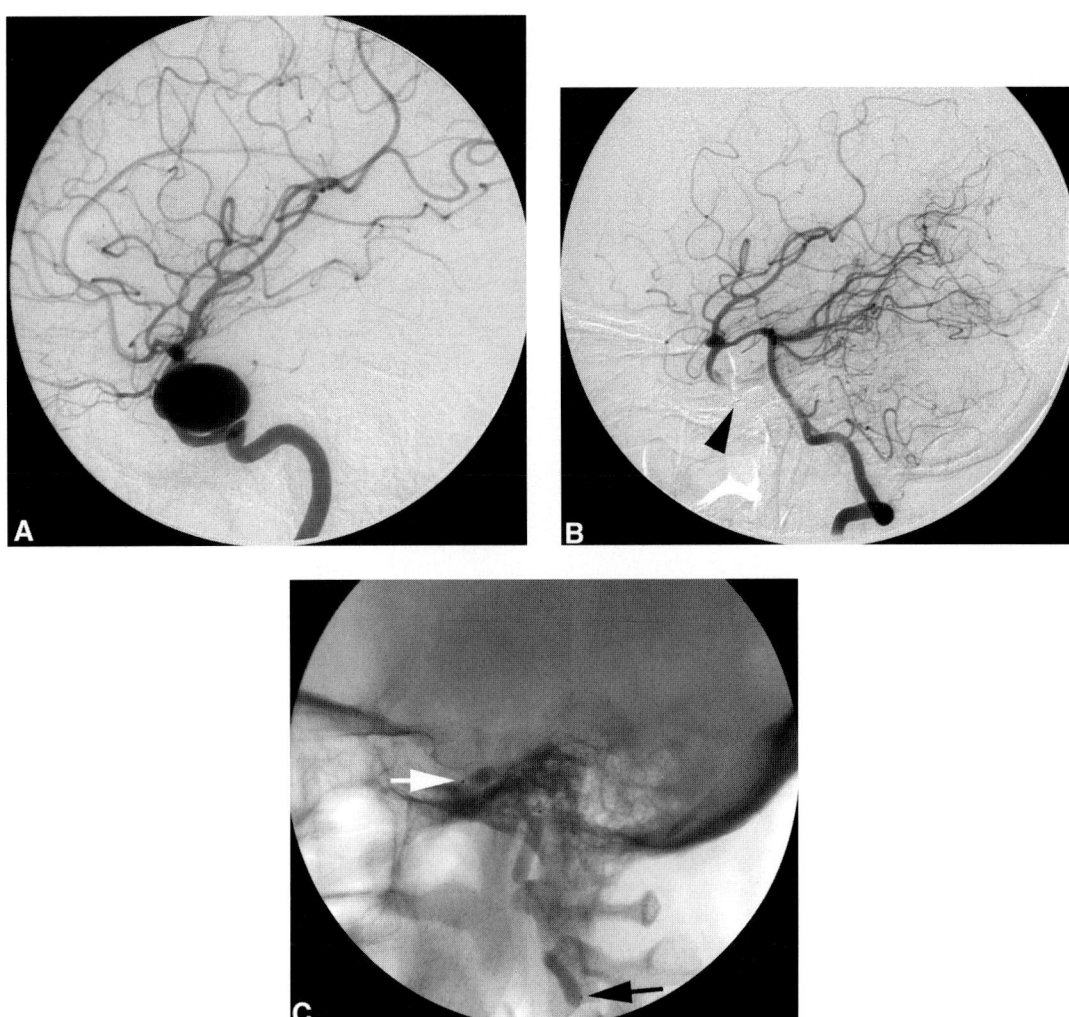

FIGURE 3.24 • *Arterial Sacrifice in the Treatment of a Cavernous Aneurysm.*
A 46-year-old female presented with severe headache and a left VI palsy related to a giant aneurysm of the left internal carotid cavernous segment. A lateral view of the aneurysm (A) shows its position to be high and close to the siphon, precluding the possibility of trapping the aneurysm with a distal balloon. There is elevation of the supraclinoid internal carotid artery due to mass-effect from the thrombosed segment of the aneurysm. A lateral view of the vertebral artery injection (B) following balloon occlusion of the right internal carotid artery shows opacification of the aneurysm mouth from the supraclinoid internal carotid artery. The marker for the uppermost balloon is indicated by the arrowhead.

A nonsubtracted image is shown in C. The uppermost balloon (white arrow) is placed around the curve of the C4–C5 segment of the internal carotid artery, the better to gain a secure grip on the arterial wall. The gold marker has become loosened within the lowest balloon (C, black arrow) and lies against the posterior wall of the balloon. Four latex balloons were placed in this patient to protect against any motion or disasters from premature deflation. Some operators prefer to use just 2 balloons for an arterial occlusion.

In a case such as this one should be vigilant against the possibility of overly rapid thrombosis of the stagnant aneurysm and escape of thrombus into the intracranial circulation. In addition to careful management and staging of patient mobilization after this procedure, it is potentially important to continue heparinization for a few days afterwards. See also Fig. 8.5.

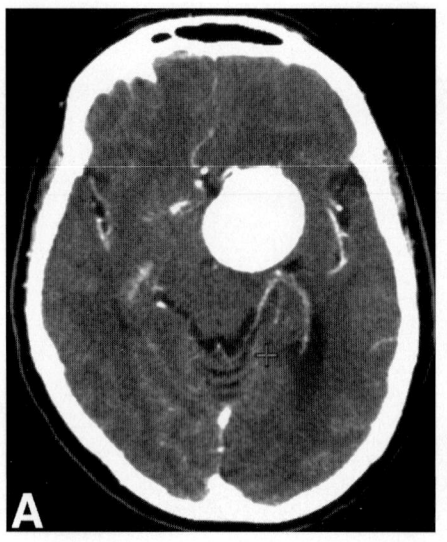 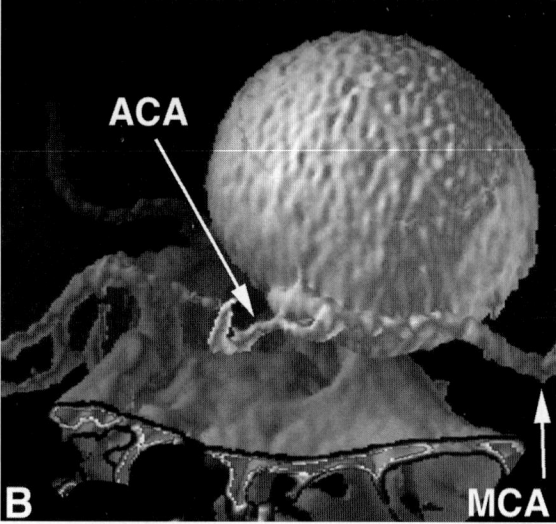

FIGURE 3.25 • *Dangers of Abrupt Aneurysm Closure in an Intracranial Giant Aneurysm.*
A 54-year-old male patient presented with moderately severe headache of some weeks' duration. A CT angiogram in axial (A) and surface-rendered mode (B, view from anterior position) demonstrated the enormous dome of the aneurysm and the displacement of the ipsilateral anterior cerebral and middle cerebral arteries. A test occlusion of the left internal carotid artery was easily tolerated by the patient. A surgical clamp was applied to the cervical internal carotid artery. Approximately 24 hours later the patient developed sudden massive intracranial hemorrhage at the site of the aneurysm. A noncontrast CT showed that most of the large dome of the aneurysm was filled with high-density thrombus, suggesting that the cause for the hemorrhage was sudden expansion of the volume of the aneurysm by the process of rapid thrombosis.
Lesson: In retrospect, one might hypothesize that anticoagulation in a patient such as this might have reduced the possibility of a postocclusion rupture.

Arterial Sacrifice in the Treatment of Subarachnoid Aneurysms

The safety of proximal arterial occlusion for treatment of intracranial aneurysms depends primarily on the patient's tolerance of the procedure from the point of view of cerebral perfusion. Most complications relate to delayed deficits from hypoperfusion. Many older case series in the published literature include large number of patients treated by intraaneurysmal deployment of balloons. As this technique is no longer used commonly, only outcome figures dealing with arterial closure need be examined.

With reference to the efficacy of proximal arterial occlusion in achieving aneurysmal thrombosis, Fox et al.[55] observed complete thrombosis of approximately half of their series of intradural aneurysms of the anterior and posterior circulations treated in this manner. In a paper on endovascular treatment of giant intracranial aneurysms, Taki et al.[59] reported on 11 patients treated by endovascular sacrifice of the parent artery. All patients showed complete thrombosis of their aneurysm (Fig. 3.25). In a large series of inoperable aneurysms referred for endovascular management reported by Higashida et al.,[60] over half were managed by arterial occlusion, with mortality rates of 3.9% and stroke rates of 5.5% and excellent long-term clinical and imaging results. Given that many of the patients in these reports had a poor clinical grade from rupture of their aneurysm prior to treatment or had giant intracranial aneurysms, these results compare

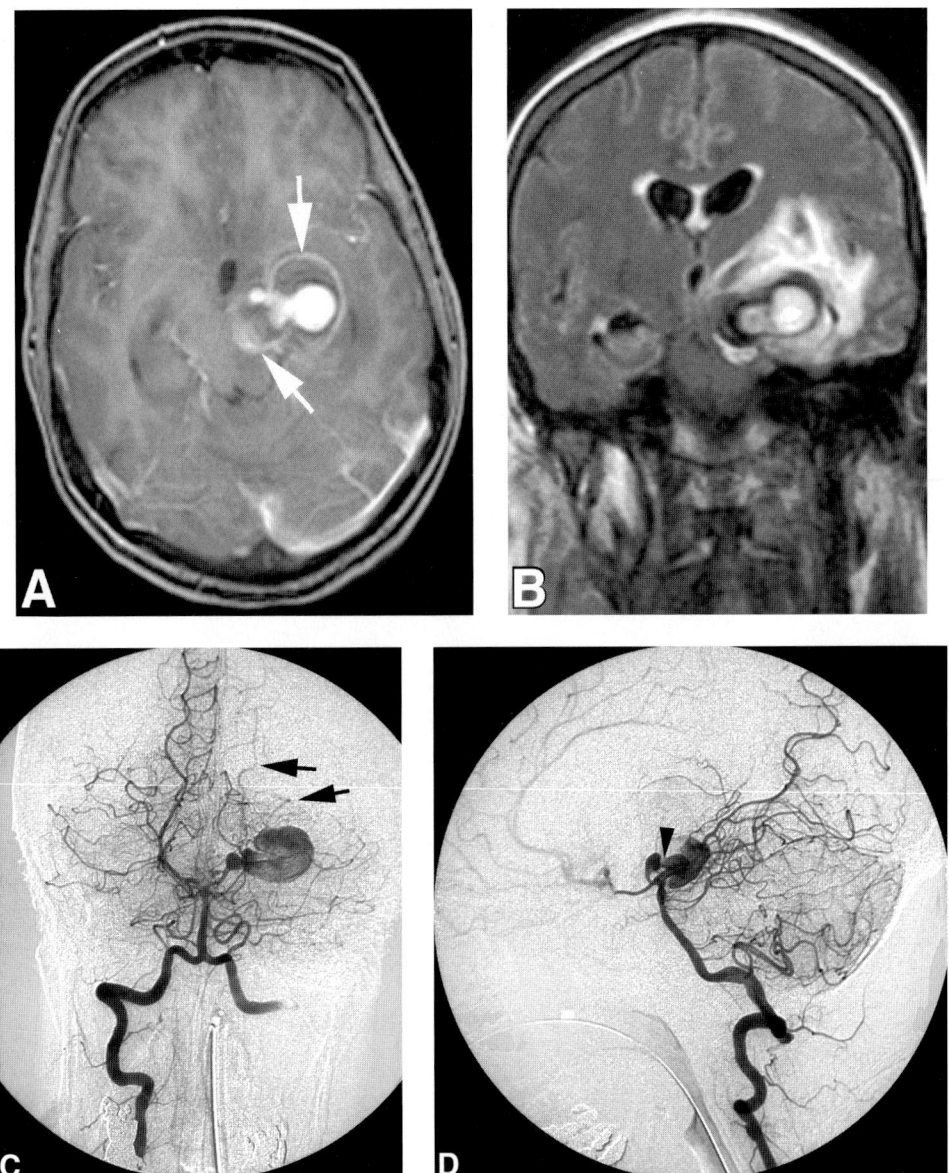

FIGURE 3.26 • *Intracranial Dissecting Aneurysm of the Left Posterior Cerebral Artery.*
A young adult female presented with midbrain compression symptoms including contralateral hemiparesis. On T1-weighted MR imaging (A) with gadolinium, the enhancing wall (arrows) of a partially thrombosed, complex, lobular aneurysm compressing the left midbrain is identified. On MR FLAIR imaging (B) extensive surrounding vasogenic edema is seen.

At angiography a bizarre aneurysm of the P2 segment of the left posterior cerebral artery is identified (C, right vertebral artery, Towne's projection; D, right vertebral artery, lateral projection). An initial bulbous segment of the aneurysm empties into a second patulous sac with a prominent jet effect seen on the lateral view (arrowhead). Slow opacification of the distal left posterior cerebral artery from the second component of the aneurysm is seen faintly on the Towne's view (arrows in C). (*Continued next page.*)

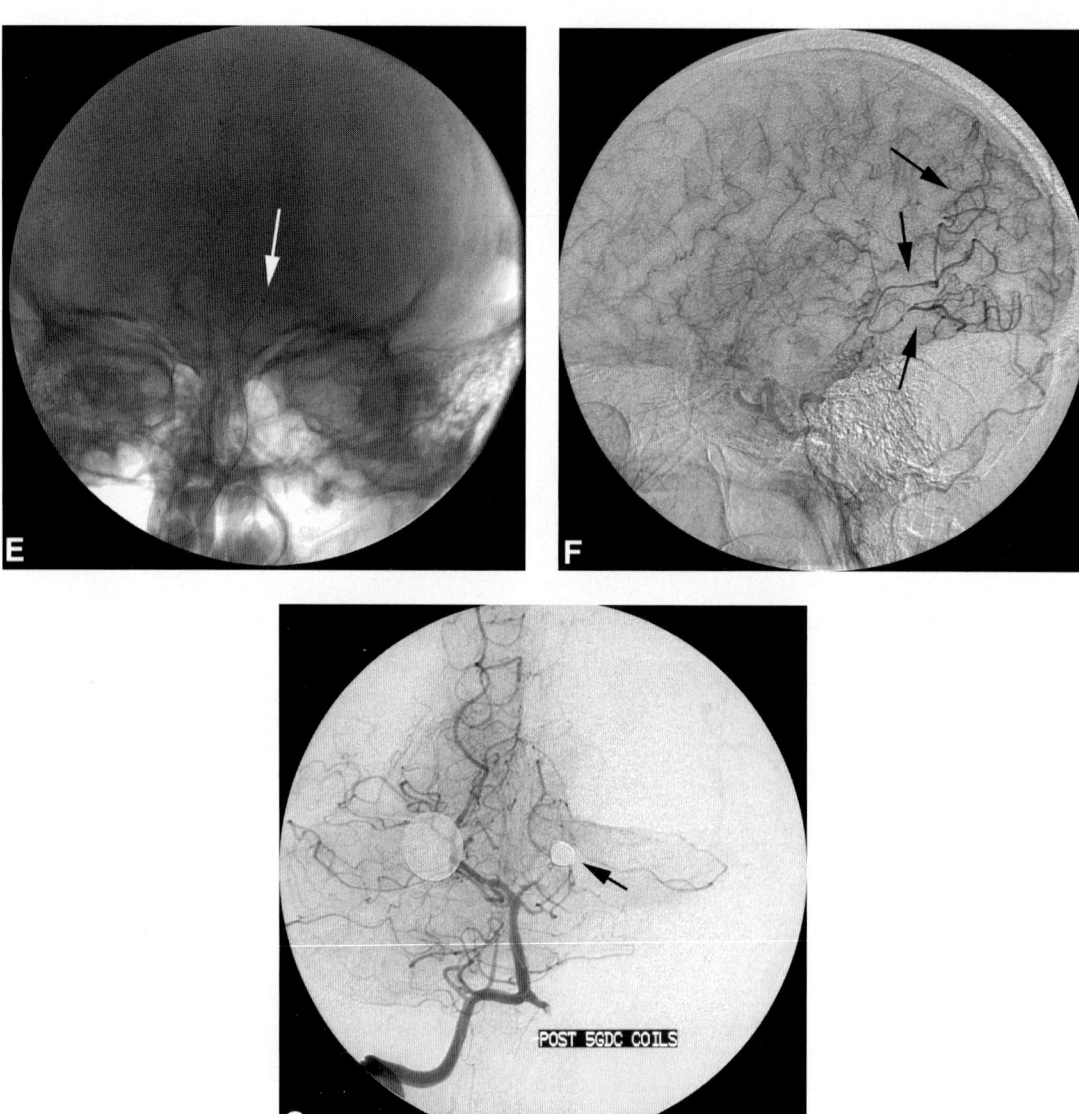

FIGURE 3.26 • *Continued.*
To determine the risk of a hemianopia following occlusion of the aneurysm, an intracranial test occlusion of the left posterior cerebral artery was conducted using an uninflated Endeavor balloon wedged into the left posterior cerebral artery (E), in association with an injection of a Tc99m radionuclide for subsequent SPECT scanning. A simultaneous injection with a second catheter was performed in the ipsilateral carotid artery, demonstrating prompt pial collaterals to the left posterior cerebral artery territory (arrows in F).

Because of multiple medical problems, occlusion of the aneurysm was delayed. Coil occlusion of the dissecting aneurysm was finally performed using GDCs (arrow in G, right vertebral artery). The left posterior cerebral artery territory tolerated the occlusion without clinical incident due to the prominent middle cerebral artery-to-posterior cerebral artery collaterals shown in image F. However, 3 days later she developed another round of septic shock with prolonged hypotension, during which her collaterals to the left posterior cerebral artery were inadequate, and she developed a left posterior cerebral artery infarction despite all the previous precautions.

very favorably with the natural history of the disease or with outcome from surgical intervention.

Intracranial Dissections and Pseudoaneurysms

Intracranial dissection may be seen following trauma, but is now well recognized as a spontaneous phenomenon presenting with subarachnoid hemorrhage or stroke. Dissections of the intracranial vessels compared with extracranial dissections are more prone to extend through the vessel wall and cause hemorrhage, due to the thinner media and adventitia of the intracranial vessels. Angiographically, the dissected segment of vessel may show a complete occlusion, a pseudoaneurysm or pouch, or a tapering of the vessel coupled with a dilatation or pseudoaneurysm called "the string and pearl" (Fig. 3.26). Because of the fragility of the walls of a dissecting pseudoaneurysm, many authors consider the risks of catheterizing such a lesion to be high. A series of 16 patients with vertebral artery dissections was treated by endovascular occlusion of the artery ($n = 15$), or occlusion of the pseudoaneurysm and preservation of the artery ($n = 1$),[61] using coils or balloons with excellent clinical and angiographic results. When the dissecting pseudoaneurysm is close to the dural margin, a high occlusion in the setting of good collateral flow will eliminate flow across the dissection and allow healing to take place. When a critical vessel arises between the site of anticipated balloon occlusion and the dissection site, more caution is necessary. Preservation of flow to the critical vessel may require a bypass procedure. Stent placement across the dissection may be an alternative too. Nevertheless, proximal arterial occlusion is still a favorable option in this circumstance in many patients, because simple reversal of flow across the dissection site will eliminate the hemodynamic factors that caused the dissection.

References

1. MULLAN S, DUDA EE, PATRONAS NJ (1980) Some examples of balloon technology in neurosurgery. *J Neurosurg* 52:321–329.
2. GUGLIELMI G, VINUELA F, SEPETKA I, MACELLARI V (1991) Electrothrombosis of saccular aneurysms via endovascular approach. Part 1: Electrochemical basis, technique, and experimental results. *J Neurosurg* 75:1–7.
3. GUGLIELMI G, VINUELA F, DION J, DUCKWILER G (1991) Electrothrombosis of saccular aneurysms via endovascular approach. Part 2: Preliminary clinical experience. *J Neurosurg* 75:8–14.
4. KING JT JR, BERLIN JA, FLAMM ES (1994) Morbidity and mortality from elective surgery for asymptomatic, unruptured, intracranial aneurysms: a meta-analysis. *J Neurosurg* 81:837–842.
5. SOLOMON RA, MAYER SA, TARMEY JJ (1996) Relationship between the volume of craniotomies for cerebral aneurysm performed at New York state hospitals and in-hospital mortality. *Stroke* 27:13–17.
6. VANNINEN R, KOIVISTO T, SAARI T, HERNESNIEMI J, VAPALAHTI M (1999) Ruptured intracranial aneurysms: acute endovascular treatment with electrolytically detachable coils—a prospective randomized study. *Radiology* 211:325–336.
7. MORET J, COGNARD C, WEILL A, CASTAINGS L, REY A (1997) Reconstruction technique in the treatment of wide-neck intracranial aneurysms. Long-term angiographic and clinical results. Apropos of 56 cases. *J Neuroradiol* 24:30–44.
8. LEVY DI, KU A (1997) Balloon-assisted coil placement in wide-necked aneurysms. Technical note. *J Neurosurg* 86:724–727.
9. RAFTOPOULOS C, MATHURIN P, BOSCHERINI D, BILLA RF, VAN BOVEN M, HANTSON P (2000) Prospective analysis of aneurysm treatment in a series of 103 consecutive patients when endovascular embolization is considered the first option. *J Neurosurg* 93:175–182.
10. JOHNSTON SC, DUDLEY RA, GRESS DR, ONO L (1999) Surgical and endovascular treatment of unruptured cerebral aneurysms at university hospitals. *Neurology* 52:1799–1805.
11. KLEIN GE, SZOLAR DH, LEBER KA, KARAIC R, HAUSEGGER KA (1997) Basilar tip aneurysm: endovascular treatment with Guglielmi detachable coils—midterm results. *Radiology* 205:191–196.
12. ESKRIDGE JM, SONG JK (1998) Endovascular embolization of 150 basilar tip aneurysms with Guglielmi detachable coils: results of the Food and Drug Administration multicenter clinical trial. *J Neurosurg* 89:81–86.
13. BAVINZSKI G, KILLER M, GRUBER A, REINPRECHT A, GROSS CE, RICHLING B (1999) Treatment of basilar artery bifurcation aneurysms by using Guglielmi detachable coils: a 6-year experience. *J Neurosurg* 90:843–852.
14. COGNARD C, WEILL A, CASTAINGS L, REY A, MORET J (1998) Intracranial berry aneurysms: angiographic and clinical results after endovascular treatment. *Radiology* 206:499–510.
15. COGNARD C, WEILL A, SPELLE L, PIOTIN M, CASTAINGS L, REY A, MORET J (1999) Long-term angiographic follow-up of 169 intracranial berry aneurysms occluded with detachable coils. *Radiology* 212:348–356.

16. GURIAN JH, VINUELA F, GUGLIELMI G, GOBIN YP, DUCKWILER GR (1996) Endovascular embolization of superior hypophyseal artery aneurysms. Neurosurgery 39:1150–1154.
17. ROY D, RAYMOND J, BOUTHILLIER A, BOJANOWSKI MW, MOUMDJIAN R, L'ESPERANCE G (1997) Endovascular treatment of ophthalmic segment aneurysms with Guglielmi detachable coils. AJNR 18:1207–1215.
18. VINUELA F, DUCKWILER G, MAWAD M (1997) Guglielmi detachable coil embolization of acute intracranial aneurysm: perioperative anatomical and clinical outcome in 403 patients. J Neurosurg 86:475–482.
19. REUL J, WEIS J, SPETZGER U, KONERT T, FRICKE C, THRON A (1997) Long-term angiographic and histopathologic findings in experimental aneurysms of the carotid bifurcation embolized with platinum and tungsten coils. AJNR 18:35–42.
20. MOLYNEUX AJ, ELLISON DW, MORRIS J, BYRNE JV (1995) Histological findings in giant aneurysms treated with Guglielmi detachable coils. Report of two cases with autopsy correlation. J Neurosurg 83:129–132.
21. MIZOI K, YOSHIMOTO T, TAKAHASHI A, NAGAMINE Y (1996) A pitfall in the surgery of a recurrent aneurysm after coil embolization and its histological observation: technical case report. Neurosurgery 39:165–168.
22. HOROWITZ MB, PURDY PD, BURNS D, BELLOTTO D (1997) Scanning electron microscopic findings in a basilar tip aneurysm embolized with Guglielmi detachable coils. AJNR 18:688–690.
23. SHIMIZU S, KURATA A, TAKANO M, TAKAGI H, YAMAZAKI H, MIYASAKA Y, FUJII K (1999) Tissue response of a small saccular aneurysm after incomplete occlusion with a Guglielmi detachable coil. AJNR 20:546–548.
24. CASTRO E, FORTEA F, VILLORIA F, LACRUZ C, FERRERAS B, CARRILLO R (1999) Long-term histopathologic findings in two cerebral aneurysms embolized with Guglielmi detachable coils. AJNR 20:549–552.
25. GRAVES VB, PARTINGTON CR, RUFENACHT DA, RAPPE AH, STROTHER CM (1990) Treatment of carotid artery aneurysms with platinum coils: an experimental study in dogs. AJNR 11:249–252.
26. GEREMIA G, HAKLIN M, BRENNECKE L (1994) Embolization of experimentally created aneurysms with intravascular stent devices. AJNR 15:1223–1231.
27. FEUERBERG I, LINDQUIST C, LINDQVIST M, STEINER L (1987) Natural history of postoperative aneurysm rests. J Neurosurg 66:30–34.
28. DRAKE CG, ALLCOCK JM (1973) Postoperative angiography and the "slipped" clip. J Neurosurg 39:683–689.
29. DRAKE CG, FRIEDMAN AH, PEERLESS SJ (1984) Failed aneurysm surgery. Reoperation in 115 cases. J Neurosurg 61:848–856.
30. LIN T, FOX AJ, DRAKE CG (1989) Regrowth of aneurysm sacs from residual neck following aneurysm clipping. J Neurosurg 70:556–560.
31. TSUTSUMI K, UEKI K, USUI M, KWAK S, KIRINO T (1999) Risk of subarachnoid hemorrhage after surgical treatment of unruptured cerebral aneurysms. Stroke 30:1181–1184.
32. GRAVES VB, STROTHER CM, DUFF TA, PERL J 2ND (1995) Early treatment of ruptured aneurysms with Guglielmi detachable coils: effect on subsequent bleeding. Neurosurgery 37:640–647.
33. BYRNE JV, MOLYNEUX AJ, BRENNAN RP, RENOWDEN SA (1995) Embolisation of recently ruptured intracranial aneurysms. J Neurol Neurosurg Psychiatry 59:616–620.
34. MALISCH TW, GUGLIELMI G, VINUELA F, DUCKWILER G, GOBIN YP, MARTIN NA, FRAZEE JG (1997) Intracranial aneurysms treated with the Guglielmi detachable coil: midterm clinical results in a consecutive series of 100 patients. J Neurosurg 87:176–183.
35. RAYMOND J, ROY D, BOJANOWSKI M, MOUMDJIAN R, L'ESPERANCE G (1997) Endovascular treatment of acutely ruptured and unruptured aneurysms of the basilar bifurcation. J Neurosurg 86:211–219.
36. BYRNE JV, SOHN MJ, MOLYNEUX AJ, CHIR B (1999) Five-year experience in using coil embolization for ruptured intracranial aneurysms: outcomes and incidence of late rebleeding. J Neurosurg 90:656–663.
37. LEMPERT TE, MALEK AM, HALBACH VV, PHATOUROS CC, MEYERS PM, DOWD CF, HIGASHIDA RT (2000) Endovascular treatment of ruptured posterior circulation cerebral aneurysms. Clinical and angiographic outcomes. Stroke 31:100–110.
38. ANONYMOUS (1998) Unruptured intracranial aneurysms—risk of rupture and risks of surgical intervention. International Study of Unruptured Intracranial Aneurysms Investigators. N Engl J Med 339:1725–1733.
39. BAXTER BW, ROSSO D, LOWNIE SP (1998) Double microcatheter technique for detachable coil treatment of large, wide-necked intracranial aneurysms. AJNR 19:1176–1178.
40. SZIKORA I, GUTERMAN LR, WELLS KM, HOPKINS LN (1994) Combined use of stents and coils to treat experimental wide-necked carotid aneurysms: preliminary results. AJNR 15:1091–1102.
41. MERICLE RA, LANZINO G, WAKHLOO AK, GUTERMAN LR, HOPKINS LN (1998) Stenting and secondary coiling of intracranial internal carotid artery aneurysm: technical case report. Neurosurgery 43:1229–1234.
42. WAKHLOO AK, LANZINO G, LIEBER BB, HOPKINS LN (1998) Stents for intracranial aneurysms: the beginning of a new endovascular era? Neurosurgery 43:377–379.
43. WILMS G, VAN CALENBERGH F, STOCKX L, DEMAEREL P, VAN LOON J, GOFFIN J (2000) Endovascular treatment of a ruptured paraclinoid aneurysm of the carotid siphon achieved using endovascular stent and endosaccular coil placement. AJNR 21:753–756.
44. RICOLFI F, LE GUERINEL C, BLUSTAJN J, COMBES C, BRUGIERES P, MELON E, GASTON A (1998) Rupture during treatment of recently ruptured aneurysms with Guglielmi electrodetachable coils. AJNR 19:1653–1658.
45. VINUELA F, DUCKWILER G, MAWAD M (1997) Guglielmi detachable coil embolization of acute intracranial aneurysm:

perioperative anatomical and clinical outcome in 403 patients. *J Neurosurg* 86:475–482.
46. Cronqvist M, Pierot L, Boulin A, Cognard C, Castaings L, Moret J (1998) Local intraarterial fibrinolysis of thromboemboli occurring during endovascular treatment of intracerebral aneurysm: a comparison of anatomic results and clinical outcome. *AJNR* 19:157–165.
47. Murayama Y, Vinuela F, Duckwiler GR, Gobin YP, Guglielmi G (1999) Embolization of incidental cerebral aneurysms by using the Guglielmi detachable coil system. *J Neurosurg* 90:207–214.
48. Klotzsch C, Nahser HC, Henkes H, Kuhne D, Berlit P (1998) Detection of microemboli distal to cerebral aneurysms before and after therapeutic embolization. *AJNR* 19:1315–1318.
49. Serbinenko FA (1974) Balloon catheterization and occlusion of major cerebral vessels. *J Neurosurg* 41:125–145.
50. Drake CG (1979) Giant intracranial aneurysms: experience with surgical treatment in 176 patients. *Clin Neurosurg* 26:12–95.
51. Drake CG (1975) Ligation of the vertebral (unilateral or bilateral) or basilar artery in the treatment of large intracranial aneurysms. *J Neurosurg* 43:255–274.
52. Graves VB, Perl J 2nd, Strother CM, Wallace RC, Kesava PP, Masaryk TJ (1997) Endovascular occlusion of the carotid or vertebral artery with temporary proximal flow arrest and microcoils: clinical results. *AJNR* 18:1201–1206.
53. Raymond J, Theron J (1986) Intracavernous aneurysms: treatment by proximal balloon occlusion of the internal carotid artery. *AJNR* 7:1087–1092.
54. Higashida RT, Halbach VV, Dowd C, Barnwell SL, Dormandy B, Bell J, Hieshima GB (1990) Endovascular detachable balloon embolization therapy of cavernous carotid artery aneurysms: results in 87 cases. *J Neurosurg* 72:857–863.
55. Fox AJ, Vinuela F, Pelz DM, Peerless SJ, Ferguson GG, Drake CG, Debrun G (1987) Use of detachable balloons for proximal artery occlusion in the treatment of unclippable cerebral aneurysms. *J Neurosurg* 66:40–46.
56. Berenstein A, Ransohoff J, Kupersmith M, Flamm E, Graeb D (1984) Transvascular treatment of giant aneurysms of the cavernous carotid and vertebral arteries. Functional investigation and embolization. *Surg Neurol* 21:3–12.
57. Vazquez Anon V, Aymard A, Gobin YP, Casasco A, Ruffenacht D, Khayata MH, Abizanda E, Redondo A, Merland JJ (1992) Balloon occlusion of the internal carotid artery in 40 cases of giant intracavernous aneurysm: technical aspects, cerebral monitoring, and results. *Neuroradiology* 34:245–251.
58. Bavinzski G, Killer M, Ferraz-Leite H, Gruber A, Gross CE, Richling B (1998) Endovascular therapy of idiopathic cavernous aneurysms over 11 years. *AJNR* 19:559–565.
59. Taki W, Nishi S, Yamashita K, Sadatoh A, Nakahara I, Kikuchi H, Iwata H (1992) Selection and combination of various endovascular techniques in the treatment of giant aneurysms. *J Neurosurg* 77:37–42.
60. Higashida RT, Halbach VV, Dowd CF, Barnwell SL, Hieshima GB (1991) Intracranial aneurysms: interventional neurovascular treatment with detachable balloons—results in 215 cases. *Radiology* 178:663–670.
61. Halbach VV, Higashida RT, Dowd CF, Fraser KW, Smith TP, Teitelbaum GP, Wilson CB, Hieshima GB (1993) Endovascular treatment of vertebral artery dissections and pseudoaneurysms. *J Neurosurg* 79:183–191.

CHAPTER 4

Extracranial Carotid and Vertebral Angioplasty and Stenting

INTRODUCTION

A paper in 1964 by Dotter and Judkins[1] marks the beginning of the history of percutaneous revascularization procedures. Their technique involved sequential dilatation of lower-extremity atherosclerotic lesions using dilators or bougies of increasing diameter passed across stenotic lesions, with favorable outcomes. A decade later the Grüntzig balloon catheter moved the field of balloon angioplasty (PTA) for iliac-femoral disease forward.[2,3] In 1980 Mullan et al.[4] used a Grüntzig balloon catheter to perform one of the first successful carotid angioplasties on a 35-year-female with fibromuscular dysplasia.[5] In the same year, Kerber et al.[6] described a successful intraoperative common carotid angioplasty performed 3 years previously. The internal carotid artery was clamped for protection of the brain during the procedure and the potential debris was flushed into the external carotid artery, making this also the first report of carotid PTA with distal protection. In 1980 again Sundt et al. reported the first successful transluminal angioplasties of basilar artery stenoses through intraoperative exposures.[7]

By the end of that decade series of carotid angioplasties sufficiently large to demonstrate that the procedure was safe and successful were being published.[8–10] Included in a 1987 paper by Kachel et al.[10] were 28 treatments of carotid and vertebral artery lesions, including four bilateral internal carotid artery treatments, with only two transient neurologic sequelae at the time of balloon inflation. In 1991 the same author[9] reported on a series of 105 patients treated successfully by PTA of the cephalic vessels with only four minor complications. Technological improvements made a big contribution to the potential of the field so that percutaneous basilar artery angioplasty, difficult in 1987, was more easily accomplished by 1992.[11,12] Although at that time there was controversy concerning whether carotid endarterectomy was an overutilized treatment for carotid disease, the field of endovascular treatment of carotid occlusive disease did not grow during the 1980s and 1990s, while the field of coronary PTA and peripheral percutaneous intervention was moving rapidly. The principal reason for this was the high standard of outcome following treatment of carotid disease with surgical endarterectomy.

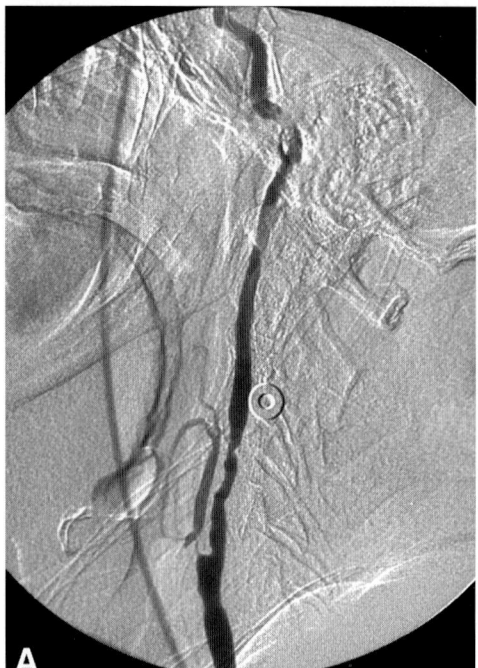 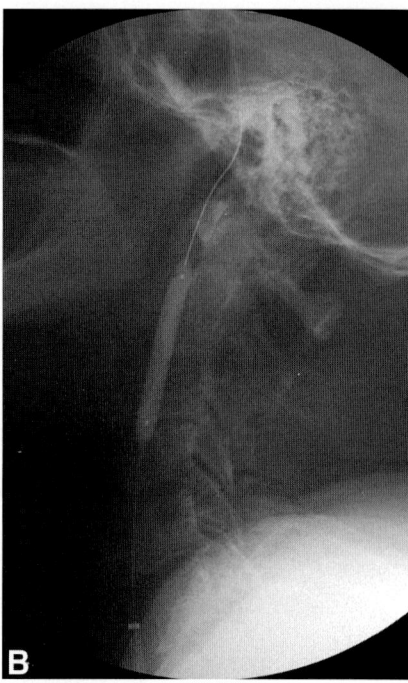

FIGURE 4.1 • *The SMART Stent (Cordis) for Carotid Artery Stenting.*
A 64-year-old male patient presented with TIA symptoms in the left hemisphere and was found to have a long segment of stenosis in the proximal left internal carotid artery (A, lateral view). Because of multiple medical problems and a contralateral internal carotid artery occlusion, he was thought to be a high risk for surgical endarterectomy. After premedication with aspirin and ticlopidine, the patient was treated by balloon angioplasty and stent placement.

After insertion of a 9F sheath, the patient was heparinized to an ACT of approximately 200–250 s and given a loading bolus of abciximab. A 9F Guider catheter (Schneider) was advanced into the left common carotid artery using the technique described in Fig. 2.30. An angioplasty was performed using an SV5 wire (Cordis) and a Savvy 6 × 40 mm balloon (Cordis) at 6 atm (B). Following this the balloon was removed and an 8 × 40 SMART stent (Cordis) was deployed satisfactorily (C, AP view, arrowheads indicate stent position). During early experience with carotid stenting, there was a tendency to postdilate mild residual narrowings such as seen in image C. However, since transcranial Doppler monitoring during such cases has demonstrated a large shower of microemboli commonly associated with postdilatation, many have abandoned postdilatation as a routine maneuver. The expansile strengths of the SMART stent (Cordis) or Wall stent (Schneider) should continue to remodel the arterial wall. If postdilatation of a stent is necessary, it is possible to do so using the parallel-balloon technique described later in this chapter. Protective devices in development will allow stent deployment and dilatation without compromise of the protection.

The femoral arterial site can be easily managed in a case such as this by predeploying a 6F Closer (Perclose) device at the time of dilation of the arteriotomy site. After the needles have been extracted the threads can be pushed to one side within a sterile gauze and a wire can be threaded back into the artery through the device to allow dilation up to the required sheath size. At the end of the procedure the suture knot is formed as usual and the arteriotomy closed with minimal effort or likelihood of complication. A covering dose of antibiotics and a liberal use of antiseptic lavage at the groin site may help to reduce any risk of infection.

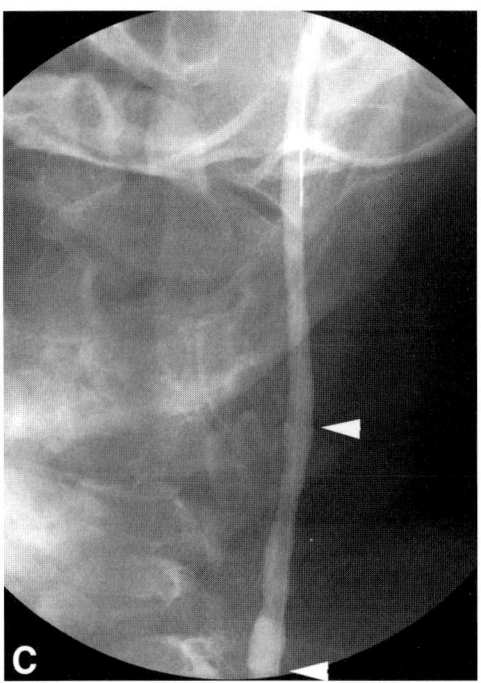

THE NORTH AMERICAN SYMPTOMATIC CAROTID ENDARTERECTOMY TRIAL

The results of the North American Symptomatic Carotid Endarterectomy Trial (NASCET)[13] have been the standard of safety and efficacy in symptomatic carotid artery intervention. However, the outcome parameters of the major symptomatic and asymptomatic carotid artery surgery studies were primarily clinical. It is likely that technological parameters, particularly intraprocedural TCD and postprocedure DWI MRI will prove a more sensitive tool. The overall rate of perioperative stroke or death in the NASCET study was 6.5%, with permanent disability or death in 2% of patients. Lesser complications included postoperative wound complications (9.3%), cranial nerve injury (8.6%), and general medical complications (8.1%).[14] It was thought that most postoperative strokes were related to acute thrombus formation at sites of denuded epithelium in the surgical bed. For symptomatic patients with >70% stenosis, carotid endarterectomy under the conditions of the NASCET study yields a 17% absolute risk reduction for ipsilateral hemispheric stroke.[15] In patients with symptomatic carotid stenosis of 50% to 69% the absolute risk reduction for ipsilateral stroke was still significant at 6.5%.

These outcome and safety figures for the various stages of the NASCET trial set a high standard which must be equaled or surpassed for endovascular treatment to become an acceptable standard of care for carotid stenosis. Until a controlled, randomized trial of endarterectomy versus endovascular treatment of carotid stenosis can be performed, a meaningful evaluation of PTA and stenting for this disease is not possible. Anecdotal reports and successful case series remain impotent in the face of the NASCET and other endarterectomy studies, except to demonstrate that conducting a randomized trial is at least a reasonable undertaking. Furthermore, the results of the NASCET study have to be understood in the context of the criteria set for the study. Patients were excluded from the study for the following reasons:

- Age >80 years in the first stage of the study
- Presence of significant intracranial stenosis
- Life expectancy <5 years
- History of ipsilateral endarterectomy
- Cardiac disease likely to cause embolism.

Surgeons too were excluded from the study if their perioperative complication rates exceeded 6%.

In other words, the results of the NASCET study or other carotid artery surgery trials cannot necessarily be generalized to the entire population of patients with carotid stenosis. Likewise, the NASCET results cannot be used validly to judge the merit of case series of carotid PTA/stent cases because these cases are, for the present, likely to be confined to the high-risk category falling outside the pale of NASCET.

Carotid Angioplasty and Stents in High-Risk Patients

Carotid artery angioplasties with and without stenting are being performed with increasing frequency

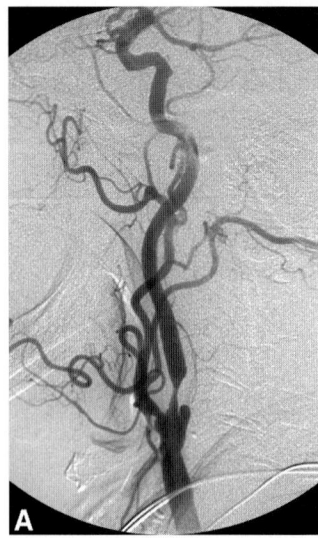 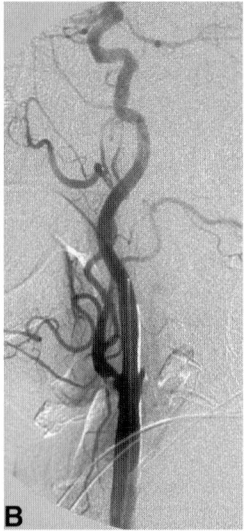

FIGURE 4.2 • *The Wall Stent (Schneider) for Carotid Artery Stenting.*
Using techniques identical to those described for the previous patient, an 8 × 40 mm Wall stent was deployed in this 64-year-old female patient with ulcerated stenosis of the left internal carotid artery (A pretreatment, B posttreatment).

at virtually all large medical centers on patients thought to represent a higher than acceptable risk for endarterectomy (Fig. 4.1–4.6). The majority of the evidence available indicates that carotid PTA and stenting offers an apparently reasonable alternative to medical or surgical therapy in patients with symptomatic disease and comorbid factors that increase the risk of endarterectomy. Mericle et al.[17] evaluated the safety and efficacy of carotid PTA and stenting in 23 patients with multiple medical risk factors and other criteria which excluded them from NASCET, including the presence of contralateral carotid occlusion. Target lesions were on average measured at 78% stenosis by NASCET criteria. The outcome of this series of patients was that 30-day mortality and stroke rates were zero. In the opinion of the authors this demonstrated an outcome better than that seen for patients with contralateral carotid occlusion in the NASCET study, in which a 14.3% rate for stroke and morbidity was found for that particular subgroup. Similar observations have been made by other groups who have established a high-volume practice for carotid stenting.[18,19] Patients with contralateral carotid occlusion were treated by stenting in a report by Mathur et al.[20] In a series of 26 patients treated, one patient (3.8%) suffered an air embolism during the diagnostic angiogram, accounting for the total periprocedural morbidity of the series.

The situation of high-surgical-risk patients treated by PTA and stenting has been evaluated in a number of other studies. A combined stroke or death rate of 4.5% was reported in 44 patients in this category by Al-Mubarak et al.[21] Despite a high proportion of patients in this study with strokes within 7 days preceding treatment or neurologic deficit within 24 hours prior to treatment, no cerebral hemorrhages due to reperfusion injury were seen. A series of 22 high-risk patients reported by Teitelbaum et al.[22] included patients with atherosclerotic disease and others with dissection flaps, pseudoaneurysms, and trauma. These patients were considered at high risk for surgical repair of the artery or endarterectomy as might be appropriate, and were referred for endovascular treatment combining stent placement with other modalities of en-

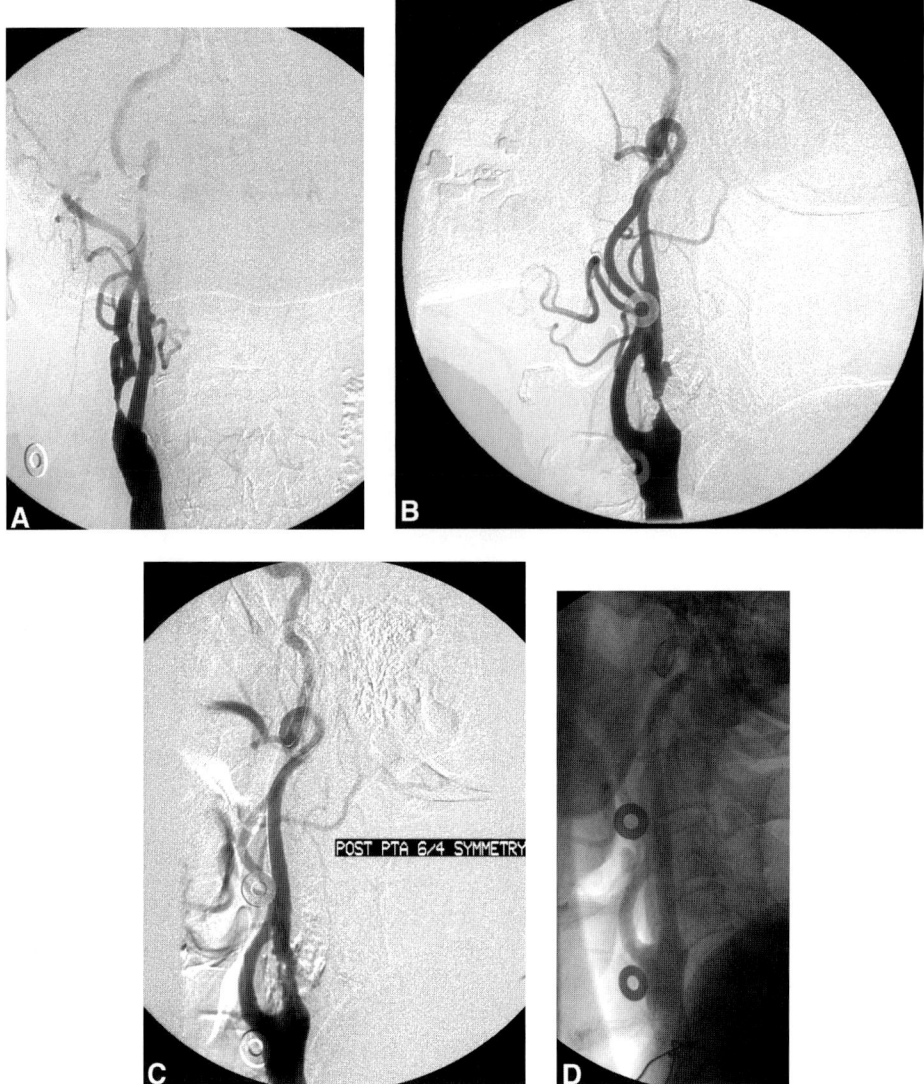

FIGURE 4.3 • *Carotid Artery Stenting with Suboptimal Result. Difficulties with Stent Sizing.*
A 72-year-old male patient was referred for angioplasty and stenting of his asymptomatic right internal carotid artery recurrent stenosis following a previous endarterectomy. His diagnostic angiogram (A, B) demonstrated a severe, ulcerated stenosis of the proximal internal carotid artery above a patulous segment of the distal common carotid artery, related to the endarterectomy site. A 6 × 40 Symmetry balloon (Meditech) was used for angioplasty with a reasonable result (C). External markers (9 mm washers) have been applied for measurement. Using the conformity of the 6-mm balloon to the arterial wall, the 6–7 mm diameter of the vessel as measured externally was confirmed. With self-expanding stents it is important not to undersize the stent, which might result in inadequate stent-wall apposition. In this patient an 8 × 40 mm Wall stent (Schneider) was deployed, which achieved a smooth result in the internal carotid artery but left a considerable length of stent in the common carotid artery without wall apposition (D). The patient tolerated the procedure well and has been asymptomatic since. Nevertheless, while this case represented an adequate result from an early excursion into the realm of carotid stenting, such a result would be better avoided. Shorter stents that are more accurate in deposition are now available and would serve this patient better by stenting only the stenotic segment of the internal carotid artery, without needing to encroach upon the common carotid artery. Another innovation in development is the idea of a funnel-shaped stent, i.e., wider at its proximal end, the better to conform to anatomic challenges such as this.

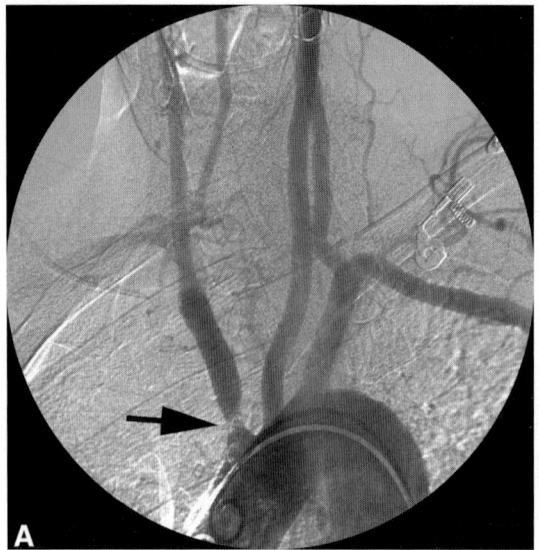 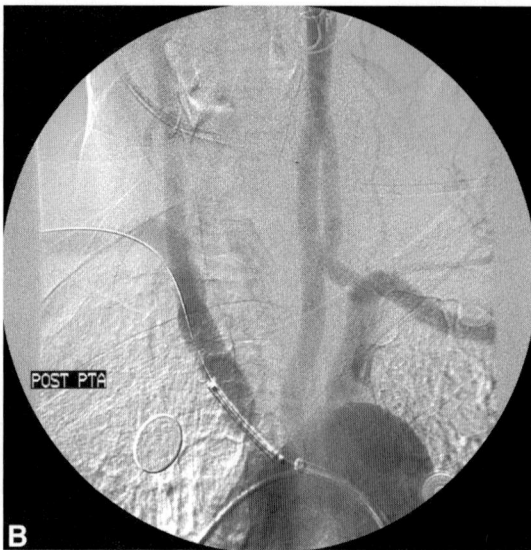

FIGURE 4.4 • *Angioplasty and Stenting of the Brachiocephalic Artery. Utility of a Combined Brachial/Femoral Approach for Wire-Stabilization.*
A 45-year-old male presented with an embolic infarct of his right middle cerebral artery. A calcified stenosis at the origin of the brachiocephalic artery was the only significant lesion identified on his angiographic work-up (A, arrow).

An 8F Shuttle sheath system (Cook) was placed in the right common femoral artery, and a 4F sheath was placed in the right brachial artery. An exchange length Bentson 0.035-in wire was passed retrogradely from the brachial artery to the aortic arch, where it was snared and extracted retrogradely via the femoral sheath. Using both ends of the wire for complete stability, angioplasty and stenting of the proximal brachiocephalic artery was thus greatly facilitated. Note also that a 5F catheter has been inserted via the left common femoral artery (B, postangioplasty) and placed on flush in the ascending aorta. This is contrived to define the sweep of the aortic curve (assisting in indicating the proximal extent of the stenosis) and to perform arch aortograms during the procedure.

After angioplasty with a Classique 6 × 20 mm balloon catheter (Meditech), a Palmaz 294 stent (Cordis) was advanced into position (B) and inflated satisfactorily using a Marshall 8 × 30 mm balloon catheter (Meditech). The Palmaz or similar balloon-expandable stents are preferable in such situations due to the absence of concern about external compression of the stent and greater accuracy of deployment, compared with self-expanding stents. On the postdeployment image (C), incomplete apposition between the distal stent and the walls of the poststenotic dilatation is evident (arrowheads). This is undesirable but could not be overcome in this particular patient. In all likelihood, the poststenotic dilated segment would have soon reversed itself into satisfactory apposition with the stent, and the result was accepted as adequate.

An alternative technique for stabilizing the wire in the brachial artery, which can sometimes be effective and avoid the need for a brachial artery puncture, is to place an exchange length stiff wire, e.g., V-18 300 cm (Meditech), distally into the subclavian artery and stabilize it there during maneuvers by inflating a sphygmomanometer cuff on the arm.

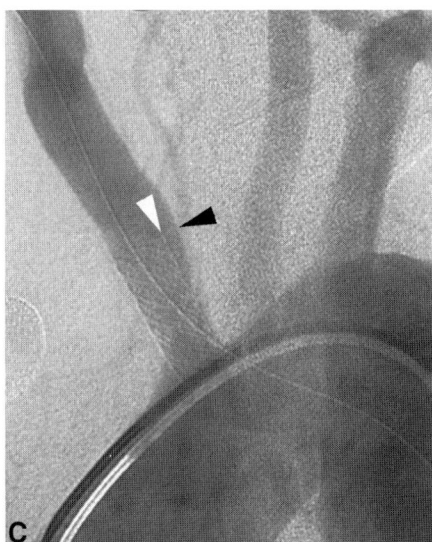

- long stenotic lesions
- multiple lesions
- advanced age of the patient

Cerebral Hyperperfusion Syndrome

Cerebral hyperperfusion syndrome is a well-recognized but uncommon complication of carotid endarterectomy with an incidence of approximately 1%.[25–28] It is related to transient hyperemia of the ipsilateral circulation after surgical reopening of the carotid artery in the setting of impaired autoregulation. Symptoms of headache, vomiting, altered mental state, seizures, focal neurological deficits, elevated intracranial pressure, and intracranial hemorrhage are typically seen. Treatment involves management of systemic blood pressure, antiseizure medication, and control of cerebral edema. If cerebral hemorrhage can be prevented, the prospects for recovery are generally good.

Cerebral hyperperfusion syndrome of varying severity has been reported following carotid endovascular revascularization.[29–30] This seems to be an uncommon event, although one series of high-risk patients demonstrated a 5% incidence of clinical events, possibly representing cerebral hyperperfusion following endovascular stenting.[32] In the small number of cases reported, the risk of hyperperfusion injury following stenting may be related to treatments involving extremely stenotic vessels or may correlate with evidence on axial imaging of small-vessel disease in the white matter or lacunar infarctions. The possibility of this potentially serious complication of carotid angioplasty and stenting is an indication of the need for close patient observation and management following the procedure.

dovascular repair. A periprocedural stroke or death rate of 27.3%, high in the opinion of the authors, was seen, but only two strokes were thought to be related to the endovascular procedure.

As of 1997 when carotid PTA and stenting was still in the early stages of acceptance, approximately 2,000 cases had been performed worldwide at the major medical institutions involved in the field.[23] Despite the early timing of this survey by Wholey et al. and the relatively early state of the technology (balloon-expandable stents being most commonly used), the technical success rate at that time was 98% with rates of restenosis (defined as stenosis >50%) at 6-month follow-up of 4.8%. A combined periprocedural stroke (minor and major) and mortality rate of 5.7% was seen, varying between 0% and 10% in different hospitals. Despite the preponderant use of balloon-expandable stents, stent deformity was seen in only 1.4% of patients. Similar results for a single-institution experience with 231 patients were reported by Mathur et al. in 1997.[74] Among the 14% of cases eligible for endarterectomy in this series, a procedure-related stroke rate of 2.7% was seen. Overall the 30-day stroke (major and minor) rate for the entire series was 6.9%. In this study, independent risk factors for procedure-related stroke included:

A Stopped Trial: Arguments against Carotid Stenting

A study sometimes quoted by authors opposed to allowing any major role for angioplasty and stenting in carotid atherosclerotic disease was published by Naylor et al. in 1998.[33] This involved a controlled, randomized trial of endarterectomy versus angio-

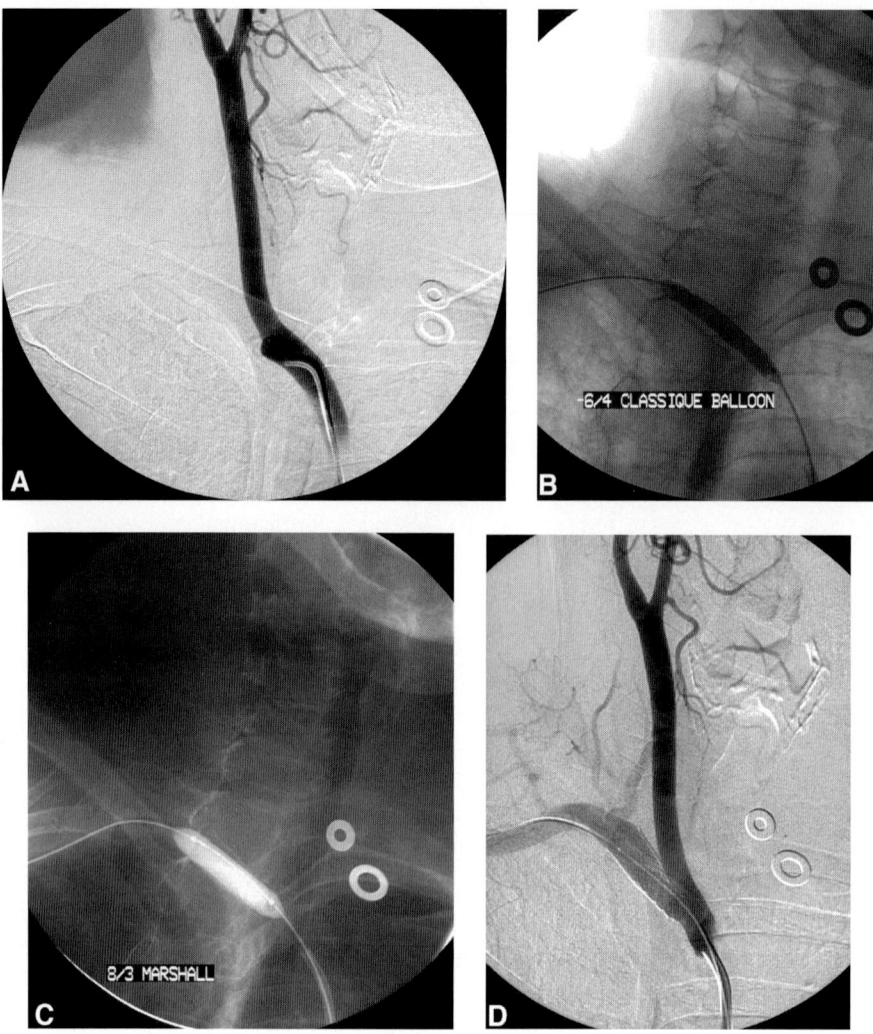

FIGURE 4.5 • *Subclavian Artery Occlusion Treated by Angioplasty and Stenting. Necessity of a Combined Brachial/Femoral Approach.*

A 65-year-old female patient presented with symptoms of subclavian steal when using her right arm for minor activities. A complete occlusion of the right subclavian artery was found during angiography, and the patient expressed a wish for an attempt at endovascular reopening of the vessel to avoid surgery. Due to the smooth surface of the occlusion (A), the occlusion could not be probed antegradely. A retrograde approach with a Terumo wire from a 5F brachial sheath was successful, and an exchange Bentson wire was advanced to the aortic arch where it was snared via a femoral approach. The Bentson wire controlled at the brachial artery and femoral artery was used to perform angioplasty with a 6 × 40 mm Classique (Meditech) balloon (B). An 8 × 20 Wall stent (Schneider) deployed a little too distally in the artery, and therefore a Palmaz stent was overlapped proximally, taking pains to avoid backing out into the origin of the right carotid artery. A postdilatation image (C) with a Marshall 8 × 30 mm (Meditech) balloon shows full expansion of both stents. The washers on the patient are external markers for measurement purposes. A final image (D) shows good stent-wall apposition.

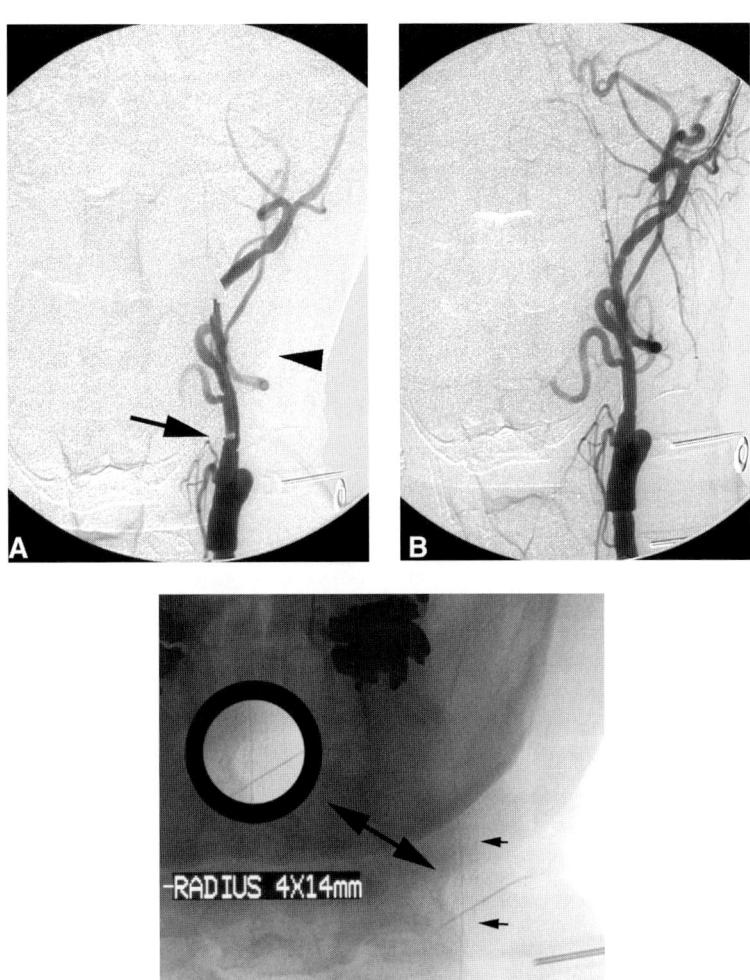

FIGURE 4.6 • *Stenting of the External Carotid Artery with a Radius Stent.*
An elderly patient with an occlusion of the right internal carotid artery suffered an asymptomatic occlusion of the left internal carotid artery following left endarterectomy. Because his collateral circulation to the anterior hemispheres relied in part on the left external carotid artery, he was referred for stent repair of a postsurgical flap causing partial stenosis of the left external carotid artery (A, arrow). The site was low in the neck (angle of the mandible indicated by the arrowhead), implying that a self-expanding stent would be preferable in such an exposed location. A Radius (Boston Scientific) 4 × 14 mm self-expanding nitinol stent was deployed across the site with a satisfactory result (B, C). A sharply defined shelf on the proximal common carotid artery is a postsurgical effect of the endarterectomy.

plasty with stenting (PTAS) for symptomatic stenotic disease in a British University hospital. The trial was stopped by the Ethics committee of the hospital when 5 of the first 7 PTAS patients suffered strokes while the first 10 endarterectomies proceeded without complications. There are a number of lessons to draw from this study. The potential for discouraging results from PTAS is very high unless issues of technique, premedication, and patient selection are addressed. Endarterectomy is a well-established technique with a large body of collective experience behind it, even when performed by trainees under supervision, as was the case in this study. A meaningful and valid trial of one technique versus the other must stipulate the conditions under which the study will be conducted. In this particular study,[33] the question of premedication with aspirin was alluded to, but doses and whether all patients were premedicated were not specified. Thienopyridine agents were not used, and postprocedure medication was not specified. Protection of the internal carotid artery during balloon angioplasty as described by Theron[8,34] was not performed. Additionally, primary stent deployment was attempted without initial balloon angioplasty. Angioplasty was used only if "resistance was noted to the passage of the stent catheter across the lesion." Presumably in this series of cases, the carotid stenosis at least in some patients was subjected to considerable shear effects during passage of the stent catheter. These factors may or may not explain the poor results of this British trial of carotid stenting, but they do represent features that underscore the need for organization and uniformity of standards in controlled trials. Until then, for those who wish to point to the apparently unacceptable risks of carotid angioplasty, there are numerous other papers which might be quoted demonstrating a point.[35] However, concerns over technical factors such as preference for a cervical puncture over a femoral one, primary stenting versus initial angioplasty, premedication with antiplatelet drugs, carotid protection, and other potential flaws are commonplace in these sources.[36,37]

Another argument raised by partisans against carotid stenting in any form is that even a controlled, randomized trial of endarterectomy versus stenting is ethically unacceptable given the excellent results of the NASCET study.[38] Ironically, this argument was also raised in opposition to enrolling patients in the NASCET study. However, definitive statements by pro-stent partisans on who should have carotid stenting for stenotic disease in preference to endarterectomy can be equally contentious and unfounded.[39]

Lessons from Coronary Artery Stenting

Fortunately, the state of background knowledge and technology involved in carotid arterial stenting is not necessarily in its infancy. The wheel has already been invented and improved upon, so to speak, particularly in the coronary vessels where stents and related devices have been improved over a number of iterations.[40] A certain amount of groundwork has already been done, and lessons have been learned in the coronary vessels that will help the field of carotid stenting get off to a safer start. However, there are also important differences between the coronary arteries on the one hand and the carotid, vertebral, and intracranial arteries on the other, wherein the fields diverge.

An important focus of concern in coronary stenting has been the study of stent-tissue interaction and prediction of in-stent restenosis. Intimal hyperplasia with proliferating smooth muscle cells and a proteoglycan-rich matrix is the predominant mechanism for post-stent coronary restenosis.[40,41] Factors identified with a likelihood of coronary in-stent restenosis include:

- Prominent thrombosis
- Deep mural injury from the balloon or another device
- Poor apposition of the stent to the wall or any cause of stagnation of flow near the stent due to native anatomy or stent design
- Underlying proliferative lesions
- Thrombosis due to plaque rupture with a large necrotic core

To ensure close apposition of the stent with the coronary arterial wall, common practice in the coronary use of stents encourages high-pressure deployment of balloon-expandable stents with pressures of 8–18 atm. Although it has been well recognized from pig models that deeper implantation of the stent into the arterial wall leads to greater medial injury and thus a greater likelihood of a myointimal proliferative response, the clinical evidence of restenosis rates favors stent placement if possible, compared with angioplasty alone. Initial comparisons of stent placement versus angioplasty demonstrated improved clinical outcomes with stenting. Restenosis rates of 22% to 31% were seen with stents and 32% to 42% following coronary angioplasty in 1994.[42,43] Since then, with improvement in technique and stent technology, restenosis rates with stenting in the coronary vessels have declined even further.

Some important ancillary technological innovations have guided research and clinical practice in coronary endovascular work:

- Intravascular ultrasound (IVUS) is particularly useful for determining the state of stent expansion and stent-to-wall apposition and the need for post-stent dilatation, the presence of lesion calcification, and evaluation of intimal dissections. It can also be used to evaluate for lesions missed by digital imaging and incomplete coverage of ostial lesions.[44]
- Atherectomy devices achieve lesion debulking and ablation with high-speed rotating heads.
- Rheolytic catheters are used for mechanical clot lysis and extraction.
- Atherectomy cutting, laser cutting, and other clot extraction catheters are avaiable.
- Beta-particle emitting stents or percutaneous gamma brachytherapy can be used.[45,46]

The role of these technologies, if any, in carotid and vertebral artery stenting can be defined in the same fashion as for the coronary vessels, i.e., in large controlled, randomized trials with stringent collection of data, control of procedural technique, and clinical and imaging follow-up.

Some aspects of the practice of coronary endovascular work are quite divergent from those relevant to the neurovascular field. For instance, it is well known that tissue response to stent placement can vary significantly between different species. The pig is a useful research subject for human coronary research, with similar vessel size lending ease of catheterization. However, the proliferative response to intimal and medial injury in the pig is very exuberant compared with the human coronary artery, making the dog a better model in some respects. Differences in the histology of the human coronary arteries and the human carotid artery and the human intracranial arteries similarly suggest that all the lessons learned in the coronary circulation may not be applicable to the neurovascular circulation. Stent deployments in the carotid bifurcation with pressures greater than 10 atm have been associated with serious and fatal cardiac arrythmias or asystole. Moreover, the relative deficiency of the intracranial arteries in elastic lamina and adventitia argues for a complete revision of technique for angioplasty and stent deployment to avoid arterial rupture. Not least in importance is the different nature of the vulnerable organ involved in neurovascular work being less resistant to the ischemic effects of particulate debris, bubbles, and other microembolic sequelae that might be of lesser significance in the heart.

The physiology of internal carotid artery flow during systole and diastole is quite different from that of the coronary circulation. This implies that among other effects, different shear stresses are experienced by the intima adjacent to the struts of a carotid stent compared with those of a coronary stent. Shear stress is known to have important effects on subcellular factors influencing intimal hyperplasia. Moreover, the pathophysiology of ischemia in the coronary circulation is different from that of the carotid circulation. Coronary ischemia is thought to be related to the hemodynamic effects of the stenotic lesion in restricting flow, while in the carotid circulation embolic epiphenomena of carotid occlusive disease are usually predominant. Therefore, the significance of in-stent restenosis might be very different in the two circulatory fields. A smoothly contoured surface with a storiform pattern of myointimal hyperplasia seen after angioplasty[41] or stent placement[47] might argue that a recurrent lesion in a carotid stent short of virtual complete obstruction of flow might not be of great embolic potential compared with an equivalent degree of stenosis due to untreated atherosclerotic disease. The significance of such recurrent stenoses might therefore not be so high. In the coronary circulation, on the other hand, a recurrent stenosis of myointimal hyperplasia has the same hemodynamic—and thus clinical—significance as an atherosclerotic lesion of similar degree.

The Significance of Microembolic Events during Endarterectomy and Angioplasty

The point has been made by Gomez and others[48] that a trial of endarterectomy with over 40 years of experience and cumulative knowledge versus endovascular techniques for stenotic carotid disease may suffer from a number of fundamental design flaws. The degree of experience and training of participants, the technical details of the procedure and the devices used, and the standardization of patient care before, during, and after the procedure all need to be factored into the design of a meaningful study. Foremost among these technical questions is whether it is possible, necessary, or desirable to protect the brain from antegrade transmission of debris and thrombus from the angioplasty site during the procedure. Theoretically, such a maneuver should protect the brain from atheromatous plaque or thrombus shorn from the arterial wall during the procedure.

It is known from intraprocedural use of transcranial Doppler imaging (TCD) in patients undergoing carotid angioplasty and stent placement that embolic phenomena occur frequently during these procedures and can persist with increased frequency compared with baseline for hours or days after the angioplasty.[49,50] Only a small fraction of these events correlates with clinically detectable deficits, and their significance remains to be defined. Discerning by TCD in vivo between microbubbles or platelet rouleaux on the one hand, and more sinister embolic material on the other is difficult. However, similar embolic events during angioplasty and stenting of carotid arteries in cadavers have been described,[47] and were found to be due to release of fragments of atherosclerotic plaque, intimal strips, and clusters of nonspecific cells ranging in size up to several millimeters. While the behavior of cadaveric tissue is probably different in many respects from the carotid arteries in living patients, these findings are cause for concern. Large showers of embolic material to the intracranial vessels during procedures that do not lead to a clinically detectable deficit by bedside examination might still be recognized as deleterious to the patient's welfare if neuropsychological testing or diffusion-weighted MRI (DWI) were factored into the evaluation process.

Embolic showers to the intracranial circulation are more frequently seen with Doppler monitoring during angioplasty than during endarterectomy.[51] Although outcome differences between carotid PTA and endarterectomy related to this observation have not been detected, this phenomenon is nevertheless of concern. It is already known that the risk of ischemic complications following carotid endarterectomy is related to the frequency of intraoperative[52] or postoperative TCD embolic events,[53] and that in cardiac surgery patients poor neuropsychological outcome is directly related to embolic load.[54,55] A prospective study of the neuropsychological outcomes of carotid angioplasty and carotid endarterectomy patients demonstrated that 20% to 25% of patients demonstrated abnormalities at 6 weeks following either procedure.[56] This outcome was thought to be related to embolic events during the procedures rather than to other factors such as prolonged ischemia from vessel clamping or balloon occlusion. The types of neuropsychological deficits described in this small group of patients by Crawley et al.[56] can have a significantly deleterious impact on a patient's quality of life, even though clinical neurological testing might be completely normal. Similarly, in a study of patients undergoing carotid endarterectomy with postoperative DWI MRI imaging, Müller et al.[57] found that intracranial Doppler-detectable embolic events are more significant than can be appreciated by clinical examination. In this study of 76 surgical patients, 34% (26 patients) had new DWI lesions following the surgical endarterectomy, of whom only 6.5% (5 patients) had clinically detectable neurological deficits. Microembolic signals were detectable during the surgical procedure by TCD in 96% of this group of patients, and the likelihood of finding a DWI lesion was proportional to the number of intraoperative embolic events. Apart from the increased sensitivity of DWI to cerebral ischemic injury, this confirms similar observations made previously using spin-echo MRI or CT in endarterectomy patients.[58–61] Such findings also correlate with prospective neurobehavioral observations in cardiac surgery patients, in whom neuropsychological outcome is inversely proportional to the number of detectable Doppler events during surgery.[62,63]

Cerebrovascular microembolic events are common during coronary interventions and are related to wire and catheter manipulation in the aorta during percutaneous procedures.[64] Clinically significant or silent microemboli of air, fat, or other matter are also common during cardiac surgery and are associated with adverse neuropsychological outcome in a large proportion of patients.[54]

In summary, the clinical outcome parameters of the large carotid artery surgery trials have been superceded by more sensitive technological parameters, TCD and DWI MRI, and by the sensitivity of formal prospective neuropsychological testing in the evaluation of carotid surgery or endovascular repair. Studies using TCD demonstrate an event rate of over 90% during carotid endarterectomy,[59,61] indicating that the NASCET study and its clinical outcomes are only a part of the larger picture of subclinical outcomes in carotid surgery. The increased sensitivity of these technologies will bring greater power to research studies comparing different interventions and will allow completion of comparison trials with smaller recruitment numbers.

Carotid Protection during Angioplasty

The techniques of carotid protection during carotid angioplasty have been pioneered by Theron and others (Figs. 4.7–4.9).[8,34,65,66] The technique consists in use of either parallel or coaxial catheter systems, one to occlude the distal artery, the other to perform the angioplasty. Debris is flushed or aspirated out from the internal carotid artery proximal to the protective balloon prior to deflation. Theron et al.[65] reported a substantial reduction in embolic and other complications (13% down to 7%) during carotid angioplasty in 259 patients using this technique compared with personal experience prior to its use. Regulatory constraints have so far limited experience with this technique in the United States.

Experience with carotid protection devices such as balloons, filters, or techniques for shunting blood from the angioplasty site to the femoral vein indicates that particulate debris is commonly extractable for the carotid artery following PTA. Atherosclerotic plaque and thrombic debris in particulate size from 50 μm to 4,000 μm can be harvested from the artery distal to the angioplasty site by use of these devices.[65] Early experience with these devices indicates a potential to reduce the number of clinically evident neurologic sequelae of carotid angioplasty and stenting by 50% compared with complication rates experienced previously with unprotected procedures.[67–71] The impact of protection devices on carotid angioplasty and stenting is likely to be highly significant, particularly in cases known to be at higher risk for clinically significant embolic events during the procedure due to the following independent risk factors:

- Lesions with a high degree >90% stenosis or echolucent appearance of ultrasound[72]
- Advanced age[24]
- Long or multiple stenoses[24,73]
- Symptomatic lesions[73]

Extracranial Vertebral Artery Angioplasty and Stenting

Extracranial atherosclerotic disease of the vertebral artery is common and is most typically seen involving or lying close to the ostium of the vertebral artery. Lesions in this location have been difficult to treat surgically. Bypass, endarterectomy, or anastomosis of the vertebral artery to the carotid artery are the surgical options.[74,75] Balloon angioplasty alone in the region of the vertebral artery ostium has also met with some clinical success. However, with limited lumen

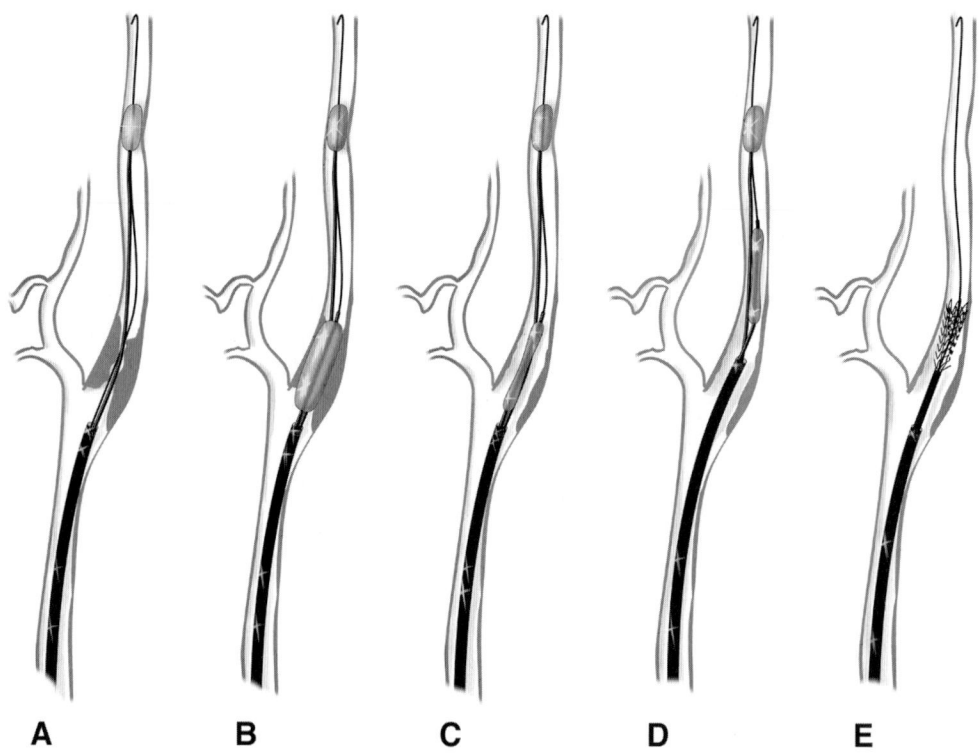

FIGURE 4.7 • *Balloon Protection during Carotid Angioplasty.*
A schematic diagram demonstrates an improvised method for carotid protection during balloon angioplasty, pending the development and trials of patented protection-exchange devices. The stenotic lesion is crossed initially with a protective compliant balloon and a parallel exchange length wire (A). The wire is used to guide the angioplasty catheter which is expanded (B), and then deflated (C). The angioplasty catheter is not withdrawn but is used as a guide for the introducer catheter, so that both slide of a piece together along the wire further up into the internal carotid artery (D). In this position the internal carotid artery can be aspirated of debris via the introducer catheter or the debris can be flushed into the external carotid artery (assuming that there are no significant collateral branches to the vertebral artery or ophthalmic artery). Usually redundant flaps on the angioplasty balloon will become entangled on the shaft of the compliant protective balloon in the lumen of the main catheter, meaning that the protective balloon must usually be removed first at this stage, then the PTA balloon. The wire is kept across the lesion and used to advance an appropriate stent (E).

A variation of this technique involves placing the tip of the wire below the compliant protective balloon on the initial image. After angioplasty the wire is removed temporarily. The internal carotid artery is flushed via the central lumen of the PTA catheter, which has been advanced above the angioplasty site. In this manner a device is kept across the angioplasty site at all times. The wire is then replaced and stent deployment undertaken.

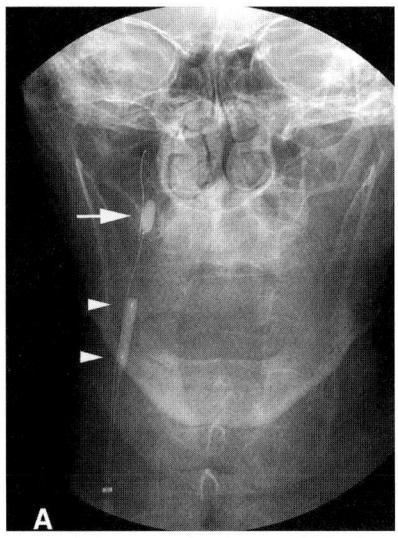 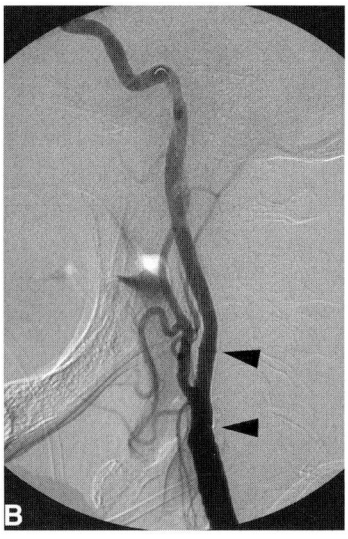

FIGURE 4.8 • *Balloon Protection during Carotid Angioplasty.*
An intraprocedural image (A) from the angioplasty phase of a carotid stent procedure in a 73-year-old male patient. The lesion has been crossed from a 9F introducer Guider catheter (Schneider) with a Balance Middle Weight 0.014-in wire (ACS) and an Endeavor balloon. A 4 × 20 mm Ranger balloon (Boston Scientific) is inflated to 12 atm (arrowheads). After withdrawal of the balloons, an 8 × 20 SMART stent (Cordis) (B, arrowheads) has been deployed across the bifurcation, covering the origin of the external carotid artery.

patency due to the high recoil nature of these lesions particularly when calcified, a high rate of restenosis following PTA and a propensity to dissect if overdilated have been seen.[76–78]

Outcome of Vertebral Artery Angioplasty and Stent Placement

For these reasons, application of stent technology to the vertebral artery has been a logical development (Figs. 4.10–4.13). Endovascular treatment of vertebral artery ostial stenosis is successful when stents are deployed in support of PTA, with prolonged patency and clinical efficacy.[79,80] Chastain et al.[81] reviewed their experience with 50 patients with symptomatic or asymptomatic unilateral or bilateral vertebral artery stenosis, treated with a variety of self-expanding and balloon-expandable coronary stents. Good clinical and angiographic results were obtained in all patients, and no direct procedure-related complications were seen. Restenosis rates of 10% were seen at 2-year follow-up. For more complex proximal subclavian artery or combined subclavian-vertebral artery lesions causing subclavian steal phenomenon, angioplasty and stent placement is also effective.

Malek et al.[82] reported on a series of 21 patients treated by endovascular stenting for symptoms of vertebrobasilar insufficiency due to proximal vertebral artery stenosis or subclavian steal phenomenon due to proximal subclavian artery stenosis. A variety of coronary stents was used including balloon-expandable GFX stents (AVE) and Palmaz stents (Johnson & Johnson) or self-expanding Wallstents (Schneider). One patient suffered a TIA within 24 hours of the procedure, another suffered from systemic sepsis from an intravenous line and developed an infection of the stent site requiring surgical extraction and arterial bypass. A third patient suffered a fatal carotid occlusion following the procedure in the vertebral artery. The remainder of the patients showed a good clinical and angio-

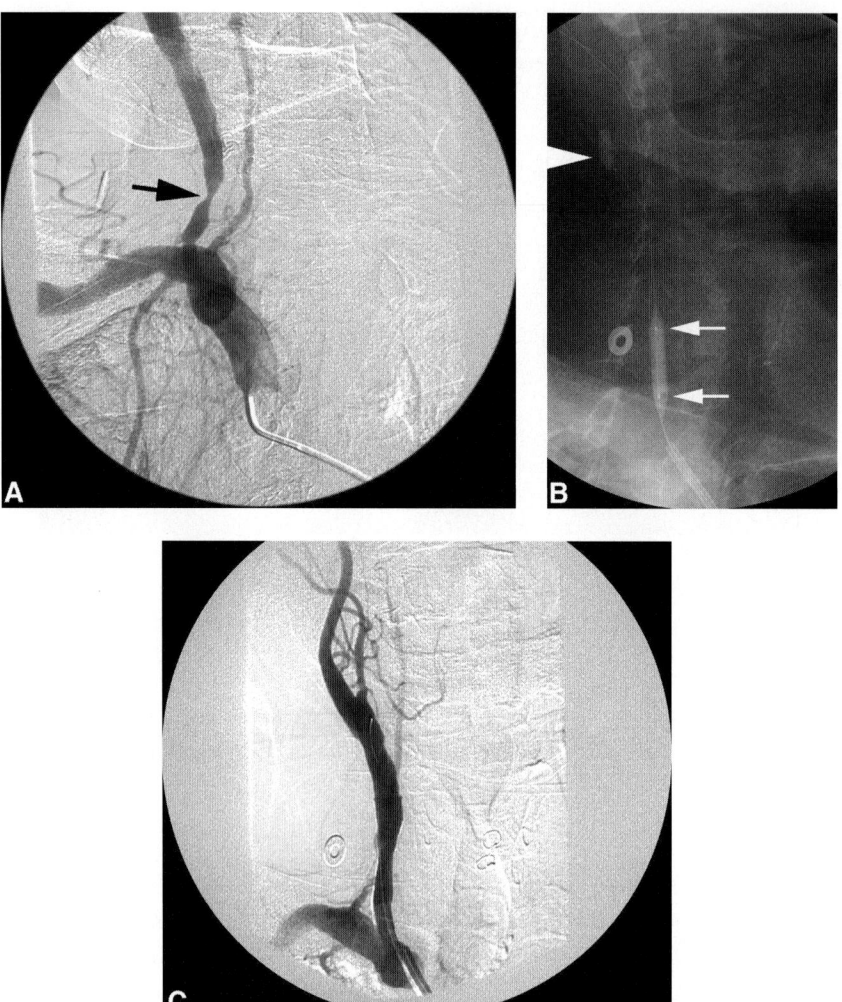

FIGURE 4.9 • *Balloon Protection of the Internal Carotid Artery and Intraprocedural Use of Transcranial Doppler Monitoring.*
A 65-year-old male patient was referred for angioplasty/stenting of a radiation-related stricture of the proximal right common carotid artery (A, arrow). Transcranial Doppler monitoring was used during the case as part of an ongoing research protocol. Using techniques described in Fig. 4.7, protection of the internal carotid artery was performed using a compliant Endeavor balloon (Target) (arrowhead in B). A 5 × 22 mm Big NC Ranger (arrows in B) is inflated to 8 atm across the lesion proximally. The external carotid artery has been used as a safe location to anchor the wire. During this phase of the procedure no embolic events were detected in the right middle cerebral artery. After deployment of an 8 × 40 SMART stent (Cordis) in the common carotid artery (during which a small number of microembolic events were identified), a moderate waist persists in the stent contour (C). To eliminate this waist, an attempt was made to postdilate the stent with an 8-mm balloon catheter. However, the tip of the balloon catheter, being a 0.035-in design, did not conform smoothly to the 0.014-in wire in use. Therefore the tip of the balloon catheter snagged on the struts of the stent as it advanced. While this could be seen on fluoroscopy, the conspicuity of the problem was visually minor. However, the acoustic response in the right middle cerebral artery was tremendous, with scores of microembolic events recorded in the space of a few seconds. Because of the TCD warnings, the attempt at postdilatation was abandoned as probably unnecessary. If the dilatation were critically important, the stent could have been crossed again with a parallel compliant balloon, which could then be used for protection of the internal carotid artery. The patient suffered no clinical deficits from the procedure and has been asymptomatic since.

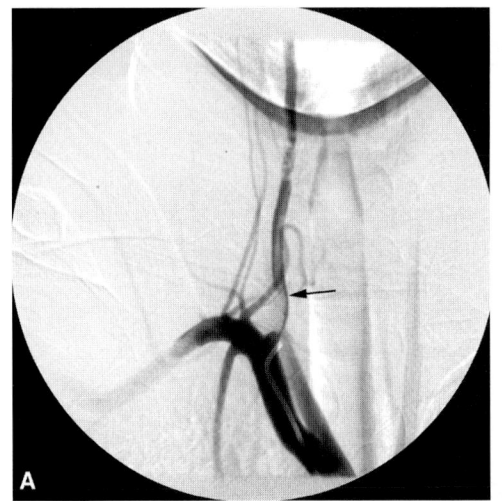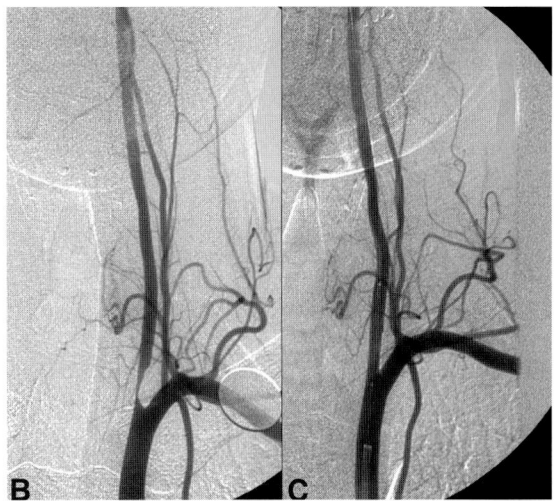

FIGURE 4.10 • *Vertebral Artery Origin Stenting with a "Slotted Tube" Stent.*
A 42-year-old female smoker presenting with a brainstem and cerebellar infarction of the territory of the right posterior inferior cerebellar artery was found to have a stenosis and yarn of thrombus in the proximal right vertebral artery (A, arrow) and a severe stenosis of the proximal left vertebral artery. For fear of dislodging a clot from the right vertebral artery, the patient was treated with anticoagulation only and suffered no further strokes. Upon return 3 months later, the right vertebral artery had proceeded to complete occlusion, while the left vertebral artery was stable (B). Following angioplasty and stenting with a 4-mm NIR stent (Boston Scientific), a satisfactory result was obtained (C).

graphic response with resolution of symptoms and improvement of stenosis from 50% to 100% before stenting to 0% to 20% following treatment. This series of patients[82] showed a 33% rate of vessel dissection from the initial angioplasty, confirming the observation made by others that ostial lesions of the vertebral artery are difficult to manage by balloon angioplasty alone.[83] Typically, lesions at the ostium of the vertebral artery have a "rubbery" quality, appearing to respond to balloon inflation with obliteration of the waist, but recoiling significantly by the time of the postangioplasty run. No complications in proximal vertebral artery angioplasty and stenting for symptomatic disease were seen in a 3-year period of follow-up in a series of seven patients reported by Piotin et al.[80]

Proximal subclavian artery lesions or subclavian tortuosity proximal to a vertebral artery stenosis can be difficult to treat from a technical point of view. Aortic arch tortuosity and other anatomic factors can make it difficult to obtain a stable position for the introducer catheter in the proximal subclavian artery or nearby in the arch. Concern for propagation of atheromatous debris into the vertebral artery with complications of posterior circulation infarction is a definite factor in some such procedures. A double-balloon technique from a transfemoral approach can be used to protect the vertebral artery while the angioplasty is in progress.[84] Sometimes the problem can be completely avoided by making a retrograde 6 Fr brachial artery approach to the vertebral artery origin. A compliant balloon can be passed retrogradely from the brachial artery and inflated in the vertebral artery while angioplasty of the subclavian artery from a transfemoral approach is being performed (Fig. 4.14). A combined approach of transfemoral angioplasty and transbrachial balloon protection of the vertebral artery has been described by Staikov et al.[85] in seven patients. The brachial approach can be used alternatively to provide stability to a transfemorally placed wire (Figs. 4.4, 4.5).

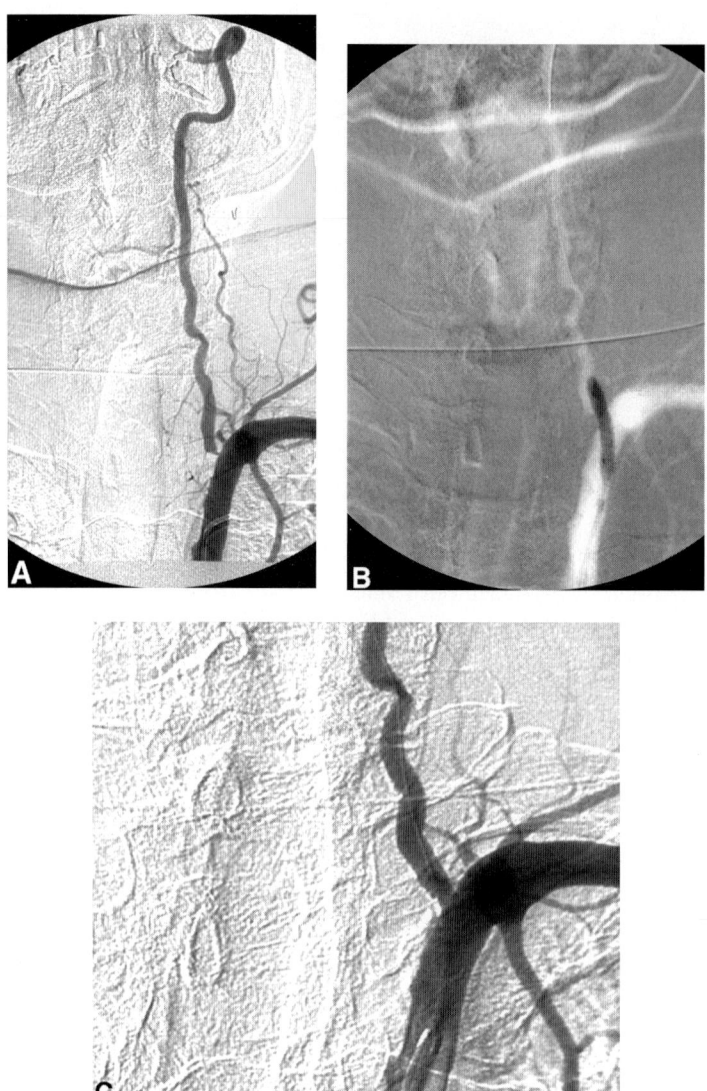

FIGURE 4.11 • *Left Vertebral Artery Angioplasty and Stenting.*
A pretreatment image (A) of the left subclavian artery in a 54-year-old male shows a severe stenosis at the origin of the left vertebral artery. Despite obliteration of the waist (B) with the angioplasty balloon (Ranger 4 × 20 mm on a 300-cm Balance ACS wire at 11 atm), virtually no effect was evident on the postangioplasty images due to vessel recoil. A 4 × 16 mm NIR stent (Boston Scientific) was inflated to 11 atm (equivalent to 4.25-mm diameter according to manufacturer specifications) and resulted in a sustained satisfactory result (C).

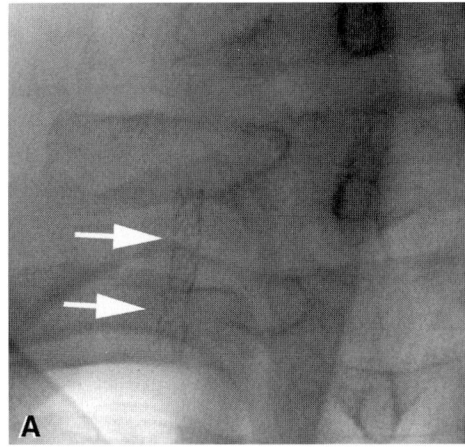 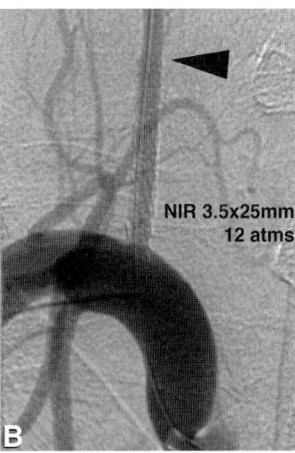

FIGURE 4.12 • *Fragmentation of a Segmented Stent at the Origin of the Right Vertebral Artery due to Arterial Motion.*
A 44-year-old male patient with occlusion of the left vertebral artery and severe stenosis of the right vertebral artery origin presented with multiple posterior circulation infarcts and insufficiency symptoms when his systolic blood pressure fell below 140 mm Hg. An excellent appearing stent deposition was obtained with a 4-mm GFX stent deployed at the origin of the right vertebral artery. He was asymptomatic following the procedure, but in preparation for major abdominal surgery for pancreatitis, a follow-up angiogram was thought prudent, lest he be vulnerable to posterior circulation ischemia from hypotension at the time of planned surgery. The AVE GFX stent showed disintegration at the right vertebral artery origin and approximately 50% restenosis 3 months following the initial procedure (A). Under fluoroscopy it was possible to see a prominent rocking motion of the right subclavian artery with the cardiac cycle, which had undoubtedly induced fatigue in the integrity of the stent. The stent site was repaired with a NIR 3.5 × 25 mm stent placed within the first stent (B, arrowhead denotes distal tip of the NIR stent). His subsequent surgery was complicated by multisystem failure, prolonged hypotension (systolic blood pressure of 50 mm Hg for several days) and supported ventilation over several weeks. However, no clinical or MRI evidence of new posterior circulation infarctions were seen despite this, and he made a full recovery without new neurological deficits.

Stent Therapy for Symptomatic Cervical Arterial Dissection

Dissections of the cervical carotid artery or vertebral artery can occur spontaneously, following injury, or in association with connective tissue disease affecting the arterial wall. When anticoagulant therapy fails or is contraindicated, options for treating the dissected artery include surgical repair, ligation, endovascular occlusion of the vessel, or more recently endovascular reconstruction of the vessel using stents. Cases of dissection with an associated pseudoaneurysm have sometimes been approached with covered endovascular stents with the intention of immediate exclusion of the pseudoaneurysm. Stents covered with autologous veins[86] or with synthetic material[87] have been used successfully in this situation, as well as noncovered stents using coils placed outside the stent for aneurysm obliteration (Fig. 12.13).[88,89] Nonaneurysmal spontaneous dissections causing occlusive or embolic complications, or dissections related to fibromuscular dysplasia or trauma have been treated successfully using stents alone (Fig. 12.14).[90–95] Following iatrogenic or spontaneous dissections of the carotid artery, Malek et

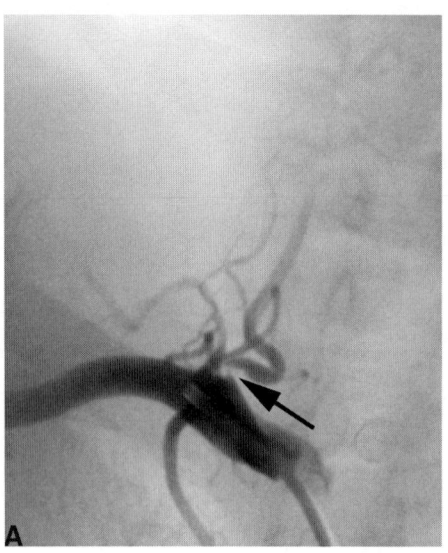 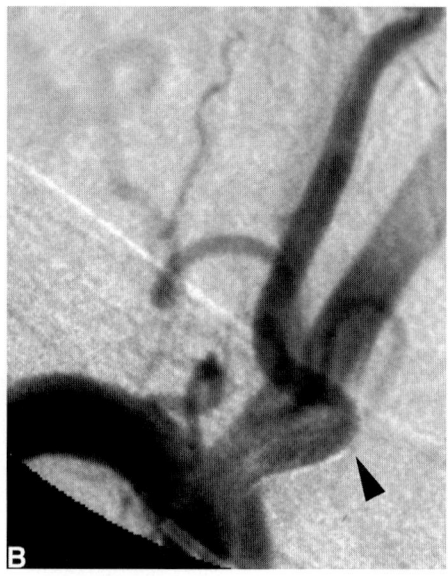

FIGURE 4.13 • *Transbrachial Approach to Vertebral Artery Stenosis.*
A 78-year-old female with symptoms of posterior circulation insufficiency and occlusion of the left vertebral artery demonstrated a severe stenosis of the right vertebral artery origin (A, arrow). Because of the angle of origin of the right vertebral artery in combination with proximal tortuosity of the great vessels, a transfemoral catheterization of the right vertebral artery was difficult. A right transbrachial approach to the stenosis via a 6F sheath allowed ease of angioplasty and stenting with an AVE GFX 4-mm stent (B, arrowhead indicates distal end of stent). A transfemoral catheter was used for making roadmaps and DSA images during the procedure.

al. have demonstrated that it is possible to navigate a microcatheter though a dissection, even in the setting of complete carotid occlusion, and reconstruct the true lumen using one or more stents.[96] Follow-up studies have sometimes shown that the presence of a noncovered stent will promote spontaneous healing of a pseudoaneurysm.[97,98] Most of these successful case reports and small case series were performed with heparinization alone without premedication of the patients with antiplatelet agents, and were performed prior to the availability of GPIIb/IIIa inhibitors.

Suggested Medication Protocol for Extracranial Stenting

- Clopidogrel 75 mg P.O. daily or ticlopidine 250 mg B.I.D. P.O. for 5 days prior to the procedure.
- Aspirin 325 mg P.O. daily for 5 days prior to the procedure.
- Heparinization during the procedure to an ACT of approximately 300 seconds, or 200 seconds or slightly higher if one intends to use GPIIb/IIIa inhibitors.
- Abciximab or eptifibatide loading dose and intravenous infusion started prior to the first angioplasty (not in universal use).
- Intraarterial papaverine (50–100 mg) and/or nitroglycerin (200–400 μg) into the target artery to reduce arterial spasm prior to initial angioplasty. This is particularly useful for the vertebral arteries or high cervical carotid artery where spasm might be problematic. However, intraarterial papaverine in an awake patient can be extremely noxious, particularly in the posterior circulation.
- Glycopyrrolate for carotid bifurcation lesions. A highly polar quaternary ammonium structure limits passage of glycopyrrolate across lipid membranes such as the blood brain barrier

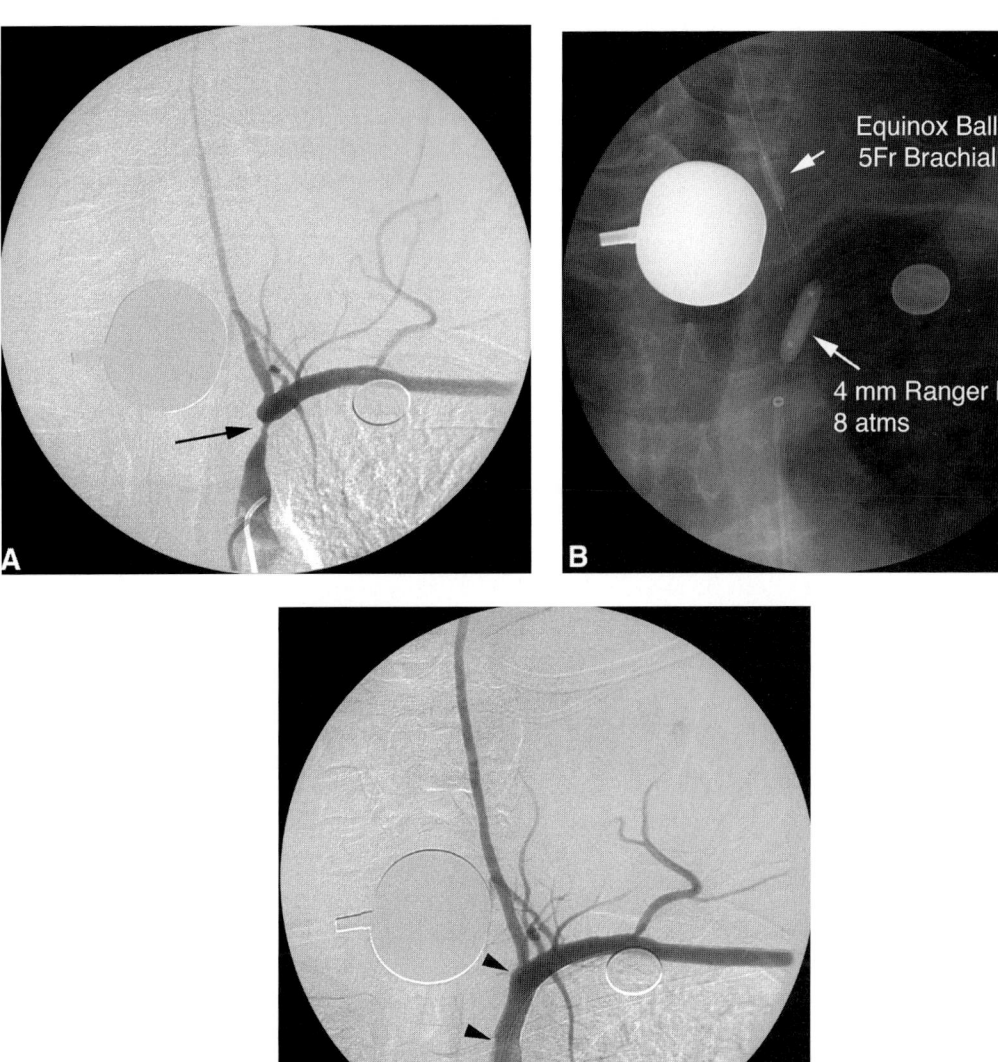

FIGURE 4.14 • *Utility of a Combined Brachial/Femoral Approach to Subclavian Stenosis.*
A diabetic 64-year-old male patient suffered from exercise-related fatigue of the left arm and symptoms of subclavian steal during activity. A severe stenosis of the left subclavian artery (A, arrow) was treated by angioplasty and stenting via a transfemoral 7F 90-cm sheath. A 5F sheath in the left brachial artery has been used to pass a compliant balloon (Equinox, MTI) retrogradely to the left vertebral artery for protection of the brain during the angioplasty with a 4-mm Ranger Balloon (B). Subsequently, an 8 × 20 mm SMART stent (Cordis) was deployed in the subclavian artery with the distal end deployed just short of the vertebral artery origin (C). With this technique any embolic threat to the posterior circulation during the procedure is eliminated.

(BBB). This is in contrast to other anticholinergic agents such as atropine or scopolamine, which do cross the BBB. Therefore using glycopyrrolate during carotid stent and angioplasty procedures to prevent vagal reflex bradycardia and hypotension may have some advantages compared with other agents, with less likelihood of confusion, delirium, and memory disruption. Typical doses for adults start with 0.1 mg intravenously, repeated after 2–3 minutes. The peripheral anticholinergic effects of glycopyrrolate can persist for up to 7 hours and include dry mouth, mydriasis, increased intraocular pressure (prompting caution in patients with glaucoma), urinary retention, and dry skin. If central CNS effects of confusion, agitation, and convulsions are seen, the effects of glycopyrrolate can be reversed by slow administration of physostigmine 0.5–5 mg intravenously.

- Postprocedure continue abciximab or eptifibatide infusions for 12 or 24 hours, respectively.
- Continue aspirin and clopidogrel or ticlopidine for at least 3–6 weeks.

References

1. Dotter CT, Judkins MP (1964) Transluminal treatment of arteriosclerotic obstruction: description of a new technique and a preliminary report of its application. *Circulation* 30:654–670.
2. Grüntzig A, Hopff H (1974) Perkutane Rekanalisation chronischer arterieller Verschlüsse mit einem neuen Dilatationskatheter. Modifikation der Dotter-Technik. *Dtsch Med Wochenschr* 99:2502–2505.
3. Grüntzig A, Kumpe DA (1979) Technique of percutaneous transluminal angioplasty with the grüntzig balloon catheter. *AJR* 132:547–552.
4. Mullan S, Duda EE, Patronas NJ (1980) Some examples of balloon technology in neurosurgery. *J Neurosurg* 52:321–329.
5. Mathias K (1977) Ein neuartiges Katheter-System zure perkutanen transluminalen Angioplastie von Karotisstenosen. *Fortschr Med* 95:1007–1011.
6. Kerber CW, Cromwell LD, Loehden OL (1980) Catheter dilatation of proximal carotid stenosis during distal bifurcation endarterectomy. *AJNR* 1:348–349.
7. Sundt TM Jr, Smith HC, Campbell JK, Vlietstra RE, Cucchiara RF, Stanson AW (1980) Transluminal angioplasty for basilar artery stenosis. *Mayo Clin Proc* 55:673–680.
8. Theron J (1987) Angioplasty of supra-aortic arteries. *Seminars Intervent Radiol* 4:331–339.
9. Kachel R, Basche S, Heerklotz I, Grossmann K, Endler S (1991) Percutaneous transluminal angioplasty (PTA) of supra-aortic arteries, especially the internal carotid artery. *Neuroradiology* 33:191–194.
10. Kachel R, Endert G, Basche S, Grossmann K, Glaser FH (1987) Percutaneous transluminal angioplasty (dilatation) of carotid, vertebral, and innominate artery stenoses. *Cardiovasc Intervent Radiol* 10:142–146.
11. Higashida RT, Hieshima GB, Tsai FY, Halbach VV, Norman D, Newton TH (1987) Transluminal angioplasty of the vertebral and basilar artery. *AJNR* 8:745–749.
12. Ahuja A, Guterman LR, Hopkins LN (1992) Angioplasty for basilar artery atherosclerosis. *J Neurosurg* 77:941–944.
13. Ferguson GG, Eliasziw M, Barr HWK, Clagett GP, Barnes RW, Wallace C, Taylor DW, Haynes B, Finan JW, Hachinski VC, Barnett HJM (1999) The North American Symptomatic Carotid Endarterectomy Trial. Surgical results in 1415 patients. *Stroke* 30:1751–1758.
14. Paciaroni M, Eliasziw M, Kappelle J, Finan JW, Ferguson GG, Barnett HJM (1999) Medical complications associated with carotid endarterectomy. *Stroke* 30:1759–1763.
15. North American Symptomatic Carotid Endarterectomy Trial Collaborators (1991) Beneficial effect of carotid endarterectomy in symptomatic patients with high-grade carotid stenosis. *N Engl J Med* 325:445–453.
16. Barnett HJM, Taylor DW, Eliasziw M, Fox AJ, Ferguson GG, Haynes RB, Rankin RN, Clagett GP, Hachinski VC, Sackett DL, Thorpe KE, Meldrum HE (1998) Benefit of carotid endarterectomy in patients with symptomatic moderate or severe stenosis. *N Engl J Med* 339:1415–1425.
17. Mericle RA, Kim SH, Lanzino G, Lopes DK, Wakhloo AK, Guterman LR, Hopkins LN (1999) Carotid artery angioplasty and use of stents in high-risk patients with contralateral occlusions. *J Neurosurg* 90:1031–1036.
18. Gasecki AP, Eliasziw M, Ferguson GG, Hachinski V, Barnett HJM (1995) Long-term prognosis and effect of endarterectomy in patients with symptomatic severe carotid stenosis and contralateral carotid stenosis or occlusion: results from NASCET. *J Neurosurg* 83:778–782.
19. Hammacher ER, Eikelboom BC, Bast TJ, De Geest R, Vermeulen FEE (1984) Surgical treatment of patients with a carotid artery occlusion and a contralateral stenosis. *J Cardiovasc Surg* 25:513–517.
20. Mathur A, Roubin GS, Gomez CR, Iyer SS, Wong PM, Piamsomboon C, Yadav SS, Dean LS, Vitek JJ (1998) Elective carotid artery stenting in the presence of contralateral occlusion. *Am J Cardiol* 81:1315–1317.
21. Al Mubarak N, Roubin GS, Gomez CR, Liu MWTJ, Lyer SS, Vitek JJ (1999) Carotid artery stenting in patients with high neurologic risks. *Am J Cardiol* 83:1411–1413.
22. Teitelbaum GP, Lefkowitz MA, Giannotta SL (1998)

Carotid angioplasty and stenting in high-risk patients. *Surg Neurol* 50:300–311.

23. WHOLEY MH, WHOLEY M, BERGERON P, DIETHRICH EB, HENRY M, LABORDE JC, MATHIAS K, MYLA S, ROUBIN GS, SHAWL F, THERON JG, YADAV JS, DORROS G, GUIMARAENS J, HIGASHIDA R, KUMAR V, LEON M, LIM M, LONDERO H, MESA J, RAMEE S, RODRIGUEZ A, ROSENFIELD K, TEITELBAUM G, VOZZI C (1998) Current global status of carotid artery stent placement. *Catheterization Cardiovasc Diag* 44:1–6.

24. MATHUR A, ROUBIN GS, IYER SS, PIAMSONBOON C, LIU MW, GOMEZ CR, YADAV JS, CHASTAIN HD, FOX LM, DEAN LS, VITEK JJ (1998) Predictors of stroke complicating carotid artery stenting. *Circulation* 97:1239–1245.

25. NIELSEN TG, SILLESEN H, SCHROEDER TV (1995) Seizures following carotid endarterectomy in patients with severely compromised cerebral circulation. *Europ J Vasc Endovasc Surg* 9:53–57.

26. ILLE O, WOIMANT F, PRUNA A, CORABIANU O, IDATTE JM, HAGUENAU M (1995) Hypertensive encephalopathy after bilateral carotid endarterectomy. *Stroke* 26:488–491.

27. BREEN JC, CAPLAN LR, DEWITT LD, BELKIN M, MACKEY WC, O'DONNELL TP (1996) Brain edema after carotid surgery. *Neurology* 46:175–181.

28. SOLOMON RA, LOFTUS CM, QUEST DO, CORRELL JW (1986) Incidence and etiology of intracerebral hemorrhage following carotid endarterectomy. *J Neurosurg* 64:29–34.

29. SCHOSER BG, HEESEN C, ECKERT B, THIE A (1997) Cerebral hyperperfusion injury after percutaneous transluminal angioplasty of extracranial arteries. *J Neurol* 244:101–104.

30. MCCABE DJH, BROWN MM, CLIFTON A (1999) Fatal cerebral reperfusion hemorrhage after carotid stenting. *Stroke* 30:2483–2486.

31. CHAMORRO A, VILA N, OBACH V, MACHO J, BLASCO J (2000) A case of cerebral hemorrhage early after carotid stenting. *Stroke* 31:792–793.

32. MEYERS PM, HIGASHIDA RT, PHATOUROS CC, MALEK AM, LEMPERT TE, DOWD CF, HALBACH VV (2000) Cerebral hyperperfusion syndrome after percutaneous transluminal stenting of the craniocervical arteries. *Neurosurgery* 47:335–343.

33. NAYLOR AR, BOLIA A, ABBOTT RJ, PYE IF, SMITH J, LENNARD N, LLOYD AJ, LONDON NJ, BELL PR (1998) Randomized study of carotid angioplasty and stenting versus carotid endarterectomy: a stopped trial. *J Vasc Surg* 28:326–334.

34. THERON J (1996) Protected carotid angioplasty and carotid stents. *Journal des Maladies Vasculaires* 21(suppl A):113–122.

35. BETTMANN MA, KATZEN BT, WHISNANT J, BRANT-ZAWADZKI M, BRODERICK JP, FURLAN AJ, HERSHEY LA, HOWARD V, KUNTZ R, LOFTUS CM, PEARCE W, ROBERTS A, ROUBIN G (1998) Carotid stenting and angioplasty: a statement for healthcare professionals from the Councils on Cardiovascular Radiology, Stroke, Cardio-Thoracic and Vascular Surgery, Epidemiology, and Prevention, and Clinical Cardiology, American Heart Association. *Circulation* 97:121–123.

36. BERGERON P, CHAMBRAN P, HARTUNG O, BIANCA S (1996) Cervical carotid artery stenosis: which technique, balloon angioplasty or surgery? *J Cardiovasc Surg* 37(suppl 1):73–75.

37. BEEBE HG (1998) Scientific evidence demonstrating the safety of carotid angioplasty and stenting: do we have enough to draw conclusions yet? *J Vasc Surg* 27:788–790.

38. YAO JS (1999) Angioplasty and stenting for carotid lesions: an argument against. *Adv Surg* 32:245–254.

39. MATHIAS KD (1999) Angioplasty and stenting for carotid lesions: an argument for. *Adv Surg* 32:225–243.

40. OESTERLE SN, WHITBOURN R, FITZGERALD PJ, YEUNG AC, STERTZER SH, DAKE MD, YOCK PG, VIRMANI R (1998) The stent decade: 1987 to 1997. Stanford Stent Summit faculty. *Am Heart J* 136:578–599.

41. CRAWLEY F, CLIFTON A, TAYLOR RS, BROWN MM (1998) Symptomatic restenosis after carotid percutaneous transluminal angioplasty. *Lancet* 352:708–709.

42. SERRUYS PW, DE JAEGERE P, KIEMENEIJ F, MACAYA CRW, HEYNDRICKX G, EMANUELSSON H, MARCO J, LEGRAND V, MATERNE P, BELARDI J, SIGWART U, COLOMBO A, GOY JJ, VAN DEN HEUVEL P, DELCAN J, MOREL MA (1994) A comparison of balloon expandable stent implantation with balloon angioplasty in patients with coronary artery disease. *N Engl J Med* 331:489–495.

43. FISCHMAN DL, LEON MB, BAIM DS, SCHATZ RA, SAVAGE MP, PENN I, DETRE KVL, RICCI D, NOBUYOSHI M, CLEMAN M, HEUSER R, ALMOND D, TEIRSTEIN PS, FISH RD, COLOMBO A, BRINKER J, MOSES J, SHAKNOVICH A, HIRSHFELD J, BAILEY S, ELLIS S, RAKE R, GOLDBERG S (1994) A randomized comparison of coronary stent placement and balloon angioplasty in patients with coronary artery disease. *N Engl J Med* 331:496–501.

44. UREN NG, SCHWARZACHER SP, METZ JA, ALDERMAN EL, ABIZAID A, FITZGERALD PG (1997) Intravascular ultrasound prediction of stent thrombosis: insights from the POST registry. *J Am Coll Cardiol* 29(suppl A):60A.

45. RUSSO RJ, MASSULO V, JANI SK, SCHATZ RA, GUARNERI EM, STEUTERMAN S (1997) Restenting versus PTCA for in-stent restenosis with or without intracoronary radiation therapy: an analysis of the SCRIPPS trial. *Circulation* 96(suppl 1):I–219.

46. TEIRSTEIN PS, MASSULLO V, JANI S, POPMA JJ, MINTZ GS, RUSSO RJ (1997) Catheter based radiotherapy to inhibit restenosis after coronary stenting. *N Engl J Med* 336:1697–1703.

47. MANNINEN HI, RASANEN HT, VANNINEN RL, VAINIO P, HIPPELAINEN M, KOSMA VM (1999) Stent placement versus percutaneous transluminal angioplasty of human carotid arteries in cadavers in situ: distal embolization and findings at intravascular US, MR imaging and histopathologic analysis. *Radiology* 212:483–492.

48. GOMEZ CR (1998) The role of carotid angioplasty and stenting. *Seminars Neurol* 18:501–511.

49. MARKUS HS, CLIFTON A, BUCKENHAM T, BROWN MM (1994) Carotid angioplasty. Detection of embolic signals during and after the procedure. *Stroke* 25:2403–2406.

50. McCleary AJ, Nelson M, Dearden NM, Calvey TA, Gough MJ (1998) Cerebral haemodynamics and embolization during carotid angioplasty in high-risk patients. Br J Surg 85: 771–774.
51. Crawley F, Clifton A, Buckenham T, Loosemore T, Taylor RS, Brown MM (1997) Comparison of hemodynamic cerebral ischemia and microembolic signals detected during carotid endarterectomy and carotid angioplasty. Stroke 28: 2460–2464.
52. Ackerstaff RGA, Moons KGM, van de Vlasakker CJW, Moll FL, Vermeulen FEE, Algra A, Spencer MP (2000) Association of intraoperative transcranial Doppler monitoring variables with stroke from carotid endarterectomy. Stroke 31:1817–1823.
53. Levi CR, O'Malley HM, Fell G, Roberts AK, Hoare MC, Royle JP, Chan A, Beiles BC, Chambers BR, Bladin CF, Donnan GA (1997) Transcranial Doppler detected cerebral microembolism following carotid endarterectomy. High microembolic signal loads predict post-operative cerebral ischaemia. Brain 120:621–629.
54. Moody DM, Bell MA, Challa VR, Johnston WE, Prough DS (1990) Brain microemboli during cardiac surgery or aortography. Ann Neurol 28:477–486.
55. Brown WR, Moody DM, Challa VR, Stump DA, Hammon JW (2000) Longer duration of cardiopulmonary bypass is associated with greater numbers of cerebral microemboli. Stroke 31:707–713.
56. Crawley F, Stygall J, Lunn S, Harrison M, Brown MM, Newman S (2000) Comparison of microembolism detected by transcranial Doppler and neuropsychological sequelae of carotid surgery and percutaneous transluminal angioplasty. Stroke 31:1329–1334.
57. Müller M, Reiche W, Langenscheidt P, Hassfeld J, Hagen T (2000) Ischemia after carotid endarterectomy: comparison between transcranial doppler sonography and diffusion-weighted mr imaging. AJNR 21:47–54.
58. Jansen C, Ramos LMP, van Heesewijk JPM, Moll FL, van Gijn J, Ackerstaff RGA (1994) Impact of microembolism and hemodynamic changes in the brain during carotid endarterectomy. Stroke 25:992–997.
59. Gaunt ME, Martin PJ, Smith JL, Rimmer T, Cherryman G, Ratliff DA, Bell PRF, Naylor AR (1994) Clinical relevance of intraoperative embolization detected by transcranial Doppler ultrasonography during carotid endarterectomy: a prospective study of 100 patients. Br J Vasc Surg 81:1435–1439.
60. Cantelmo NL, Babikian VL, Samaraweera RN, Gordon JK, Pochay VE, Winter MR (1998) Cerebral microembolism and ischemic changes associated with carotid endarterectomy. J Vasc Surg 27:1024–1031.
61. Müller M, Behnke S, Walter P, Omlor G, Schimrigk K (1998) Microembolic signals and intraoperative stroke in carotid endarterectomy. Acta Neurologica Scandinavica 97: 110–117.
62. Stump DA, Brown WR, Moody DM (1999) Microemboli and neurologic dysfunction after cardiovascular surgery. Seminars Cardiothorac Vasc Anesth 3:47–54.
63. Pugsley W, Klinger L, Paschalis C, Treasure T, Harrison M, Newman S (1994) The impact of microemboli during cardiopulmonary bypass on neuropsychological functioning. Stroke 25:1393–1399.
64. Bladin CF, Bingham L, Grigg L, Yapanis AG, Gerraty R, Davis SM (1998) Transcranial Doppler detection of microemboli during percutaneous transluminal coronary angioplasty. Stroke 29:2367–2370.
65. Theron JG, Payelle GG, Coskun O, Huet HF, Guimaraens L (1996) Carotid artery stenosis: treatment with protected balloon angioplasty and stent placement. Radiology 201: 627–636.
66. Albuguerque FC, Teitelbaum GP, Lavine SD, Larsen DW, Giannotta SL (2000) Balloon-protected carotid angioplasty. Neurosurgery 46:918–923.
67. Henry M, Amor M (1999) The safety and efficacy of the PercuSurge GuardWire in the treatment of carotid stenosis: European multicenter trial. 11th Transcatheter Cardiovascular Therapeutics Meeting, Washington, DC.
68. Ohki T, Parodi JC, Bates M, Rabin J, Goldstein K, Veith FJ (1999) The need for protection device during carotid artery stenting. 11th Transcatheter Cardiovascular Therapeutics Meeting, Washington, DC.
69. Ohki T, Veith FJ (1998) The potential of the PercuSurge Guardwire to prevent embolic events in endovascular interventions. Endocardiovascular Multimedia Magazine 2(1):33–38.
70. Henry M, Amor M, Henry I (1999) Carotid stenting with cerebral protection. First clinical experience using the PercuSurge Guardwire system. J Endovasc Surg 6:321–331.
71. Parodi J (1999) Cerebral protection: initial experience with three different devices. Presented at 12th International Symposium on Endovascular Therapy, Miami.
72. Ohki T, Marin M, Lyon R, Berdejo GL, Soundararajan K, Ohki M, Yuan JG, Faries PL, Wain RA, Sanchez LA, Suggs WD, Veith FJ (1998) Ex vivo human carotid artery bifurcation stenting: correlation of lesion characteristics with embolic potential. J Vasc Surg 27:463–471.
73. Qureshi AI, Luft AR, Janardhan V, Suri FK, Sharma M, Lanzino G, Wakhloo AK, Guterman LR, Hopkins LN (2000) Identification of patients at risk for periprocedural neurological deficits associated with carotid angioplasty and stenting. Stroke 31:376–382.
74. Spetzler RF, Hadley MN, Martin NA (1987) Vertebrobasilar insufficiency. Part 1: Microsurgical treatment of extracranial vertebrobasilar disease. J Neurosurg 66:648–661.
75. Imperato AM (1985) Vertebral artery reconstruction: a nineteen-year experience. J Vasc Surg 2:626–634.
76. Vitek JJ (1989) Subclavian artery angioplasty and the origin of the vertebral artery. Radiology 170:407–409.
77. Courtheoux P, Tournade A, Theron J, Henriet JP, Maiza D, Derlon JM, Perlouze G, Evrard C (1985) Transcuta-

neous angioplasty of vertebral artery atheromatous ostial strictures. *Neuroradiology* 27:259–264.
78. MOTARJEME A, KEIFER JW, ZUSKA AJ (1981) Percutaneous transluminal angioplasty of the vertebral arteries. *Radiology* 139:715–717.
79. STOREY GS, MARKS MP, DAKE M, NORBASH AM, STEINBERG GK (1996) Vertebral artery stenting following percutaneous transluminal angioplasty. Technical note. *J Neurosurg* 84:883–887.
80. PIOTIN M, SPELLE L, MARTIN JB, WEILL A, RANCUREL G, ROSS IB, RUFENACHT DA, CHIRAS J (2000) Percutaneous transluminal angioplasty and stenting for the proximal vertebral artery for symptomatic stenosis. *AJNR* 21:727–731.
81. CHASTAIN HD, CAMPBELL MS, IYER S, ROUBIN GS, VITEK J, MATHUR A, AL-MUBARAK NA, TERRY JB, YATES V, KRETZER K, ALRED D, GOMEZ CR (1999) Extracranial vertebral artery stent placement: in-hospital and follow-up results. *J Neurosurg* 91:547–552.
82. MALEK AM, HIGASHIDA RT, PHATOUROS CC, LEMPERT TE, MEYERS PM, GRESS DR, DOWD CF, HALBACH VV (1999) Treatment of posterior circulation ischemia with extracranial percutaneous balloon angioplasty and stent placement. *Stroke* 30:2073–2085.
83. MOTARJEME A (1996) Percutaneous transluminal angioplasty of supra-aortic vessels. *J Endovasc Surg* 3:171–181.
84. NASIM A, SAYERS RD, BELL PRF, BOLIA A (1994) Protection against vertebral artery embolization during proximal subclavian artery angioplasty. *Europ J Vasc Surg* 8:362–363.
85. STAIKOV IN, DO DD, REMONDA L, MATTLE H, BAUMGARTNER R, SCHROTH G (1999) The site of atheromatosis in the subclavian and vertebral arteries and its implication for angioplasty. *Neuroradiology* 41:537–542.
86. MAROTTA TR, BULLER C, TAYLOR D, MORRIS C, ZWIMPFER T (1998) Autologous vein-covered stent repair of a cervical internal carotid artery pseudoaneurysm: technical case report. *Neurosurgery* 42:408–412.
87. NICHOLSON A, COOK AM, DYET JF, GALLOWAY JM (1995) Case report: Treatment of a carotid artery pseudoaneurysm with a polyester covered stent. *Clin Radiol* 50:872–873.
88. PEREZ-CRUET MJ, PATWARDHAN RV, MAWAD ME, ROSE JE (1997) Treatment of dissecting pseudoaneurysm of the cervical internal carotid artery using a Wall stent and detachable coils: case report. *Neurosurgery* 40:622–625.
89. KLEIN GE, SZOLAR DH, RAITH J, FRUHWIRTH H, PASCHER O, HAUSEGGER KA (1997) Posttraumatic extracranial aneurysm of the internal carotid artery: combined endovascular treatment with coils and stents. *AJNR* 18:1261–1264.
90. HUANG A, BAKER DM, AL-KUTOUBI A (1996) Endovascular stenting of internal carotid artery false aneurysm. *Europ J Endovasc Surg* 12:375–377.
91. HONG MK, SATLER LF, GALLINO R, LEON MB (1997) Intravascular stenting as a definitive treatment of spontaneous carotid artery dissection. *Am J Cardiol* 79:538.
92. BEJJANI GK, MONSEIN LH, LAIRD JR, SATLER LF, STARNES BW, AULISI EF (1999) Treatment of symptomatic cervical carotid dissections with endovascular stents. *Neurosurgery* 44:755–760.
93. DEOCAMPO J, BRILLMAN J, LEVY DI (1997) Stenting: a new approach to carotid dissection. *J Neuroimag* 7:187–190.
94. DUKE BJ, RYU RK, COLDWELL DM, BREGA KE (1997) Treatment of blunt injury to the carotid artery by using endovascular stents: an early experience. *J Neurosurg* 87:825–829.
95. MARKS MP, DAKE MD, STEINBERG GK, NORBASH AM, LANE B (1994) Stent placement for arterial and venous cerebrovascular disease: preliminary experience. *Radiology* 191:441–446.
96. MALEK AM, HIGASHIDA RT, PHATOUROS CC, LEMPERT TE, MEYERS PM, SMITH WS, DOWD CF, HALBACH VV (2000) Endovascular management of extracranial carotid artery dissection achieved using stent angioplasty. *AJNR* 21:1280–1292.
97. HOROWITZ MB, MILLER G, MEYER Y, CARSTENS G, PURDY PD (1996) Use of intravascular stents in the treatment of internal carotid and extracranial vertebral artery pseudoaneurysms. *AJNR* 17:693–696.
98. MANNINEN HI, KOIVISTO T, SAARI T, MATSI PJ, VANNINEN RL, LUUKKONEN M, HERNESNIEMI J (1997) Dissecting aneurysms of all four cervicocranial arteries in fibromuscular dysplasia: treatment with self-expanding endovascular stents, coil embolization, and surgical ligation. *AJNR* 18:1216–1220.

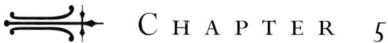

CHAPTER 5

Intracranial Angioplasty and Stenting

INTRODUCTION

The application of endovascular technology to the treatment of severe intracranial atherosclerotic occlusive disease derives from the recognition of the grave prognosis for such patients once they become symptomatic and from the lack of an established mode of effective treatment. It is thought, based on various sources, that intracranial atherosclerotic stenotic lesions carry a risk of stroke of 7% to 56% per year and a strong correlation with high risk of death from ischemic heart disease, but the studies supporting these assumptions are mostly small and retrospective or nonrandomized in methodology.[1–5] The efficacy of medical treatment of such lesions with antiplatelet therapy and/or warfarin is not yet firmly established, and external carotid artery to internal carotid artery surgical bypass does not seem to be effective for most patients.[6] A small, retrospective study of warfarin versus aspirin in the treatment of intracranial stenosis indicates a slightly greater efficacy from warfarin in symptomatic patients. Rates of major vascular events of 8.4% (stroke 3.6%) with warfarin and 18.1% (stroke 10.4%) per year with aspirin were seen.[7] Evidence supporting a slightly greater efficacy for warfarin compared with antiplatelet medication was also seen in an observational study of symptomatic intracranial atherosclerotic disease, in which a 31% and 55.8% risk of ischemic events was seen in patients taking warfarin or antiplatelet agents, respectively.[5] Follow-up studies indicate that intracranial atherosclerotic disease once detected is also likely to have a progressive course.[5,8] In summary, the prospective management of a patient with severe intracranial atherosclerotic disease, particularly once it becomes symptomatic, is still a dilemma.

The question of endovascular intervention for intracranial atherosclerotic disease generally arises only when a symptomatic patient fails on medical therapy and has persistent strokes or symptoms of intracranial vascular insufficiency. Part of the reason for withholding endovascular techniques until all medical therapy has failed may be related to the initially cautionary results of intracranial angioplasty when intracranial stenting was not possible. Early case reports using cruder balloons than are now available also reported a risk of intraprocedural vessel rupture, vasospasm, dissection, or death in 10% to 33% of patients,[9–15] a risk that must still be taken seriously with more modern materials. Compared with the extracranial arteries, the intracranial arteries are considerably smaller and have a mural composition deficient in adventitia and external elastic lamina.[16,17] This places them at serious risk for vessel rupture due to even minor oversizing of balloons during PTA (Fig. 5.1).

CLINICAL EFFICACY OF INTRACRANIAL BALLOON ANGIOPLASTY

If procedural complications can be avoided, intracranial PTA for symptomatic stenotic disease resistant to medical therapy seems to be effective at improving the clinical status of the patient, the angiographic appearance of the vessel, and distal perfusion of the brain. The apparent risk of stroke in symptomatic patients seems to be reduced by PTA, and neurologic symptoms such as crescendo TIAs or episodic insufficiency seem to be significantly improved in published series.

- Marks et al.[12] reported a group of 23 patients treated by intracranial PTA followed over a mean period of 3 years and found a 3.2% annual rate of stroke in the target territory.
- Connors and Wojack[11] treated a group of 50 symptomatic patients with intracranial PTA and found a rate of 8% late restenosis (3–12 month follow-up), all amenable to effective retreatment, and no major strokes in the target territory posttreatment.
- Callahan and Berger[13] found no significant recurrent disease or symptoms over a 16-month period in patients with an initially successful outcome from intracranial PTA.
- Nahser et al.[18] treated a group of 20 patients with intracranial atherosclerotic vertebrobasilar stenoses. Using angioplasty alone, they reported a 86% procedural success with complete resolution of symptoms of posterior circulation ischemia. One patient (5%) experienced a permanent ischemic complication. On follow-up a 14% rate of restenosis over a period of 3–18 months was seen.

FIGURE 5.1 • *Sometimes Angioplasty Alone Is Safer Than Stent Placement.*

A 68-year-old male presented with severe persistent symptoms of vertebrobasilar insufficiency. At angiography the left vertebral artery was completely occluded, and collateral circulation via the posterior communicating arteries was marginal. A severe stenosis of the distal intradural right vertebral artery distal to the origin of the right posterior inferior cerebellar artery (A, lateral view, arrow) was identified as a potentially treatable lesion. However, a CT scan at that level demonstrated prominent calcification at the site of the stenosis, which is reason for concern about the state of compliance of the arterial wall (B, CT scan nonenhanced, arrow). This implies a risk of intraprocedural rupture.

The lesion was crossed with a Balance Middle Weight (ACS) wire and dilated to 8 atm with a 1.5-mm Ranger balloon (Boston Scientific) without much improvement in flow. A 2-mm Ranger balloon was then inserted and a prominent waist was seen on the balloon until the pressure reached 11.5 atm in the course of inflation over many minutes (C, lateral roadmap image during angioplasty). The elimination of the waist on the balloon happened very quickly over a small pressure increment. The resulting angiogram showed much improved flow to the basilar artery, but a severe dissection of the basilar artery was now present (D, arrowheads postangioplasty).

Despite a prolonged attempt to stent the dissected site with a number of coronary stents and wires, the lesion could not be reached easily. Out of fear of rupturing the vessel with excessive force and manipulation, the procedure was abandoned when it was clear that the dissection did not seem to be worsening, at least during the period of observation. The patient was asymptomatic following the procedure and was discharged on antiplatelet medications and coumadin. A year later, a follow-up angiogram (E, AP view; F, lateral view) showed complete healing of the angioplasty site with maintenance of flow.

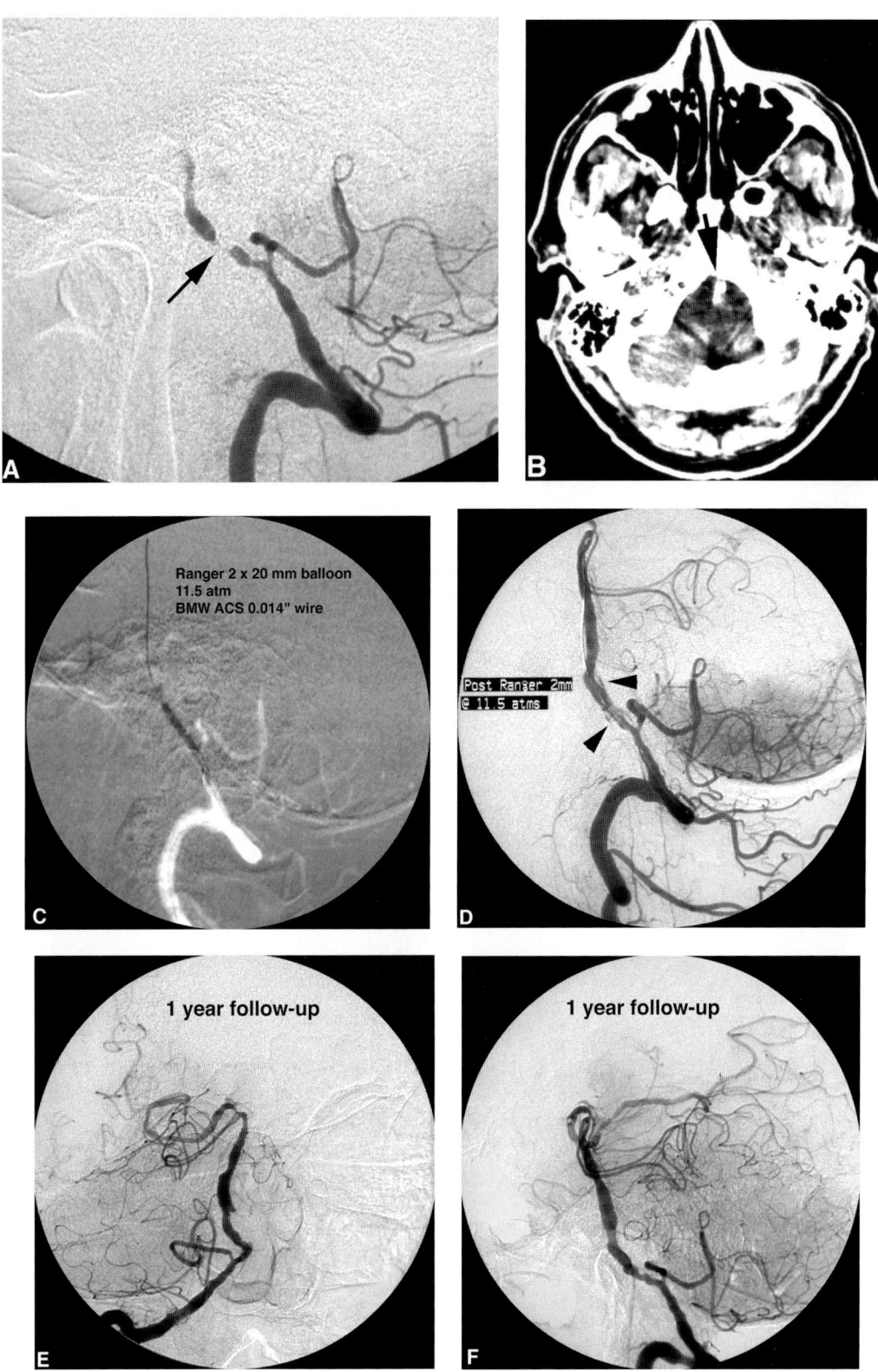

INTRACRANIAL ANGIOPLASTY AND STENTING

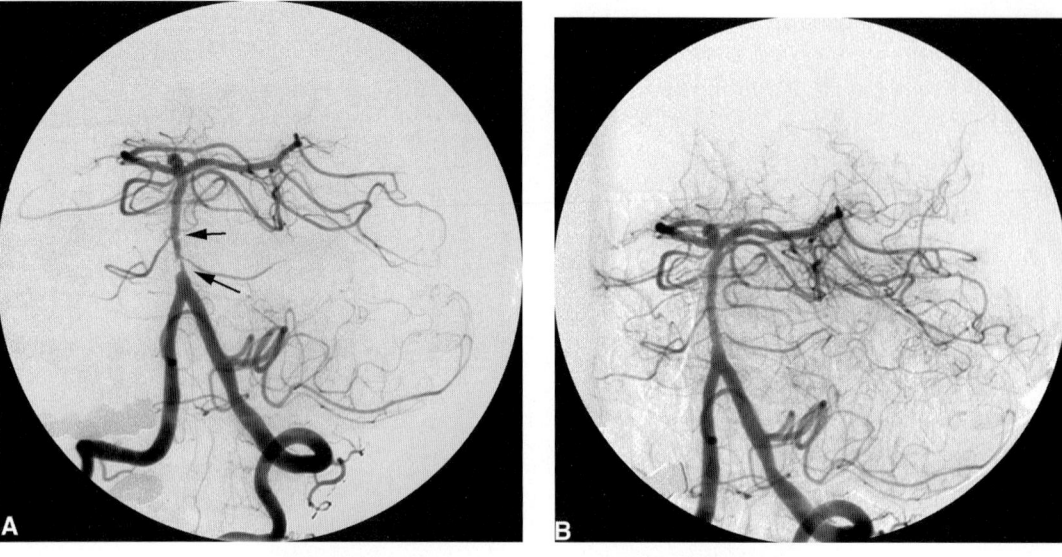
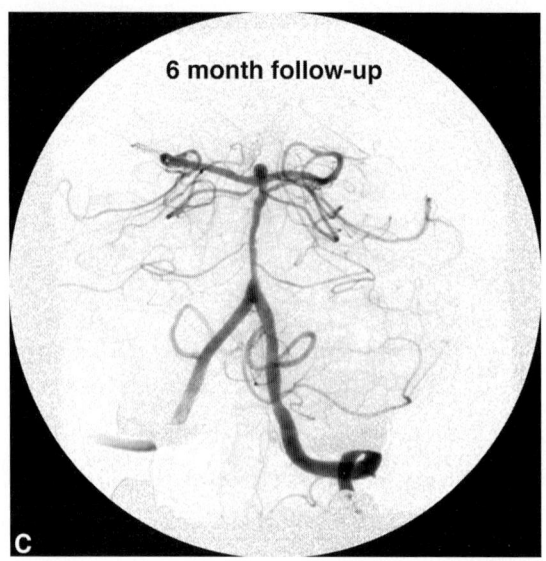

FIGURE 5.2 • *Short-Term Restenosis of Type B Lesion Following Angioplasty and Stent Placement.* A 67-year-old female patient with recurrent symptoms of posterior circulation ischemia with failure of coumadin therapy was referred for angioplasty and stent treatment. The pretreatment image (A) demonstrates that a focal lesion is present in the proximal basilar artery with a more extensive lesser degree of atherosclerotic narrowing. Despite an excellent immediate response (B) to angioplasty and stent placement (3-mm AVE GFX2 stent), a 6-month follow-up angiogram demonstrates approximately 40% in-stent restenosis (C). Although the patient is asymptomatic at this time, the long-term outcome in patients with intracranial restenosis following stenting remains to be defined. An incidental basilar tip aneurysm was not treated. Case courtesy of Frank Huang-Hellinger MD PhD, Orlando, Florida.

- Improved angiographic appearance of the vessel and improved clinical status can be shown to correlate with improved cerebral perfusion following intracranial PTA.[19,20]

The incidence of intracranial atherosclerotic disease is higher in some ethnic groups, and there is a growing experience reported from Japan on the use of intracranial PTA for this disease. The appearance of the lesion itself has been used successfully by Mori et al. to classify patients according to likelihood of a successful angioplasty.[21,22] The likelihood of a successful coronary angioplasty has been correlated with the classification of the stenotic lesion, with Type A lesions having best results, Type B an intermediate risk, and Type C responding least to PTA in the coronary literature (Table 5.1).

Mori et al. reported a clinical success rate of 92%, 86%, and 33% for PTA of intracranial lesions of Type A, B, and C, respectively, in a series of 42 patients.[21] At 1-year follow-up restenosis rates of 0%, 33%, and 100% were seen, respectively. Additionally, the long-term clinical outcome of these patients correlated with the lesion morphology (Figs. 5.2, 5.3). Patients with Type A lesions had an 8% risk of major stroke, while those with Type C lesions had a 56% risk.

Risks of Intracranial Balloon Angioplasty

The risks of intracranial PTA for atherosclerotic disease have decreased with growing experience in the field, improved materials and balloon-catheters, and the advent of glycoprotein IIb/IIIa inhibitor agents for prevention of acute thrombosis. Mori et al.[21] found that technical success at reopening a lesion was less likely with Type C lesions. Probing an intracranial occlusion with a wire carries a high risk of vessel perforation, but wire perforations or ruptures can occur in other patients with nonocclusive stenoses too. It is known from the coronary literature that an understanding of the arterial wall as a viscoelastic solid will enhance the safety of PTA and reduce the risk of rupture. The response of a viscoelastic solid to a shear stress is dependent upon the rate of application. Therefore, an abrupt stress is more likely to cause a fracture line to develop in the structure of the solid, e.g., abruptly bending a stick of butter, whereas a slow application causes gradual deformity. This phenomenon has been applied successfully in the coronary arteries, and a prolonged slow (15 minute) balloon inflation compared

TABLE 5.1
CLASSIFICATION OF INTRACRANIAL STENOTIC LESIONS[21] MODIFIED FROM SCHEME FOR CORONARY ARTERIES[23]

Type A
Discrete, length <5 mm (10 mm for coronary arteries)
Concentric or moderately eccentric
Angulation <45°
Smooth contour
Calcification not prominent
Non-ostial
Not completely occlusive
Absence of thrombus
No major side-branch involvement

Type B
Tubular 5–10 mm (10–20 mm for coronary arteries)
Eccentric
Moderate tortuosity
Angulation 45°–90°
Irregular contour
Moderate/heavy calcification
Total occlusion <3 months old
Ostial location
Situated at a bifurcation
Some thrombus present

Type C
Diffuse >10 mm in length (>20 mm for coronary arteries)
Severe tortuosity
Angulation >90°
Total occlusion >3 months old

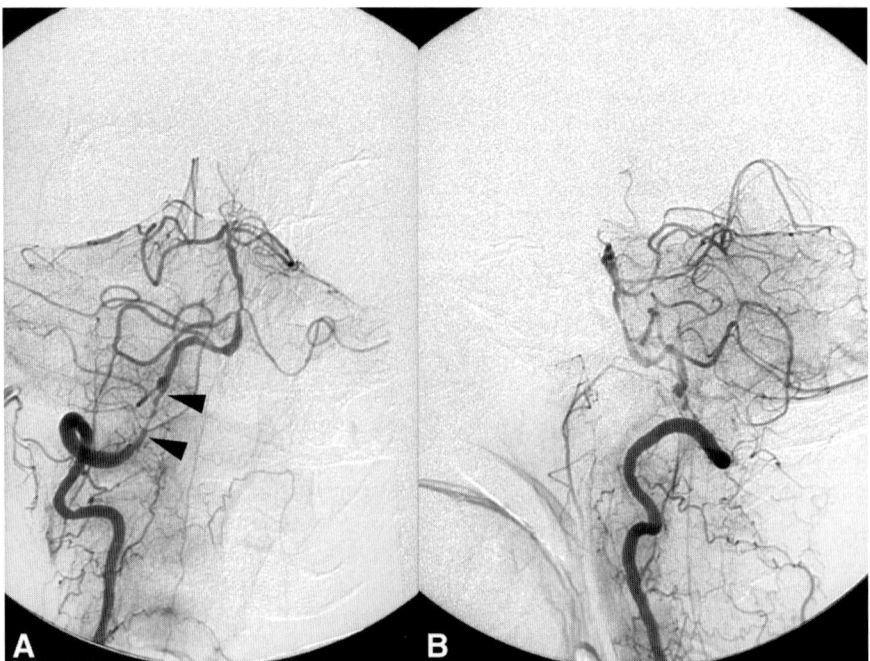

FIGURE 5.3 • *Example of Long-Term Restenosis in Response to Angioplasty Alone with Type C Stenotic Lesions.*
An 82-year-old female patient suffered dizzy spells with even minimal neck extension for a period of months and had suffered a number of falls in the recent weeks. Angiography showed a long-segment of stenotic disease in the right vertebral artery superimposed on an appearance of diffuse atherosclerotic disease (arrowheads in A, Caldwell projection; B, lateral projection).

Due to vessel tortuosity, balloon angioplasty was conducted via a right brachial artery approach using a 6F Envoy (Cordis) catheter, a Traverse 0.014-in 300-cm wire, and sequential Photon (Guidant) 1.5-mm and 2-mm balloons at 6 atm. The resulting images (C and D postangioplasty) showed improved velocity of flow from the vertebral artery to the basilar artery, and an attempt at stenting was not performed due to the small caliber of the vessels involved.

Although the patient remained symptom-free for 6 weeks afterwards, she returned with recurrent, but milder, symptoms of posterior circulation insufficiency. A repeat diagnostic angiogram showed recurrent long-segment disease in the intradural vertebral artery (E).

with a number of abrupt, short (1 minute) inflations has been found to result in fewer procedural dissections (3% versus 9%), higher angiographic success at vessel reopening (95% versus 89%), and less residual stenosis (35% versus 38%).[24] This knowledge has been applied by Connors and Wojack in their personal experience over 9 years of evolving technique.[11] Using a technique of slow inflation of an undersized balloon, they reduced their dissection rate for intracranial PTA from 75% to 14%, and reduced their procedural complication rate accordingly. Their improved procedural and clinical outcome was also associated with incorporation of use of glycoprotein IIb/IIIa inhibitors into their protocol as well as rigorous premedication of the patient in advance of the procedure.

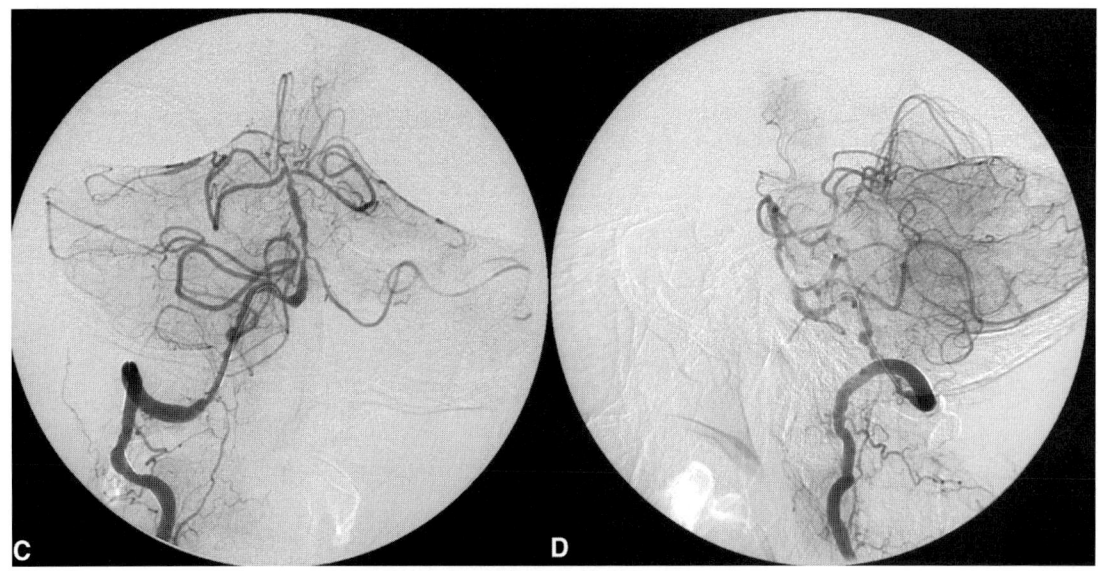
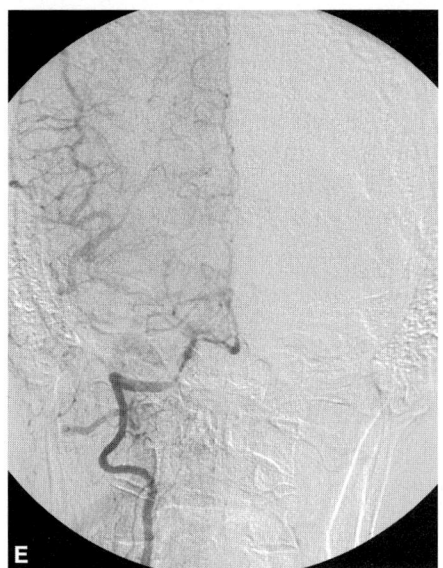

With the recognition that coronary stents are now capable of accessing the intracranial circulation, the question becomes whether intracranial PTA will be safer if supported by stent deployment, emulating the coronary experience. Certainly, for acute vessel closure due to abrupt dissection following PTA, stent deployment is essential to restore flow immediately (Fig. 5.4). Stents may prevent subacute postprocedural closure and may improve long-term patency, but this has not been established. However, the experience of even one intracranial occlusive dissection is enough to convince some operators of the benefit of primary stenting of intracranial lesions whenever possible, particularly in the petrous and cavernous segments of the internal carotid artery.[25,26]

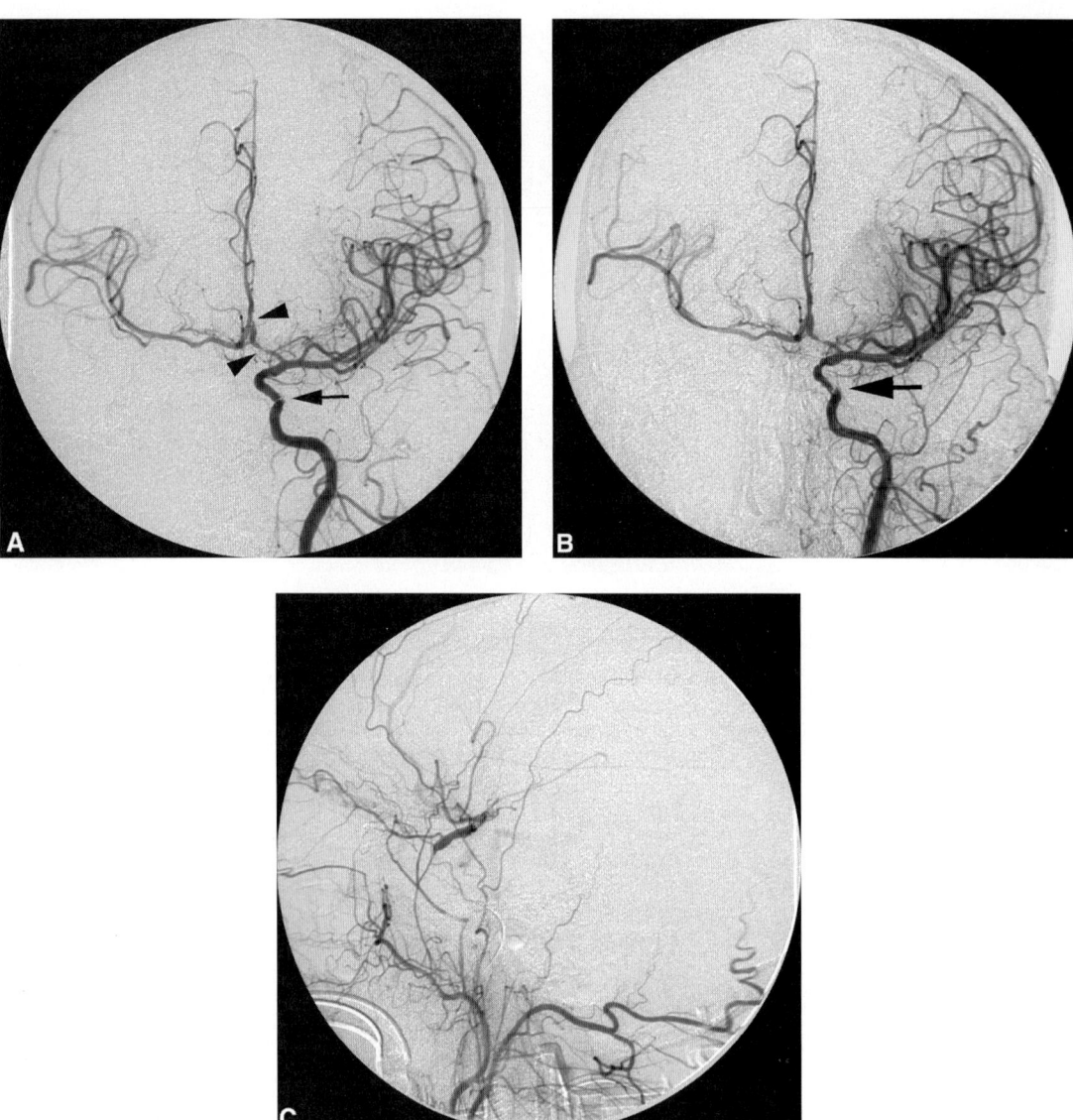

FIGURE 5.4 • *Risks of Angioplasty without Stenting.*
A 42-year-old male patient presented with bihemispheric infarctions. Angiography demonstrated a complete closure of the right internal carotid artery, a stenosis of the cavernous segment of the left internal carotid artery (A, pretreatment, arrow), and multiple intracranial stenotic areas (A, arrowheads). Because of his acute infarctions in the right hemisphere, surgical opinion was in favor of waiting a period of time before performing a bypass to the right hemisphere. However, on heparin he showed evidence of recurrent neurologic events and fluctuating deficits. As an interim measure, it was thought that an angioplasty of the left internal carotid artery cavernous stenosis might help to improve flow globally, while the patient was awaiting surgery.

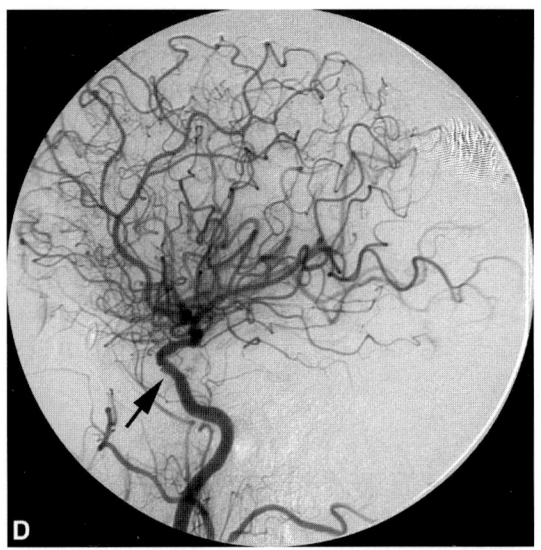

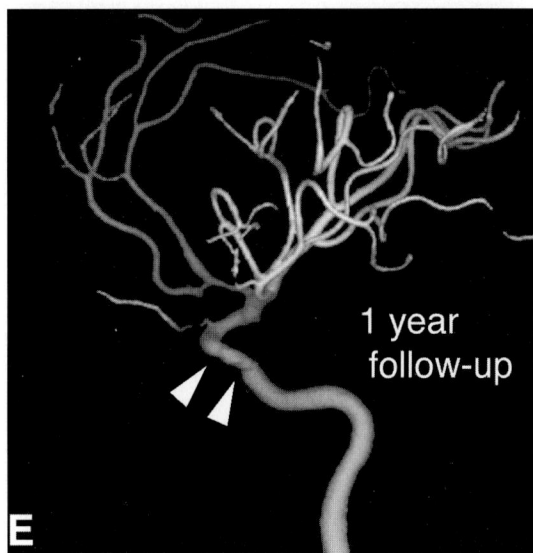

Angioplasty was performed with a 2.5-mm Surpass balloon (Boston Scientific) and a 3-mm Ranger (Boston Scientific) balloon at <6 atm of pressure. However, a dissection was apparent on the postangioplasty images (B, postangioplasty, arrow), and the vessel proceeded to complete closure within a matter of minutes (C, lateral view postangioplasty). It is important during angioplasty not to remove the wire from a vessel until one is completely satisfied with the results of the procedure. In this case maintaining the wire position following the angioplasty was pivotal to the subsequent rescue procedure. A GFX 3.5 × 8 mm stent (AVE) was advanced along the wire and inflated to 6 atm and immediately reopened the artery (D). The patient made an uneventful recovery from the procedure and subsequently had a successful bypass to the right internal carotid artery. At follow-up 12 months later, 3D angiography (E, arrowheads) demonstrates no change in the smoothly contoured left internal carotid artery stent site.

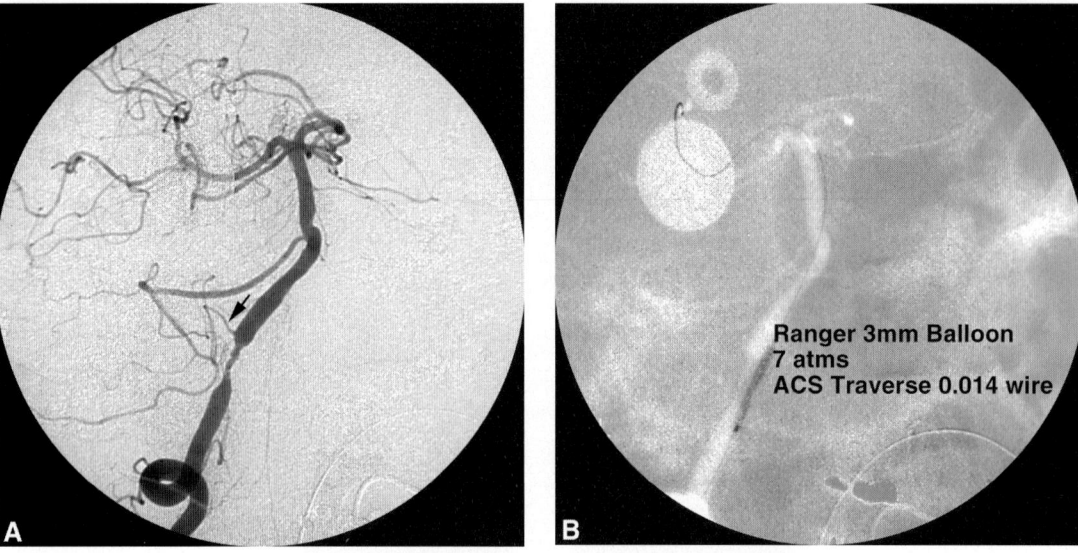
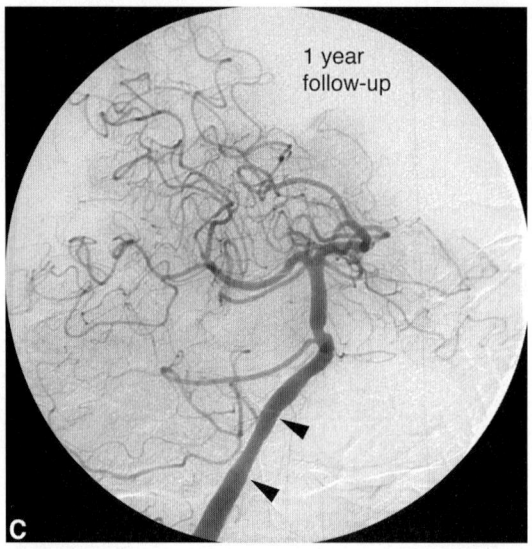

FIGURE 5.5 • *Coverage ("Jailing") of the Posterior Inferior Cerebellar Artery with a Stent at 1-Year Follow-up.*
A 43-year-old male patient presented with crescendo TIA-like symptoms of the posterior circulation with persistence of symptoms after heparinization. Angiography demonstrated an 8-mm long (Type B) lesion just proximal to the right posterior inferior cerebellar artery (A, arrow). Angioplasty was undertaken with a 2-mm Ranger balloon followed by a 3-mm Ranger balloon (Boston Scientific) at 7 atm over an ACS Traverse wire (B, intraprocedural roadmap). Following this a 4 × 12 mm GFX (AVE) stent was deployed slowly to 7 atm across the stenotic site, covering the origin of the posterior inferior cerebellar artery. The patient made an uneventful neurological recovery. He was premedicated with clopidogrel, aspirin, papaverine, nitroglycerin, heparin, and abciximab as described in the text. The case was performed under general anes-

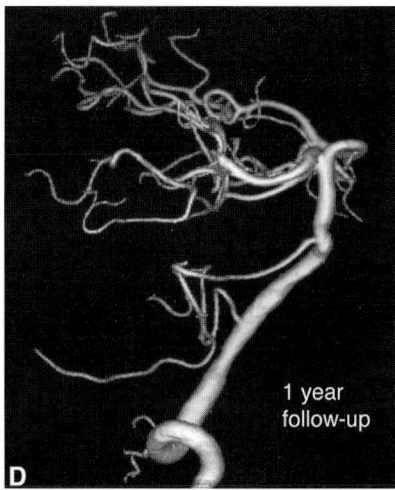

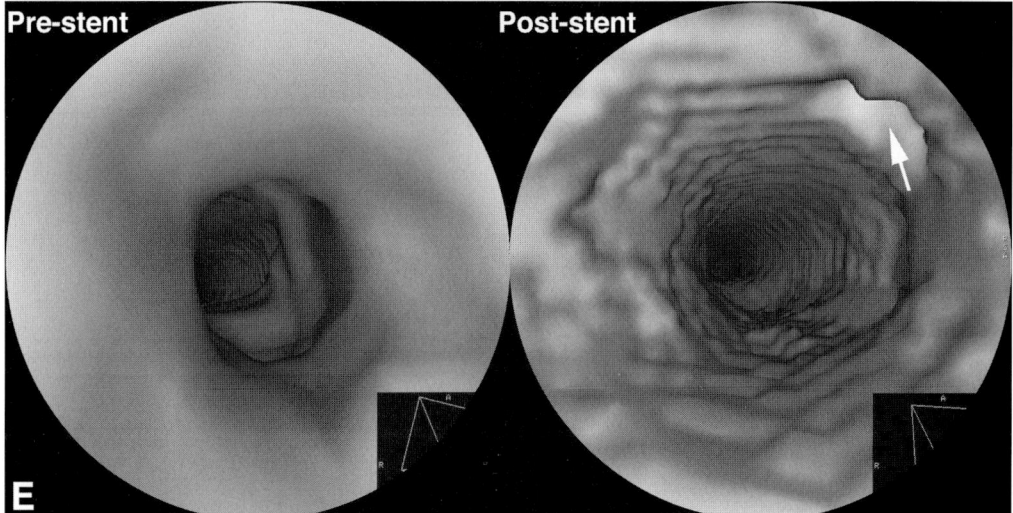

thesia, during which there were difficulties with intubation. As a result of the difficulties with tongue retraction and the administration of antiplatelet agents, the patient suffered an intraglossal hematoma persisting for a few days, which did not compromise his airway.

At 1-year follow-up the patient continues to be asymptomatic (C, arrowheads indicate stent position). The surface-rendered 3D view (D) also demonstrates the smoothly contoured healing of the site. Pre- and post-stent endoluminal images (E) demonstrate the endovascular remodeling effect of the stent and the preservation of the posterior inferior cerebellar artery (white arrow).

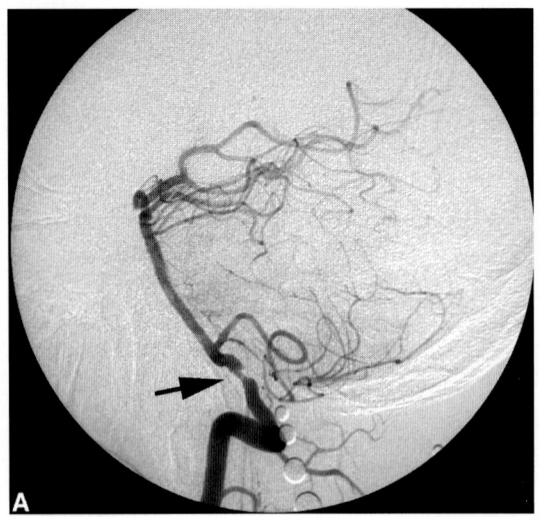 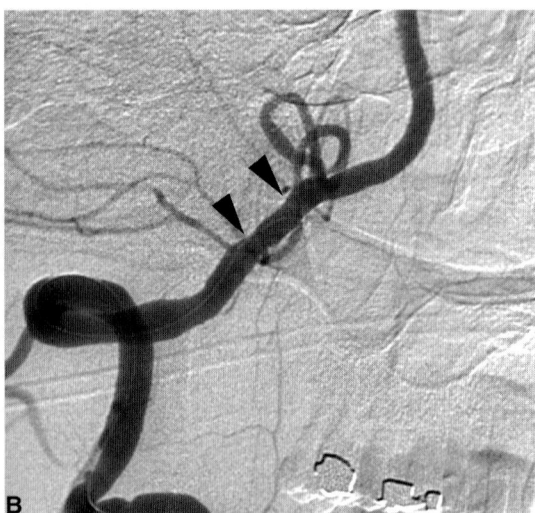

FIGURE 5.6 • *Stent of Intradural Right Vertebral Artery.*
After a successful thrombolysis for complete basilar artery thrombosis at an outside hospital (see Fig. 13.1), a 45-year-old male patient was referred for evaluation of bilateral severe intracranial vertebral artery stenosis. He had sustained cerebellar infarctions and a small brainstem infarction from the episode of thrombosis, but was doing well neurologically with mild deficits. The right vertebral artery was larger than the left, and it was decided to treat that vessel first. The pretreatment lateral view (A) shows a stenosis (arrow) of the intradural segment of the right vertebral artery proximal to the right posterior inferior cerebellar artery. Measuring ball-bearings are placed on the field of view for sizing purposes, starting at 3 mm and increasing by 1-mm increments.

The case was performed with predeployment of a 6F Closer (Perclose) device in the right common femoral artery, and the arteriotomy site was then expanded to an 8F sheath. A 7F Lumax catheter (Cook) with a matching dilator was used to catheterize the right vertebral artery. This was chosen with the assumption that the smooth transition from dilator to catheter would be less traumatic to the artery than alternative 6F or 7F catheters. However, a smaller introducer size would probably have been perfectly adequate.

After insertion of the sheath the patient was given a bolus of eptifibatide and was heparinized to an ACT of 200–230 s. Because of his 2-day-old infarctions in the posterior fossa, the heparinization was carefully monitored and the lower renal dose of eptifibatide (135 μg/kg bolus and 2 μg/kg per minute infusion) was administered out of concern for hemorrhagic complications. An accelerated loading dose of clopidogrel (300-mg) and aspirin (325 mg) was given the night before in preparation for the procedure. The artery was treated prophylactically with intraarterial papaverine (50 mg) and nitroglycerin (300 μg) before crossing the lesion with a 300-cm Choice PT wire (Boston Scientific). The stenosis was then crossed with an AVE 4 × 9 mm S670 stent inflated to 6 atm slowly with the result seen in image B (arrowheads indicate stent position). Notice that the wire in B has slipped back inadvertently to the level of the stent, and that despite premedication spasm has occurred in the upper cervical vertebral artery. The left vertebral artery was not treated on this occasion. The patient tolerated the procedure without incident and continued to make recovery after discharge home.

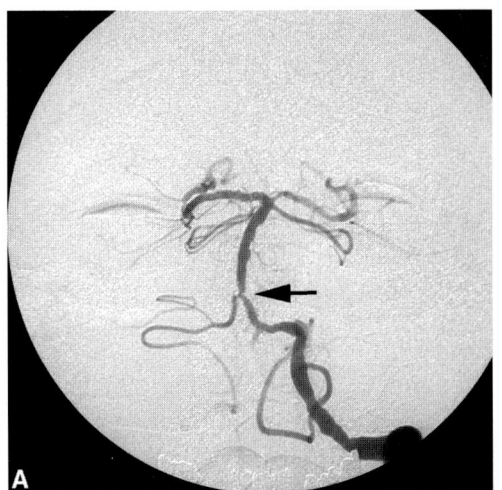
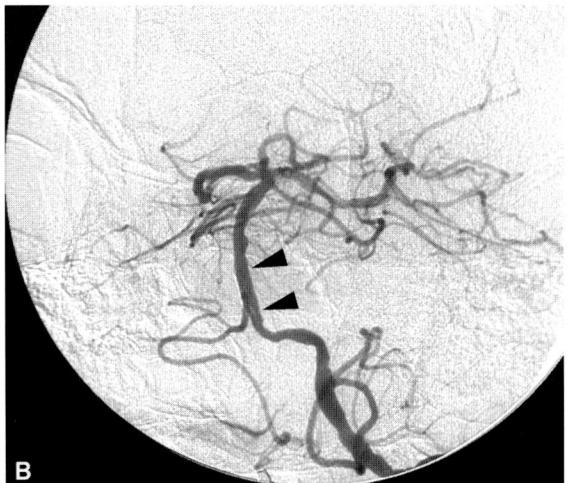
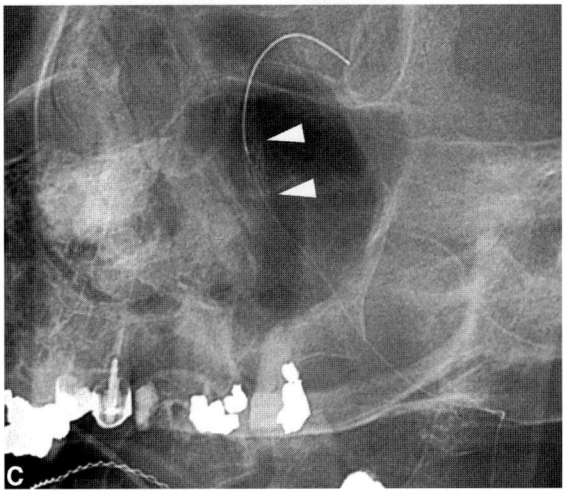

FIGURE 5.7 • *Basilar Artery Stenting with Coverage of the Right AICA-PICA Origin.*
A 66-year-old male patient presented with signs and symptoms of vertebro-basilar insufficiency despite optimal therapy with antiplatelet drugs and coumadin. Angiography demonstrates the likely culprit lesion to be his known mid-basilar stenosis at the origin of the right anterior inferior cerebellar artery, which had progressed since being imaged previously (A, arrow).

After premedication with clopidogrel and aspirin the case was performed under general anesthesia. A 6F Brite-Tip sheath (Cordis) was used for access to the left vertebral artery. A bolus of abciximab followed by a 12-hour infusion was started after the sheath was inserted, and the ACT was raised to 250 s with heparin. The lesion was crossed with an ACS Traverse 300-cm 0.014-in wire and dilated slowly with a 2 × 20 mm Ranger balloon and a 2.5 × 20 Ranger (Boston Scientific) balloon inflated to 6 atm. A 3 × 8 mm GFX2 stent (AVE) was then deployed uneventfully (B) in a position where it covered the origin of the cerebellar artery side-branches. This resulted in a satisfactory appearance of opening of the vessel without compromise of the side-branch (arrowheads in B indicate stent site). A nonsubtracted view (C) is provided as a reminder that an oblique view to remove bone artifact can assist enormously in visualizing the stent.

The patient awoke from anesthesia intact without any symptoms. However, the next day after discontinuation of the abciximab infusion the patient developed hemidysesthesia and hemiparesis of a waxing and waning character. It was thought likely that this was related to intermittent compromise of a brainstem perforator artery. After a bolus of heparin and elevation of blood pressure, his symptoms subsided within a few hours of onset without permanent deficit. He was discharged on clopidogrel and aspirin and has been asymptomatic since.

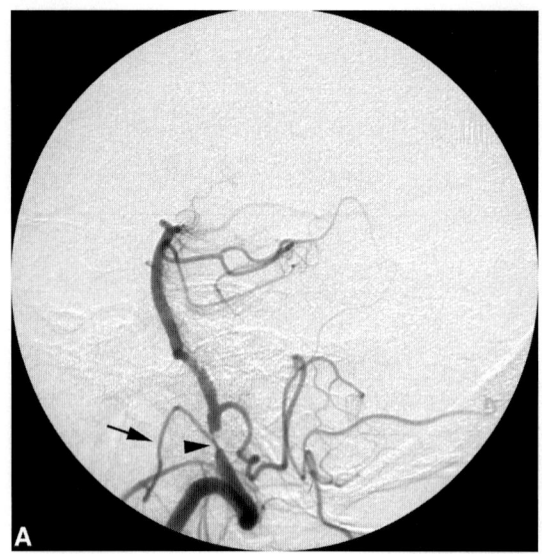 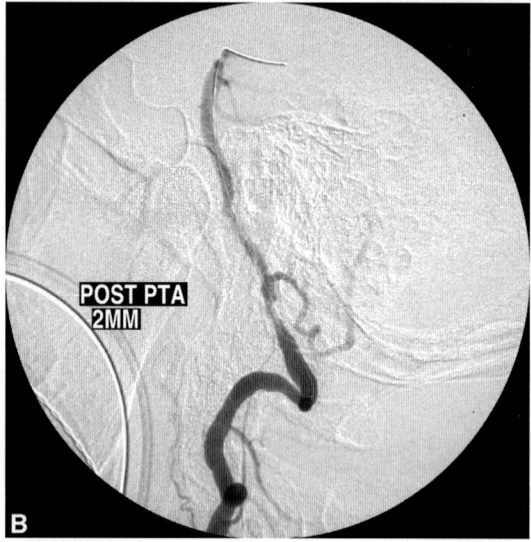

FIGURE 5.8 • *Stenting of the Intradural Left Vertebral Artery.*
A 48-year-old male patient with multiple small posterior circulation infarcts progressing over a 2-week period despite heparinization was referred for angioplasty and stenting. The right vertebral artery was occluded at the right posterior inferior cerebellar artery. The intradural left vertebral artery (A, lateral view pretreatment) shows a severe stenosis proximal to the left posterior inferior cerebellar artery (arrowhead). Due to the presence of an ipsilateral external carotid artery stenosis, there is retrograde filling of the hypoglossal branch of the ascending pharyngeal artery (arrow) overlying the stenotic lesion.

The patient was premedicated with clopidogrel and aspirin for 3 days and heparinized to an ACT of 200–250 s. Despite his acute and subacute infarctions, the use of abciximab during and after the case did not cause any hemorrhagic or other complications.

The left vertebral artery was catheterized with a 6F Brite-Tip sheath (Cordis) and the lesion was crossed with a 300-cm ACS Balance wire. Angioplasty of the lesion was performed with a 2 × 20 mm (B) and a 3 × 20 Ranger (Boston Scientific) balloon inflated slowly to <4 atm (C).

An AVE GFX 4 × 12 mm stent was advanced with great difficulty, ultimately requiring use of a Mailman 300-cm 0.014-in wire (ACS) for extra support. The posttreatment 3D image. (D) shows the stent position marked with arrowheads, while angiographic follow-up 3 months later shows minimal asymptomatic intimal growth through the struts (E, arrows).

INTRACRANIAL STENT DEPLOYMENT FOR ATHEROSCLEROTIC DISEASE

Intracranial deployment of coronary stents either with primary intent or as an emergency procedure following dissection from PTA seems to be feasible, safe, and clinically effective.[26–35] Several coronary stents have been found sufficiently flexible to reach different regions of the intracranial circulation, including the Gianturco-Roubin-2 stent,[31] and the Palmaz-Schatz stent,[26] but the greatest ease of use has been found with the Arterial Vascular Engineering (AVE) series of stents, most recently the AVE S670 stent and the Guidant Tetramultilink stent.[29,36] In the limited experience with intracranial stenting for atherosclerotic disease, late restenosis or occlusion of side-branch perforators does not seem to be a major problem (Figs. 5.5–5.9).

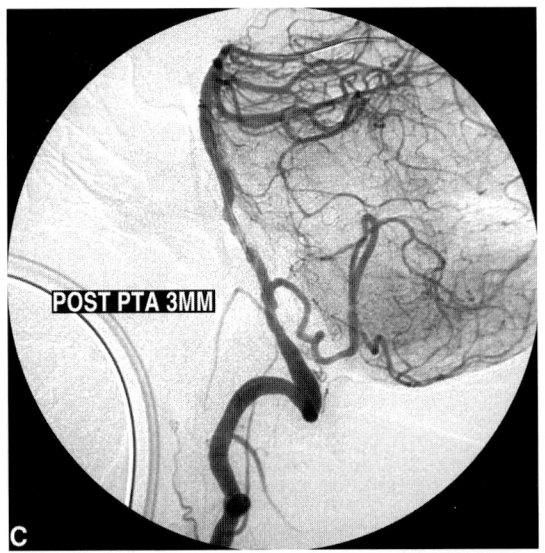
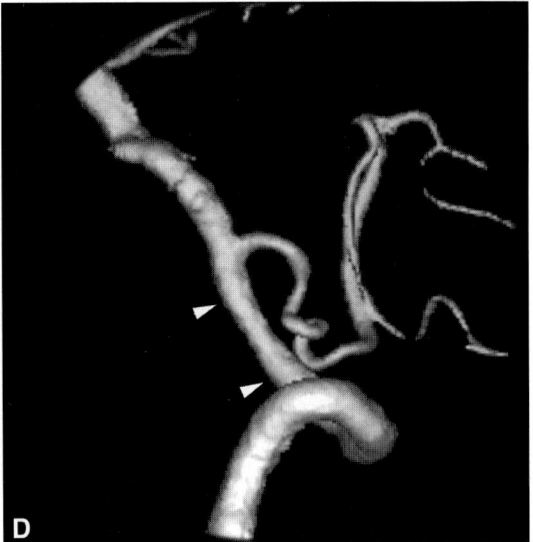
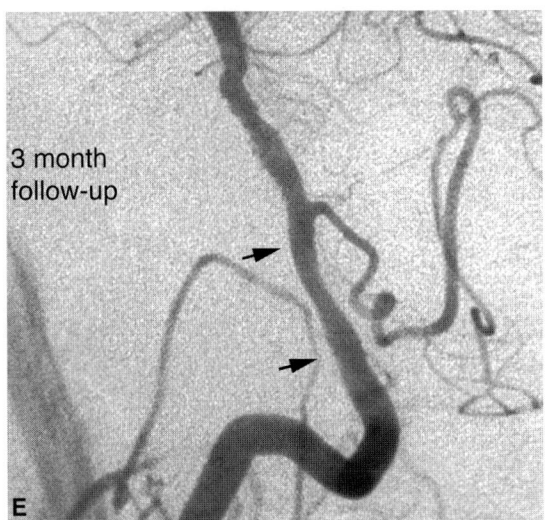

Building on their experience with 1-year restenosis rates of 33% and 100% for Type B and Type C lesions, respectively, following balloon angioplasty, Mori et al.[27] demonstrated 0% restenosis on short-term follow-up for similar lesions following balloon angioplasty followed by stent placement. In a consecutive series of eight successful angioplasties with stenting of the intracranial vessels, no complications were encountered and no ischemic strokes were seen in the relevant territories over a follow-up period of 6 months.

Suggested Medication Protocol for Intracranial Stenting

- Clopidogrel 75 mg P.O. daily or ticlopidine 250 mg B.I.D. P.O. for 5 days prior to the procedure.

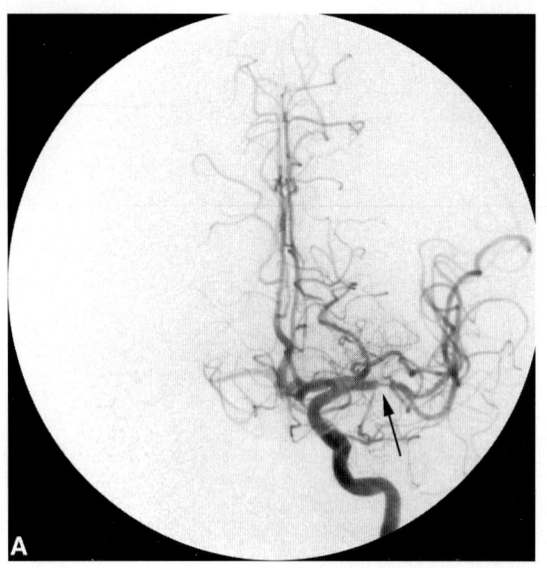
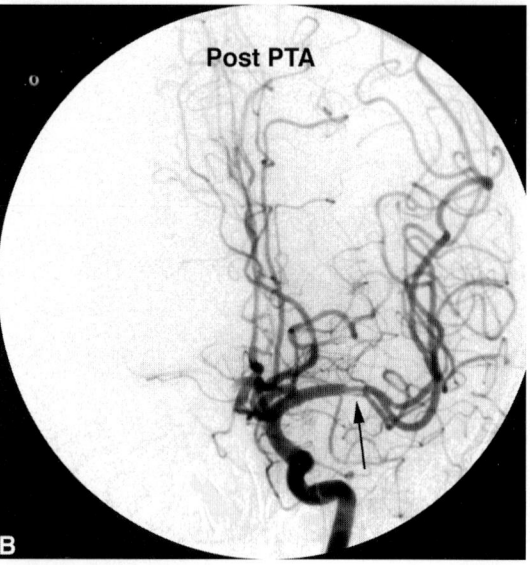
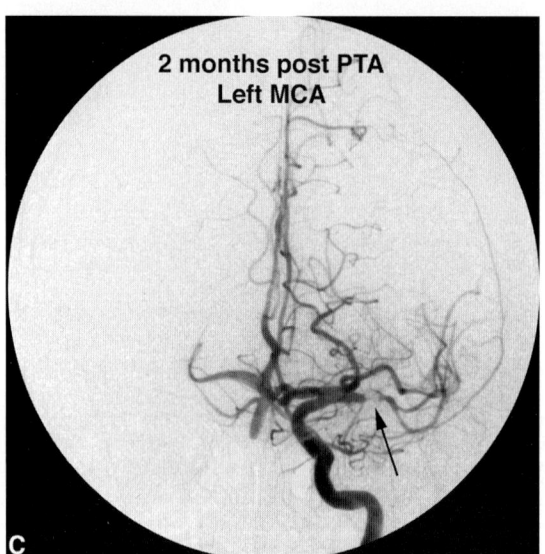

FIGURE 5.9 • *Middle Cerebral Artery Stent Placement Following Short-Term Failure of Response to Angioplasty.*
A 72-year-old female presenting with stuttering ischemic symptoms of the left hemisphere demonstrated a severe intracranial stenosis of the distal left M1 segment (A, arrow). Following angioplasty alone (B) stenosis persists (arrow) but is much improved, with a probable dissection evident on the image. However, the patient returned 2 months later with a symptomatic recurrent stenosis of the angioplasty site (C, arrow).

An intraprocedural roadmap shows a 3 mm GFX2 (AVE) stent being advanced into the stenotic site (D), with a satisfactory subsequent angiographic appearance (E). Note the preservation of flow in the lateral lenticulostriate branches (arrow in E). The patient tolerated the procedure well without further incident.

Case courtesy of Frank Huang-Hellinger MD PhD, Orlando, Florida.

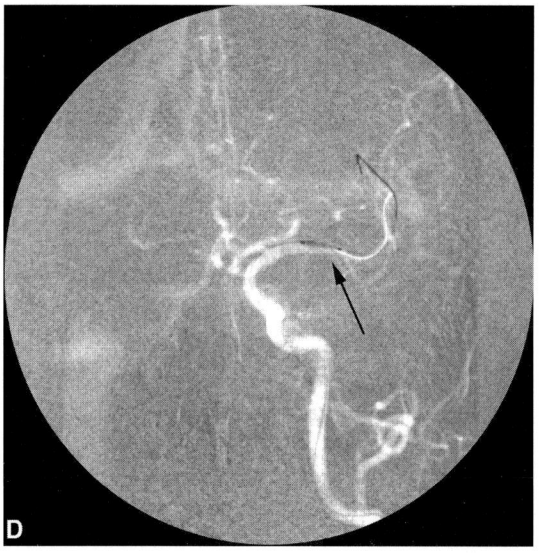
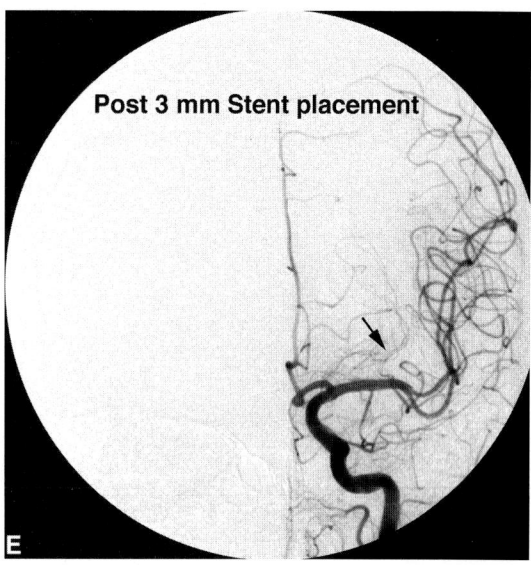

- Aspirin 325 mg P.O. daily for 5 days prior to the procedure.
- Heparinization during the procedure to an ACT of 200 seconds or slightly higher.
- Abciximab or eptifibatide loading dose and intravenous infusion started prior to the first angioplasty (not in universal use).
- Intraarterial papaverine (50–100 mg) and/or nitroglycerin (200–400 μg) into the target artery to reduce arterial spasm prior to initial angioplasty.
- Postprocedure continue abciximab or eptifibatide infusions for 12 or 24 hours, respectively (not in universal use).
- Continue aspirin and clopidogrel or ticlopidine for at least 3–6 weeks.

References

1. Craig DR, Meguro K, Watridge C, Robertson JT, Barnett HJM, Fox AJ (1982) Intracranial internal carotid artery stenosis. *Neurology* 13:825–828.
2. Marzewski DJ, Furlan AJ, St Louis P, Little JR, Modic MT (1982) Intracranial internal carotid artery stenosis: long-term prognosis. *Stroke* 13:821–824.
3. Wechsler LR, Kistler JP, Davis KR, Kaminski MJ (1986) The prognosis of carotid siphon stenosis. *Stroke* 17:714–718.
4. Bogousslavsky J, Barnett HJM, Fox AJ, Hachinski VC, Taylor W (1986) Atherosclerotic disease of the middle cerebral artery. *Stroke* 17:1112–1120.
5. Thijs VN, Albers GW (2000) Symptomatic intracranial atherosclerosis. Outcome of patients who fail antithrombotic therapy. *Stroke* 55:490–497.
6. EC/IC Bypass Study Group (1985) Failure of extracranial-intracranial arterial bypass to reduce the risk of ischemic stroke: results of an international randomized trial. *N Engl J Med* 313:1191–1200.
7. Chimowitz MI, Kokkinos J, Strong J, Brown MB, Levine SR, Silliman S, Pessin MS, Weichel E, Sila CA, Furlan AJ, Kargman DE, Sacco RL, Wityk RJ, Ford G, Fayad PB (1995) The Warfarin-Aspirin Symptomatic Intracranial Disease Study. *Neurology* 45:1488–1493.
8. Akins PT, Pilgram TK, Cross DT 3rd, Moran CJ (1998) Natural history of stenosis from intracranial atherosclerosis by serial angiography. *Stroke* 29:433–438.
9. Higashida RT, Tsai FY, Halbach VV, Dowd CF, Hieshima GB (1993) Cerebral percutaneous transluminal angioplasty. *Heart Dis Stroke* 2:497–502.
10. Volk EE, Prayson RA, Perl J (1997) Autopsy finding of fatal complications of posterior cerebral circulation angioplasty. *Arch Pathol Lab Med* 121:738–740.
11. Connors JJ, Wojak JC (1999) Percutaneous transluminal angioplasty for intracranial atherosclerotic lesions: evolution of technique and short-term results. *J Neurosurg* 91:415–423.
12. Marks MP, Marcellus M, Norbash AM, Steinberg GK, Tong D, Albers GW (1999) Outcome of angioplasty for atherosclerotic intracranial stenosis. *Stroke* 30:1065–1069.

13. Callahan AS, Berger BL (1997) Balloon angioplasty of intracranial arteries for stroke prevention. *J Neuroimag* 7:232–235.
14. Takis C, Kwan ES, Pessin MS, Jacobs DH, Caplan LR (1997) Intracranial angioplasty: experience and complications. *AJNR* 18:1661–1668.
15. Terada T, Higashida RT, Halbach VV, Dowd CF, Nakai E, Yokote H, Itakura T, Hieshima GB (1996) Transluminal angioplasty for arteriosclerotic disease of the distal vertebral and basilar arteries. *J Neurol Neurosurg Psych* 60:377–381.
16. Lee RM (1995) Morphology of cerebral arteries. *Pharmacol Ther* 66:149–173.
17. Scott GE, Neubuerger KT, Denst J (1960) Dissecting aneurysms of intracranial arteries. *Neurology* 10:22–27.
18. Nahser HC, Henkes H, Weber W, Berg-Dammer E, Yousry TA, Kühne D (2000) Intracranial vertebrobasilar stenosis: angioplasty and follow-up. *AJNR* 21:1293–1301.
19. Touho H, Takaoka M, Ohnishi H, Furuoka N, Karasawa J (1995) Percutaneous transluminal angioplasty for severe stenosis of the posterior cerebral artery: case report. *Surg Neurol* 43:42–47.
20. Touho H, Ohnishi H, Karasawa J, Furuoka N, Komatsu T (1994) Percutaneous transluminal angioplasty for acute stroke due to stenosis of major cerebral vessels: report of two cases. *Surg Neurol* 41:362–367.
21. Mori T, Fukuoka M, Kazita K, Mori K (1998) Follow-up study after intracranial percutaneous transluminal cerebral balloon angioplasty. *AJNR* 19:1525–1533.
22. Mori T, Mori K, Fukuoka M, Arisawa M, Honda S (1997) Percutaneous transluminal cerebral angioplasty: serial angiographic follow-up after successful dilatation. *Neuroradiology* 39:111–116.
23. Ryan TJ, Bauman WB, Kennedy JW, Keriakes DJ, King SB, McCallister BD, Smith SC, Ullyot DJ (1993) Guidelines for Percutaneous Transluminal Coronary Angioplasty. A Report of the American College of Cardiology/American Heart Association Task Force on Assessment of Diagnostic and Therapeutic Cardiovascular Procedures. *J Am Coll Cardiol* 22:2033–2054.
24. Ohman EM, Marquis JF, Ricci DR, Brown RIG, Knudtson ML, Kereiakes DJ, Samaha JK, Margolis JR, Niederman AL, Dean LS, Gurbel PA, Sketch MH, Wildermann NM, Lee KL, Califf RM (1994) A randomized comparison of the effects of gradual prolonged versus standard primary balloon inflation on early and late outcome. Results of a multicenter clinical trial. *Circulation* 89:1118–1125.
25. Gomez CR (1998) The role of carotid angioplasty and stenting. *Sem Neurol* 18:501–511.
26. Dorros G, Cohn JM, Palmer LE (1998) Stent deployment resolves a petrous carotid artery angioplasty dissection. *AJNR* 19:392–394.
27. Mori T, Kazita K, Chokyu K, Mima T, Mori K (2000) Short-term arteriographic and clinical outcome after cerebral angioplasty and stenting for intracranial vertebrobasilar and carotid atherosclerotic occlusive disease. *AJNR* 21:249–254.
28. Feldman RL, Trigg L, Gaudier J, Galat J (1996) Use of coronary Palmaz-Schatz stent in the percutaneous treatment of an intracranial carotid artery stenosis. *Cath Cardiovasc Diag* 38:316–319.
29. Morris PP, Martin EM, Regan J, Braden G (1999) Intracranial deployment of coronary stents for symptomatic atherosclerotic disease. *AJNR* 20:1688–1694.
30. Al-Mubarak N, Gomez CR, Vitek JJ, Roubin GS (1998) Stenting of symptomatic stenosis of the intracranial internal carotid artery. *AJNR* 19:1949–1951.
31. Phatouros CC, Higashida RT, Malek AM, Smith WS, Mully TW, DeArmond SJ, Dowd CF, Halbach VV (1999) Endovascular stenting of an acutely thrombosed basilar artery: technical case report and review of the literature. *Neurosurgery* 44:667–673.
32. Lanzino G, Fessler RD, Miletich RS, Guterman LR, Hopkins LN (1999) Angioplasty and stenting of basilar artery stenosis: technical case report. *Neurosurgery* 45:404–407.
33. Lanzino G, Wakhloo AK, Fessler RD, Hartney ML, Guterman LR, Hopkins LN (1999) Efficacy and current limitations of intravascular stents for intracranial internal carotid, vertebral, and basilar artery aneurysms. *J Neurosurg* 91:538–546.
34. Lanzino G, Guterman LR, Hopkins LN (1999) The case for stenting. *Clin Neurosurg* 45:249–255.
35. Gomez CR, Misra VK, Liu MW, Wadlington VR, Terry JB, Tulyapronchote R, Campbell MS (2000) Elective stenting of symptomatic basilar artery stenosis. *Stroke* 31:95–99.
36. Mori T, Kazita K, Seike M, Nojima Y, Mori K (1999) Successful cerebral artery stent placement for total occlusion of the vertebrobasilar artery in a patient suffering from acute stroke. Case report. *J Neurosurg* 90:955–958.

CHAPTER 6

Endovascular Treatment of Vasospasm

INTRODUCTION

Cerebral vasospasm of the major arterial vessels at the base of the brain can occur acutely and usually transiently at the time of subarachnoid hemorrhage or in a delayed manner peaking at 10–14 days later. As a clinical problem vasospasm is most commonly encountered following aneurysmal subarachnoid hemorrhage, but can also be seen following other causes of bleeding including trauma, arteriovenous malformations, and tumors.[1] The exact pathophysiology of vasospasm is uncertain but involves the products of clot degradation in the basal cisterns, especially oxyhemoglobin.[2]

Increasing availability of superoxide radicals in the days following subarachnoid hemorrhage leads to activation of protein kinase C. It is hypothesized that activation of protein kinase C causes an inhibition in the production of prostacyclin (a vasodilating agent) and an increase in the production of vasoconstricting prostaglandins. The imbalance between vasodilating and vasoconstricting messengers may cause the sustained vasospasm seen following subarachnoid hemorrhage.[3,4] Increased production of protein kinase C also leads to excessive intracellular availability of free calcium in the smooth muscle, causing phosphorylation of contractile proteins.[5] Thus calcium antagonists, particularly nimodipine, have become part of the standard treatment in subarachnoid hemorrhage patients to prevent or mitigate the severity of vasospasm.

An alternative focus of research is the hypothesis that vasospasm may be the result of a local depletion of nitric oxide (NO) due to the absorbtefacient properties of subarachnoid hemorrhage.[6] Nitric oxide is an important tonic dilator of cerebral arteries by virtue of its activation of cyclic guanosine monophosphate (cGMP). Inactivation of NO by oxyhemoglobin or superoxide radicals may be the mechanism by which posthemorrhage vasospasm is induced. Vasospasm could therefore be treated by administration of NO donor agents such as sodium nitroprusside, among others.[7,8]

Another branch of the interrelated biochemical sequelae of subarachnoid hemorrhage is the increased availability of endothelin (ET-1), a potent vasoconstrictor, an increase that may be related to the decreased availability of NO and cGMP. Endothelin-1 levels rise in response to shear stress, hypoxia, catecholamines, insulin, and angiotensin II and are counteracted by nitric oxide through the intermediary role of endothelin-3, prostaglandin E_2, and prostacyclin.[9] Cisternal injections of ET-1 can induce angiographic changes similar in appearance to vasospasm in animals, and plasma concentrations of ET-1 correlate strongly with the risk of vasospasm and ischemic deficits.[10] Endothelin and NO may play a counterbalancing role in normal arterial tone.[11] Inhibition of endothelin synthesis or endothelin receptors is a potential mode of therapy under investigation for cerebral vasospasm, complications of myocardial ischemia, and postischemic renal failure.[12]

Not all patients with cerebral vasospasm are symptomatic. Vasospasm can be seen angiographically in 30% to 70%[13,14] of patients following subarachnoid hemorrhage, of whom about half become symptomatic. The likelihood of patients becoming symptomatic has decreased since the introduction of prophylactic calcium antagonists in all subarachnoid hemorrhage patients.[15] Of those who become symptomatic, approximately 50% will develop infarction or die as a direct result of the vasospasm if not treated. More aggressive Triple H therapy (hemodilution, hypertension, hypervolemia) can improve the outcome of symptomatic patients. Nevertheless, among patients who survive an ictus of subarachnoid hemorrhage, 15% or more may die or sustain significant neurological injury as a result of delayed vasospasm despite maximal therapy. The International Cooperative Study on the timing of aneurysm surgery demonstrated that 13.5% of patients who survived an aneurysmal bleed later died or became disabled from vasospasm, and that vasospasm accounts for 39% of subsequent disability.[16] Because vasospasm is a transient phenomenon lasting a few days to a week at its most critical level, such outcomes are potentially avoidable in some patients with earlier and more aggressive treatment for vasospasm.

The mechanism of neurological injury with vasospasm is now accepted to be ischemic, as demonstrated by studies using positron emission tomography (PET) and single photon emission computed tomography (SPECT).[17,18] These studies demonstrate alterations in regional cerebral blood flow (rCBF) and increased oxygen extraction in territories affected by proximal vasospasm, effects that can be partially reversed by endovascular and maximal medical therapy. Studies of vasospastic patients undergoing treatment with papaverine and balloon angioplasty by monitoring jugular bulb oxygenation and degree of lactic acidosis confirm that the fundamental element of this disease state is cerebral ischemia.[19] The onset of ischemia is usually gradual and is heralded by focal deficits such as hemiplegia, aphasia, confusion, or hemisensory deficits in the anterior circulation. In the posterior circulation typically altering levels of consciousness or problems with dysarthria, diplopia, or ataxia can be seen. These early clinical signs of onset of vasospasm may initially be completely reversible with amplification of medical therapy. The reversibility of clinical signs of early vasospasm by such bedside measures has meant that endovascular therapy for vasospasm was therefore reserved for patients who progressed to more severe and later levels of vasospasm. However, there is a growing opinion that earlier endovascular intervention at the time of initial onset of significant vasospasm may have a greater role to play in addition to standard medical management.

Risk Factors for Vasospasm

The risk of vasospasm is proportional to the volume of subarachnoid blood present. The Fisher Scale[20] rated the degree of blood in the subarachnoid space on the CT scan at initial presentation and found a correlation with the likelihood of onset of subsequent vasospasm. Female patients and patients who smoke have also been found to have an increased risk of significant vasospasm following subarachnoid hemorrhage.[21-23] Cigarette smoking as a risk factor independent of the Fisher CT scale at presentation increases the likelihood of clinically significant vasospasm by a factor of 2.5, and is also associated with presentation with subarachnoid hemorrhage at a younger age.

Diagnosis of Vasospasm

The preferred method for detection of vasospasm is with routine monitoring of cerebral blood flow using transcranial Doppler monitoring (TCD) introduced by Aaslid et al. in 1982.[24] Normal values for velocity of flow in all of the major intracranial arteries have been established, although velocities can be increased by concurrent Triple-H therapy:

- Middle cerebral artery: 90–120 cm/s (approximately)
- Anterior cerebral artery: 80–110 cm/s
- Posterior cerebral artery: 60–90 cm/s[25]

A sudden rise in velocity readings on the TCD above 120 cm/s is suspicious for onset of vasospasm. At velocities between 120 and 200 cm/s the severity of vasospasm can sometimes be difficult to judge clinically. The Lindegaard carotid index attempts to eliminate the effects of hemodynamic factors related to medical therapy by evaluating the ratio between middle cerebral artery TCD velocity and extracranial internal carotid velocity.[26] A carotid index of greater than 3 or intracranial velocities greater than 120 cm/s are usually predictive of spasm at angiography, although the degree of spasm can be variable. Ratios of 5 or velocities of greater than 200 cm/s have a greater positive predictive value for the spasm being severe at angiography. However, frequently the results of TCD monitoring can be difficult to interpret, and clinical evaluation of the patient remains an important component of decision making. Vora et al.[27] found that TCD values between 120 cm/s and 200 cm/s had a weak predictive value and thus were not dependable in this range.

Long-Term Histologic Effects of Vasospasm

Microstructural changes in the arterial wall occur over a period of days in the setting of severe vasospasm. Because these effects have an adverse impact on the compliance of the arterial wall and responsiveness to vasodilator agents, they are of concern in the endovascular treatment of vasospasm. Animal and human studies have shown areas of thickening and discontinuation of the elastic lamina, smooth muscle vacuolation and myonecrosis, migration of myointimal cells to the intimal surface, periadventitial inflammation, and ultimately medial and subendothelial fibrosis in spastic cerebral arteries following subarachnoid hemorrhage.[28–32] These sequelae have an impact on the risks and efficacy of endovascular treatment of vasospasm. It is a well-recognized phenomenon that vasospastic vessels become less responsive to the dilator effects of papaverine over the course of many days of endovascular treatment of vasospasm. It is likely, although not demonstrable in humans, that the decreasing responsiveness of the vessels to papaverine correlates with the histologic changes described above. It is also likely that the decreasing compliance of the arterial wall in response to these microstructural changes requires that greater stress be applied to the wall of the vessel during balloon angioplasty (PTA) for relief of vasospasm. The increased balloon pressure required for effective PTA in this circumstance probably translates into greater risk of arterial rupture during the procedure.

Although these concerns are partially speculative for human patients, rat and monkey experiments confirm the hypothesis that decreasing responsiveness to papaverine over the course of a vasospastic episode correlates with histologic changes.[33] Fujiwara et al.[34] studied the effects of papaverine in monkey subjects in which vasospasm had been induced by experimentally contrived subarachnoid hemorrhage. The monkeys were studied 3 and 7 days following the subarachnoid hemorrhage. They were found to have greater responsiveness to papaverine by TCD and angiographic criteria at 3 days than at 7 days, and this correlated with histologic changes of intimal corrugation and muscular hypertrophy of the middle cerebral artery. The dilation induced by papaverine was almost completely eliminated in both groups 24 hours later. This argues inauspiciously for the efficacy of papaverine therapy alone in humans, in whom studies have consistently demonstrated the evanes-

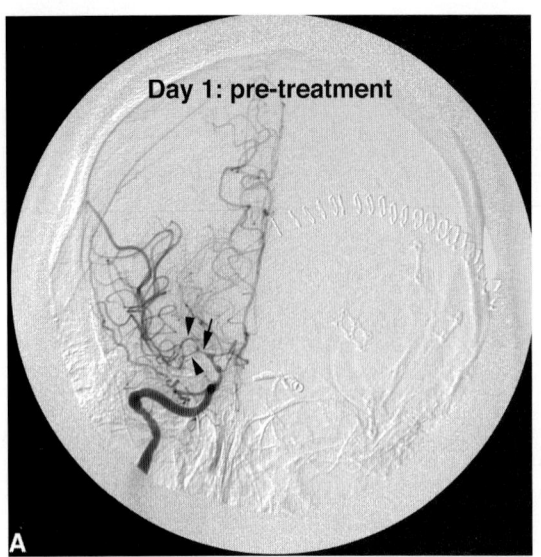
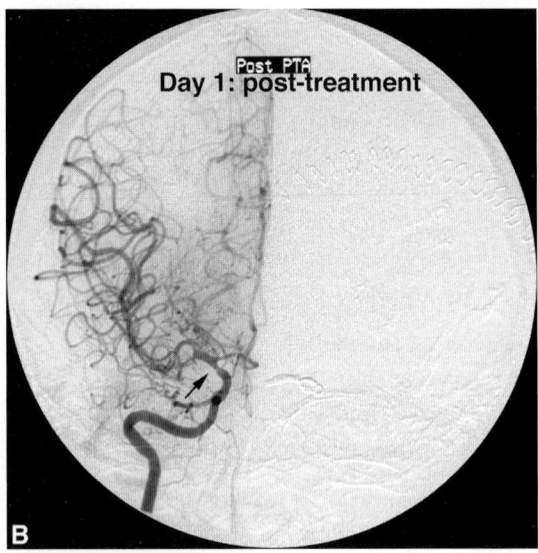
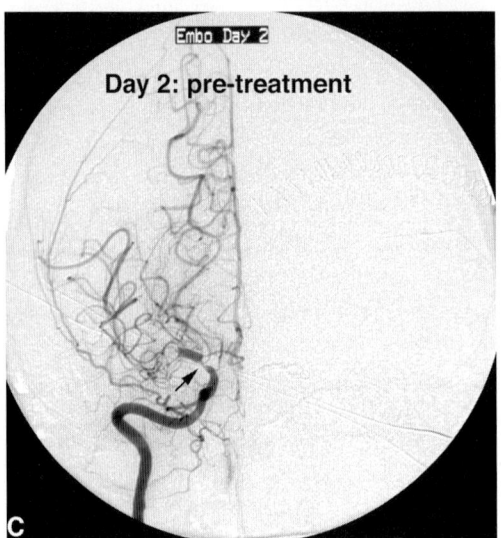

FIGURE 6.1 • *Durability of the Vessel Response to Balloon Angioplasty Compared with Papaverine.* A 35-year-old female patient was treated for vasospasm over the course of 5 days with balloon angioplasty and papaverine infusions. On day 1 (A) extreme vasospasm is evident proximally (arrow) and distally (arrowheads) in the circle of Willis, and was treated with proximal vessel angioplasty and papaverine infusion with a reasonable result (B). The arrow in image B at the end of day 1 points to an area of vessel that responded well to papaverine and which was therefore skipped during balloon angioplasty.

On the next day (C) it is clear that only the segments treated with the balloon on the previous day have had a durable response. The short segment of the supraclinoid internal carotid artery skipped over during balloon PTA on the previous day demonstrates severe recurrent spasm (arrow) in contrast to the vessel proximally and distally, areas that were treated with balloon PTA on day 1.

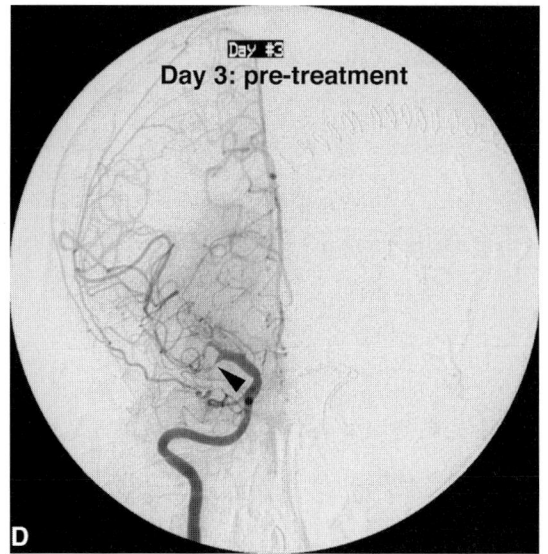
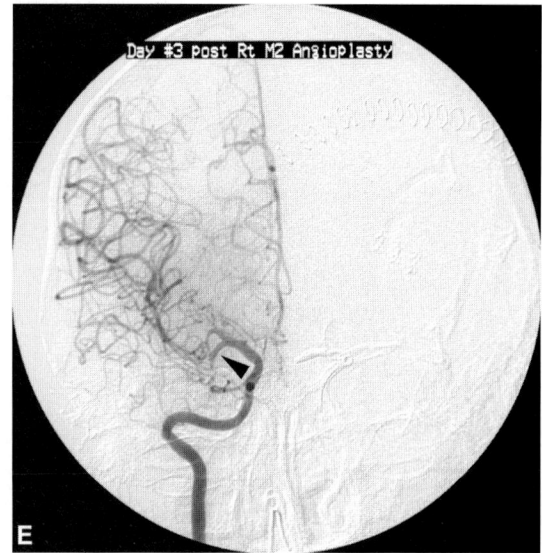
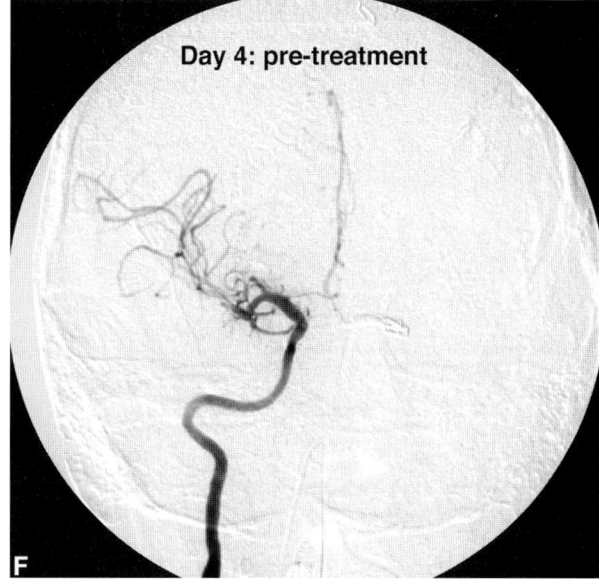

On the start of day 3 (D) the proximal vessels are now showing an enduring response, whereas the distal vessels (arrowhead), hitherto treated only with papaverine, have severely recurrent spasm. The inferiorly directed M2 branch was specifically targeted for balloon PTA at least along its proximal course (E, arrowhead). On the start of day 4 (F), only those vessel segments treated by balloon PTA continue to demonstrate an enduring response.

This case in its angiographic evolution and ultimate poor clinical outcome demonstrates the evanescent, and perhaps illusory, response of the spastic vessels to papaverine and the need for more aggressive distal vessel angioplasty early in the course of treatment in such patients.

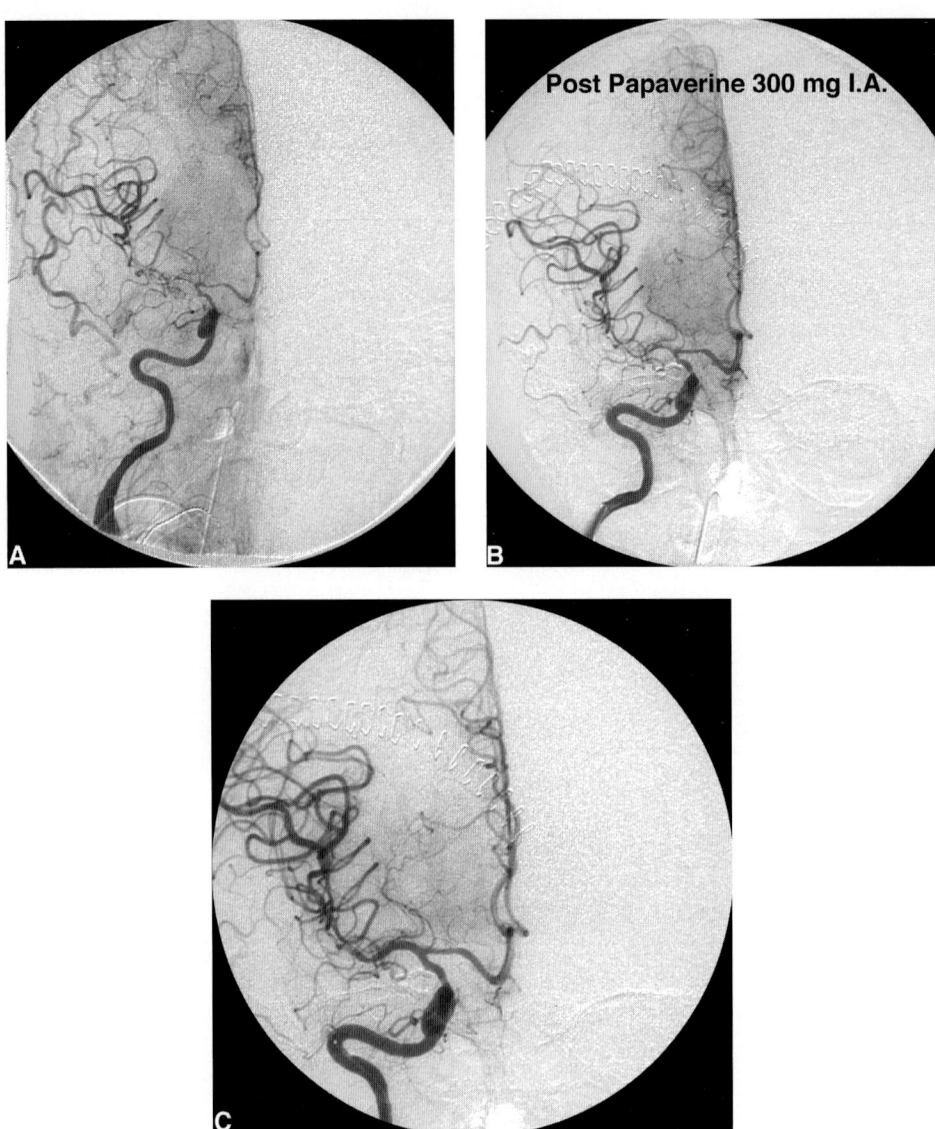

FIGURE 6.2 • *Relative Efficacy of Papaverine Versus Balloon Angioplasty.*
A 64-year-old female with symptomatic vasospasm demonstrates extreme vasospasm of the intracranial vessels (A). After supraclinoid infusion of papaverine 300 mg, there is some improvement (B). However, the increment of improvement following balloon angioplasty of the supraclinoid carotid and M1 segment is substantial (C). Furthermore, one can expect the changes wrought by balloon angioplasty to be more sustained than those related to papaverine alone.

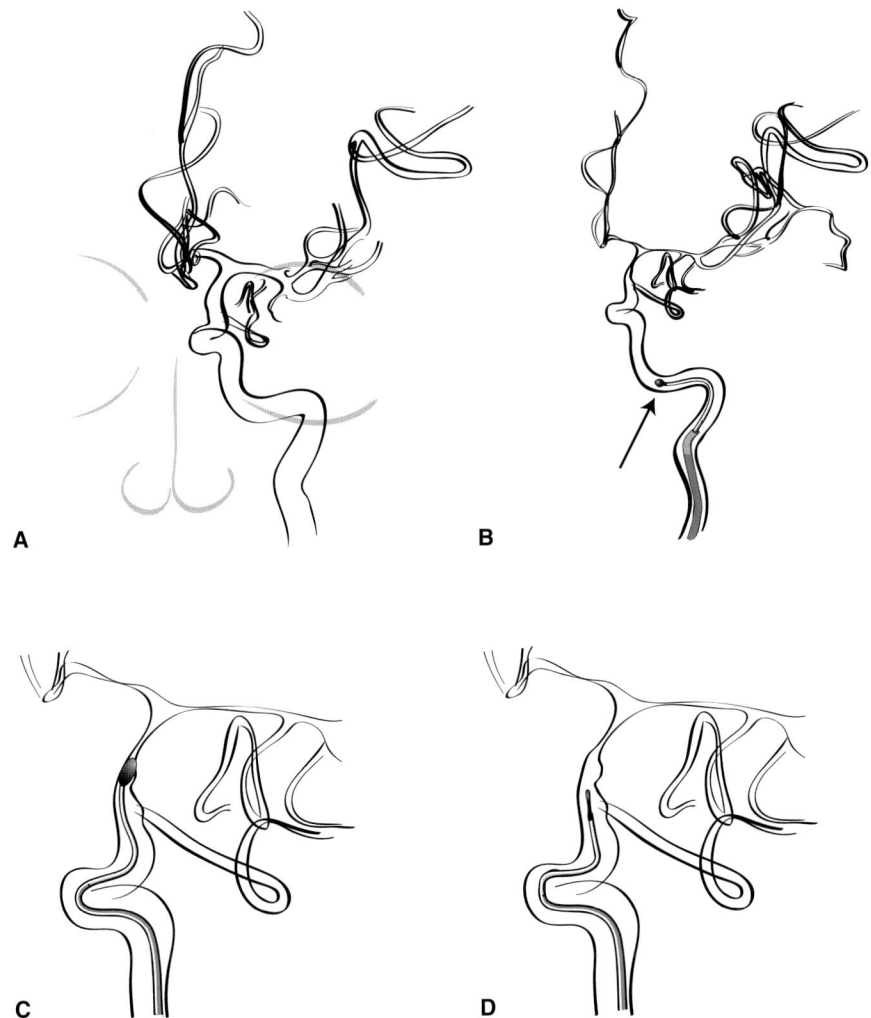

FIGURE 6.3 • *Using a Compliant Endeavor Balloon for Proximal-to-Distal Vasospasm Angioplasty.* Diagrams based on an actual case illustrate the technique for gentle repetitive angioplasty with small increments of balloon pressure. Some authors have promoted a distal-to-proximal approach for angioplasty for vasospasm, allowing the balloon to float distally before inflating it, and then working back to the proximal vessels. Often, however, the vessels are so spastic that even small balloons cannot enter them easily. Image A represents the patient at the time of the diagnostic angiogram 1 week previously. It is very important to have the previous angiogram in the angiography suite so as to avoid PTA of hypoplastic or previously small vessels.

Using the illustrated proximal-to-distal approach, the first inflation of the Endeavor balloon (Target) is made in a safe area of the vessel, e.g., petrous segment or cervical segment, to confirm the correct functioning of the balloon mechanism, visibility of the contrast, and ease of deflation. The balloon is then inflated minimally and allowed to float distally until it wedges itself in the proximal end of the spastic segment. In the supraclinoid location illustrated in C, it is vitally important to be sure that the balloon is not wedged in a hypoplastic posterior communicating artery or the anterior choroidal artery. A small increment of pressure, barely discernible to the eye, is applied slowly, and the balloon is deflated and pulled proximally, reinflated a little, and the procedure is repeated. Intermittent digital runs can be performed to monitor progress. The procedure must be done slowly to stretch rather than rupture the vessel. Although most experience with intracranial balloon angioplasty has been gained with the blind-ending Endeavor balloon, it almost certainly will be supplanted for this purpose by the wire-directed compliant balloons now available.

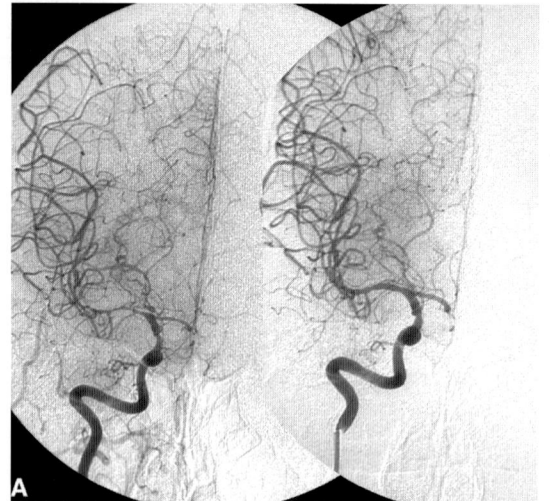 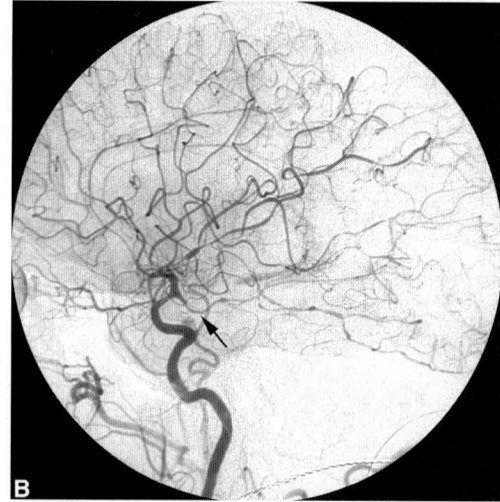

FIGURE 6.4 • *Balloon Angioplasty of the Proximal Circle of Willis. Always Be Absolutely Certain Where the Balloon Is before Inflating.*
Using the principles illustrated in Fig. 6.3, gentle balloon angioplasty was conducted in a 34-year-old female with idiopathic postpartum subarachnoid hemorrhage followed by symptomatic vasospasm. Pre- and posttreatment images (PTA and papaverine) of the right internal carotid artery demonstrate substantial improvement in the angiographic appearance of perfusion of the right hemisphere (A).

In the left carotid tree (B, lateral, pretreatment) severe proximal and peripheral vasospasm is present, raising the question of an underlying arteritis as the cause for her angiogram negative subarachnoid hemorrhage. Note the position of the spastic posterior communicating artery. Devices have a remarkable capacity to seek inadvertently the posterior communicating artery, and this can represent a hazard for rupture during balloon angioplasty if one thinks on an AP roadmap that the balloon is still within the supraclinoid carotid artery.

In this patient the balloon's inclination to seek the posterior communicating artery was used to perform a very diffident PTA in that vessel (C, roadmap image). Note the extremely low degree of inflation of the balloon (arrow in C) in contrast to the degree of inflation used in the right middle cerebral artery (D, roadmap, arrow). Posttreatment images (E) of the left internal carotid artery show the substantial proximal improvement in the posterior communicating artery and posterior cerebral artery.

cence, less than 24 hours, of the papaverine response.[35] Canine experiments with vasospasm have suggested that the therapeutic effect of papaverine may be as short as 10 minutes[36] to 2 hours.[37]

Early Endovascular Intervention for Vasospasm

With increased experience of endovascular treatment for cerebral vasospasm, many centers are moving toward a more aggressive and early approach to treatment. Zubkov et al. from St. Petersburg who first described the technique of intracranial PTA for vasospasm recommends treatment with PTA early, before the spasm becomes florid and the patient's condition more tenuous.[38] Therefore at many neurosurgical centers, instead of a trial of escalation of Triple-H therapy with calcium antagonists alone in response to a spasm-related deficit in the hope that endovascular therapy can

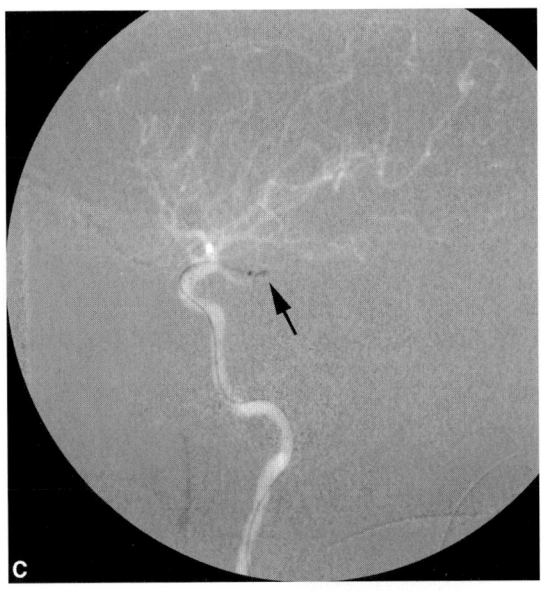
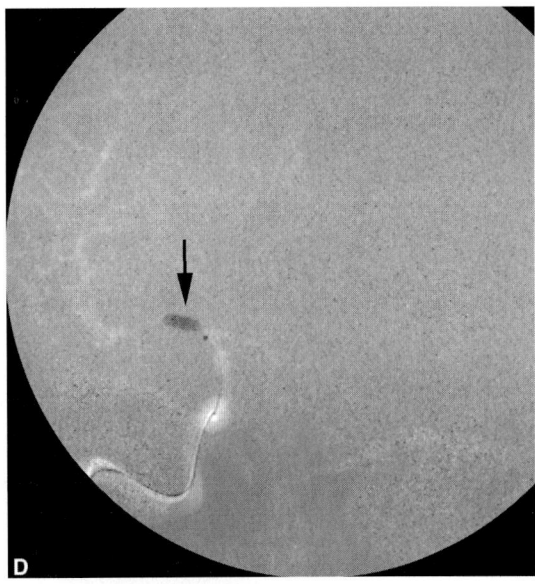
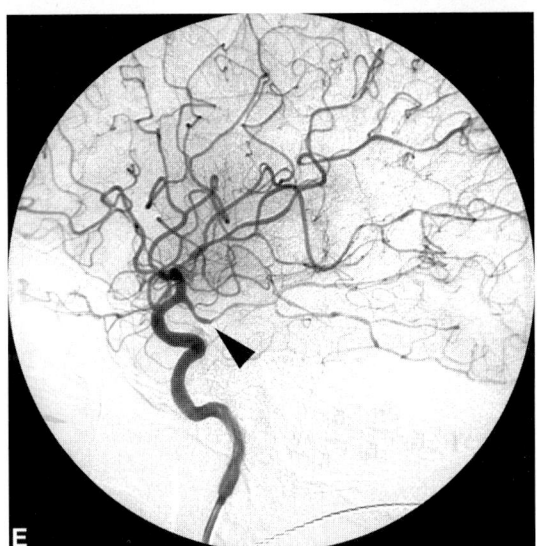

be avoided, patients are brought immediately to the endovascular suite for therapy under general anesthetic. There has also been a recognition that papaverine therapy alone may be inadequate or insufficient as a mode of endovascular treatment,[39–41] with a greater emphasis being placed on balloon angioplasty as the more effective means of achieving durable reversal of vasospasm.[42–45]

Rosenwasser et al.[45] demonstrated that patients treated within a 2-hour window of onset of vasospasm by endovascular PTA and papaverine infusion had an improved long-term outcome compared with patients treated later or equivalently ill patients treated by medical therapy alone. They and other authors have observed that the improvements in vessel caliber and peripheral perfusion wrought with PTA are more enduring than the transient improvements seen with papaverine infusions.[45–48] The ischemic effects of vasospasm are graduated in degree initially, and therefore a functional deficit

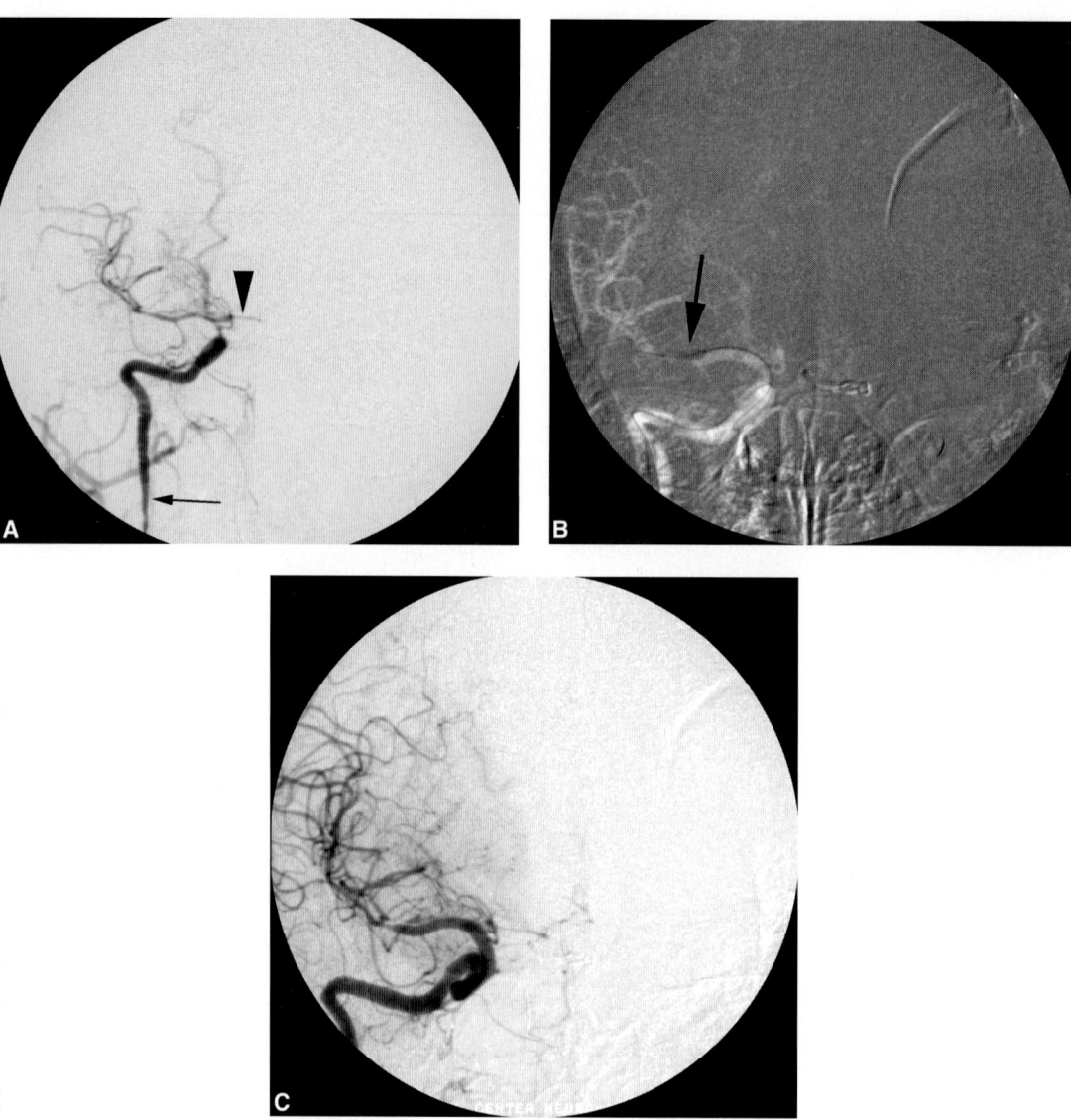

FIGURE 6.5 • *Wire-Directed Commodore Balloon (Cordis) for Vasospasm.*
A right internal carotid angiogram (A) in a 36-year-old postpartum patient with subarachnoid hemorrhage illustrates a number of important points. First, the threadlike anterior cerebral artery (arrowhead) must not be assumed to be in spasm. A prior angiogram showed it to be a hypoplastic vessel. Balloon angioplasty of such a vessel would have a high risk of rupture. Second, extreme vasospasm of the cervical internal carotid artery (arrow), even though the patient is under general anesthesia, is commonly seen in subarachnoid hemorrhage patients with cerebral vasospasm. This predisposes to the risk of dissection during long cases or to induction of ischemia through undetected interruption of flow to the hemisphere due to overlooked vasospasm at the catheter tip. One must be especially vigilant to monitor for catheter-related vasospasm during such cases.

A roadmap image (B) during the case demonstrates the Commodore balloon (Cordis) inflating at the M1/M2 junction. The postdilation images (C) demonstrate the immediate efficacy of balloon angioplasty. Distal flow seemed to be significantly improved, and therefore the spasm at the origin of the M2 segments was not pursued on this occasion.

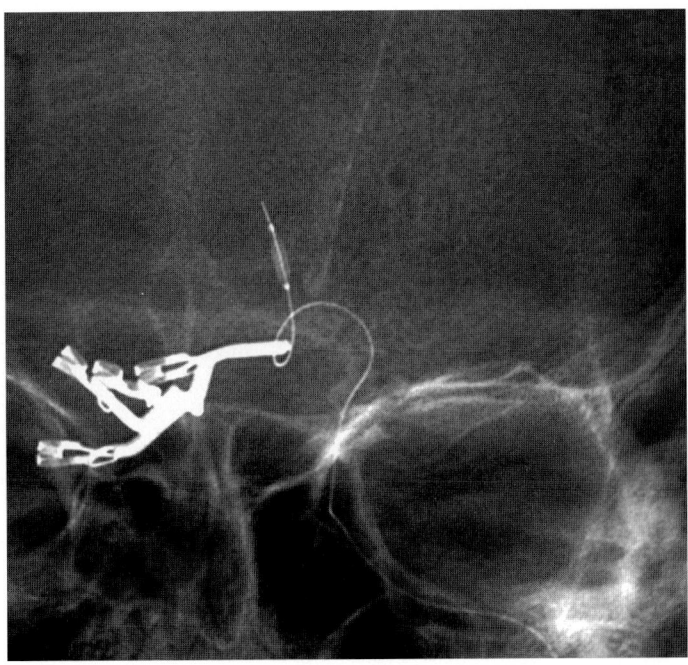

FIGURE 6.6 • The Sentry balloon (Target) inserted over a 0.010-in wire also demonstrates excellent visibility and performance with consistent ease of access to the distal vessels, as in this case of uncomplicated A2 angioplasty. Inflation of the balloon is minimal due to the extremely small size and delicacy of the vessels involved.

does not immediately imply an irreversible ischemic injury to the brain, even in the setting of low attenuation on the CT scan. Partially ischemic brain territories can become edematous on CT, an effect sometimes reversed by endovascular therapy without development of infarction. Even beyond the 2-hour window described by Rosenwasser et al. there is potential for effective endovascular therapy. Bejjani et al.[49] found that patients treated within 24 hours of onset of symptoms related to ischemia had a generally favorable outcome, as did some patients treated even later. Prevention of extension of ischemia to other territories and rescue of the noninfarcted ischemic penumbra probably accounts for their favorable results. Frequently, a pretreatment CT demonstrating hypodensities related to vasospastic ischemia can be difficult to interpret. The risk of reperfusion hemorrhage in an infarction following PTA is fairly low, and one might incline to give the patient the benefit of aggressive therapy as

a general rule to increase the likelihood of avoiding completed infarction in suspected territories. Even proponents of xenon-enhanced CT acknowledge that perfusion criteria for infarcted tissue versus ischemic injury established in other patient groups might not be applicable in vasospastic patients.[50]

It has been found in canine studies that prophylactic balloon PTA performed before the onset of vasospasm can prevent its development, presumably through some disruptive effect on the mural smooth muscle.[51] Prophylactic use of PTA has been used in a small series of patients with Fisher Grade 3 subarachnoid hemorrhage.[52] This series of patients subsequently had an outcome of only mild vasospasm with favorable rates of neurologic improvement. However, one patient died in this series from a complication related to the procedure, a ruptured posterior inferior cerebellar artery following patient motion and roadmap misregistration. Absolute immobility of the patient,

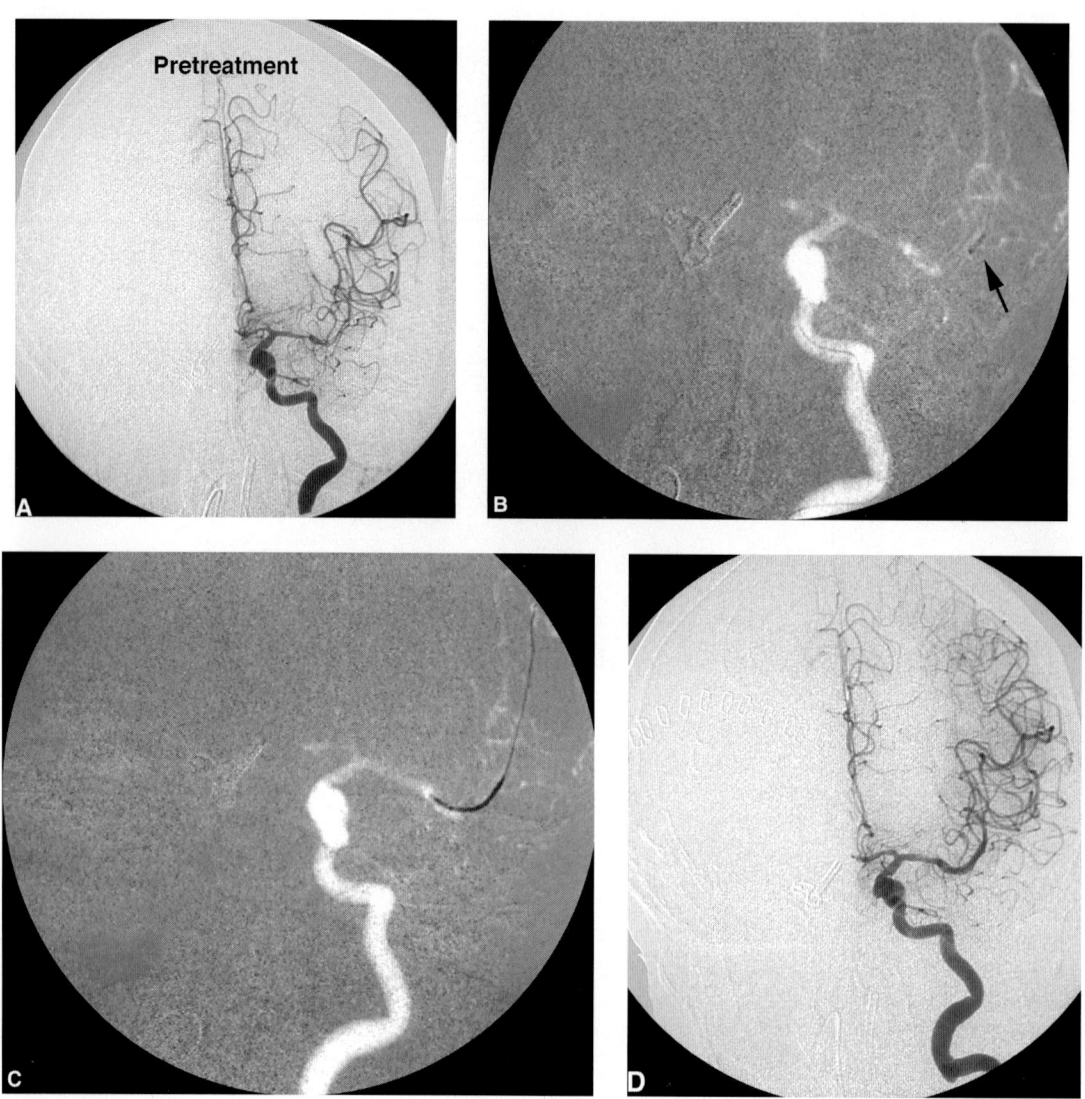

FIGURE 6.7 • *Distal Vessel Angioplasty.*
A 76-year-old female patient with severe vasospasm of the intracranial left internal carotid artery (A) was treated with proximal and distal segment angioplasty using a variety of balloons. An Endeavor balloon, stiffened and curved with a 0.010-in wire, was used to dilate the M1 and M2 segments (B, roadmap, arrow) and the A1 segment. Residual areas of spasm in the proximal M2 segments were then treated with a 2 × 10 mm Fastealth balloon (Target) over a 0.014-in Fasdasher wire (C). This wire was used in preference to the obturating Valve wire, so as to assure distal decompression of the balloon through leakage around the wire. The posttreatment image (D) shows the improved segments. The Fastealth balloon has been eclipsed by newer less rigid wire-directed balloons that have become available since this case was performed. Note that in all images the degree of inflation is minimal and that extreme deference is paid throughout to the size and fragility of the intracranial vessels.

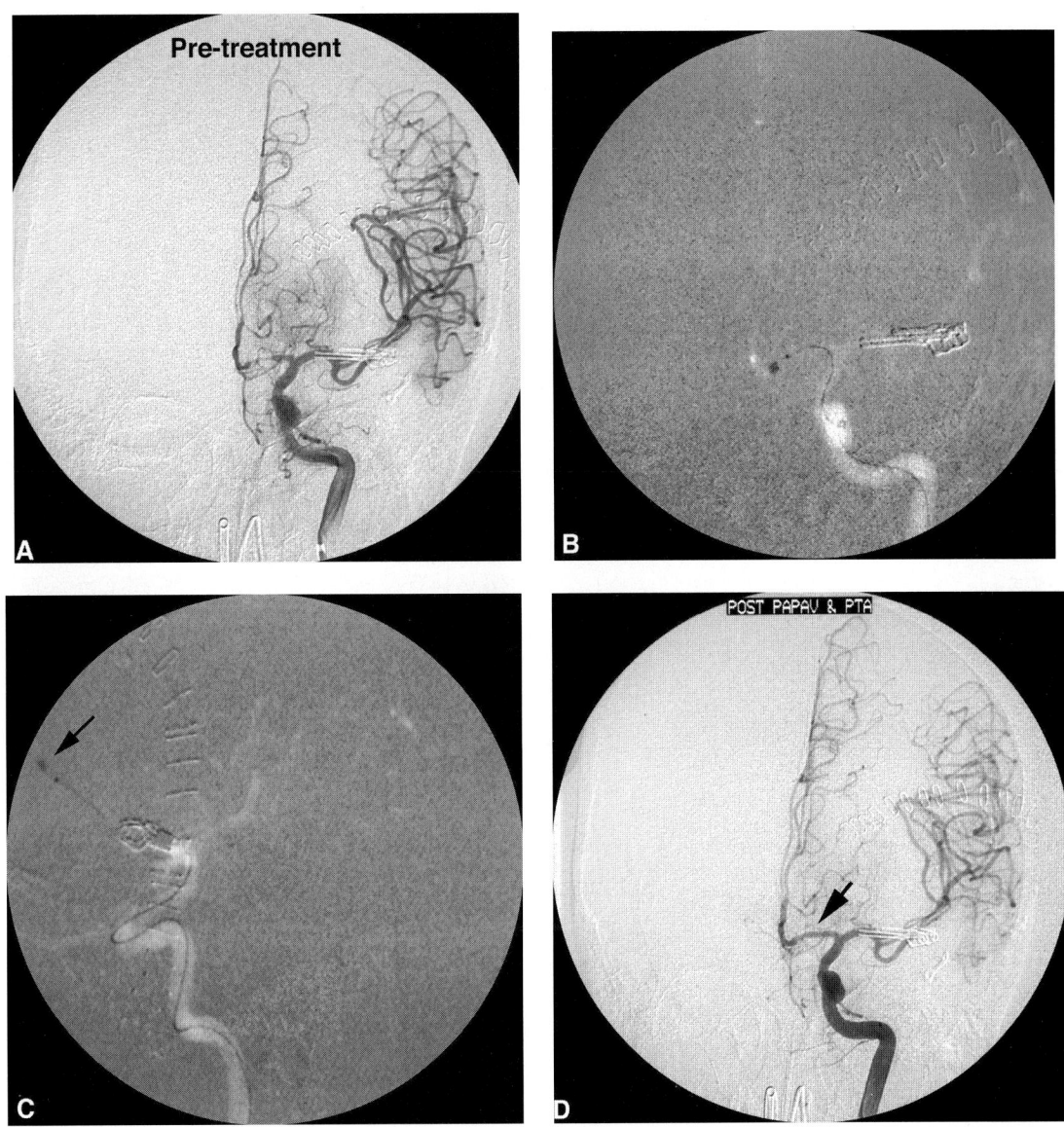

FIGURE 6.8 • *Distal Vessel Angioplasty.*
In this patient a left middle cerebral artery aneurysm has been clipped with loss of a branch of the left middle cerebral artery. Severe intracranial spasm of the anterior cerebral artery in particular (A) was treated by a combination of papaverine and balloon PTA, including the A1 segment (B, roadmap in AP projection) and the A2 segment (C, lateral view roadmap) with improvement in flow (D). Note the extremely low state of inflation of the balloon in all instances.

FIGURE 6.9 • A 45-year-old female referred for intracranial angioplasty following subarachnoid hemorrhage treated by coil embolization of a right posterior communicating aneurysm and an anterior communicating aneurysm. The images demonstrate various uses of the Endeavor balloon during vasospasm therapy. The pretreatment image (A) shows extensive spasm of the anterior cerebral artery and middle cerebral artery. With use of a curved 0.010-in wire within the balloon, both M2 segments were reached proximally (B, C). However, severe anterior cerebral artery spasm persisted refractory to papaverine (D).

Two balloons were used in a parallel manner, with one in the middle cerebral artery used to deflect the other into the A1 segment (E) to achieve a satisfactory result (F). A variant of this technique would be to deflect papaverine exclusively into the A1 segment by brief occlusion of the M1 segment with a balloon while infusing papaverine proximally. Wire-directed balloons now have a greater success rate at accessing the A1 segment for angioplasty and are the device of choice for these vessels (see Fig. 6.6).

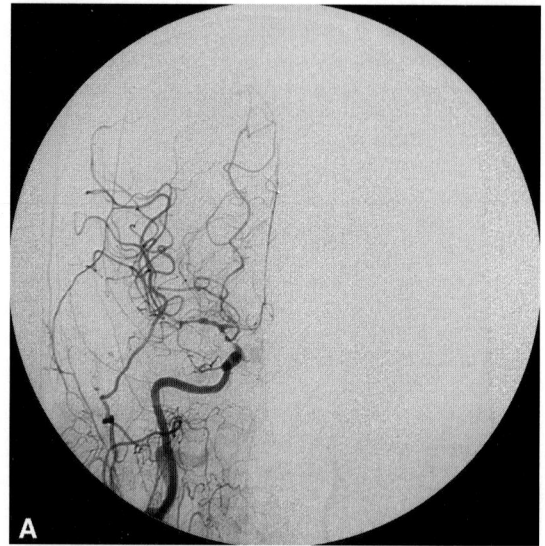

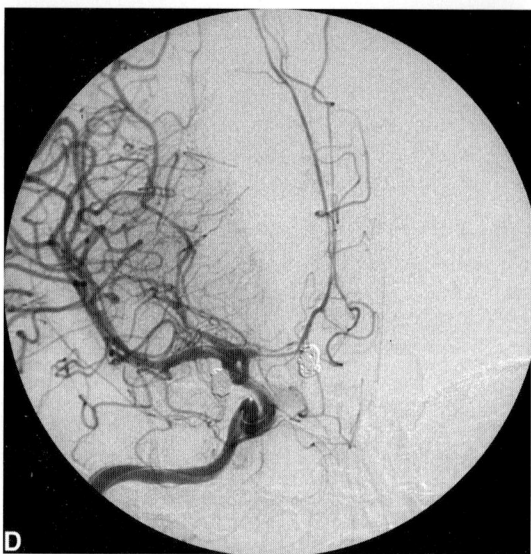

preferably under general anesthetic, is enormously important for these procedures.

Papaverine versus Balloon Angioplasty

It is recognized from anecdotal experience and published clinical case series that the therapeutic effect of PTA is preferable in some respects to that of intraarterial papaverine infusion alone (Figs. 6.1–6.6). Segments of vessel treated by balloon PTA are much less likely to require repeated treatment compared with those treated with papaverine.[44] The first report of intracranial PTA for vasospasm was by Zubkov et al. from then Leningrad, using latex balloons.[53] The major concern with intracranial PTA is the risk of catastrophic hemorrhage from vessel rupture due to excessive balloon distension, and isolated case reports of intraprocedural vessel rupture have earned the procedure a reputation more fearsome than its due.

However, an assumption that papaverine infu-

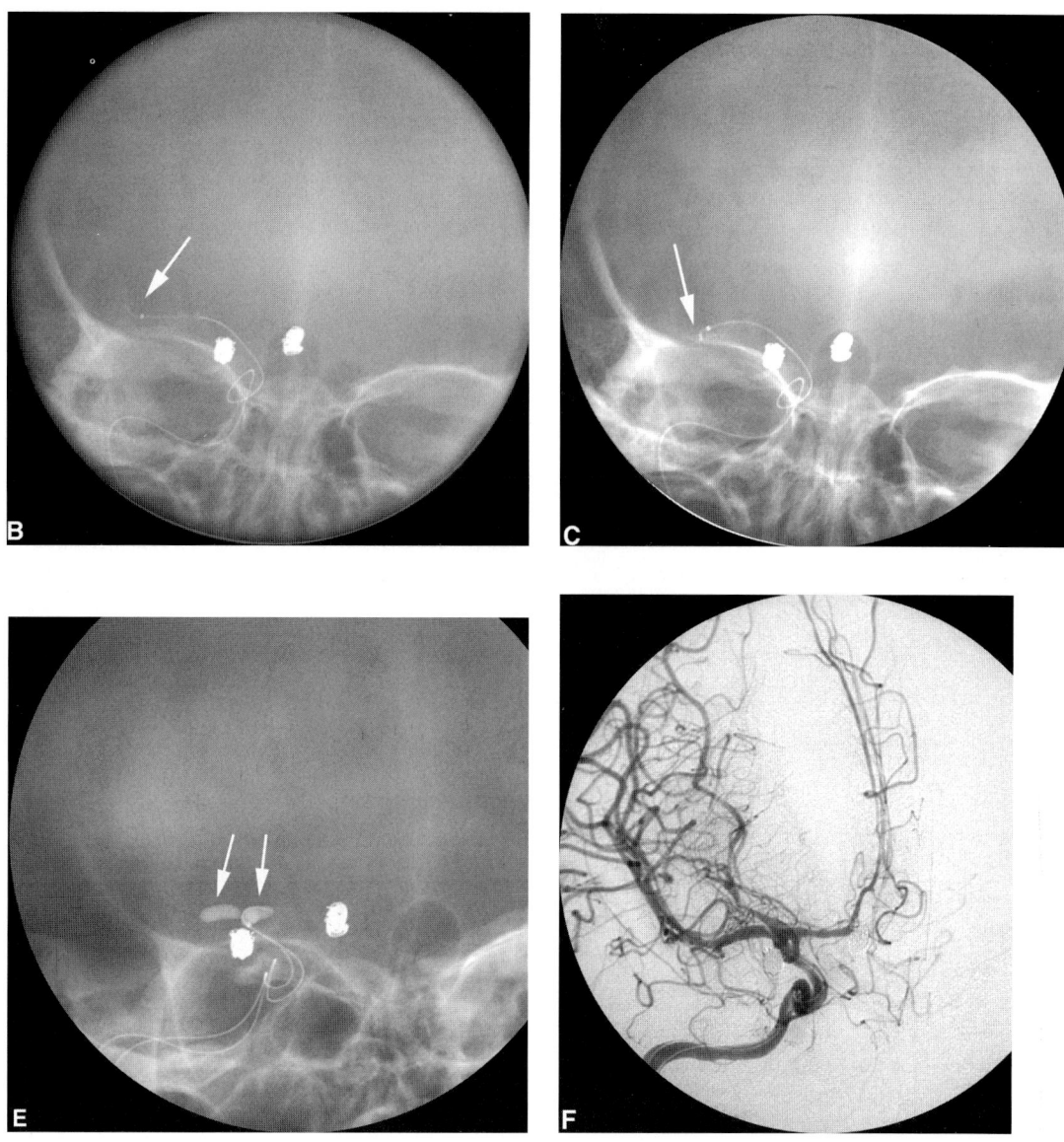

sions alone might be safer although a little less effective than PTA has not been demonstrated. Terada et al.[54,55] have reported more side effects from papaverine infusions than from aggressive balloon PTA, even when venturing into the M2 segment of the middle cerebral artery with the balloon (Figs. 6.7–6.9). Katoh et al.[56] reported improved outcome following PTA in patients with vasospasm compared with those treated with papaverine or with conservative treatment and had more serious procedural complications with papaverine. It is not currently known for certain whether papaverine infusions alone improve ultimate patient outcome to a degree that warrants the risks associated with this therapy.[39–41] Balloon PTA, on the other hand, works for vasospasm by forcefully tearing and stretching the collagen fibers of the arterial wall.[47] The margin of safety during intracranial PTA between therapeutic efficacy in achieving this effect and excessive force resulting in arterial rupture is known to be very narrow in some patients by anybody who has ever witnessed an intraprocedural arterial rupture.[57] Particular care is warranted adjacent to any site of recent aneurysmal rupture even if the aneurysm is secure with clips or coils, or at sites of arterial bifurcation where medial wall defects tend to be found.[58]

Elliott et al.[48] compared papaverine therapy alone with PTA in combination with papaverine in patients with vasospasm. Balloon angioplasty was more likely to result in a greater sustained angiographic improvement and a greater sustained diminution in TCD velocities in treated vessels (45% diminution in velocity). The effects of papaverine on TCD velocity (20% diminution in TCD velocity) were less than those seen with PTA and tended to have vanished by the next day, requiring repetition of the papaverine infusion or PTA of the targeted vessel. Greater improvements with rCBF on SPECT too were seen in this study with PTA than with papaverine alone, correlating with the TCD results.

Papaverine

Papaverine is a benzylisoquinoline alkaloid derived either from morphine or by a synthetic process. Its usefulness in neurointerventional procedures is due to its strong antispasmodic effect on the smooth muscle wall of large- and medium-sized arteries. It can be administered intraarterially for treatment of severe vasospasm following subarachnoid hemorrhage in doses up to 300 mg per arterial tree. Smaller doses of 50–100 mg can be given intraarterially to relieve catheter-related vasospasm.

Papaverine is supplied as a colorless fluid in 10-ml vials containing 300 mg of papaverine. Usually for neurointerventional procedures it is diluted to a total volume of 100 ml with saline for intraarterial injections (3 mg/ml), at rates of 9 mg or less per minute.

Side Effects and Risks of Papaverine

- Arterial injury with repeated procedures
- Crystal formation and embolic complications
- Elevation of intracranial pressure
- Hemorrhagic reperfusion of infarcted territories
- Central and systemic autonomic effects

Intraarterial papaverine infusions are not an entirely benign and risk-free alternative to PTA for treatment of vasospasm. In view of its questionable efficacy, the following factors must be considered.

First, a complete infusion of 300 mg per arterial tree at 9 mg/min takes at least 30 minutes, during which time the introducer catheter in the internal carotid artery can be the cause of significant arterial injury. This risk is greatest in vasospastic patients who are subjected to a sustained hyperdynamic cardiovascular drive by Triple-H therapy. This increases the shear stress on the carotid wall and exaggerates the motion of the introducer catheter against the intima during the cardiac cycle. Performed daily over the course of 3–5 days of repeated papaverine treatments, the cumulative risk of a catheter-related dissection becomes substantial.

The immediate physical and pharmacological effect of papaverine in the internal carotid artery or vertebral artery can be extremely dangerous in certain circumstances. Under conditions of mixing with other drugs, serum, heparin, or contrast agents, crystallization of papaverine in sizes of 50–100 μm can be identified in vitro.[59] Paradoxical aggravation of intracranial spasm has been seen in patients and in animals.[60] Retinal artery embolization with monocular blindness with infusions made in the cervical internal carotid artery is another complication best avoided.[59,61–65] To avoid risks of this nature, papaverine infusions are therefore usually performed above the ophthalmic artery.

Papaverine infusions can cause a severe and dangerous elevation of intracranial pressure (ICP) during treatment.[66] Even patients with an initially low ICP and a slow rate of papaverine infusion can demonstrate ICP rises of up to 60 mm Hg, and increases of 10 mm Hg or more correlate with significant adverse change in the patient.[67] This sometimes responds to a slowing of the rate of infusion, but occasionally can be so severe and immediate that resumption of the infusion cannot be performed safely. The ICP effects of papaverine can occasionally be muted or prevented by administration of intravenous mannitol during or before the procedure. However, it is vitally important during papaverine therapy to monitor the ICP and mean arterial pressure (MAP) carefully. When the difference between the two, i.e., the cerebral perfusion pressure (CPP), approaches 60 mm Hg or below, then cerebral perfusion will be severely compromised. The ICP effect of papaverine can be most severe in patients who have already sustained large areas of infarction with cerebral edema. These patients may have an additional risk of hemorrhagic transformation of infarcted territories from reperfusion under conditions of hyperdynamic therapy.

Papaverine infusions in the posterior circulation even with general anesthetic very commonly cause systemic and neurologic complications which, while usually transient, can be life-threatening. These phenomena are probably due to the immediate effects of papaverine on the brainstem. Typically autonomic instability, hypertension or hypotension, alterations in heart rate, mydriasis, nystagmus, and even loss of respiratory drive can be seen.[68] These procedures are best performed under general anesthetic therefore, with adequate warning given to the anesthetic team. Papaverine can cause peripheral side effects with prolongation of the PR interval on EKG, extreme perspiration, or hypotension.

References

1. MAYBERG MR (1998) Cerebral vasospasm. *Neurosurg Clin North Am* 9:615–627.
2. DIETRICH HH, DACEY RG (2000) Molecular keys to the problems of cerebral vasospasm. *Neurosurgery* 46:517–530.
3. PASQUALIN A (1998) Epidemiology and pathophysiology of cerebral vasospasm following subarachnoid hemorrhage. *J Neurosurg Sci* 42:15–21.
4. FINDLAY JM, MACDONALD RL, WEIR BK (1991) Current concepts of pathophysiology and management of cerebral vasospasm following aneurysmal subarachnoid hemorrhage. *Cerebrovasc Brain Metabol Rev* 3:336–361.
5. TAKENAKA K, YAMADA H, SAKAI N, ANDO T, NAKASHIMA T, NISHIMURA Y (1991) Induction of cytosolic free calcium elevation in rat vascular smooth-muscle cells by cerebrospinal fluid from patients after subarachnoid hemorrhage. *J Neurosurg* 75:452–457.
6. WOLF EW, BANERJEE A, SOBLE-SMITH J, DOHAN FC JR, WHITE RP, ROBERTSON JT (1998) Reversal of cerebral vasospasm using an intrathecally administered nitric oxide donor. *J Neurosurg* 89:279–288.
7. THOMAS JE, ROSENWASSER RH, ARMONDA RA, HARROP J, MITCHELL W, GALARIA I (1999) Safety of intrathecal sodium nitroprusside for the treatment and prevention of refractory cerebral vasospasm and ischemia in humans. *Stroke* 30:1409–1416.
8. YAMAMOTO S, NISHIZAWA S, YOKOYAMA T, RYU H, UEMURA K (1997) Subarachnoid hemorrhage impairs cerebral blood flow response to nitric oxide but not to cyclic GMP in large cerebral arteries. *Brain Res* 757:1–9.
9. LEVIN ER (1995) Endothelins. *N Engl J Med* 333:356–363.
10. JUVELA S (2000) Plasma endothelin concentrations after aneurysmal subarachnoid hemorrhage. *J Neurosurg* 92:390–400.
11. ALABADI JA, TORREGROSA G, MIRANDA FJ, SALOM JB, CENTENO JM, ALBORCH E (1997) Impairment of the modulatory role of nitric oxide on the endothelin-1-elicited contraction of cerebral arteries: a pathogenetic factor in cerebral vasospasm after subarachnoid hemorrhage? *Neurosurgery* 41:245–252.
12. SOBEY CG, FARACI FM (1998) Subarachnoid haemorrhage: what happens to the cerebral arteries? *Clin Exp Pharmacol Physiol* 25:867–876.
13. KASSELL NF, PEERLESS SJ, DURWARD QJ, BECK DW, DRAKE CG, ADAMS HP (1982) Treatment of ischemic deficits from vasospasm with intravascular volume expansion and induced arterial hypertension. *Neurosurgery* 11:337–343.
14. HUNT WE, HESS RM (1968) Surgical risk as related to time of intervention in the repair of intracranial aneurysms. *J Neurosurg* 28:14–20.
15. PICKARD JD, MURRAY GD, ILLINGWORTH R, SHAW MD, TEASDALE GM, FOY PM, HUMPHREY PR, LANG DA, NELSON R, RICHARDS P, ET AL. (1989) Effect of oral nimodipine on cerebral infarction and outcome after subarachnoid haemorrhage: British aneurysm nimodipine trial. *Br Med J* 298:636–642.
16. KASSELL NF, TORNER JC, HALEY EC JR, JANE JA, ADAMS HP, KONGABLE GL (1990) The International Cooperative Study on the Timing of Aneurysm Surgery. Part 1: Overall management results. *J Neurosurg* 73:18–36.
17. POWERS WJ, GRUBB RL JR, BAKER RP, MINTUN MA, RAICHLE ME (1985) Regional cerebral blood flow and metabolism in reversible ischemia due to vasospasm. Determination by positron emission tomography. *J Neurosurg* 62:539–546.
18. LEWIS DH, ESKRIDGE JM, NEWELL DW, GRADY MS, COHEN WA, DALLEY RW, LOYD D, GROTHAUS-KING A, YOUNG P, WINN HR (1992) Brain SPECT and the effect of cerebral angioplasty in delayed ischemia due to vasospasm. *J Nucl Med* 33:1789–1796.

19. Fandino J, Kaku Y, Schuknecht B, Valavanis A, Yonekawa Y (1998) Improvement of cerebral oxygenation patterns and metabolic validation of superselective intraarterial infusion of papaverine for the treatment of cerebral vasospasm. *J Neurosurg* 89:93–100.
20. Fisher CM, Kistler JP, Davis JM (1980) Relation of cerebral vasospasm to subarachnoid hemorrhage visualized by computerized tomographic scanning. *Neurosurgery* 6:1–9.
21. Winn HR, Richardson AE, Jane JA (1977) The long-term prognosis in untreated cerebral aneurysms: I. The incidence of late hemorrhage in cerebral aneurysm: a 10-year evaluation of 364 patients. *Ann Neurol* 1:358–370.
22. Weir BK, Kongable GL, Kassell NF, Schultz JR, Truskowski LL, Sigrest A (1998) Cigarette smoking as a cause of aneurysmal subarachnoid hemorrhage and risk for vasospasm: a report of the Cooperative Aneurysm Study. *J Neurosurg* 89:405–411.
23. Lasner TM, Weil RJ, Riina HA, King JT Jr, Zager EL, Raps EC, Flamm ES (1997) Cigarette smoking-induced increase in the risk of symptomatic vasospasm after aneurysmal subarachnoid hemorrhage. *J Neurosurg* 87:381–384.
24. Aaslid R, Markwalder TM, Nornes H (1982) Noninvasive transcranial Doppler ultrasound recording of flow velocity in basal cerebral arteries. *J Neurosurg* 57:769–774.
25. Bartels E, Fuchs HH, Flugel KA (1995) Color Doppler imaging of basal cerebral arteries: normal reference values and clinical applications. *Angiology* 46:877–884.
26. Lindegaard KF, Bakke SJ, Sorteberg W, Nakstad P, Nornes H (1986) A non-invasive Doppler ultrasound method for the evaluation of patients with subarachnoid hemorrhage. *Acta Radiologica—Supplementum* 369:96–98, 1986
27. Vora YY, Suarez-Almazor M, Steinke DE, Martin ML, Findlay JM (1999) Role of transcranial Doppler monitoring in the diagnosis of cerebral vasospasm after subarachnoid hemorrhage. *Neurosurgery* 44:1237–1248.
28. Hughes JT, Schianchi PM (1978) Cerebral artery spasm. A histological study at necropsy of the blood vessels in cases of subarachnoid hemorrhage. *J Neurosurg* 48:515–525.
29. Smith RR, Clower BR, Grotendorst GM, Yabuno N, Cruse JM (1985) Arterial wall changes in early human vasospasm. *Neurosurgery* 16:171–176.
30. Ohkawa M, Fujiwara N, Tanabe M, Takashima H, Satoh K, Kojima K, Irie K, Honjo Y, Nagao S (1996) Cerebral vasospastic vessels: histologic changes after percutaneous transluminal angioplasty. *Radiology* 198:179–184.
31. Kobayashi H, Ide H, Aradachi H, Arai Y, Handa Y, Kubota T (1993) Histological studies of intracranial vessels in primates following transluminal angioplasty for vasospasm. *J Neurosurg* 78:481–486.
32. Fujiwara N, Ohkawa M, Tanabe M, Irie K, Nagao S (1994) The effect of PTA on cerebral vessels in experimental vasospasm: a histopathological study. *Nippon Igaku Hoshasen Gakkai Zasshi—Nippon Acta Radiologica* 54:378–388.
33. Kazan S (1998) Effects of intra-arterial papaverine on the chronic period of cerebral arterial vasospasm in rats. *Acta Neurologica Scandinavica* 98:354–359.
34. Fujiwara N, Honjo Y, Ohkawa M, Tanabe M, Irie K, Nagao S, Takashima H, Satoh K, Kojima K (1997) Intraarterial infusion of papaverine in experimental cerebral vasospasm. *AJNR* 18:255–262.
35. Milburn JM, Moran CJ, Cross DT3, Diringer MN, Pilgram TK, Dacey RGJ (1998) Increase in diameters of vasospastic intracranial arteries by intraarterial papaverine administration. *J Neurosurg* 88:38–42.
36. Nagai H, Noda S, Mabe H (1975) Experimental cerebral vasospasm. Part 2: effects of vasoactive drugs and sympathectomy on early and late spasm. *J Neurosurg* 42:420–428.
37. Kuwayama A, Zervas NT, Shintani A, Pickren KS (1972) Papaverine hydrochloride and experimental hemorrhagic cerebral arterial spasm. *Stroke* 3:27–33.
38. Zubkov YN, Alexander LF, Smith RR, Benashvili GM, Semenyutin V, Bernanke D (1994) Angioplasty of vasospasm: is it reasonable? *Neurol Res* 16:9–11.
39. Kallmes DF, Jensen ME, Dion JE (1997) Infusing doubt into the efficacy of papaverine. *AJNR* 18:263–264.
40. Polin RS, Hansen CA, German P, Chadduck JB, Kassell NF (1998) Intra-arterially administered papaverine for the treatment of symptomatic cerebral vasospasm. *Neurosurgery* 42:1256–1264.
41. Polin RS, Kassell NF (1998) Treatment of vasospasm. *J Neurosurg* 88:933.
42. Eskridge JM, Newell DW, Winn HR (1994) Endovascular treatment of vasospasm. *Neurosurg Clin North Am* 5:437–447.
43. Eskridge JM, Song JK (1997) A practical approach to the treatment of vasospasm. *AJNR* 18:1653–1660.
44. Eskridge JM, McAuliffe W, Song JK, Deliganis AV, Newell DW, Lewis DH, Mayberg MR, Winn HR (1998) Balloon angioplasty for the treatment of vasospasm: results of first 50 cases. *Neurosurgery* 42:510–516.
45. Rosenwasser RH, Armonda RA, Thomas JE, Benitez RP, Gannon PM, Harrop J (1999) Therapeutic modalities for the management of cerebral vasospasm: timing of endovascular options. *Neurosurgery* 44:975–979.
46. Le Roux PD, Newell DW, Eskridge J, Mayberg MR, Winn HR (1994) Severe symptomatic vasospasm: the role of immediate postoperative angioplasty. *J Neurosurg* 80:224–229.
47. Yamamoto Y, Smith RR, Bernanke DH (1992) Mechanism of action of balloon angioplasty in cerebral vasospasm. *Neurosurgery* 30:1–5.
48. Elliott JP, Newell DW, Lam DJ, Eskridge JM, Douville CM, Le Roux PD, Lewis DH, Mayberg MR, Grady MS, Winn HR (1998) Comparison of balloon angioplasty and papaverine infusion for the treatment of vasospasm following aneurysmal subarachnoid hemorrhage. *J Neurosurg* 88:277–284.
49. Bejjani GK, Bank WO, Olan WJ, Sekhar LN (1998) The efficacy and safety of angioplasty for cerebral vasospasm after subarachnoid hemorrhage. *Neurosurgery* 42:979–986.
50. Pistoia F, Horton JA, Sekhar L, Horowitz M (1991) Imag-

ing of blood flow changes following angioplasty for treatment of vasospasm. *AJNR* 12:446–448.
51. MEGYESI JF, FINDLAY JM, VOLLRATH B, COOK DA, CHEN MH (1997) In vivo angioplasty prevents the development of vasospasm in canine carotid arteries. Pharmacological and morphological analyses. *Stroke* 28:1216–1224.
52. MUIZELAAR JP, ZWIENENBERG M, RUDISILL NA, HECHT ST (1999) The prophylactic use of transluminal balloon angioplasty in patients with Fisher Grade 3 subarachnoid hemorrhage: a pilot study. *J Neurosurg* 91:51–58.
53. ZUBKOV YN, NIKIFOROV BM, SHUSTIN VA (1984) Balloon catheter technique for dilatation of constricted cerebral arteries after aneurysmal SAH. *Acta Neurochirurgica* 70:65–79.
54. TERADA T, NAKAMURA Y, YOSHIDA N, KURIYAMA T, ISOZAKI S, NAKAI K, ITAKURA T, HAYASHI S, KOMAI N (1993) Percutaneous transluminal angioplasty for the M2 portion vasospasm following SAH: development of the new microballoon and report of cases. *Surg Neurol* 39:13–17.
55. TERADA T, KINOSHITA Y, YOKOTE H, TSUURA M, NAKAI K, ITAKURA T, HYOTANI G, KURIYAMA T, NAKA Y, KIDO T (1997) The effect of endovascular therapy for cerebral arterial spasm, its limitation and pitfalls. *Acta Neurochirurgica* 139:227–234.
56. KATOH H, SHIMA K, SHIMIZU A, TAKIGUCHI H, MIYAZAWA T, UMEZAWA H, NAWASHIRO H, ISHIHARA S, KAJI T, MAKITA K, TSUCHIYA K (1999) Clinical evaluation of the effect of percutaneous transluminal angioplasty and intra-arterial papaverine infusion for the treatment of vasospasm following aneurysmal subarachnoid hemorrhage. *Neurol Res* 21:195–203.
57. LINSKEY ME, HORTON JA, RAO GR, YONAS H (1991) Fatal rupture of the intracranial carotid artery during transluminal angioplasty for vasospasm induced by subarachnoid hemorrhage. Case report. *J Neurosurg* 74:985–990.
58. NEWELL DW, ESKRIDGE JM, MAYBERG MR, GRADY MS, WINN HR (1989) Angioplasty for the treatment of symptomatic vasospasm following subarachnoid hemorrhage. *J Neurosurg* 71:654–660.
59. MATHIS JM, DENARDO AJ, THIBAULT L, JENSEN ME, SAVORY J, DION JE (1994) In vitro evaluation of papaverine hydrochloride incompatibilities: a simulation of intraarterial infusion for cerebral vasospasm. *AJNR* 15:1665–1670.
60. CLYDE BL, FIRLIK AD, KAUFMANN AM, SPEARMAN MP, YONAS H (1996) Paradoxical aggravation of vasospasm with papaverine infusion following aneurysmal subarachnoid hemorrhage. Case report. *J Neurosurg* 84:690–695.
61. CLOUSTON JE, NUMAGUCHI Y, ZOARSKI GH, ALDRICH EF, SIMARD JM, ZITNAY KM (1995) Intraarterial papaverine infusion for cerebral vasospasm after subarachnoid hemorrhage. *AJNR* 16:27–38.
62. NUMAGUCHI Y, ZOARSKI GH (1998) Intra-arterial papaverine treatment for cerebral vasospasm: our experience and review of the literature. *Neurologia Medico-Chirurgica* 38:189–195.
63. MATHIS JM, JENSEN ME, DION JE (1997) Technical considerations on intra-arterial papaverine hydrochloride for cerebral vasospasm. *Neuroradiology* 39:90–98.
64. MATHIS JM, DENARDO A, JENSEN ME, SCOTT J, DION JE (1994) Transient neurologic events associated with intraarterial papaverine infusion for subarachnoid hemorrhage-induced vasospasm. *AJNR* 15:1671–1674.
65. KALLMES DF, MCGRAW JK, EVANS AJ, CLOFT HJ, MATHIS JM, HERGENROTHER R, JENSEN ME, DION JE (1998) Effects of systemic heparinization on the thrombogenicity of hydrophilic and nonhydrophilic catheters in a swine model. *Neuroradiology* 40:530–535.
66. MCAULIFFE W, TOWNSEND M, ESKRIDGE JM, NEWELL DW, GRADY MS, WINN HR (1995) Intracranial pressure changes induced during papaverine infusion for treatment of vasospasm. *J Neurosurg* 83:430–434.
67. CROSS DT 3RD, MORAN CJ, ANGTUACO EE, MILBURN JM, DIRINGER MN, DACEY RGJ (1998) Intracranial pressure monitoring during intraarterial papaverine infusion for cerebral vasospasm. *AJNR* 19:1319–1323.
68. BARR JD, MATHIS JM, HORTON JA (1994) Transient severe brain stem depression during intraarterial papaverine infusion for cerebral vasospasm. *AJNR* 15:719–723.

Chapter 7

Dural Arteriovenous Malformations

RISKS OF DURAL ARTERIOVENOUS MALFORMATIONS ARE RELATED TO IMPACT ON THE VENOUS SYSTEM

Dural arteriovenous fistulas or malformations (dAVM) represent 10% to 15% of intracranial arteriovenous malformations and occur most commonly in the posterior fossa along the sigmoid and transverse sinuses.[1] The second most common location is the cavernous sinus, where they are sometimes referred to as "indirect carotid cavernous fistulas." Various classification schemes for dAVMs have been canvassed, but classification can be simplified by considering the impact of the dAVM on the venous system.[2–4] Only those dAVMs with low or moderate flow with antegrade drainage into dural sinuses and without evidence of disturbance of venous flow in the connected venous sinuses or adjacent veins can be considered benign. All others must be considered potential causes of current or future venous hypertension (Fig. 7.1), venous infarction, or intracranial hemorrhage. The risk of imminent complications can be estimated by the degree of reversal of dural sinus venous flow, state of retrograde opacification and ectasia of the parenchymal veins, and the degree of restriction on the venous drainage.

Dural arteriovenous malformations are usually acquired lesions presenting in adulthood,[5,6] although presumed congenital fistulas of the dura are sometimes seen in children.[7] Acquired dAVMs in adults are thought likely to represent the effects of recanalization following an episode of dural sinus thrombosis, but can also be seen following head trauma.[8] The clinical significance of dAVMs spans the range from mildly irritating nocturnal awareness of a bruit on one end to life-threatening intracranial hemorrhage and venous hypertension on the other. The precise location of the dAVM, the arterial feeders involved, and the volume of shunting present are usually secondary considerations in the management of these lesions (Figs. 7.2–7.4). The principal pathophysiologic concern is the state of the receiving venous field on the distal end of the dAVM. Large dAVMs with a florid angiographic appearance of prompt antegrade venous drainage and no effect on the intradural venous physiology may be inconsequential to the patient. If the patient can tolerate the bruit related to such lesions, they are often best left untreated. Alternatively, in a different patient a tiny dural AVF too small to generate a bruit but with a restricted venous field and intradural drainage may be the cause of a fatal intracranial bleed.

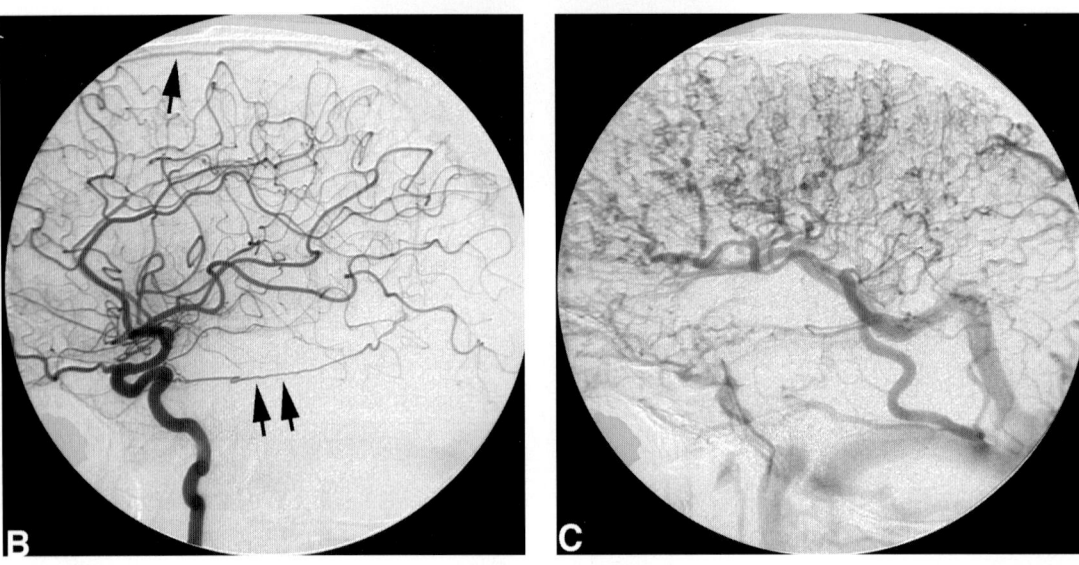

FIGURE 7.1 • *Severe Intracranial Venous Hypertension due to an Extensive Bilateral dAVM.*
A 47-year-old male patient complaining of chronic severe headaches demonstrated signs of extensive venous congestion on a T1 weighted contrast-enhanced MRI (A). The right internal carotid artery angiogram (B, arterial phase, lateral view) shows enlargement of the anterior artery of the falx (arrow) and the marginal tentorial artery (double arrow). The venous phase (C) of the same injection shows a grossly disordered appearance of the superficial and deep veins, with no opacification of the superior sagittal sinus. The left internal carotid artery injection (D, AP projection) demonstrates a markedly enlarged fistulous branch (arrow) from the left middle meningeal artery arising from the left ophthalmic artery, an origin that precluded reasonably safe catheterization of the vessel.

Multiple large fistulas from the external carotid arteries on each side were catheterized retrogradely from the venous side and embolized with coils. Image E (AP projection) demonstrates an injection made retrogradely into one of the fistulous branches of the right middle meningeal artery. However, success was limited due to the extensive branches involved, and skeletonization of the superior sagittal sinus was eventually necessary.

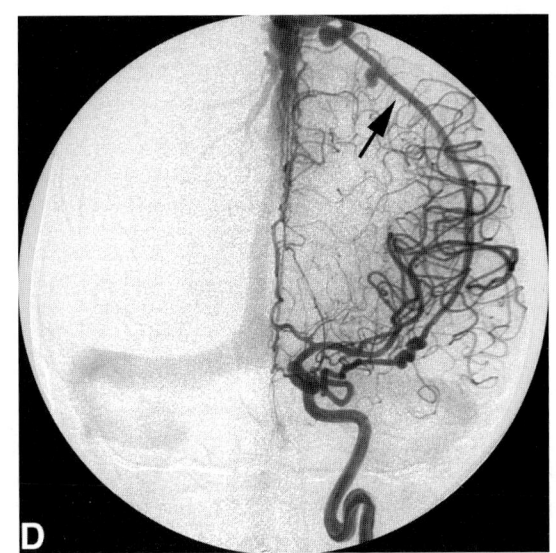
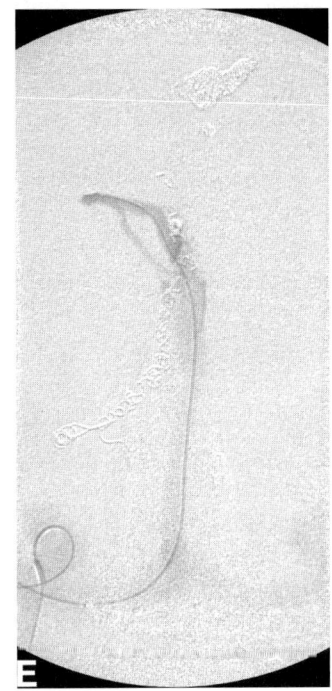

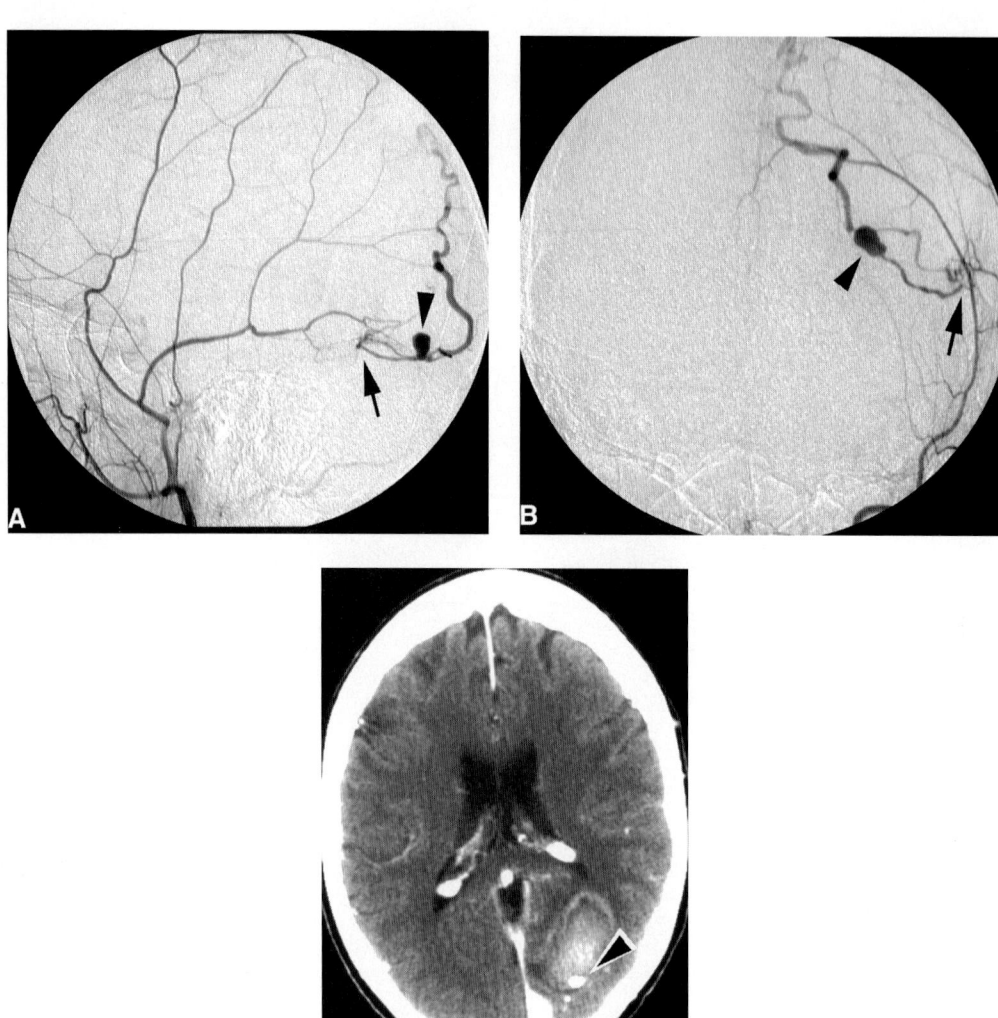

FIGURE 7.2 • *The Size of the Arterial Feeders and the Volume of Flow in a Dural AVM Are Often Not Predictive of Risk.*

A 76-year-old female presented with a large intraparenchymal hemorrhage. An angiogram was performed to rule out the possibility of a brain AVM. A subtle, slowly flowing abnormality of the left middle meningeal artery was noticed and a selective injection showed a tiny rete of dAVM (arrow) in the posterior territory of the middle meningeal artery (A, lateral projection; B, Towne's projection). The dAVM drains through constrained brain parenchymal veins, one of which demonstrated a varix or rupture point (arrowhead) within the left occipital lobe. After embolization of the dAVM with a single column of dilute histoacryl, an axial CT (C) shows that the pseudoaneurysm with a small amount of histoacryl (arrowhead in C) within lies directly within the occipital hematoma.

Rarely, dAVMs can be seen in association with tumors, e.g., glioblastoma multiforme. In a case such as this, follow-up of the patient for resolution of the hematoma would be a prudent step to avoid the rare instance of overlooking a masked tumor.

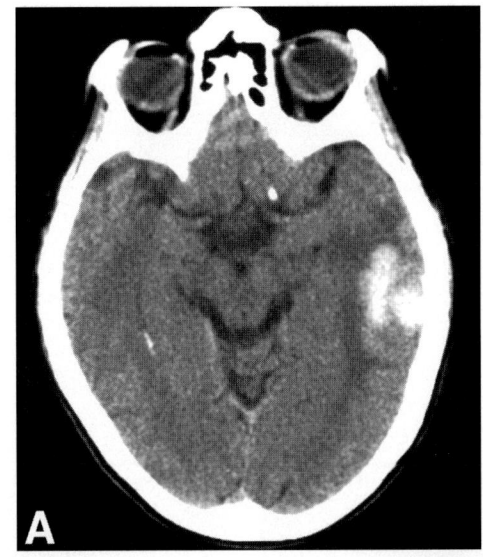

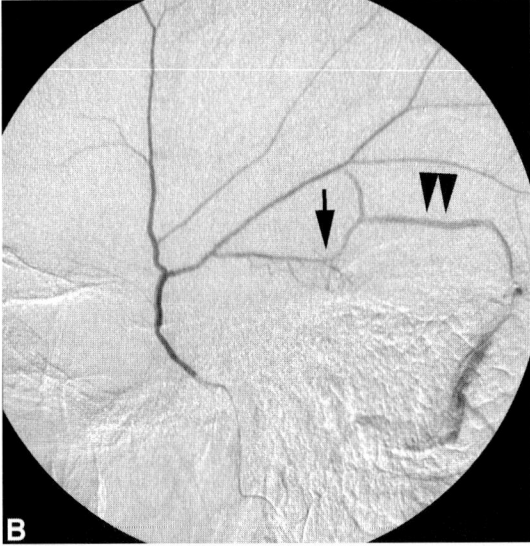

FIGURE 7.3 • *The Venous Field Determines the Significance of a dAVM.*
A similar case to Fig. 7.2. An elderly female presented with a left temporal lobe hemorrhage (A). A small dAVF (B, lateral angiographic view) of the left middle meningeal artery (arrow) drains via a posterior temporal parenchymal vein (double arrowheads) to the left transverse sinus. This was successfully eliminated with a single injection of dilute histoacryl performed distally in the vessel, i.e., close to the fistula site.

Proximal injections in the middle meningeal artery involve risks to the petrous branch (connecting with the VIIth nerve), and risks to the orbital collaterals of the middle meningeal artery (connecting to the ophthalmic artery).

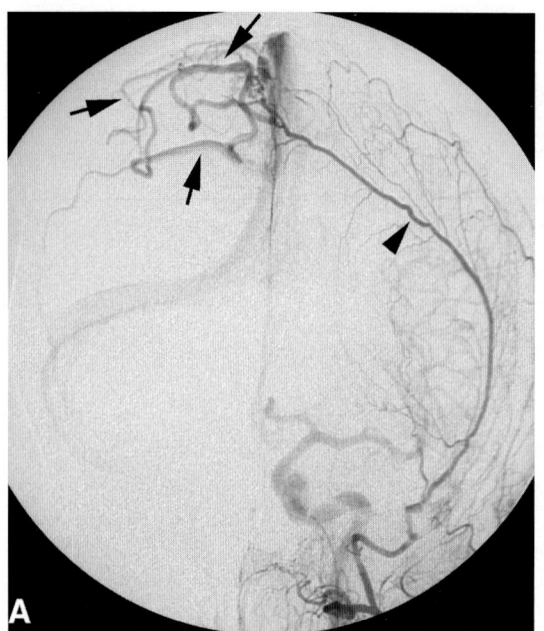 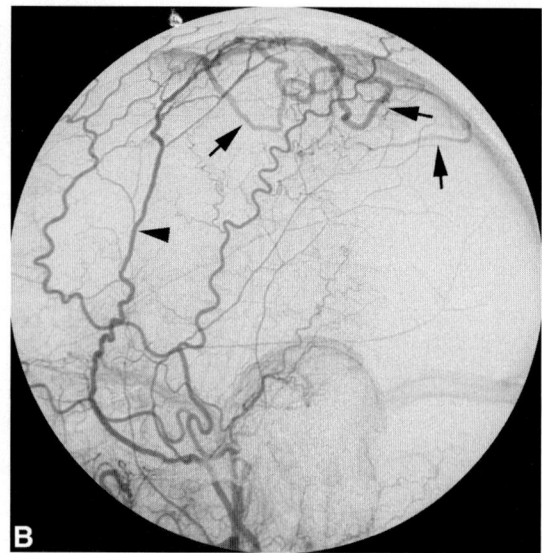

FIGURE 7.4 • A 58-year-old male patient presented with severe persistent and worsening headaches over many months. An angiogram at an outside hospital with bilateral common carotid injections was thought initially to be normal, but closer inspection demonstrated very fleeting opacification of a venous structure over the calvarium. The patient did not have a bruit. On the suspicion of a dAVM a repeat superselective angiogram was performed (A, Towne's projection, left external carotid artery injection; B, lateral view), showing that the relatively slowly flowing dAVM was fed almost predominantly by the left middle meningeal artery (arrowhead) and drained via parasagittal parenchymal veins (arrows) on the right side. The vessels could not be catheterized to a point sufficiently distal to allow safe histoacryl injection, and a skeletonization procedure was eventually performed with good results.

Clinical Presentation of Dural Arteriovenous Malformations

Patients presenting with dAVMs may be asymptomatic or may have complaints only of a bruit most audible at night. More serious symptoms are related to the state of alteration of flow in the affected venous field. Elevated venous pressure with diversion of venous flow and elevation of intracranial pressure may present with headache, symptoms of pseudotumor cerebri, or even with dementia. Focal venous hypertension in an orbit presents with proptosis, chemosis, ophthalmoplegia, secondary glaucoma, and diplopia. Venous hypertension of the posterior fossa may present with cerebellar signs, brain-stem dysfunction, hydrocephalus, or ataxia (Fig. 7.5). When the venous flow is diverted into the spinal veins, a cranial dAVM can present with signs and symptoms identical to those of a spinal vascular malformation or can mimic the presentation of a spinal tumor. Dural AVMs with intradural venous drainage may present with headache, seizure, intracranial subarachnoid or intraparenchymal hemorrhage, or focal neurologic signs.[9] Although there is evidence that many acquired dAVMs are related to recanalized segments of dural sinus thrombosis, there are also case reports documenting the appearance of dAVMs in proximity to more grave conditions such as primary brain tumors. Therefore, the possibility of an underlying primary neoplasm may have to be considered in some rare patients in whom the abnormalities on the initial MRI may not be

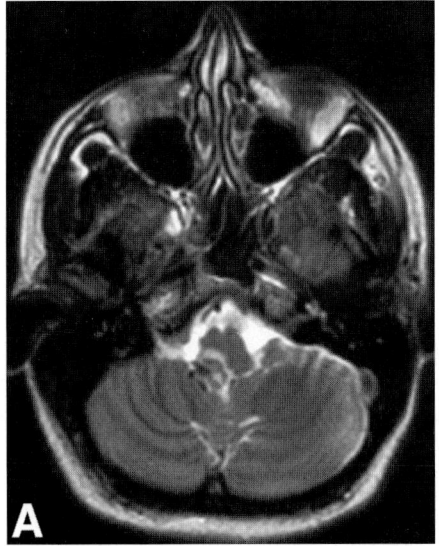 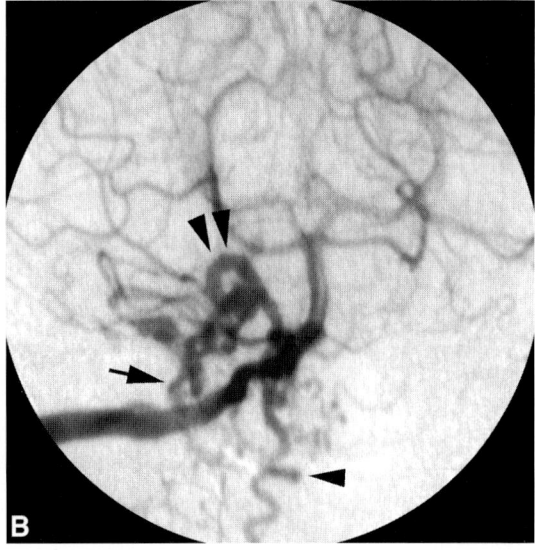

FIGURE 7.5 • *Dural AVM of the Foramen Magnum.*
A 39-year-old female presented with subarachnoid hemorrhage and a right lateral medullary syndrome. Abnormal flow voids, medullary edema, and mass-effect are seen on the MRI T2 weighted images (A). A right vertebral artery (B) injection demonstrates a dural AVM from the C1 branch (arrow) of the vertebral artery opacifying a large subarachnoid varix (double arrowhead) and draining to a spinal vein inferiorly (arrowhead). Attempts to embolize the lesion were unsuccessful, and it was isolated and eliminated surgically.

completely related to intraparenchymal hemorrhage and venous hypertension.

Dural AVMs in children tend to be complex and extensive. They may present with a clinical appearance similar to that seen with Vein of Galen malformations with advanced signs of elevated and sustained intracranial pressure, failure to thrive, hydrocephalus, brain "atrophy," congestive heart failure, and psychosocial retardation.[7]

Therefore, although they are uncommon lesions, dAVMs are a disorder to bear in mind in the clinical and angiographic evaluation of patients without an obvious alternative cause for intracranial bleeding or who present with signs compatible with venous hypertension. An index of suspicion requiring thorough angiographic evaluation is often necessary to detect these lesions as the location and its neurologic effects may often be physically remote from one another. For example, a patient presenting with myelopathy might not prompt consideration of a dAVM of the cavernous sinus as the first consideration, but evaluation of the cranial circulation should be part of the spinal angiographic evaluation of such patients.

CAROTID-JUGULAR COMPRESSION PROTOCOL

Where treatment of a dAVM is not necessary, it should be avoided. In the absence of neurologic complications, elevated intraocular pressure, or angiographic signs of intracranial complications, a trial of carotid artery compression may be worthwhile to eliminate otherwise uncomplicated complaints of bruit (Fig. 7.6). Spontaneous regression of dAVMs can occur in a minority of patients, and it is possible that this phenomenon can be enhanced by having the patient compress the carotid and jugular vein of the side of the lesion until the bruit is eliminated using the contralateral hand. Patients and their family members must be taught the need for the patient only to do this with the contralat-

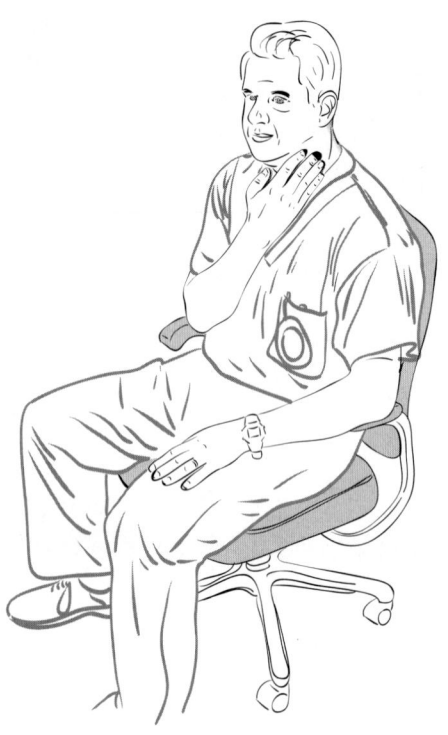

FIGURE 7.6 • *Technique of Carotid-Jugular Compression.*
An obliging neuroradiology fellow demonstrates the technique of carotid-jugular compression for promotion of spontaneous thrombosis of dAVM. The key instructions to patients and families are:
- Compression is performed only by the patient, not a family member, and only with the contralateral hand.
- The patient sits in a comfortable chair from which he/she will not tumble if faintness occurs.
- The thumb of the compressing hand is held away from the skin to prevent inadvertent bilateral carotid compression.
- The elbow of the compressing arm is free, not propped up, so that it will fall away if hemispheric ischemia and extremity weakness intervene.
- The compression is performed in such a manner as to eliminate the patient's awareness of bruit.

eral hand in a free position to facilitate falling of the hand in the event of hemispheric ischemia. Therefore, the patient is instructed to do this in a sitting position. Emphasis is also placed on avoiding inadvertent compression of the contralateral carotid artery with the thumb. Compression is started for 10-second periods several times per hour, working up to 30 seconds or longer. Using this protocol Halbach et al. have seen a response rate of up to 30% in uncomplicated dural AVMs of the cavernous sinus and transverse sinuses.[10,11]

INDICATIONS FOR TREATMENT

Endovascular or surgical treatment for patients with dAVMs on the basis of bruit alone should usually be performed only for patients with absolutely intolerable symptoms. Virtually all patients with neurologic symptoms or signs, elevated intraocular pressure, or papilledema require immediate aggressive treatment.[12] An ophthalmology evaluation prior to intervention is invariably prudent when there is ocular involvement. This documents the baseline reading of the intraocular pressure and serves as a marker of the efficacy of treatment. Temporizing pharmacological management of secondary glaucoma and evaluation of the visual fields is very important for patients with dAVMs of the cavernous sinus.

The angiographic appearance alone of a dAVM can also be an indication for urgent treatment even in the absence of clinical complications. This is true when there is evidence of intradural venous drainage with its attendant risks of intracranial hemorrhage or elevated ICP.

The surgical exploration and management of dAVMs tends to be difficult and bloody due to the profusion of small vessels in the vicinity of the lesion. The treatment of choice is endovascular management in most patients (Fig. 7.7). However, there are some patients in whom surgical exploration and "skeletonization" of a segment of dural sinus is necessary. This involves isolating the sinus from all its afferent arterial sources of input, while preserving venous flow within. Combined operating-room endovascular and surgical management for complex lesions may be necessary in certain

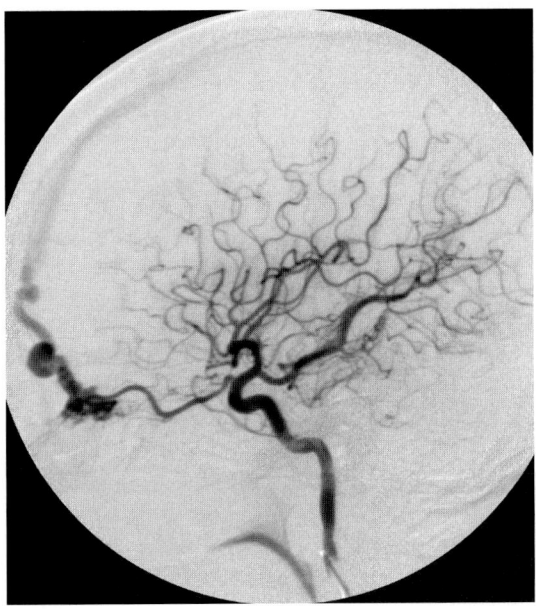

FIGURE 7.7 • *Dural AVM of the Cribriform Plate.* A middle-aged patient presenting with headache demonstrates a dAVM of the cribriform plate arising from ethmoidal branches of the ophthalmic artery, draining to the superior sagittal sinus. These lesions most commonly present with subarachnoid hemorrhage due to the fragility of the veins in this area. Due to the unreasonable risks of embolization in the ophthalmic artery, dAVMs in this region are almost always approached surgically.

Endovascular Treatment of Dural AVMs

There are three main routes of endovascular approach to a dAVM: transvenous, transarterial, and transorbital.

Transvenous Embolization of Dural AVMs

The transvenous approach to a dAVM was pioneered by Mullan.[13] It is now the preferred treatment in the majority of patients and is usually executed from a transfemoral approach. Occasionally a jugular vein or facial vein puncture is necessary. The transvenous approach involves catheterization of the segment of diseased sinus with a microcatheter and occluding the segment, usually with fibered coils. It is important to explore and consider the effects of this occlusion on adjacent normal tissue first as the risks can be considerable if the consequences are overlooked (Figs. 7.8, 7.9). Typically, a segment of the transverse sinus or sigmoid sinus may be involved, and occluding that segment with endovascular devices will eliminate the fistula. However, the effects of this maneuver on an ipsilateral vein of Labbé or a vein from the posterior fossa can be momentous if a venous infarction or hemorrhage occurs (Figs. 7.10, 7.11). Furthermore, if the distal transverse sinus is to be occluded, one must first ascertain that reversal of flow in the proximal transverse sinus is well tolerated by the patient. Test occlusion with a temporary balloon and measurement of venous pressures in the sinuses may be appropriate in certain patients. Ironically, it is those patients who are least severely affected by the dAVM that these perils most threaten. This is because uncomplicated dAVMs allow continued antegrade venous outflow in the diseased segment of sinus. More severe dAVMs with reversal of venous flow and venous hypertension will have tested and encouraged the patient's capacity for collateral venous outflow by the time of presentation for treatment. Therefore, the greatest complications with endovascular transvenous treatment of dAVMs tend to happen with lesions of a milder state where inadvertent therapeutic occlusion of routes of normal venous outflow is induced.

Where the entire diseased segment of sinus cannot be occluded safely, selective transvenous catheterization and coil embolization of the fistula itself can sometimes be accomplished (Fig. 7.12).[14] In other patients transarterial catheterization may be possible, or surgical alternatives may have to be evaluated.

The presence of dural sinus stenoses either at the site of disease or remote from the disease can have a profoundly deleterious effect on the pattern of venous hypertension found with a dAVM or affecting the feasibility of transvenous embolization. A proximal venous stenosis, for example, may impede venous flow, worsening the state of venous hypertension.[12] A new approach to this situation is to open the sinus with transvenous stents to allow decompression

patients, such as for an isolated segment of diseased sinus requiring surgical exposure for endovascular access.

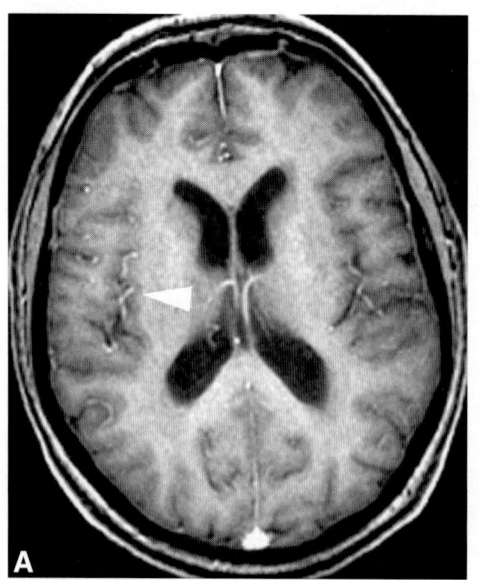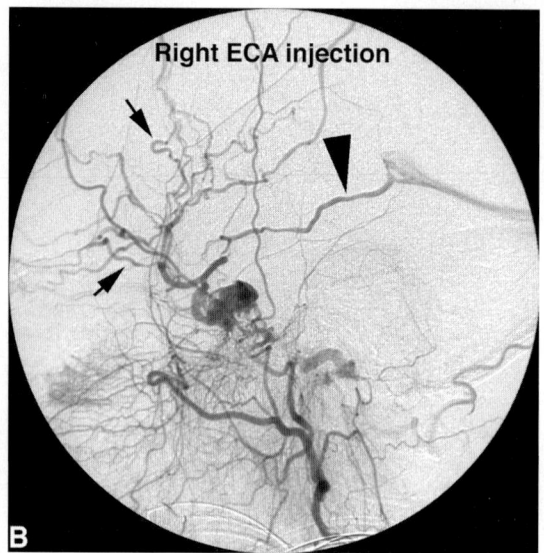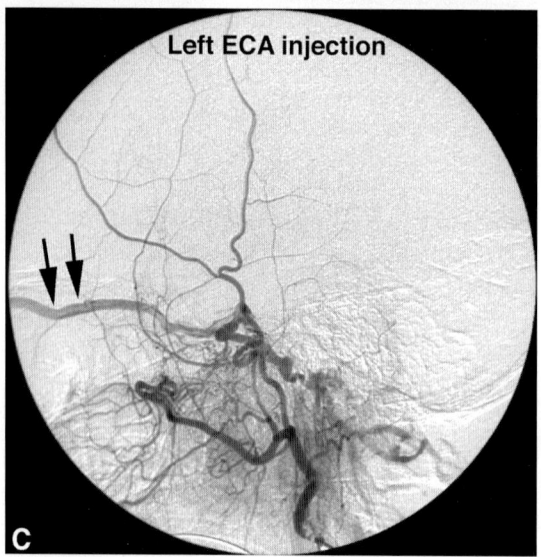

FIGURE 7.8 • *Strategic Planning of Transvenous Embolization Is Important to Avoid Disasters.*
A 47-year-old female patient complaining of headaches and a red left eye was evaluated by MRI (A). The most subtle asymmetry (arrowhead) of contrast enhancement in the right Sylvian fissure was noted, raising the question of a dural AVM with intraparenchymal venous drainage. This was confirmed with subsequent angiography (B, lateral projection of right external carotid artery injection) in which parenchymal drainage of a cavernous dAVM is seen to the Sylvian and frontal superficial veins (arrows) and to the deep basal vein of Rosenthal (arrowhead). The left external carotid artery injection (C, lateral projection) also causes opacification of the left superior ophthalmic vein (double arrow), correlating with the clinical signs of the disease.

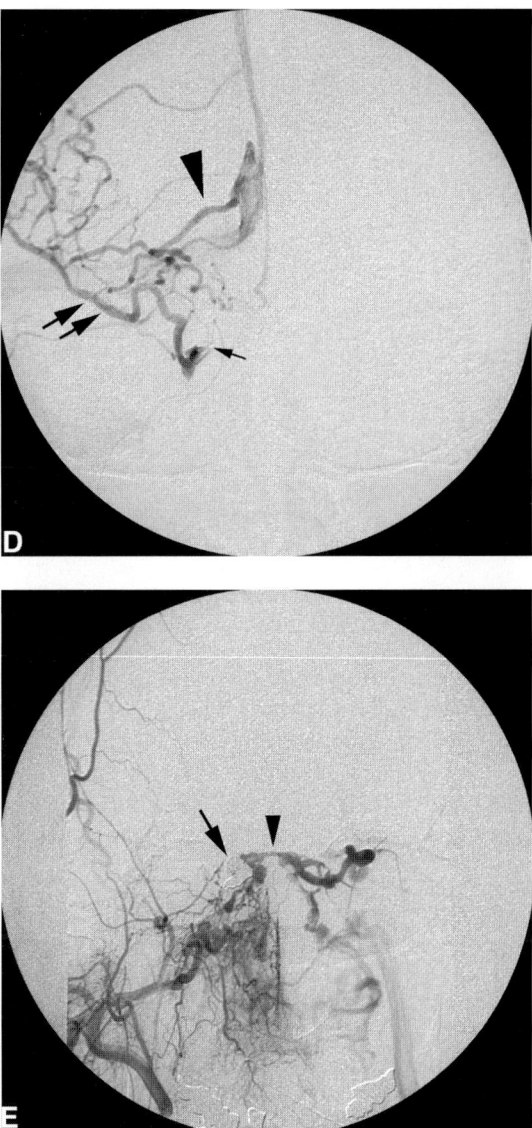

A potential danger exists in this case in that if one were to indiscriminately pack the cavernous sinuses with coils, one might block alternative routes of outflow and cause increased flow into the parenchymal veins. This would almost certainly cause catastrophic complications. A Towne's projection (D) of the microcatheter injection in the right cavernous sinus shows that the catheter (small arrow) is right at the connection between the cavernous sinus and the hazardous veins to the frontal lobe (double arrow) and the deep veins (arrowhead). Coiling is commenced at this location. After the initial coiling eliminates hazardous venous flow (E, AP view, arrow indicates initial deposition of coils), an interim right external carotid artery injection shows that the venous drainage remaining is all directed across the midline (arrowhead) to the left cavernous sinus and left superior ophthalmic vein. The remainder of the right and left cavernous sinuses could then be packed uneventfully, resulting in elimination of the lesion.

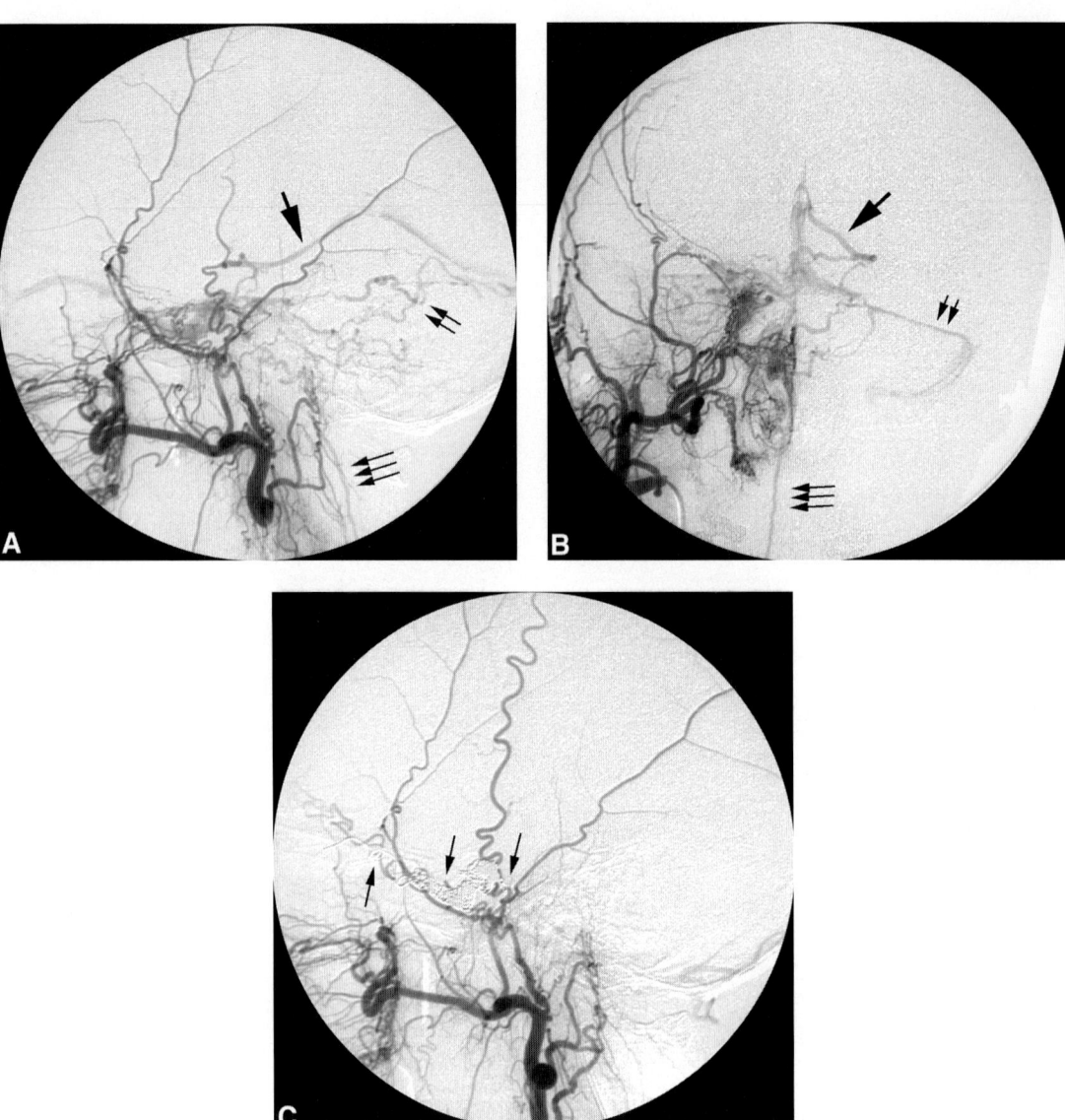

FIGURE 7.9 • *Dural AVM of the Cavernous Sinuses with Deep Parenchymal Drainage.*
A dAVM with extensive bilateral arterial feeders from the internal carotid arteries and external carotid arteries demonstrates deep venous drainage on the right external carotid artery injection (A, lateral projection; B, AP projection). Venous outflow involves the anterior spinal vein (triple arrows), left superior petrosal sinus and cerebellar veins (double arrows), and left basal vein of Rosenthal (arrow).

After transvenous coil embolization of the cavernous sinuses (including some errant placement of coils in the left superior ophthalmic vein) complete elimination of venous shunting was seen from all sources (C, lateral projection of right external carotid angiogram posttreatment).

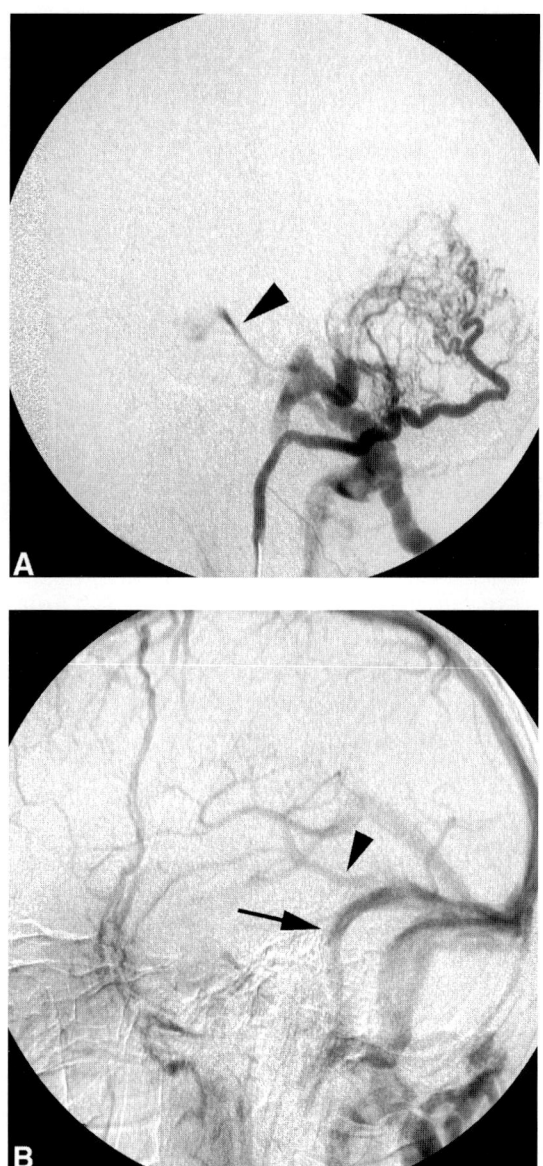

FIGURE 7.10 • *Dural AVM of the Left Transverse Sinus with Antegrade Venous Flow.*
A 58-year-old male presented with headache, intermittent redness of the left eye, and a left-sided bruit. A left occipital artery injection (A) demonstrates an extensive dAVM of the left transverse sinus with antegrade flow into the ipsilateral sigmoid sinus and reflux into the inferior petrosal sinus (arrowhead), which probably explained his intermittent left orbital symptoms. The important information in this patient is on the venous phase of the left internal carotid artery injection (B, lateral projection). This view has been purposely skewed to separate the sigmoid sinuses. The left sigmoid sinus continues to flow antegrade (arrow) through the diseased segment with a prominent afferent vein of Labbé (arrowhead). Although this patient probably would tolerate a transvenous occlusion of the sigmoid sinus distal to the vein of Labbé, the consequences if he could not would be monumental. In consideration of this risk, it was finally decided to perform a surgical skeletonization of the sinus with intraoperative angiography and diligent preservation of the vein of Labbé. This resulted in uneventful elimination of his symptoms.

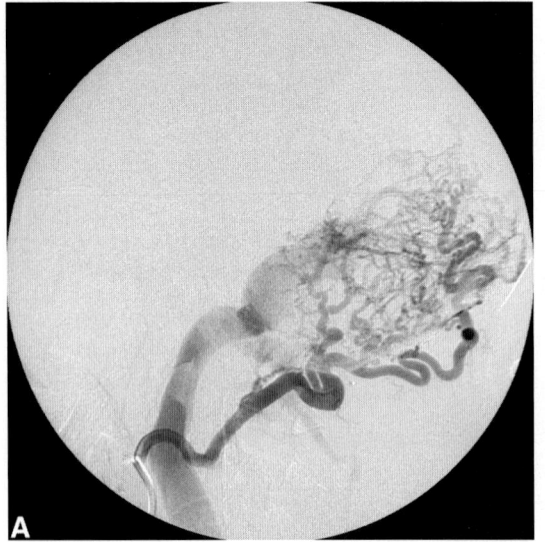 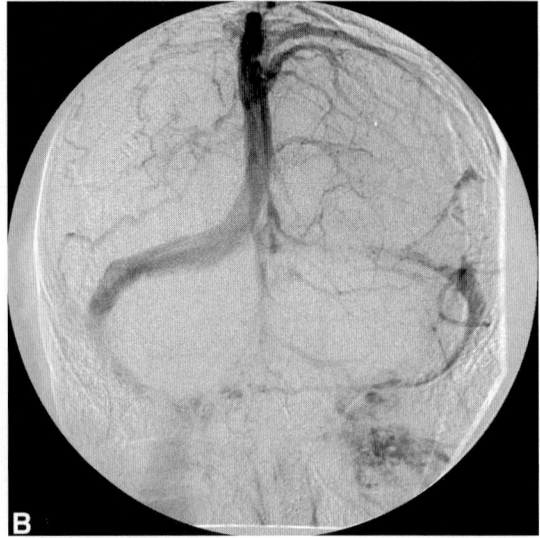

FIGURE 7.11 • *Dural AVM of the Right Sigmoid Sinus with Antegrade Parenchymal Venous Drainage.* A 66-year-old male presenting with an irritating bruit on the right side of his head demonstrates a florid dAVM of the distal right transverse sinus and sigmoid sinus (A, right occipital artery injection, lateral view). Both cerebral hemispheres and the posterior fossa (B, venous phase of left carotid injection) drain antegrade through the dominant right transverse sinus compared with the smaller left transverse sinus. One should be extremely careful about performing transvenous occlusion procedures in patients such as this. The likelihood of calamitous venous infarctions is high, and the non-life-threatening nature of his disease at this time must be kept in focus. Palliative transarterial embolization was performed with histoacryl on this patient with some improvement in symptoms. With histoacryl or any embolic agent in the occipital artery, dangers include skin necrosis from aggressive embolization, facial nerve (VIIth) palsy from injury to the vasa nervorum of the stylomastoid canal, and embolic injury to the posterior circulation through the C1 and C2 anastomoses to the ipsilateral vertebral artery.

of the venous system. The durability of lumen patency in stents within the venous sinuses is not yet established, however.

Transarterial Embolization of Dural AVMs

In general, transarterial embolization of dAVMs tends to be ineffective and unsatisfactory. This is because of the complexity of the lesions in many patients and the need to use relatively bland embolic agents near the skull base if injury to the vasa nervorum of the cranial nerves is to be avoided. However, PVA and Gelfoam sponge tend to have a high likelihood of recanalization in these disorders[15] and are usually discouraged except for palliative use. On the other hand, Gelfoam powder, alcohol, and acrylate adhesive represent a great risk to the cranial nerves around the foramen magnum or cavernous sinus, and carry a risk of tissue necrosis even when used distally near the scalp. There are some patients in whom other options do not exist, and transarterial embolization to reduce flow may be necessary. Direct needle puncture of a distal occipital artery can sometimes be useful when the vessel is too tortuous to catheterize distally, a frequent problem with this artery.

Transorbital Embolization of Dural AVMs of the Cavernous Sinus

In unusual situations, the only available route of access to the cavernous sinus may be via the su-

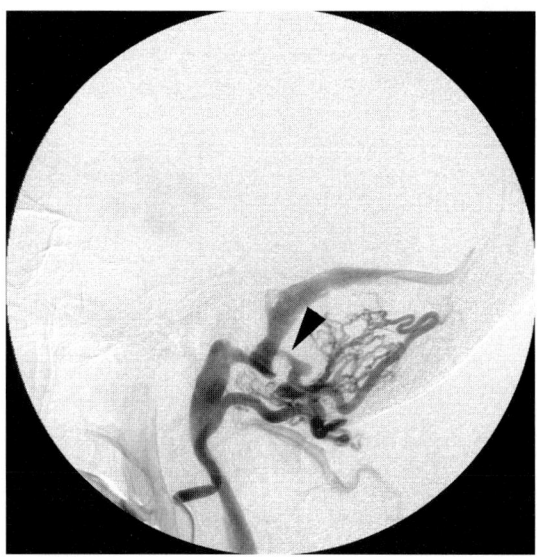

FIGURE 7.12 • *Anatomy of a Transverse Sinus dAVM Favoring Transvenous Embolization.*
Unlike the patient in Fig. 7.10 this patient with a similar diagnosis shows a dAVM of the left transverse sinus in which all of the flow reaches the sinus through a single venous tributary (arrowhead). This lends itself very satisfactorily to transvenous coil embolization of this single channel while preserving the ipsilateral sigmoid sinus.

perior ophthalmic vein.[9,16] When venous pressure in the superior ophthalmic vein is elevated due to the effects of a dAVM, the vein is easily ruptured and the consequential intraorbital hematoma can be severe. Therefore a transorbital approach to a dAVM of the cavernous sinus is most safely performed by a combined procedure involving surgical exposure of the vein and application of ties proximal and distal to the site of venous puncture. The vein can then be catheterized with a microcatheter or a sheath (Fig. 8.8). The surgical exposure and catheterization of the superior ophthalmic vein is not an easy procedure, and a vein that appears very large and distended on the angiogram can be surprisingly elusive and diminutive in the surgical field. For patients in whom no alternative exists, this approach can be very effective. The dAVM can be occluded by delivery of fibered coils or balloons in this manner.

Complications of Transvenous Embolization of the Cavernous Sinus

Surprisingly, cranial nerve deficits following a coil embolization of the cavernous sinus are uncommon. The most vulnerable nerve is the abducens nerve (VI), which is vulnerable to injury in Dorelo's canal during catheterization of the inferior petrosal sinus. Perforation of the dura resulting in intradural or subdural hemorrhage can also occur but is rare. Pituitary injury from wire trauma or the osmotic effects of contrast injury is also possible and has been reported with transarterial embolizations in this vicinity, but seems to be rare with transvenous catheterization. Commonly, in the course of embolization of a dAVM in the cavernous sinus, many injections of contrast will be made to evaluate the progress of treatment. When there is drainage to the ophthalmic veins, this can affect the appearance of the eye afterwards. Even though venous distension around the eye is markedly improved immediately following a successful treatment, the appearance of edema of the sclera can be paradoxically worse. This effect is transient and quickly resolves. Perforation of one of the ophthalmic veins with a microwire can happen during catheterization. As long as the leak is sealed quickly with coils, the resulting hematoma is unlikely to threaten vision and should resolve within a few days.

Transvenous Catheterization of the Cavernous Sinus in the Absence of an Inferior Petrosal Sinus

The most common route of transvenous catheterization from the femoral vein to the cavernous sinus is via the inferior petrosal sinus (Figs. 7.13). When the initial diagnostic angiograms demonstrate no evidence of an inferior petrosal sinus, it may still be possible to gain the ipsilateral cavernous sinus through this route by probing with a wire. The hydrophilically coated wires are especially adept at this, and hydrophilically coated microcatheters are most suited for following the course of the wire afterwards. This maneuver requires a great deal of patience and some educated guesswork on where to pursue probing with the microwire. It probably in-

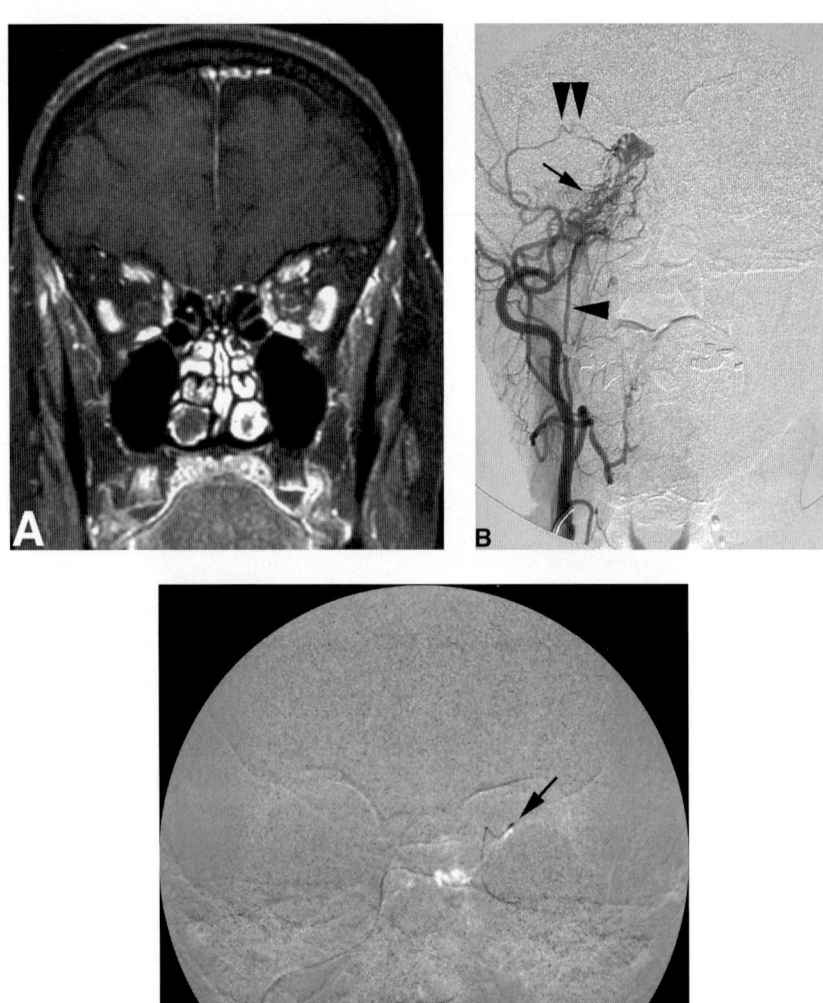

FIGURE 7.13 • *Dural AVM of the Cavernous Sinus. Bilateral Catheterization of the Cavernous Sinus from the Right Side.*
A 67-year-old female patient presented with chemosis and redness of the left eye. An MRI examination (A) demonstrated asymmetric prominence of vessels around the left optic nerve and subtle edema of the left extraocular muscles. Although the clinical signs of the dAVM were on the left side, the dAVM was bilateral and extensive. The right external carotid angiogram, for example, demonstrated a profusion of enlarged arterial feeders to the right cavernous sinus (B) from the right middle meningeal artery (double arrowhead), the internal maxillary artery (arrow) and the ascending pharyngeal artery (arrowhead).

A left-sided inferior petrosal sinus could not be found. The left cavernous sinus was catheterized from the right inferior petrosal sinus across the midline (C, AP roadmap). The arrow points to the guide-wire in the left superior ophthalmic vein advanced from the right inferior petrosal sinus.

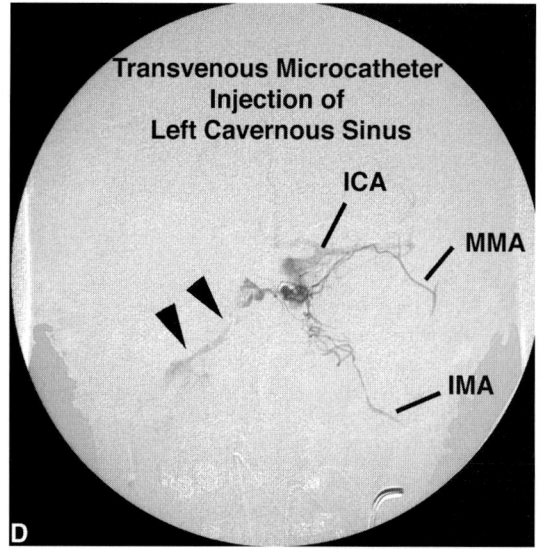
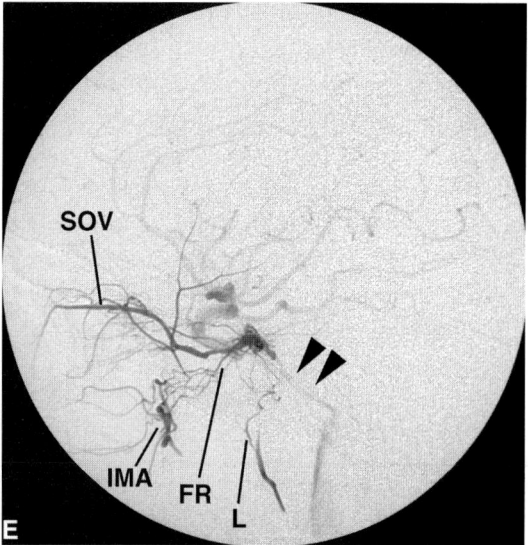
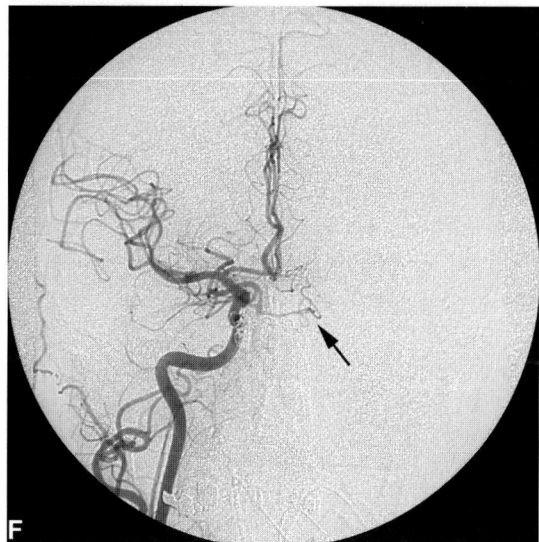

A hand-injection was performed in the left cavernous sinus (D, AP projection; E, lateral projection). The effect of this injection causes transient reflux into the laceral branch of the left ascending pharyngeal artery (L), the artery of the foramen rotundum (FR) opacifying the left internal maxillary artery (IMA), the left internal carotid artery (ICA), and the left superior ophthalmic vein (SOV). The right inferior petrosal sinus is identified by the double arrowhead. This was not a hard injection. It demonstrates the ease with which anastomoses in the region of the inferolateral trunk and elsewhere can communicate during embolization procedures.

After packing of both cavernous sinuses with fibered microcoils, a right common carotid injection (F) demonstrates only a single dural branch (arrow) from the right internal carotid artery to the left cavernous sinus with persistent but extremely slow opacification of the left superior ophthalmic vein. This progressed to complete thrombosis on follow-up angiography one month later.

volves risk of injury to the VIth nerve or risk of dural perforation, but these complications are not common. This maneuver is usually preferable and easier than alternative routes via the superior petrosal sinus, ophthalmic veins, or surgical exposure of the cavernous sinus. In the event of failure to probe a channel along the inferior petrosal sinus, the contralateral inferior petrosal sinus may be patent, and access to the diseased side can be gained via a retroclival or transsellar venous channel.

Radiotherapy for Dural Arteriovenous Malformations

Some success has been reported with the use of gamma knife therapy for dAVMs of the cavernous sinus.[17,18] A success rate of over 90% in slow flow dAVMs was reported by Barcia-Saloria et al.[19,20] using doses of 30–40 Gy with resolution of the dAVM in a period of 2–7 months following treatment. However, many of the cases illustrated in these reports show lesions that are very small or extremely slow in character. The impact of spontaneous resolution of such lesions in the patients treated with irradiation is not known. Rates of spontaneous resolution for dAVMs of 36% or higher have been observed without any treatment in this disorder.[15] In the experience of Barcia-Salorio et al.[19] radiation therapy is probably less likely to be effective in states of higher flow.

References

1. Newton TH, Cronqvist S (1969) Involvement of the dural arteries in intracranial arteriovenous malformations. Radiology 93:1071–1078.
2. Borden JA, Wu JK, Shucart WA (1995) A proposed classification for spinal and cranial dural arteriovenous fistulous malformations and implications for treatment. J Neurosurg 82:166–179.
3. Cognard C, Gobin YP, Pierot L, Bailly AL, Houdart E, Casasco A, Chiras J, Merland JJ (1995) Cerebral dural arteriovenous fistulas: clinical and angiographic correlation with a revised classification of venous drainage. Radiology 194:671–680.
4. Davies MA, TerBrugge K, Willinsky R, Coyne T, Saleh J, Wallace MC (1996) The validity of classification for the clinical presentation of intracranial dural arteriovenous fistulas. J Neurosurg 85:830–837.
5. Houser OW, Cambell JK, Cambell RJ, Sundt TM (1979) Arteriovenous malformations affecting the transverse dural venous sinus: an acquired lesion. Mayo Clin Proc 54:651–661.
6. Chaudhary MY, Sachdev VP, Cho SH, Weitzer I, Puljic S, Huang YP (1982) Dural arteriovenous malformations of the major venous sinuses: an acquired lesion. AJNR 3:13–19.
7. Burrows PE, Lasjaunias PL, Ter Brugge KG, Flodmark O (1987) Urgent and emergent embolization of lesions of the head and neck in children: indications and results. Pediatrics 80:386–394.
8. Komiyama M, Nakajima H, Nishikawa M, Kan M (1998) Traumatic carotid cavernous sinus fistula: serial angiographic studies from the day of trauma. AJNR 19:1641–1644.
9. Lee AG, Miller NR (1999) Neuroophthalmology of arteriovenous malformations. Neurosurg Clin 10:667–681.
10. Halbach VV, Higashida RT, Hieshima GB, Goto K, Norman D, Newton TH (1987) Dural fistulas involving the transverse and sigmoid sinuses: results of treatment in 28 patients. Radiology 163:443–447.
11. Halbach VV, Higashida RT, Hieshima GB, Reicher M, Norman D, Newton TH (1987) Dural fistulas involving the cavernous sinus: results of treatment in 30 patients. Radiology 163:437–442.
12. Ishii K, Goto K, Ihara K, Hieshima GB, Halbach VV, Bentson JR, Shirouzu T, Fukumura A (1987) High-risk dural arteriovenous fistulae of the transverse and sigmoid sinuses. AJNR 8:1113–1120.
13. Mullan S (1979) Treatment of carotid-cavernous fistulas by cavernous sinus occlusion. J Neurosurg 50:131–144.
14. Mironov A (1998) Selective transvenous embolization of dural fistulas without occlusion of the dural sinus. AJNR 19:389–391.
15. Barrow DL, Spector RH, Braun IF, Landman JA, Tindall SC, Tindall GT (1985) Classification and treatment of spontaneous carotid-cavernous sinus fistulas. J Neurosurg 62:248–256.
16. Miller NR, Monsein LH, Debrun GM, Tamargo RJ, Nauta HJ (1995) Treatment of carotid-cavernous sinus fistulas using a superior ophthalmic vein approach. J Neurosurg 83:838–842.
17. Pierot L, Poisson M, Jason M, Pontvert D, Chiras J (1992) Treatment of type D dural carotid-cavernous fistula by embolization followed by irradiation. Neuroradiology 34:77–80.
18. Bitoh S, Hasegawa H, Fujiwara M, Nakao K (1982) Irradiation of spontaneous carotid-cavernous fistulas. Surg Neurol 17:282–286.
19. Barcia-Salorio JL, Soler F, Barcia JA, Hernandez G (1994) Radiosurgery of carotid-cavernous fistulae. Acta Neurochirurgica—Supplementum 62:10–12.
20. Barcia-Salorio JL, Soler F, Barcia JA, Hernandez G (1994) Stereotactic radiosurgery for the treatment of low-flow carotid-cavernous fistulae: results in a series of 25 cases. Stereotactic Func Neurosurg 63:266–270.

Chapter 8

Carotid Cavernous Fistulas

Introduction

All dural arteriovenous malformations near the cavernous sinus are classified by some authors under the general category of carotid cavernous fistulas. Within this generalization, readers will sometimes be referred to the Barrow[1] classification:

- Type A—direct shunts from the internal carotid artery to the cavernous sinus.
- Type B—fistulas between the meningeal branches of the internal carotid artery and the cavernous sinus.
- Type C—dural shunts between the meningeal branches of the external carotid artery and the cavernous sinus.
- Type D—fistulas between the meningeal branches of both the internal carotid artery and the external carotid artery to the cavernous sinus.

However, as described in Chapter 7, the identity of the arterial feeders to dAVMs is usually of little consequence. Therefore, a dichotomous separation of direct carotid cavernous fistulas (CCF), i.e., type A, from dural arteriovenous malformations of the cavernous sinus, i.e., types B, C, and D, is a more helpful and pragmatic discrimination.

Direct carotid cavernous fistulas usually have a different pathogenesis from dural arteriovenous malformations, being either posttraumatic or related to spontaneous rupture of a preexisting cavernous aneurysm. The size of the laceration in a direct fistula is often relatively large, and this frequently has relevance to the techniques of treatment. Dural arteriovenous malformations, on the other hand, indiscriminately involve any of the small dural branches of the cavernous sinus. The presentation and symptoms can be similar in both types of patients, and the same principles of urgent care can apply when elevated intracranial venous pressure or intraocular pressure is present.

Early Treatments for Carotid Cavernous Fistulas

Prior to the advent of modern transvascular embolization techniques, the therapeutic options for high-flow CCFs were limited. Since the 1930s, the possibility of transarterial embolization of autologous muscle fragments had been examined to close arteriovenous fistulas,[2,3] but this was an obviously hazardous procedure. Supraclinoid ligation of the internal carotid artery with or without "trapping" of the fistula was the surgical alternative.[4] Occasionally, the two techniques were combined. A supraclinoid ligation was followed by proximal embolization of muscle fragments and then with proximal ligation of the internal carotid artery.[5] In the 1970s surgical exposure of the cavernous sinus followed by direct electrothrombosis of the venous structures with needles or wires passing a current of 0.2–1.0 mA for a few minutes was attempted by a number of centers.[6–8] Although the technique was successful, significant complications to the internal carotid artery or adjacent cranial nerves were frequent.

ENDOVASCULAR TREATMENT OF CAROTID CAVERNOUS FISTULAS

Transvenous treatment of CCFs and dAVMs of the cavernous sinus was pioneered by Sean Mullan at the University of Chicago.[7] This innovation derived from work by Prolo and Hanbery[9] and Serbinenko,[10] who described the techniques of intracranial balloon detachment with preservation of parent vessel flow in CCFs and other disorders.

Occlusion of the venous side of the fistula either by a transarterial, transvenous, or transorbital approach has become the mainstay of endovascular approach to CCFs. Higashida et al.[11] reported that in 88% of a large series of 206 patients with traumatic tears of the carotid artery, it was possible to preserve the parent vessel and close the fistula on the venous side. In the remaining patients therapeutic closure of the parent artery was necessary. An 80% rate of parent-artery preservation with balloon occlusion of CCFs was reported also by Debrun et al.[12] Complicated or inaccessible fistulas have occasionally been treated by surgical exposure of the carotid artery or of the venous structures, allowing access for balloon or coil placement.[12,13] Another alternative for access to the cavernous sinus is a retrograde approach through the ophthalmic vein or even the facial vein.[14]

The advantages of endovascular treatment of CCFs include the ability to close the fistula rapidly in an acutely ill or hemodynamically compromised patient. When performed under local anesthesia this allows monitoring of the patient's neurologic status in the event that arterial sacrifice and trapping of the fistula become necessary. When a complete transection of the internal carotid artery is present or when the laceration is very large, complete safe closure of the fistula with balloons or coils is difficult, and such cases have generally required trapping of the lesion with arterial closure.[11] It is likely that stent technology using either uncovered stents with coil packing outside the stent or covered stents to occlude the fistula will allow preservation of the parent artery in a greater number of such patients in the future.

INDICATIONS FOR TREATMENT

Direct CCFs occur as a consequence of spontaneous rupture of a preexisting cavernous carotid aneurysm or following skull base trauma with laceration of one or both internal carotid arteries. Therefore the size of the fistula is almost invariably substantial. While spontaneous resolution of a direct fistula can occur, this is uncommon, and almost all of these lesions require treatment. Spontaneous rupture of an aneurysm is usually an isolated event, but posttraumatic patients frequently have other injuries, including intracranial hemorrhage or contusions. This raises the question of timing of endovascular treatment because of the risks associated with heparinization or antiplatelet agents desirable during endovascular procedures. Sometimes a delay in treatment is prudent, and this will often allow a "maturation" of the fistula to occur. Usually, this means that the fistula will enlarge or that progressive venous distension will occur, rendering subsequent balloon or coil embolization a little more technically easy. However, delay of treatment in the main involves prolongation of risk for the patient. Early treatment is the best prevention of delayed complications such as intracranial hemorrhage.

Indications for urgent treatment of CCFs include any signs of elevated intracranial venous pressure, intradural venous drainage from the fistula, restriction of venous drainage, rapidly progressive

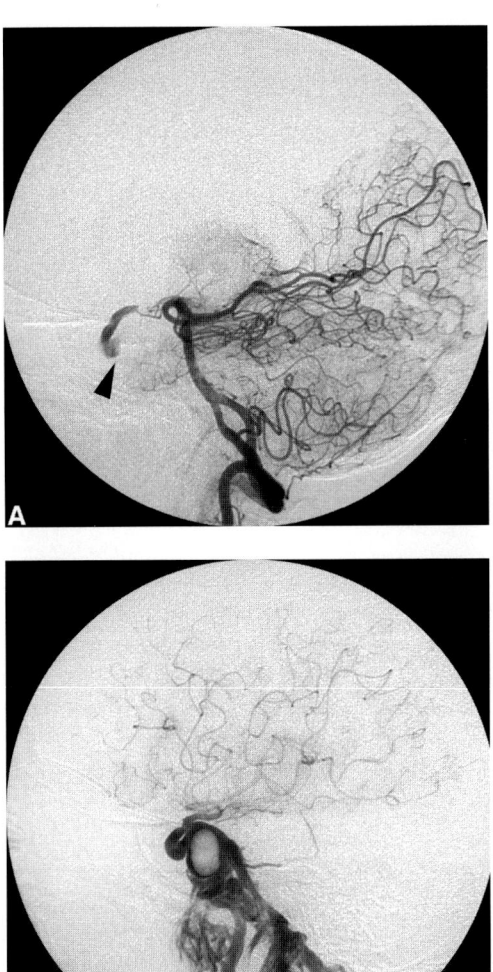

FIGURE 8.1 • *Balloon Inflation in a CCF.*
An injection in an alternative artery can give indirect opacification of a CCF, and because the volume of flow is less than with a direct injection, a more precise localization of the fistula can be achieved. In this vertebral artery injection in an 81-year-old female (A) the internal carotid artery opacifies retrogradely to the distal horizontal cavernous segment (arrowhead indicates the upper/distal end of the fistula). Knowing the precise location of the fistula can be very important while navigating the balloon.

An intraoperative DSA run from the treatment session (B) demonstrates that the silicone DSB has been inflated to full recommended volume on the venous side of the fistula, but the fistula is far from sealed. This is a frustrating and common situation in the treatment of large CCFs. An option probably best avoided is to overinflate the balloon. This would probably involve a risk of premature deflation. A larger balloon might accomplish the task. Alternatively, this first balloon could be detached in a semi-inflated state, leaving room on the venous side for a second balloon. Failing all of these options, the fistula might be approached from the venous side. The inferior petrosal sinus is large in this case, and access should not be problematic. If the patient can tolerate it, the carotid artery might be sacrificed on this side by trapping the fistula with balloons above and below. In this patient a slightly larger balloon was successful at closing the fistula and preserving the internal carotid artery.

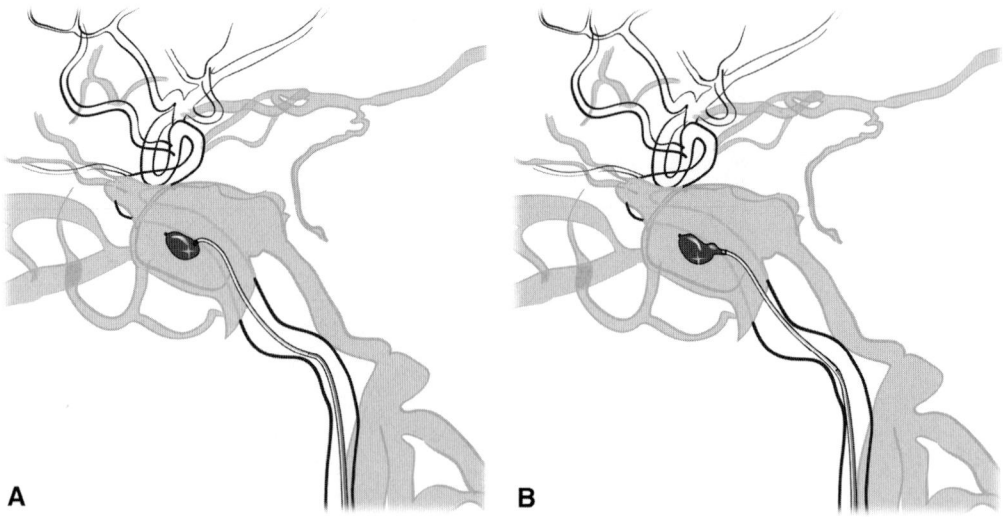

FIGURE 8.2 • *Safety Balloon Technique for CCF Embolization I.*
A tense moment always comes during balloon detachment in a CCF or other locations. The dangers include balloon motion forwards or backwards, or premature deflation. A technique that greatly enhances the ease and safety of balloon deployment within a CCF is illustrated. The problem is demonstrated where a single balloon is floated into the fistula and inflated to the point of complete fistula occlusion (A). Upon retraction of the microcatheter on the balloon, the arterial rent is sufficiently large that the balloon begins to retract with the microcatheter (B) with attendant risks of arterial compromise or even distal migration. These problems are avoided by stabilizing the detachable balloon in the fistula at the time of detachment with a nondetachable balloon in the artery (C). The microcatheter can be withdrawn from the detachable balloon with impunity (D), leaving the fistula site secure (E).

This technique can be conducted through a single catheter as illustrated in Fig. 3.15. It is very important, however, to avoid any possibility of pushing the detachable balloon off its microcatheter within the shaft of the introducer catheter. This could happen easily by pushing on the nondetachable balloon-catheter at an ill-chosen moment. Therefore the detachable balloon must remain in fluoroscopic view above the tip of the introducer catheter while the nondetachable balloon is advancing. The detachable balloon should be extruded from the introducer catheter and held near the fistula or in it, while the nondetachable balloon-catheter is being advanced from the groin to the fistula.

proptosis, diminishing visual acuity, intracranial hemorrhage, or neurologic symptoms.[15] Additionally, any evidence of varix formation in the cavernous sinus with extension of a distended vein or varix into the subarachnoid space is a harbinger of subarachnoid or intraparenchymal hemorrhage, indicating a need for urgent treatment. Protrusion of a distended vein into the sphenoid sinus through a skull fracture represents a serious risk of exsanguinating epistaxis. Therefore, any report of epistaxis in a patient with a CCF should be considered a potential emergency. Clinical symptoms of headache, retroorbital pain, and signs of fluctuating levels of consciousness and papilledema may be indications of rising intracranial pressure, likewise constituting an indication for urgent treatment. Some authors have considered the hemodynamic sump of the CCF to be potentially injurious to the brain with "steal" phenomenon resulting in ischemic injury.[16] A more common mechanism for ischemic injury to the brain in CCF patients is the invariable dissection that occurs with any carotid

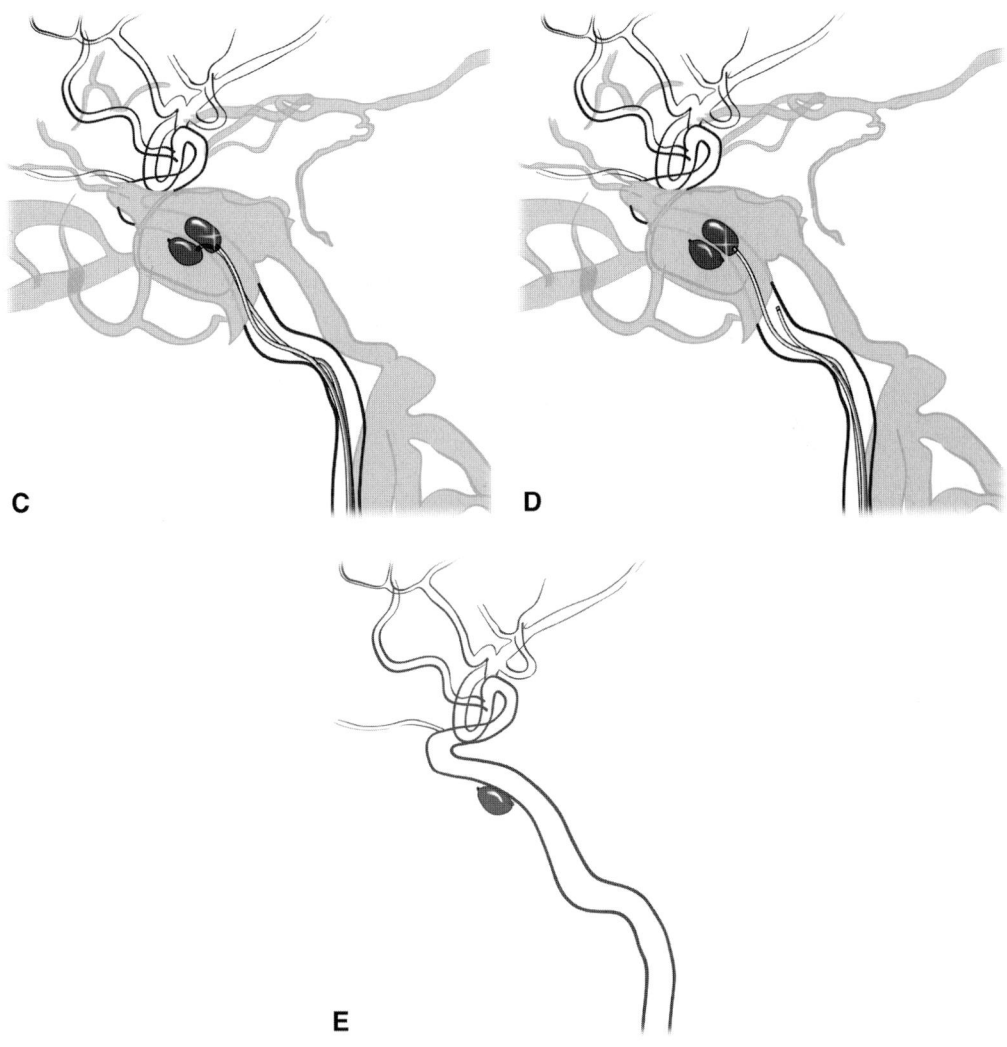

laceration. This can result in carotid occlusion with infarction when collateral circulation is inadequate, or can be a source of thromboembolic infarction. A corollary of the "steal" phenomenon that can be seen, however, is the possibility of normal perfusion pressure breakthrough hemorrhage or cerebral edema when abrupt closure of long-standing carotid or vertebral artery fistulas is executed.[17] In patients who have had a large fistula of many years' standing, upon balloon closure of the fistula immediate onset of headache, vertigo, focal deficits, or signs of brain edema and incipient herniation can be seen, which can be reversible when the balloon is deflated. Staged or slow closure of the fistula is advised in such patients to prevent this serious complication.

Materials and Methods

Several embolic agents have been used for occluding arteriovenous fistulas of the cranial vessels including balloons, liquid adhesives, coils,

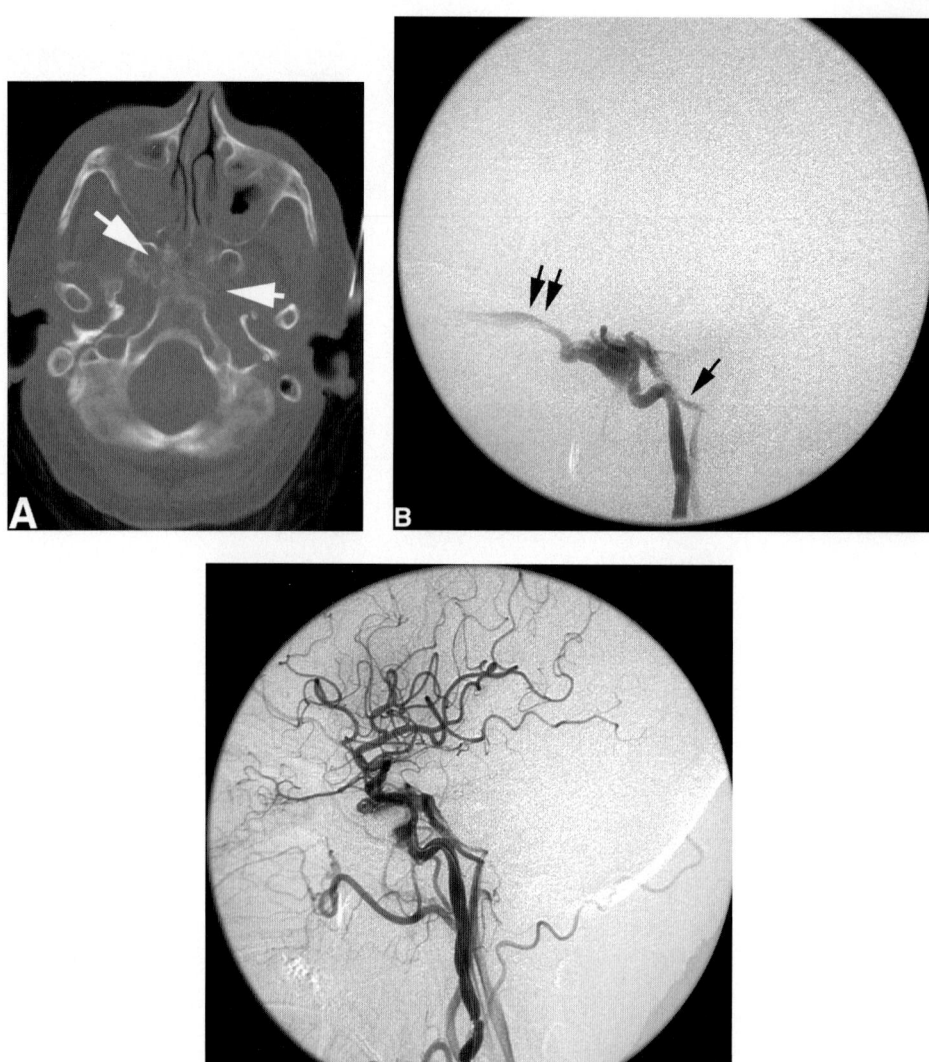

FIGURE 8.3 • *Safety Balloon Technique II.*
An elderly female patient sustained skull fractures in an automobile accident followed by onset of bilateral proptosis and a loud bruit. A CT examination (A) showed, among other injuries, a fracture of the body of the sphenoid bone (arrows), a typical finding in such patients.

The left internal carotid artery angiogram (B, lateral view) prior to treatment shows no antegrade flow in the intracranial circulation from this artery. This could represent an occlusion above the fistula, but reflux from the collateral arteries back to the fistula was present. Nevertheless, the patient's demonstrated tolerance of elimination of the left carotid artery from the cranial circulation implies that a therapeutic occlusion of the left internal carotid artery could be performed quickly in an urgent situation without fear of cerebral hypoperfusion. A large venous sac in the left cavernous sinus opacifies the ipsilateral superior ophthalmic vein (double arrow) and the inferior petrosal sinus (single arrow).

A single silicone balloon was floated into the fistula on an extended-tip microcatheter and inflated. Despite several attempts, a satisfactory balloon inflation could not be obtained that would seal the fistula and preserve the internal carotid artery at the same time (C).

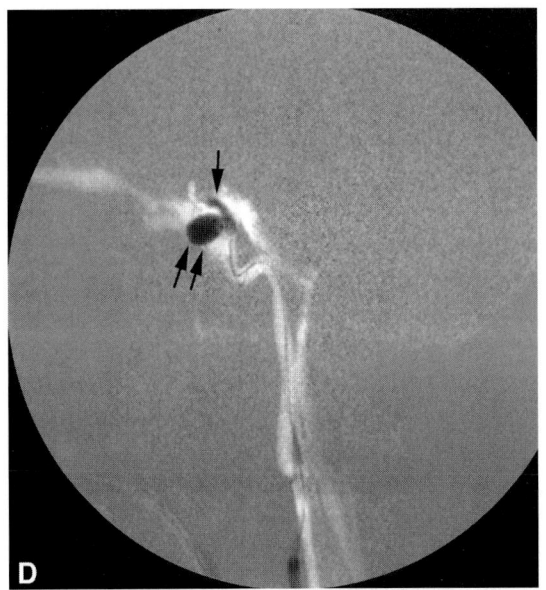
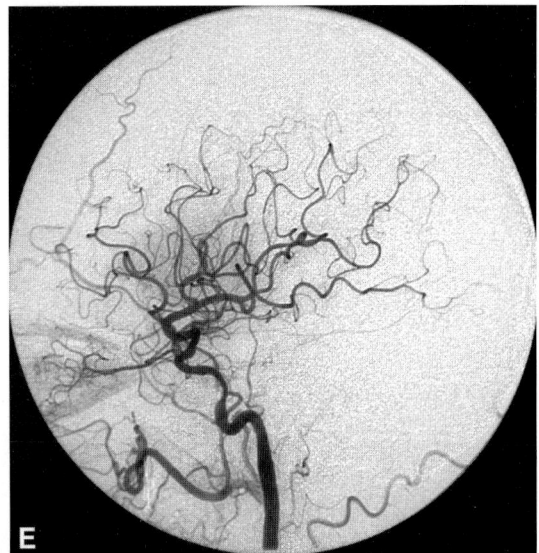
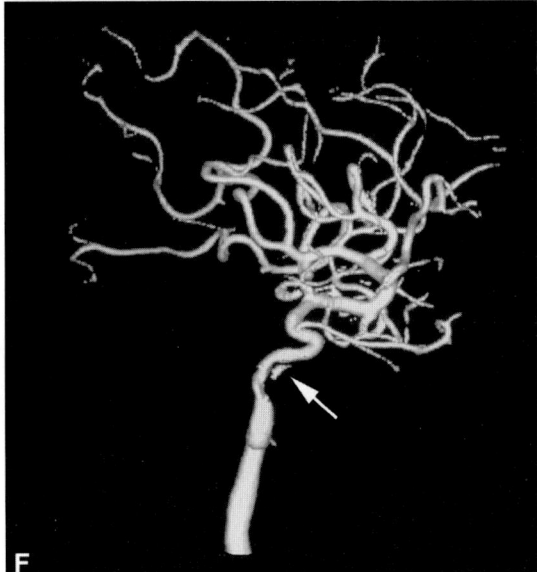

Subsequently, a nondetachable Endeavor balloon (Target) was placed parallel to the detachable balloon and inflated within the artery prior to inflating the detachable balloon. A procedural roadmap (D) shows the safety balloon (arrow) describing the curve of the carotid artery and preserving its integrity while the detachable balloon (double arrow) is inflated.

The final run (E) after deposition of the balloon shows a reasonable outcome with minimal compromise of the carotid lumen at the balloon site. A small pseudoaneurysm of the internal carotid artery can be seen through the balloon.

The 3D final image (F) also demonstrates the small residual pseudoaneurysm (arrow) without overlying balloon artifact. Such residua are common, given the genesis of the condition. Antiplatelet therapy and heparin following the procedure are generally considered prudent.

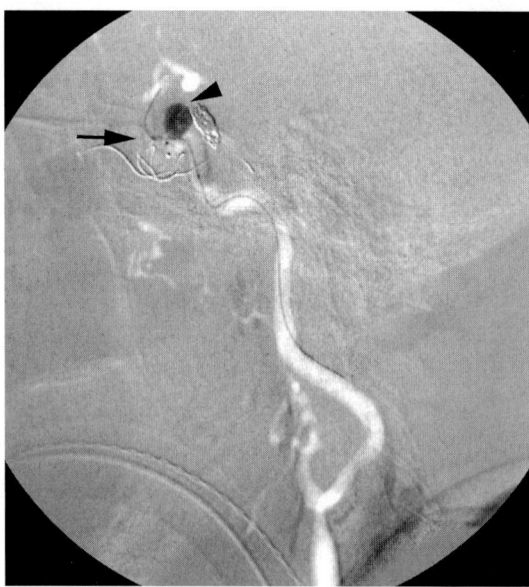

FIGURE 8.4 • *Safety Balloon Technique III.*
In this patient with a treatment protocol similar to that of the case in Fig. 8.3, an Equinox (MTI) balloon (arrow) has been advanced into the artery over a 0.010-in wire. The DSB is inflated successfully within the fistula (arrowhead). Because of this patient's proximal carotid bifurcation disease, seen on this roadmap image, there was initial reluctance to treat the patient transarterially. Therefore, artifact from a failed attempt at transvenous coiling of the fistula is present on the image. However, the flow was heavier than could be stanched by fibered coils. This transarterial procedure was, therefore, conducted from the left common carotid artery.

sutures, and more recently covered and uncovered stents.

Detachable Latex and Silicone Balloons

From the point of view of duration of the procedure and cumulative experience with CCF treatment, the preferred mode of treatment is transarterial embolization of the fistula with a detachable balloon, allowing preservation of the carotid artery. The ideal repair of an artery is one in which a single balloon is floated on a microcatheter through the fistula to the venous side, inflated, and detached, forming a seal on the laceration. Most CCFs are treated in this manner with a singleton balloon, while occasionally multiple balloons are necessary. A follow-up study over 10 years of 87 patients treated with latex or silicone balloons for CCF demonstrated no evidence of late complications related to the balloons themselves or recurrence of the fistula.[18,19] A long-term pseudoaneurysm rate of 30% following balloon deposition in a CCF has been observed by some authors, but any clinical risk associated with this phenomenon does not appear to be substantial.[20]

Lewis et al.[19] reported a complication rate of approximately 4% in a consecutive series of 100 patients treated for CCF with silicone or latex balloons. Complications appeared to be related to heparinization for the procedure or clot formation around the catheter system. A high rate of preservation of the internal carotid artery (75%) was observed with good outcome of treatment in general. Although alternative approaches and materials for CCF embolization have been developed, transarterial embolization with detachable balloons remains the preferred method.[1,12,21]

Techniques of Balloon Placement

Detachable balloons can be mounted on a variety of microcatheters and advanced up the carotid artery in a deflated state. Minimal inflation of the balloon can allow the microcatheter-balloon combination to become flow-directed. Care is necessary to avoid inflation of the balloon within the carotid artery when the traction holding the balloon on the microcatheter is low. This could lead to premature detachment. As the balloon approaches the fistula, it frequently encounters turbulence in the arterial flow. This can be seen fluoroscopically as a trembling of the balloon, indicating that the fistula is close by. By slight inflation of the balloon, it can be encouraged to pop through the fistula to the venous side, where it is progressively inflated until closure of the fistula is confirmed fluoroscopically by arterial injections (Fig. 8.1). Ideally, a profile view of the

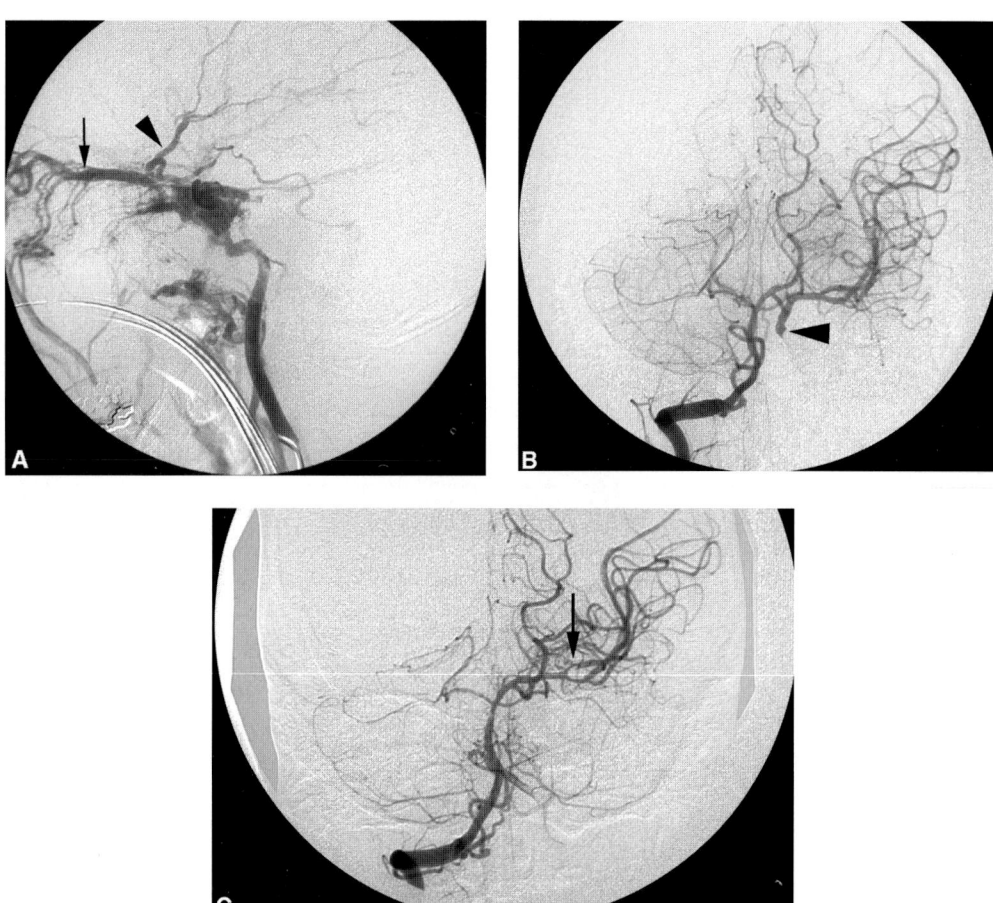

FIGURE 8.5 • *Embolic Complications Following CCF Treatment.*
A 22-year-old female was involved in a high-speed automobile accident and sustained multiple injuries requiring splenectomy, liver repair, and multiple other procedures. A bruit was audible over her proptotic left eye, and a direct light reflex was absent in the left eye. The trauma team taking care of the patient was reluctant to countenance an immediate treatment of her presumed CCF because the use of heparin would be involved.

However, compromises were made because of planned departmental absences, and this proved providential. The left internal carotid artery angiogram (A, lateral view, left carotid injection) shows that the fistula was very large with drainage to the superior ophthalmic vein (arrow). No intracranial arterial flow was present; instead retrograde opacification of the left middle cerebral vein (arrowhead) was present, placing the patient at risk for intracranial venous hemorrhage or infarctions if treatment were further delayed.

Despite placement of 3 silicone balloons in the fistula, the fistula could not be closed. Considerations of use of a covered or noncovered stent to reconstruct and preserve the artery in a patient so young were stymied by cautions about her brain contusions and other injuries. Therefore, the left carotid artery was sacrificed using balloons. The right vertebral artery injection following occlusion (B, Towne's projection) shows reflux to the topmost balloon (arrowhead) sitting below the left ophthalmic artery.

Because of her multiple injuries, there was reluctance to heparinize the patient, which would be an otherwise routine precaution following a procedure such as this. Five days following the treatment while making steady recovery, she was abruptly noted to be intermittently dysphasic and paretic on the right side. An emergency angiogram (C, right vertebral injection, Towne's view) shows a saddle-embolus (arrow) astride the left middle cerebral bifurcation (compare with same projection in image B). Fortunately, with heparinization her neurologic status improved thereafter without evidence of an infarction in the left hemisphere. Although she has since made an excellent clinical recovery, she did not regain vision in the left eye.

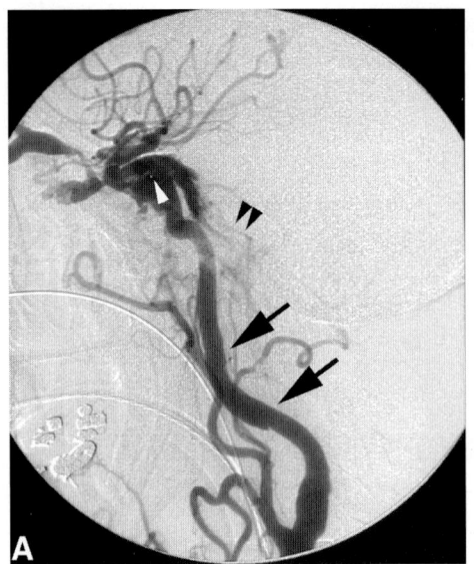 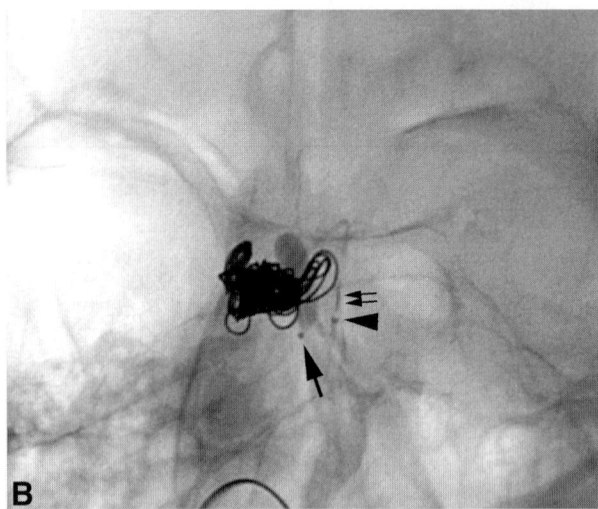

FIGURE 8.6 • *Combination of Techniques in CCF Treatment.*
A 56-year-old male patient sustained a dissection of the right internal carotid artery and a large CCF of the right cavernous carotid artery following a car crash. After stabilization of multiple other injuries, his proptosis having worsened in the interim, he was referred for endovascular occlusion of the fistula. A latex balloon was floated up the carotid artery and inflated uneventfully within the fistula, detached, and the microcatheter withdrawn. However, the next morning while the patient's eye looked much improved, the loud bruit was again audible over his right brow. A plain film of the skull confirmed that the balloon had deflated prematurely, and a second treatment was planned.

The pretreatment images on day 2 (A, lateral view) showed the dissection of the cervical internal carotid artery (arrows), and resumption of flow within the fistula with drainage to the superior ophthalmic vein and inferior petrosal sinus (arrowheads). The metallic marker from the deflated latex balloon is still present (white arrowhead), giving assurance that it has not shifted to a hazardous location.

To avoid another transarterial procedure across the dissection, an attempt was made to coil-occlude the fistula transvenously. A number of concerns became prominent: First, the rent in the carotid artery was so large that the first GDC placed within the sinus from a transvenous microcatheter prolapsed into the carotid artery and was quickly dragged into the ipsilateral middle cerebral artery. Second, the possibility arose that the transvenous coils could push the deflated latex balloon back into the internal carotid artery, causing a cerebral embolus.

To avoid these possibilities, but persisting with the transvenous treatment, an Endeavor (Target) balloon was floated up the carotid artery and inflated across the fistula intermittently during coil deposition. Image B shows the balloon with its proximal marker (arrow) in the carotid artery. The proximal marker of the microcatheter (single arrowhead) and detachment marker of the fibered GDC (double arrow) within the inferior petrosal sinus project nearby. Incidentally, the coil is pushed too far in on this picture. The detachment marker (double arrow) should be retracted until it touches the proximal microcatheter marker (arrowhead).

This combined balloon technique proved very helpful in this patient, because as the case progressed, the deposition of coils within the cavernous sinus began to enclose the carotid artery. Without the balloon it would have been impossible to know whether some of the coils were making their way into the arterial lumen. The final image (C, lateral view) shows the obscuration of the carotid artery by coil artifact. Minimal fistulous flow persists (arrow) but is so slow that it could be safely assumed that it would eventually thrombose, which was the case.

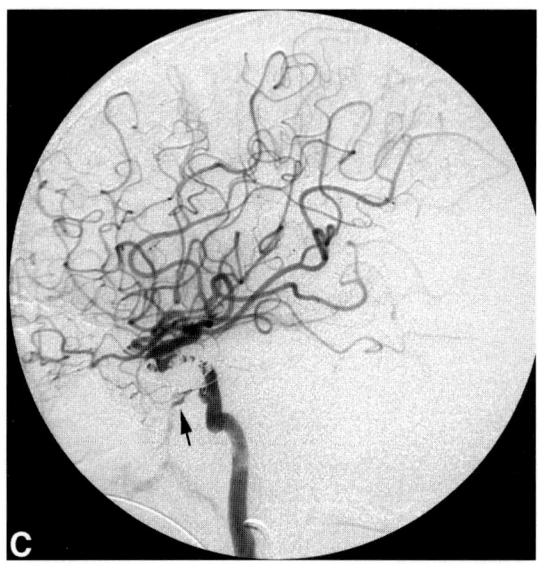

artery and balloon is desirable to prevent inflation of the balloon partially within the artery before detachment is performed.

Particular dangers exist at the time of balloon detachment, mainly related to traction of the microcatheter on the balloon and the risk of pulling it back into the artery. Therefore, a nondetachable "safety" balloon can be used to provide countertraction in the artery during withdrawal of the microcatheter (Figs. 8.2–8.4, 8.5).[22] Partial deflation of the detachable balloon at the time of detachment can also occur when the volume of the balloon is particularly critical. This can sometimes be prevented by inflating a tiny extra drop of contrast into the balloon prior to detachment to allow for loss of a drop of contrast from the balloon valve at the time of traction.

Coil Embolization of Carotid Cavernous Fistulas

Coil embolization of a CCF represents an effective and safe alternative for treatment when transarterial balloon embolization is not possible. Transarterial balloon embolization of CCFs fails or encounters insurmountable technical obstacles in 5% to 10% of cases.[23] Coils are a slower and more expensive method, however, involving greater financial costs, longer procedure time, and greater radiation exposure.[24] Fibered thrombogenic GDC or standard GDC can be placed via a microcatheter directly into the cavernous sinus in a very controlled fashion from a transarterial or transvenous approach (Figs. 8.6, 8.7). Transvenous access can be gained from a standard transfemoral approach via the inferior or superior petrosal sinuses, via a transorbital exposure of the ophthalmic veins, or by direct surgical exposure of the cavernous sinuses.[23] When the underlying lesion is a preexisting cavernous aneurysm and a transarterial coil embolization of the aneurysm is planned, nonfibered coils are a safer material because the potential for thromboembolic cerebral complications with fibered coils in the arterial system is probably higher. When the laceration of the internal carotid artery is very large, prolapse of coils from a transvenous approach into the artery can occur. In such cases the artery can be protected by an intermittently inflated arterial balloon similar to the technique used for aneurysm reconstructive therapy.[25]

Because the progressive occlusion of a CCF with coils (or a dAVM of the cavernous sinus) is a gradual process, some risks must be anticipated that may not exist when occluding a CCF with a single balloon. In particular, diversion of the venous flow into a deep parenchymal vein can occur inadvertently in the course of a coiling procedure and can result in hemorrhagic complications. Additionally, dural perforations with subarachnoid hemorrhage can occur during the catheterization process.[26]

Transorbital Approach to Carotid Cavernous Fistulas

A retrograde approach to the cavernous sinus via the ophthalmic vein is possible and can be effective in patients for whom alternatives do not exist (Fig. 8.8). This is a technically more challenging procedure with particular risks. Surgical exposure of the vein by an ophthalmic surgeon with control of the vein proximal and distal to the point of puncture with vascular slings is the key to the safety of this approach.[27] The danger lies in losing control of the

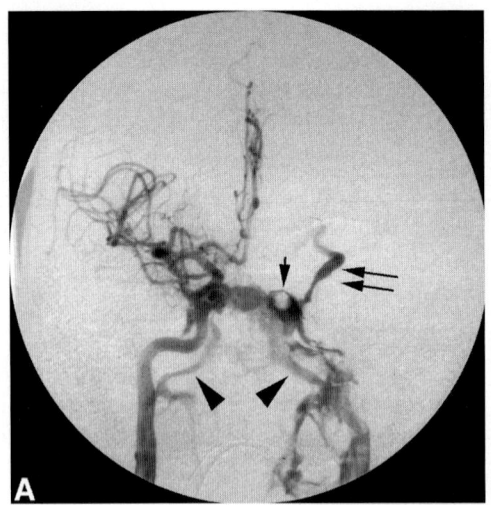
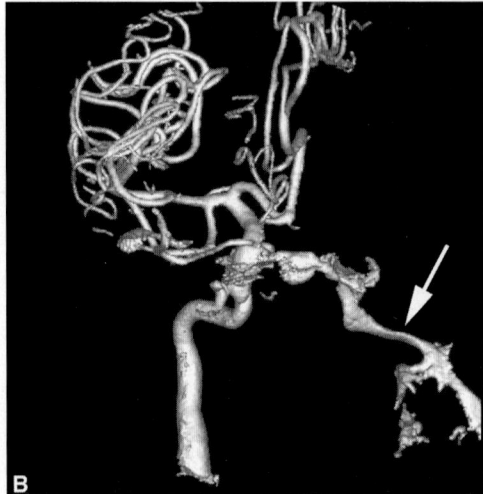
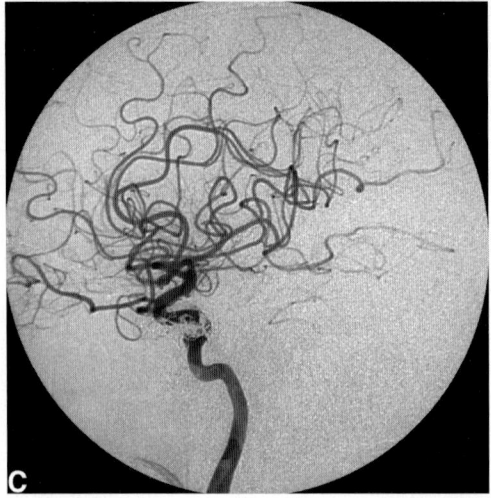

FIGURE 8.7 • *Air-bag Injury in a 58-Year-Old Male Patient.*
This patient was driving at 35 miles per hour, lost control of his car, and hit a wall causing deployment of his airbag. His apparent injuries were minimal and he was discharged from hospital the next day. Two weeks later his left eye became alarmingly proptotic. He noticed a bruit, and over the course of a 24-hour period he lost vision completely in the left eye.

An emergency angiogram showed that although his blindness was on the left, the CCF was from his right carotid artery (A). Drainage is referred to the left superior ophthalmic vein (double arrow). Outflow from that point was restricted, explaining the alarming appearance of his left eye. Both inferior petrosal sinuses (arrowheads) participate in the venous outflow too. The lucency within the left cavernous sinus (small single arrow) is the nonopacified left internal carotid artery seen end-on.

Despite the relatively large fistula present, a balloon could not be navigated into the right cavernous sinus over many hours of attempts. A 3D view from a right carotid injection (B) shows the relative ease of access from the left inferior petrosal sinus (arrow) to the right cavernous sinus. This route was used for a coil-packing procedure of the right cavernous sinus, which resulted in prompt elimination of the fistula (C, final lateral view). The patient quickly recovered vision in the left eye, and two weeks following treatment had 20/25 vision with complete resolution of his proptosis.

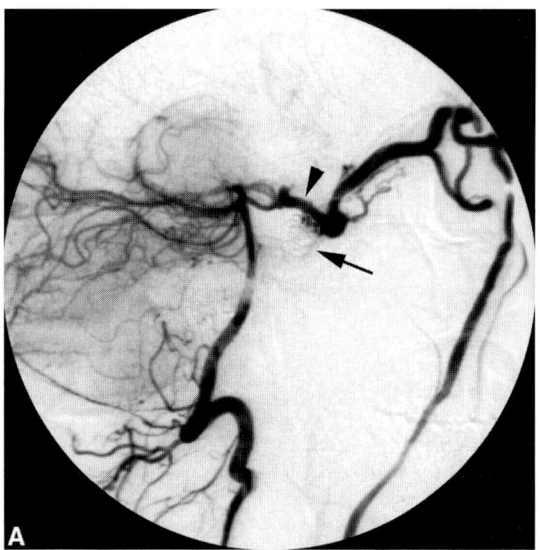

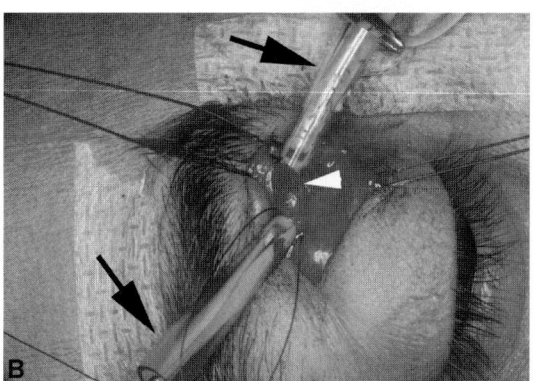
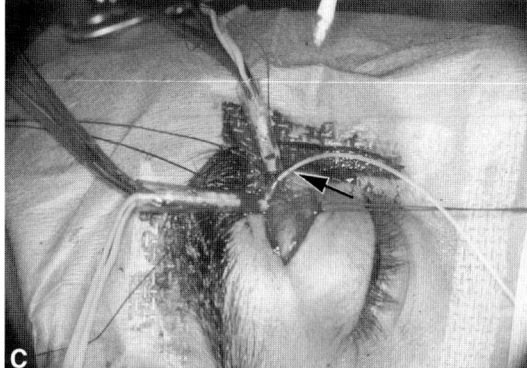

FIGURE 8.8 • *Transorbital Venous Catheterization for Treatment of CCF.*
A 34-year-old male patient presented with right-sided proptosis following an assault. An occlusive dissection of the right internal carotid artery precluded a direct transarterial approach to his CCF, but a coiling procedure from the posterior circulation via the right posterior communicating artery was initially successful. Two weeks later however, his bruit returned. A repeat angiogram (A, lateral view of left vertebral artery injection) demonstrated that recanalization from the supraclinoid right internal carotid artery (arrowhead) past the nidus of coils (arrow) had taken place.

A retrograde transorbital approach to the recanalized fistula was performed under general anesthesia. The right superior ophthalmic vein (white arrowhead in B) was isolated and secured with vascular ties (black arrows in B) proximally and distally. The eyeball is protected by a colored guard. A microcatheter over a wire was then threaded retrogradely into the vein (black arrow in C). The upper vascular tie was loosened slightly to accommodate retrograde passage of the microcatheter and then tightened anew. (*Continued on following page.*)

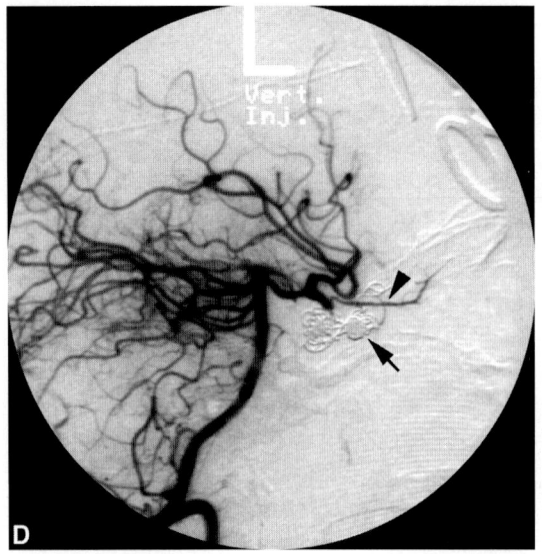 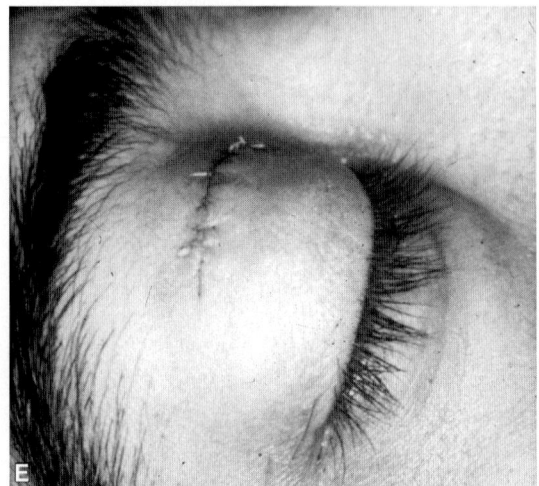

FIGURE 8.8 • *Continued.*
A second nidus of coils was placed retrogradely into the fistula (arrow in D, lateral view, left vertebral injection), resulting in elimination of the fistula. The ophthalmic artery (arrowhead) still flows antegradely from the supraclinoid carotid artery. The postoperative photograph (E) shows the excellent external postsurgical appearance of the eyelid.

Case conducted in collaboration with Dr. Joseph Rubin, Massachusetts Eye and Ear Infirmary, Boston, MA.

puncture site with profuse hemorrhage into the orbit. The vein can be punctured directly with a microcatheter or with an intravenous cannula with a hemostatic valve. The cannula acts as a sheath for the microcatheter.

The transorbital approach[28,29] can be used for retrograde occlusion of the cavernous sinus either by coils or balloons. Balloons are more difficult to steer retrogradely against the stream of flow and require a larger introducer device than a microcatheter for coil placement.

References

1. BARROW DL, SPECTOR RH, BRAUN IF, LANDMAN JA, TINDALL SC, TINDALL GT (1985) Classification and treatment of spontaneous carotid-cavernous sinus fistulas. *J Neurosurg* 62:248–256.
2. BROOKS B (1930) The treatment of traumatic arteriovenous fistula. *South Med J* 23:100–106.
3. WANISSORN R (1970) Mechanism of experimental muscle embolization of the carotid cavernous fistula and fate of emboli. *J Neurosurg* 32:344–348.
4. HAMBY WB, GARDNER WJ (1933) Treatment of pulsating exopthalmos with report of two cases. *Arch Surg* (Chicago) 27:676–685.
5. JAEGER R (1949) Intracranial aneurysms. *South Surg* 15:205–217.
6. MULLAN S (1974) Experiences with surgical thrombosis of intracranial berry aneurysms and carotid cavernous fistulas. *J Neurosurg* 41:657–670.
7. MULLAN S (1979) Treatment of carotid-cavernous fistulas by cavernous sinus occlusion. *J Neurosurg* 50:131–144.
8. ISHIKAWA M, HANDA H, TAKI W, YONEDA S (1982) Management of spontaneous carotid-cavernous fistulae. *Surg Neurol* 18:131–139.
9. PROLO DJ, HANBERY JW (1971) Intraluminal occlusion of a carotid cavernous fistula with a balloon catheter. Technical Note. *J Neurosurg* 35:237–242.
10. SERBINENKO FA (1974) Balloon catheterization and occlusion of major cerebral vessels. *J Neurosurg* 41:125–145.
11. HIGASHIDA RT, HALBACH VV, TSAI FY, NORMAN D, PRIBRAM HF, MEHRINGER CM, HIESHIMA GB (1989) Interventional

neurovascular treatment of traumatic carotid and vertebral artery lesions: results in 234 cases. *AJR* 153:577–582.
12. DEBRUN GM, VINUELA F, FOX AJ, DAVIS KR, AHN HS (1988) Indications for treatment and classification of 132 carotid-cavernous fistulas. *Neurosurgery* 22:285–289.
13. BATJER HH, PURDY PD, NEIMAN M, SAMSON DS (1988) Subtemporal transdural use of detachable balloons for traumatic carotid-cavernous fistulas. *Neurosurgery* 22:290–296.
14. TENG MM, LIRNG JF, CHANG T, CHEN SS, GUO WY, CHENG CC, SHEN WC, LEE LS (1995) Embolization of carotid cavernous fistula by means of direct puncture through the superior orbital fissure. *Radiology* 194:705–711.
15. HALBACH VV, HIESHIMA GB, HIGASHIDA RT, REICHER M (1987) Carotid cavernous fistulae: indications for urgent treatment. *AJR* 149:587–593.
16. IIDA K, UOZUMI T, ARITA K, NAKAHARA T, OHBA S, SATOH H (1995) Steal phenomenon in a traumatic carotid-cavernous fistula. *J Trauma-Inj Infect Crit Care* 39:1015–1017.
17. HALBACH VV, HIGASHIDA RT, HIESHIMA GB, NORMAN D (1987) Normal perfusion pressure breakthrough occurring during treatment of carotid and vertebral fistulas. *AJNR* 8:751–756.
18. LEWIS AI, TOMSICK TA, TEW JM JR, LAWLESS MA (1996) Long-term results in direct carotid-cavernous fistulas after treatment with detachable balloons. *J Neurosurg* 84:400–404.
19. LEWIS AI, TOMSICK TA, TEW JM JR (1995) Management of 100 consecutive direct carotid-cavernous fistulas: results of treatment with detachable balloons. *Neurosurgery* 36:239–244.
20. MORET J (1995) Management of 100 consecutive direct carotid-cavernous fistulas: results of treatment with detachable balloons. *Neurosurgery* 36:245.
21. BARROW DL, FLEISCHER AS, HOFFMAN JC (1982) Complications of detachable balloon catheter technique in the treatment of traumatic intracranial arteriovenous fistulas. *J Neurosurg* 56:396–403.
22. MASARYK TJ, PERL J 2ND, WALLACE RC, MAGDINEC M, CHYATTE D (1999) Detachable balloon embolization: concomitant use of a second safety balloon. *AJNR* 20:1103–1106.
23. HALBACH VV, HIGASHIDA RT, HIESHIMA GB, HARDIN CW, YANG PJ (1988) Transvenous embolization of direct carotid cavernous fistulas. *AJNR* 9:741–747.
24. SINILUOTO T, SEPPANEN S, KUURNE T, WIKHOLM G, LEINONEN S, SVENDSEN P (1997) Transarterial embolization of a direct carotid cavernous fistula with Guglielmi detachable coils. *AJNR* 18:519–523.
25. MORRIS PP (1999) Balloon reconstructive technique for the treatment of a carotid cavernous fistula. *AJNR* 20:1107–1109.
26. BARNWELL SL, O'NEILL OR (1994) Endovascular therapy of carotid cavernous fistulas. *Neurosurg Clin North Am* 5:485–495.
27. MILLER NR, MONSEIN LH, DEBRUN GM, TAMARGO RJ, NAUTA HJ (1995) Treatment of carotid-cavernous sinus fistulas using a superior ophthalmic vein approach. *J Neurosurg* 83:838–842.
28. COURTHEOUX P, LABBE D, HAMEL C, LECOQ P, JAHARA M, THERON J (1987) Treatment of bilateral spontaneous dural carotid-cavernous fistulas by coil and sclerotherapy. *J Neurosurg* 66:468–470.
29. MILLER NR (1998) Severe vision loss and neovascular glaucoma complicating superior ophthalmic vein approach to carotid-cavernous sinus fistula. *Am J Ophthalmol* 125:883–884.

CHAPTER 9

Balloon Test Occlusion and Postocclusion Patient Care

INTRODUCTION

Therapeutic occlusion of an internal carotid artery or vertebral artery is an accepted alternative treatment for inoperable aneurysms, fistulas, pseudoaneurysms, dissections, or as part of the treatment of neck and skull-base tumors when less radical alternatives cannot be applied. Arterial occlusion can be performed as part of a surgical procedure or can be accomplished endovascularly using coils or balloons. Preoperative test occlusion of the carotid artery is necessary in all but the most urgent cases in order to avoid complications of hemodynamic ischemia following permanent occlusion. Approximately 80% to 90% of the general population can tolerate sudden occlusion of an internal carotid artery without hemodynamic complications provided that no other adverse factors affecting the patient's hemodynamic status prevail.[1,2] With careful postocclusion management of patients' hemodynamic status, mean arterial pressure, and state of hydration, the percentage of the population that can undergo permanent safe occlusion of an internal carotid artery can be raised even higher.

VERTEBRAL ARTERY TEST OCCLUSION

Generally, test occlusion of the vertebral artery is conducted only when there is some concern about the adequacy of collateral flow from the posterior communicating arteries and the contralateral vertebral artery. Test occlusion of the posterior circulation does not lend itself well to corroborative imaging techniques involving radiotracers to evaluate perfusion. Therefore, testing in the posterior circulation is usually conducted using only clinical and angiographic parameters. For temporary and permanent occlusions of the vertebral artery, it is usually desirable or necessary to eliminate inflow above the balloon from the C1 or C2 anastomoses. In the case of temporary occlusions this flow could lead to a false-negative test. After permanent occlusions, inflow from these side branches could shear thrombus from the distal stump into the intracranial circulation. Therefore, vertebral artery occlusions are usually performed between the C1 branch and the dural margin.

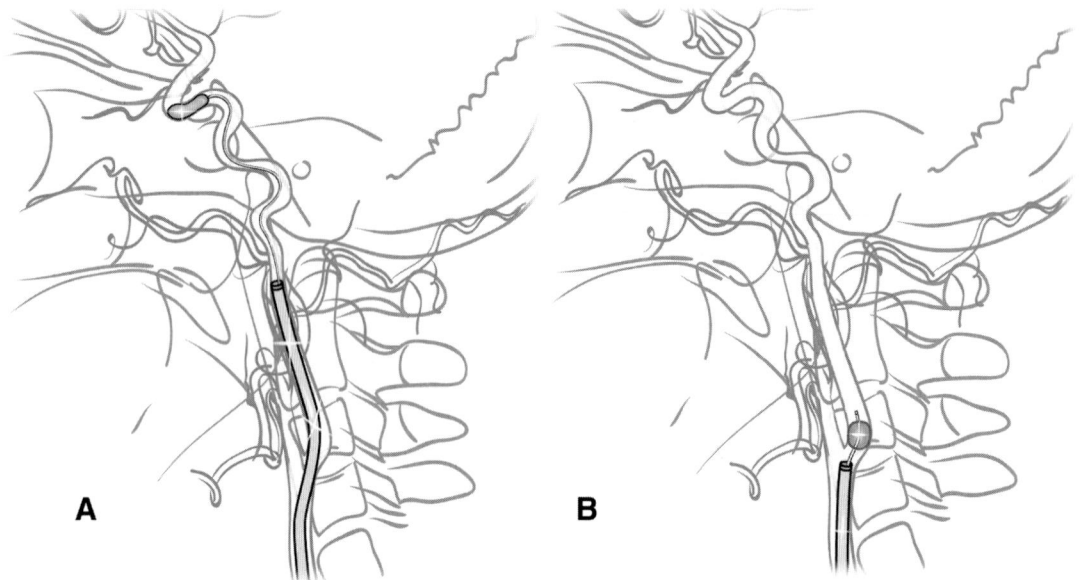

FIGURE 9.1 • *The Two Generally Used Techniques of Test Occlusion of the Internal Carotid Artery Are Illustrated.*
In image A a soft compliant balloon is placed in the distal carotid artery proximal to the ophthalmic artery and inflated until complete occlusion of the artery is achieved. The patient is heparinized systemically, and heparinized flush runs through the introducer catheter lower in the neck.

In B a double-lumen balloon catheter (e.g., 5F Meditech occlusion balloon) occludes the proximal artery. A central lumen used for wire guidance is available after removal of the wire for flushing distally in the carotid artery with heparinized flush. It is important with both techniques to ascertain and check continually for balloon competence during the procedure, lest a false-negative result of the test be obtained due to undetected resumption of carotid flow.

Techniques of Internal Carotid Artery Test Occlusion

There is great variety in the approach to how test occlusions of the internal carotid artery should be conducted. There is no established consensus on the use of a hypotensive challenge during the test occlusion, or what period of time constitutes an adequate test. Acquisition of objective data such as transcatheter measurement of stump pressure in the internal carotid artery above the occluding balloon has not yielded definitive guidelines.[3] Corroborative perfusion imaging in association with the test occlusion, such as technetium-99m-hexamethyl-propyleneamine oxine (Tc-99m HMPAO) SPECT,[4,5] transcranial Doppler testing,[6] or stable xenon/computed tomography (xe/CT)[7,8] are routinely used at some medical centers, but these are not in universal use.[9] There is also no consensus on how best to manage a patient who tolerates a test occlusion clinically but who develops a deficit with an additional hypotensive challenge or who appears to have an asymmetry only on perfusion imaging. Some neurointerventionalists prefer to place greatest reliance on the clinical tolerance of the patient and the angiographic evidence of collateral flow, while others consider an asymmetry on perfusion imaging to represent a contraindication to elective arterial occlusion.

Balloon test occlusion of the internal carotid artery is conducted under full heparinization (ACT >300 seconds). Premedication of the patient with

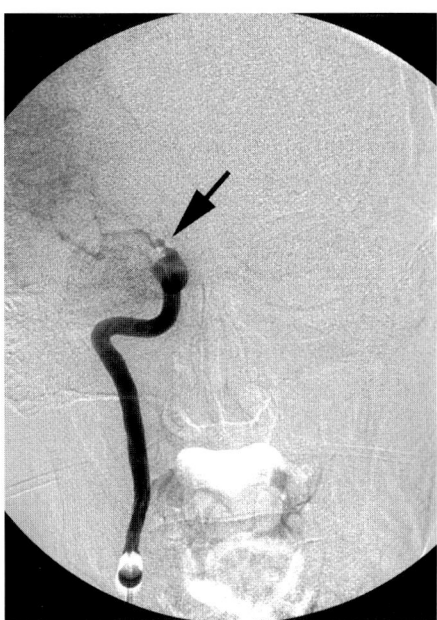

FIGURE 9.2 • *Prompt Washout of Contrast above the Balloon.*
In this patient an injection is made through the central lumen of the balloon catheter during test occlusion. This confirms the competence of the proximal balloon and also gives an indication of the immediacy of washout from collateral channels in the Circle of Willis (arrow). This is a reassuring angiographic sign early in the test that the patient will tolerate the occlusion period. To avoid intimal injury from prolonged contrast stasis, the stagnant cervical internal carotid artery should be cleansed with heparinized saline after this injection.

antiplatelet agents to reduce further the risk of thromboembolic complications might also be considered if it does not affect adversely any surgical plans for the patient. Recommended periods of test occlusion vary from 10–20 minutes of normotension followed by 10–20 minutes of induced hypotension.[2,10]

Balloon placement during the test occlusion depends on the type of equipment with which one is familiar (Figs. 9.1–9.3). A soft compliant balloon is necessary to minimize any risk of iatrogenic dissection from the procedure which can be seen in 0% to 6% of patients in some series.[10,11] Despite heparinization of the patient, clot formation in the stagnant artery proximal and distal to the balloon is a potential for disastrous complications. To reduce this possibility, two approaches are used:

- A nondetachable silicone balloon is placed high in the internal carotid artery just proximal to the ophthalmic artery while an introducer catheter is used to perfuse the internal carotid artery proximal to the balloon with heparinized saline.[11] Rare complications specific to this site of balloon placement can include cavernous sinus syndrome related to ischemia of the paracavernous cranial nerves,[12] or tearing of the artery, resulting in a cavernous sinus fistula.
- Alternatively a wire-directed double-lumen catheter with a larger balloon is placed proximally in the internal carotid artery, allowing lavage of the internal carotid artery distal to the balloon with heparinized saline while an introducer catheter in the common carotid artery perfuses proximally.[10] With excessive distal flushing of heparinized saline, dysfunction of the paracavernous cranial nerves, facial pain, or symptoms of ocular ischemia can occasionally be seen but are invariably transient.[13]

While the balloon is inflated, clinical testing of the patient is conducted using such clinical parameters as can be tested periodically within the confines imposed by conditions of the neuroangiographic suite. Testing of hand grip, foot flexion and extension, language, memory, orientation, facial expression, and pronator drift are generally feasible in most patients. An intravenous injection of radionuclide tracer is given soon after occlusion of the internal carotid artery is confirmed (Fig. 9.4). Again, no firm guidelines exist on when to administer the radionuclide. Using measurements of carotid stump pressure during test occlusion, Barker et al.[14] observed an evolution in the autoregulatory response over a period of some minutes following the occlusion, indicating that administration of radionuclide immediately following occlusion may fail to reflect the more stable state of autoregulation seen at 15 minutes following occlusion. Careful monitoring of the patient's vital signs is important lest the test be conducted

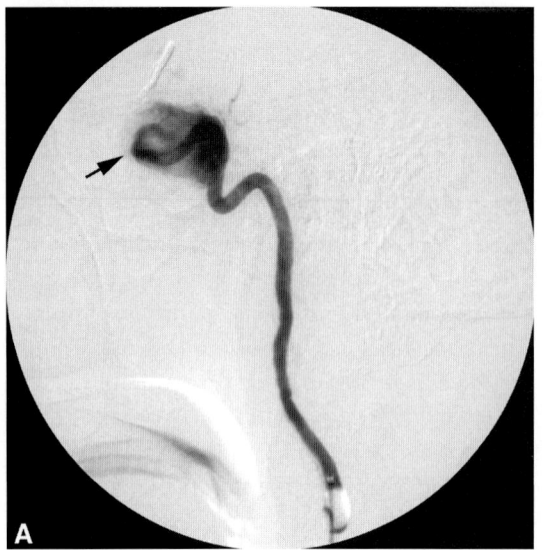 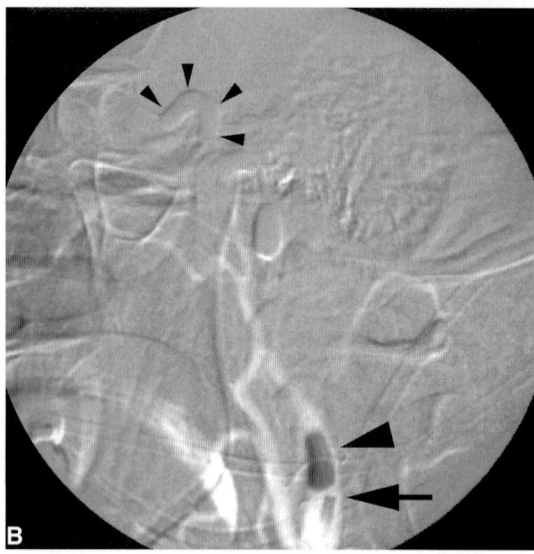

FIGURE 9.3 • *Diagnostic Information during a Test Occlusion.*
In this 35-year-old female presenting with headaches, a test occlusion of the right internal carotid artery was conducted in preparation for occlusion of the artery, after a giant cavernous aneurysm was discovered. The injection made via the occlusion balloon catheter (A) shows the neck and origin of the aneurysm better than could be seen on any of the previous diagnostic images. The neck (arrow) is high in the cavernous segment, extending posteriorly from the siphon. If balloon coverage of the ophthalmic artery is to be avoided, this finding precludes the possibility of placing a balloon distal to the aneurysm for trapping.

The patient had an allergy to latex. A proximal balloon occlusion using silicone balloons was performed uneventfully. The roadmap (B) of the balloon placement shows the position of the uppermost balloon (arrowheads) and the lowest balloon (larger arrowhead). The uppermost balloon is deliberately curved around the C4–C5 segment of the cavernous carotid artery for greater stability. The introducer catheter (arrow) is being used to stabilize the lowest balloon by giving countertraction against the microcatheter during detachment. The lowest balloon is placed a little above the common carotid bifurcation for two reasons. First, the possibility of a sustained carotid body reflex bradycardia and hypotension can be avoided by placing the balloon a little away from the carotid body. If this autonomic complication happens, percutaneous puncture of the offending balloon may be necessary. Second, lower in the internal carotid artery where the vessel is funnel-shaped and smooth in a young adult, such as this patient, it is difficult for the balloon to avoid slipping back down the artery into the common carotid artery.

Sequential plain films (C, D) of the neck after the procedure show shift of the lowest balloon (white arrow) over a period of 2 days. Fortunately, the other balloons did not move. In retrospect, the lower balloons should have been inflated more. Silicone balloons have a greater tendency to move after detachment than latex balloons. A surgical clip projects at the site of previous clipping of a left internal carotid bifurcation aneurysm.

A follow-up angiogram of the left carotid artery 6 months later (E) demonstrated a growing aneurysm of the left posterior communicating artery, which had not been previously present. Hemodynamic stress changes following vessel closure can sometimes, it is thought, induce aneurysm formation. This may be particularly the case in patients with a propensity for aneurysm formation, as this young patient demonstrated. This is fortunately a fairly uncommon complication. The new aneurysm was clipped.

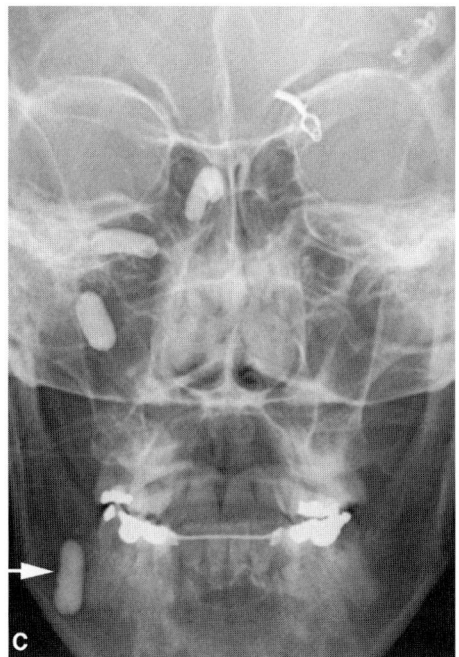
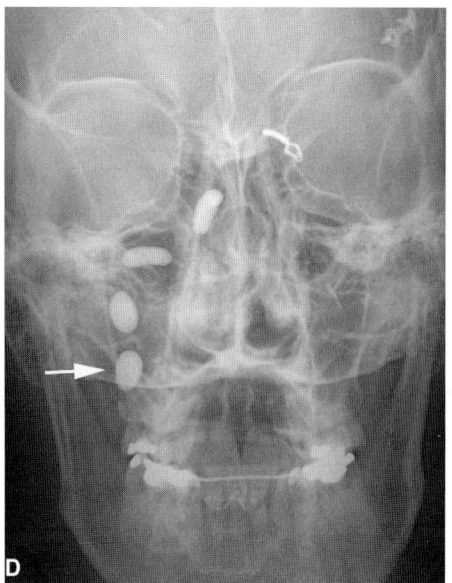
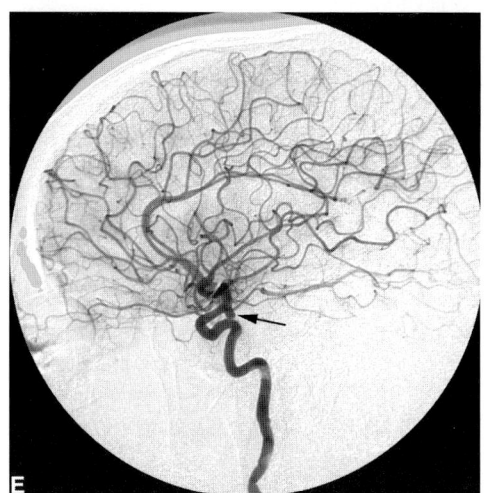

inadvertently under relatively hypertensive conditions, which might result in a false-negative outcome. An alternative maneuver to consider might involve administering the radionuclide during the hypotensive challenge portion of the test. However, as stated previously there is no consensus on how best to manage patients who demonstrate clinical evidence of ischemia only during hypotension or who demonstrate an imaging-based asymmetry only.

COMPLICATIONS OF BALLOON TEST OCCLUSION

Published symptomatic complication rates for test occlusion of the internal carotid artery vary between 0% and 4% with additional rates of up to 2% more for asymptomatic complications.[2,10,11] Most complications involve dissecting injuries to the internal carotid artery and/or thromboembolic procedural complications. Most published complications resulted in a favorable long-term outcome for the patient or were related to a need to execute a permanent occlusion of the internal carotid artery under emergent circumstances at the same session despite the inauspicious outcome of the test occlusion.

Patient Management Following Permanent Internal Carotid Artery Occlusion

Clinical experience with permanent therapeutic occlusion of an internal carotid artery suggests that delayed ischemic complications can occur for a period of days following the procedure. Some of these complications may be embolic, and consideration might therefore be given to the use of a heparin protocol for a period of days following the occlusion to slow the process of thrombosis in the distal stump (Fig. 8.5).

Delayed ischemic deficits following permanent internal carotid artery occlusion are probably also likely to be related to hypoperfusion, particularly in patients in whom there is preocclusion evidence of a marginal state of collateral flow to the ipsilateral hemisphere (Fig. 9.4). For example, patients who clinically tolerate a test occlusion but demonstrate impairment of perfusion on SPECT or xe/CT are presumed to be at greater risk for delayed complications, but this is not always the case. In these and all patients following permanent arterial sacrifice, a graduated protocol of patient management over a period of 3–4 days is probably prudent to avoid excessive early stress on the adjusting autoregulatory system. The following protocol has had favorable success in avoiding delayed ischemic complications and in immediately reversing such deficits when they occur:

- Patient admission to the neurointensive care unit for 2–4 days following therapeutic carotid sacrifice.
- Patient flat in bed for 24–48 hours followed by

FIGURE 9.4 • *Balloon Occlusion for Cavernous Aneurysms.*

A 46-year-old female patient presented with right III and VI palsy with headache and was found to have two aneurysms of the right cavernous segment (A, lateral view, right carotid). A SPECT study was performed with 32 mCi of Tc99m tracer injected intravenously during the test occlusion of the right internal carotid artery and imaged afterwards. This demonstrated a 14% asymmetry of tracer activity in the right hemisphere compared with the left (arrow in B). However, she tolerated the test occlusion clinically.

The configuration of the upper aneurysm precluded the possibility of trapping the aneurysms, and consequently a proximal occlusion with four silicone balloons was performed without clinical incident. A plain film of the neck the next day (C), however, showed that the lowest balloon, previously placed just above the right carotid bifurcation, has advanced up the neck a little. This is an ever-present danger with balloons, and therefore it is generally safer to err on the side of placing too many balloons rather than too few.

The patient's postocclusion management was conducted as described in the text. However, on the third day when sitting in bed it was noted that the patient had a pronator drift of the left arm and weakness of the left foot. She was placed flat in bed, hydrated vigorously to raise her blood pressure, and heparinized. She responded immediately with no evidence of permanent infarction. An embolus from the aneurysms or the carotid stump is a possibility to explain these events. However, the immediacy of her response to lying flat in bed was very clear. In view of the 14% asymmetry on her test occlusion SPECT scan (B), her collateral circulation might have been borderline in adequacy. In either event, her course and management point to the critical role that postocclusion care plays in preventing postocclusion complications.

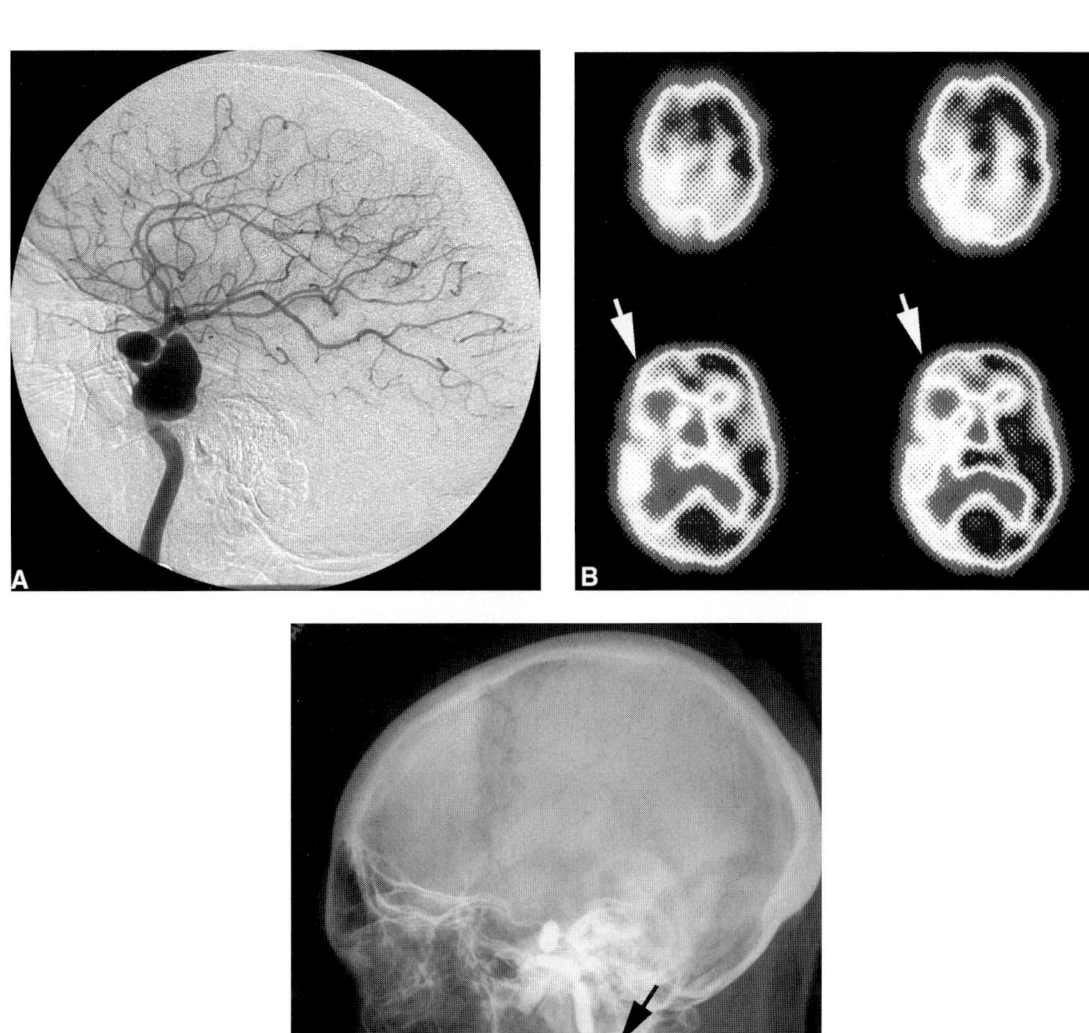

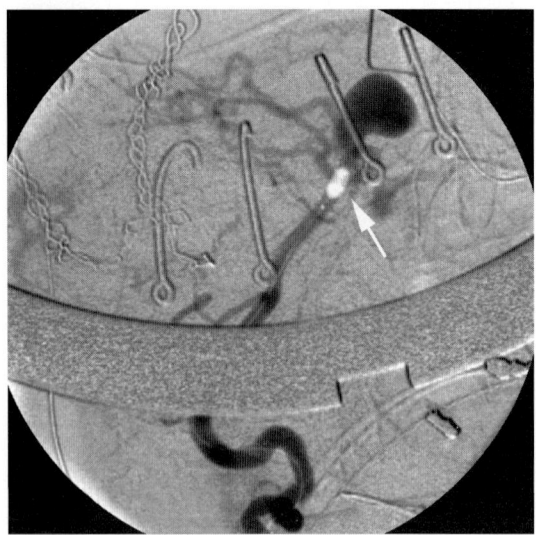

FIGURE 9.5 • *Intraoperative Test Occlusion.* Some neurosurgeons like the deflating effect that a proximal occlusion has on a tense aneurysm. A balloon placed proximally in the basilar artery (arrow) on this intraoperative roadmap image shows the balloon close to the basilar tip aneurysm at the level of the superior cerebellar arteries. It is currently unknown whether a surgical procedure such as this represents a smaller risk than coil embolization to the patient with an unruptured aneurysm with a well-defined neck, as demonstrated. Randomized trials are needed.

gradual elevation of the head of the bed by increments of 30° to 40° per day. Potentially ischemic symptoms are managed by immediately placing the patient flat in bed and by elevating systemic pressure with fluid boluses to improve cerebral perfusion pressure.
- Vigilant monitoring and management of the patient's hydration for maintenance of mean arterial pressure.
- Heparinization at high- or low-dose regimens for prevention of thromboembolic complications.
- For patients with particularly marginal perfusion of the ipsilateral hemisphere or where delayed ischemic complications do not respond immediately to bedside measures described above, placement of an arterial line and administration of intravenous pressor agents or oral fludrocortisone may be necessary.

INTRAOPERATIVE ARTERIAL OCCLUSION

Some neurosurgeons find that intraoperative assistance with temporary arterial occlusion during aneurysm clipping can be very helpful (Fig. 9.5). Proximal occlusion of the artery renders a large aneurysm softer and more pliable during clip application. A variation on this technique is to use a double-lumen balloon catheter so that suction decompression of the artery can further decrease intraaneurysmal pressure and improve the ease of manipulation of the aneurysm. However, there is no good soft-tipped balloon catheter available at present for this purpose. As the central wire must be removed to allow suction decompression, which must perforce be conducted without fluoroscopic assistance during aneurysm clipping, there are hazards in this procedure that must be considered. Suction of the unprotected catheter-tip has a high likelihood of impacting itself against an intimal surface and inducing an arterial dissection. Furthermore, most surgeons are apprehensive about heparinization of the patient during surgery, and arterial occlusion with an endovascular device during the intraoperative period probably carries an even higher risk than usual of thromboembolic complications. Nevertheless, published accounts of this technique and outcomes have been favorable.[15,16]

REFERENCES

1. ECKERT B, THIE A, CARVAJAL M, GRODEN C, ZEUMER H (1998) Predicting hemodynamic ischemia by transcranial Doppler monitoring during therapeutic balloon occlusion of the internal carotid artery. *AJNR* 19:577–582.
2. MATHIS JM, BARR JD, JUNGREIS CA, YONAS H, SEKHAR LN, VINCENT D, PENTHENY SL, HORTON JA (1995) Temporary balloon test occlusion of the internal carotid artery: experience in 500 cases. *AJNR* 16:749–754.
3. KURATA A, MIYASAKA Y, TANAKA C, OHMOMO T, YADA K, KAN S (1996) Stump pressure as a guide to the safety of permanent occlusion of the internal carotid artery. *Acta Neurochirurgica* 138:549–554.
4. MONSEIN LH, JEFFERY PJ, VAN HEERDEN BB, SZABO Z, SCHWARTZ JR, CAMARGO EE, CHAZALY J (1991) Assessing adequacy of collateral circulation during balloon test occlusion of the internal carotid artery with 99mTc-HMPAO SPECT. *AJNR* 12:1045–1051.

5. PETERMAN SB, TAYLOR A JR, HOFFMAN JC JR (1991) Improved detection of cerebral hypoperfusion with internal carotid balloon test occlusion and 99mTc-HMPAO cerebral perfusion SPECT imaging. *AJNR* 12:1035–1041.
6. SORTEBERG A, SORTEBERG W, BAKKE SJ, LINDEGAARD KF, BOYSEN M, NORNES H (1997) Cerebral haemodynamics in internal carotid artery trial occlusion. *Acta Neurochirurgica* 139:1066–1073.
7. LINSKEY ME, JUNGREIS CA, YONAS H, HIRSCH WL JR, SEKHAR LN, HORTON JA, JANOSKY JE (1994) Stroke risk after abrupt internal carotid artery sacrifice: accuracy of preoperative assessment with balloon test occlusion and stable xenon-enhanced CT. *AJNR* 15:829–843.
8. ERBA SM, HORTON JA, LATCHAW RE, YONAS H, SEKHAR L, SCHRAMM V, PENTHENY S (1988) Balloon test occlusion of the internal carotid artery with stable xenon/CT cerebral blood flow imaging. *AJNR* 9:533–538.
9. ECKARD DA, PURDY PD, BONTE FJ (1992) Temporary balloon occlusion of the carotid artery combined with brain blood flow imaging as a test to predict tolerance prior to permanent carotid sacrifice. *AJNR* 13:1565–1569.
10. STANDARD SC, AHUJA A, GUTERMAN LR, CHAVIS TD, GIBBONS KJ, BARTH AP, HOPKINS LN (1995) Balloon test occlusion of the internal carotid artery with hypotensive challenge. *AJNR* 16:1453–1458.
11. MEYERS PM, THAKUR GA, TOMSICK TA (1999) Temporary endovascular balloon occlusion of the internal carotid artery with a nondetachable silicone balloon catheter: analysis of technique and cost. *AJNR* 20:559–564.
12. LOPES DK, MERICLE RA, WAKHLOO AK, GUTERMAN LR, HOPKINS LN (1998) Cavernous sinus syndrome during balloon test occlusion of the cervical internal carotid artery. Report of two cases. *J Neurosurg* 89:667–670.
13. RUSSELL EJ, GOLDBERG K, OSKIN J, DARLING C, MELEN O (1994) Ocular ischemic syndrome during carotid balloon occlusion testing. *AJNR* 15:258–262.
14. BARKER DW, JUNGREIS CA, HORTON JA, PENTHENY S, LEMLEY T (1993) Balloon test occlusion of the internal carotid artery: change in stump pressure over 15 minutes and its correlation with Xenon CT cerebral blood flow. *AJNR* 14:587–590.
15. SHUCART WA, KWAN ES, HEILMAN CB (1990) Temporary balloon occlusion of a proximal vessel as an aid to clipping aneurysms of the basilar artery and paraclinoid internal carotid arteries: technical note. *Neurosurgery* 27:116–119.
16. BAILES JE, DEEB ZL, WILSON JA, JUNGREIS CA, HORTON JA (1992) Intraoperative angiography and temporary balloon occlusion of the basilar artery as an adjunct to surgical clipping: technical note. *Neurosurgery* 30:949–953.

CHAPTER 10

Spine

VERTEBROPLASTY

Originally described for the treatment of painful vertebral fractures related to vertebral body hemangiomas, percutaneous vertebroplasty has attracted increasing attention in the treatment of pathologic vertebral fractures related to osteoporosis, and various tumors of the spine.[1,2] The aim of the treatment is two-fold: pain relief and prevention of further fracture and vertebral collapse.

Percutaneous vertebroplasty consists of injecting a radioopaque preparation of polymethylmethacrylate (PMMA) into a vertebral body via a large-bore needle to stabilize the bone, thus relieving pain. The cement strengthens the internal structure of the vertebral body, thus preventing further loss of height and exacerbation of symptoms. Although controlled trials of the procedure have not been performed, clinical and safety results from open trials and case series indicate a significant impact from the procedure on the lives of most patients on whom this procedure has been performed.

Studies in cadavers have demonstrated that vertebral bodies strengthened by techniques of vertebroplasty have a greater ability to withstand the crushing effect of an axial load.[3,4] Cadaveric studies have also shown that Cranioplastic, the preparation of polymethylmethacrylate most commonly used for vertebroplasty, while not as strong as Simplex P or Osteobond, is still very effective at restoring vertebral body stiffness.[5] Cranioplastic may have other advantages, particularly with reference to viscosity of the preparation and injectability, that make it suitable for vertebroplasty procedures.[3]

Vertebroplasty for Osteoporotic Compression Fractures

Osteoporosis is a disorder of demineralization of bone leading to increased skeletal fragility. Osteoporosis affects 30% of postmenopausal white females in the United States and is only slightly less prevalent in some other racial groups.[6] With advanced demineralization osteoporosis can lead to fractures with minimal trauma. Osteoporotic fractures, particularly hip fractures, are associated with significant morbidity and mortality, and because this condition is common, the cumulative economic impact of osteoporosis is very high. The lifetime risk of a vertebral osteoporotic fracture in a white female over age 50 is 16% with a national cost of $746 million for the United States in 1995.[6] Contrary to popular belief, vertebral fractures are common in men too, but due to lower life expectancy the cumulative risk in white males over age 50 is 5%. Furthermore, the pain suffered by individual patients with osteoporotic fractures is frequently relentless and severe, with few effective treatment options beyond bed rest, analgesics, external braces, or calcitonin therapy. The emotional and psychosocial impact of the pain and immobility associated with vertebral osteoporotic fractures is difficult to quantify in economic terms, but it has been recognized as a significant and highly prevalent problem.[7,8]

Vertebroplasty seems to be an effective and safe therapy for patients immobilized or discomfited by relentless pain from osteoporotic compression fractures. A group of 29 osteoporotic patients (47 vertebral bodies) treated by Jensen et al.[9] and followed over a mean period of 9 months showed that 90% of patients experienced significant relief of pain and increased mobility within 24 hours of the procedure. Three patients (10%) experienced no relief. Apart from two rib fractures related to prone positioning during the procedure, no clinically significant complications were observed. The procedure appears to be equally effective in osteoporotic fractures related to chronic corticosteroid therapy.[10]

Similar results were seen by Cortet et al.,[11] who treated 16 patients with a total of 20 vertebral fractures. Patient rating scales for pain, mobility, mood, and social isolation were improved significantly within 3 days of the procedure, and the effect was sustained at 6-month follow-up. No significant complications were seen. The authors estimated that the efficacy of pain relief was between 44% and 88%, with variable degrees of diminution of analgesic medication following the procedure. Deramond et al.[12] achieved substantial relief of pain and improved mobility within 24 hours of the procedure in 80 patients treated over a 10-year period. Immediate results were excellent in 90% of cases with sustained improvement observed during long-term follow-up.

Vertebroplasty for Vertebral Hemangioma

Vertebral hemangiomas are common incidental findings (12%) on axial imaging and are usually of no consequence to the patient. However, occasionally vertebral hemangiomas can be aggressive, as identified by clinical or imaging changes. Back pain or deficits following spine or nerve-root compression can be seen clinically. Imaging characteristics of aggressive behavior include:

- a pattern of expansion with indistinct borders
- evolution of an associated soft tissue mass
- extension into the neural arch
- involvement of the entire vertebral body
- irregular honeycomb pattern
- diminishing fat content on CT or MRI
- extension into the epidural space

Percutaneous vertebroplasty was first described for treatment of vertebral hemangiomas associated with pain and aggressive change.[1] Over 90% of patients have complete or near-complete relief of pain with no recurrence of the hemangioma following vertebroplasty.[12] In patients with neurologic deficits due to vertebral collapse or compromise of the spinal canal, vertebroplasty can be performed safely as a preoperative measure aimed at stabilization and reduction of blood loss.[13] This technique may be particularly useful in patients with hemangiomas and other vascular tumors of the spine, in whom preoperative particle embolization is forestalled by propinquity of the spinal arteries.

Vertebroplasty for Aggressive and Malignant Spinal Tumors

Vertebroplasty may have a beneficial effect in the stabilization and analgesia of vertebral bodies weakened by osteolytic metastatic tumors and myeloma. Deramond et al.[12] reported an 80% improvement in quality-of-life parameters such as analgesic use and mobility in 101 such patients following vertebroplasty. In contrast to the analgesic effects of radiation therapy for such tumors, vertebroplasty offers the added benefit of strengthening the weakened spine with the hope that future imminent fractures can be averted. In addition to the mechanical effects of the cement, some of the therapeutic effect of the procedure could be related to the exothermic nature of the cement's hardening process, or to the myelinoclastic effects of the solvent.

In a series of 40 patients with osteolytic metastatic disease or myeloma, Martin et al.[2] observed a significant relief or elimination of pain in over 80% of patients. The degree of relief of pain was not related to the percentage of filling of the vertebral body with cement, and improvement in pain was seen even with less than 25% filling of the vertebra, as reckoned by postprocedure CT. These and other authors speculated that placebo effect alone, while still a possibility, was difficult to invoke as an explanation of the analgesic effect of the procedure. The patients in this particular series seem to have had a uniformly excruciating spectrum of pain symptoms prior to treatment. The authors considered that the meager physical buttress provided by the cement in some of their patients in the setting of substantial pain relief pointed to the possibility that the vascular, chemical, and thermal effects of the cement within the tumor may have an extremely important role.

Weill et al.[14] treated a group of 37 patients with malignant disease of the spine metastatic from a wide variety of primary sources. The treatments were predominantly aimed at analgesia alone or analgesia with spinal stabilization. Again, these authors observed a significant pain response in 94% of their patients within the first week, and this effect was sustained in 65% to 73% of patients during the course of a year of follow-up. Eleven of the patients in this series were treated with spine stabilization as a treatment goal, and in the course of over a year of follow-up no displacement of treated vertebral bodies was seen. These authors commented that the analgesic effects of vertebroplasty are therefore comparable to those of local palliative radiation therapy.[15,16] However, vertebroplasty and other effective therapies for such patients including radiation therapy and/or surgical decompression and stabilization are not mutually exclusive.

Risks and Complications from Vertebroplasty

Complications from vertebroplasty are uncommon, at least in the published literature, and can be related to a number of factors:

- Systemic toxicity of the cement solvent. A mild pyrexia within 24 hours can be seen in some patients following orthopedic procedures, which may be related to the cement solvent. However, systemic effects of the solvent monomer seem to be rare or nonexistent due to the small volume of cement used during vertebroplasty compared with operative orthopedic procedures.[17]
- Local mechanical effects of the cement injection causing foraminal nerve-root compression, spinal compression, or esophageal dysphagia in the cervical region.[14]
- Local hemorrhage in coagulopathic or anticoagulated patients[18].
- Thermal effects of the cement causing neural injury. This is a theoretical consideration in most patients and is probably only a factor in those patients with direct spine or root compression. Cadaveric studies of the exothermic effects of injected PMMA have shown temperature elevations within the vertebral body as high as 73°C, but canal temperatures above 41°C were not seen.[19]
- Spinal or nerve-root injury due to needle misplacement or misadventure such as pedicle fracture during needle insertion.
- Venous embolization of cement to the lungs.[20]
- Fat liquefaction and mobilization due to direct physical pressure within the vertebral body and the thermal effect of the cement on adjacent marrow, causing fat embolization. Fat embolization following orthopedic procedures involving pressurized injections of PMMA can be seen occasionally with severe neurological complications. The prevalence of subclinical fat embolization during orthopedic procedures is not known for sure but may be as high as 8%.[21,22,23] This is a potential area of concern for vertebroplasty patients, particularly when multiple levels are treated during the same treatment session.
- Infection. Most authors recommend a systemic dose of antibiotics at the time of the procedure. Some also add a vial of Tobramycin 1.2 g to the powder mix before mixing in the liquid monomer, although this is less frequently done now than when the procedure was new.
- Stress fractures of ribs or other bones due to the prolonged nature of the procedure with the patient in an unwonted position.[9]

- Alteration of spinal mechanics with induction of stress fractures in adjacent vertebral bodies following the procedure, possibly exacerbated by sudden augmentation of general patient mobility. However, a retrospective study by Jensen et al. found no convincing evidence for increased fracture rates adjacent to vertebroplasty sites compared with more remote vertebral bodies.[24]

By far the commonest sources of clinically significant complications are those related to local cement extrusion into undesirable positions, indicating that complications are most effectively avoided by procedural technique. In osteoporotic compression fractures where the cortical margins of the vertebral body are preserved, procedural containment of the cement is fairly easy, and clinically detectable complications due to undesirable glue extrusion are seen in <2% of patients.[11] In procedures for hemangiomas the risk of clinical complications is slightly higher (2% to 5%), and for tumorous conditions of the spine this figure is closer to 10% due to the absence of a containing cortical margin.[12,14,25] Symptomatic local extrusions of cement can be treated successfully with analgesic medication and steroid therapy when the cement mass is minor. Surgical excision and decompression can sometimes be necessary when the offending extrusion is in the spinal canal.

The risk of spinal compromise from vertebroplasty is probably most severe in those patients with tumoral compromise or fractures of the posterior cortical margin of a cervical or thoracic vertebral body. Additionally, needle placement and cement injections become more technically difficult when the degree of vertebral collapse exceeds 65% to 70%.[10] However, in the opinion of Weill et al.[14] these imaging findings do not represent an absolute contraindication to the procedure, but rather an admonition toward procedural caution. Minor cement leaks toward the paravertebral veins, intervertebral disc space, neural foramina, or epidural venous plexus are common during these procedures, seen in 38%[14] to 72%[26] of patients, but remain asymptomatic in the overwhelming majority of cases. More clinically serious extrusions of cement are rare and are more likely to be seen with hypervascular metastatic destruction of the vertebral body cortical margins. The importance of adequate opacification of the cement prior to injection and biplane fluoroscopic monitoring of the injection is recognized in reports of symptomatic and asymptomatic pulmonary embolization of cement in some patients.[9,20]

Exposure to Methylmethacrylate Vapors

The volatile nature of the liquid monomer used during vertebroplasty and orthopedic procedures is an environmental concern for personnel involved. Methylmethacrylate exposure in very high concentrations has been linked with acute pulmonary toxicity, liver necrosis, and carcinogenicity. Many individuals are extremely sensitive to the vapor of the monomer and quickly develop a lingering headache, anorexia, and a sense of malaise from even brief exposure during medical procedures. These difficulties can be reduced by forceful ventilation of the room with fans or extractors during the procedure. Chilling the monomer during the procedure may also decrease its volatility as well as prolonging the working time of the mixture. Cloft et al.[27] examined the potential exposure of operating personnel during vertebroplasty procedures by using air-sampling pumps. The results obtained were below the level of sensitivity of the detectors used (4.88 parts per million), and thus well below the published recommended standard of safety at 100 ppm for methylmethacrylate exposure over an 8-hour day. However, the sampling method used by Cloft et al. took place over the course of an hour. Using a similar volume of orthopedic cement McLaughlin et al.[28,29] observed a vapor concentration of 277 ppm at the time of mixing at the level of the operator's mask. The air concentrations fell quickly thereafter. Exposure to methylmethacrylate vapors can be reduced by using a commercially available closed system for mixing of powder and liquid components.

Patient Selection and Screening

The best results with vertebroplasty are obtained with judicious patient selection. The following recommendations augur a more favorable outcome:

- Point tenderness on physical examination over the suspected site of pain.
- Evidence of physiologic stress in the vertebral body in question as represented by activity on a nuclear bone scan or edema on T2-weighted MRI examination.
- Height preservation in the vertebral body >30% of estimated baseline.
- Extreme caution should be exercised in patients with compromise by tumor or fracture of the posterior cortical margin of the vertebral body. For this reason a preprocedure CT scan is virtually imperative.
- Avoidance of unnecessary procedures. With conservative management, medications, and brace support the pain from acute compression fractures settles down in 3–4 weeks in over 60% of patients anyway. Delaying the procedure in the setting of acute fractures may be a prudent policy.

Techniques

A number of excellent detailed technical descriptions of the techniques of vertebroplasty have been published.[9,10,12,25,30] As described above, the efficacy of the technique is not manifestly dependent upon the degree of vertebral body filling, and therefore all technique modifications are generally aimed at avoiding complications, particularly misadventurous cement extrusion.

Approach of the Needle

Needles must be of the disposable kind due to the permanence of the cement adherent to the needle (Fig. 10.1).

- Cervical spine: an anterolateral approach with CT guidance using a 13 G or 15 G bone biopsy needle. The foremost concern is avoidance of the carotid artery and jugular vein.
- Thoracic spine: a 13 G needle placed using a transpedicular route to avoid pleural injury.
- Lumbar spine: an 11 G or 13 G needle placed via a transpedicular or posterolateral approach. Most authors prefer the transpedicular approach. Avoidance of transgression of the medial border of the pedicle is the priority. Leakage of cement back along the needle track is common, and if the medial cortex is compromised, extrusion of cement into the spinal canal is unavoidable. Ideally, as the needle makes its way through the pedicle, if it sweeps from lateral to medial within the pedicle, it will access its destination within the vertebral body closer to the midline. In this location, an injection of methylmethacrylate has a greater chance of permeating the entire vertebral body, and thus a contralateral needle placement can be avoided.

Depending on the preferences of the operator a number of needles can be placed in different levels either unilaterally or bilaterally prior to mixing the cement, or each level can be treated separately. The advantage of multilevel treatment is the restriction on time available for mixing and using the cement. With multiple needles placed one could maximize the utility of a single mixing preparation. The advantage of treating one level at a time is the ability to concentrate exclusively on the anatomy of that level and to position the biplane equipment accordingly.

Venogram

When the needle has been inserted to the junction of the anterior and middle third of the vertebral body, an injection of nonionic water-soluble contrast is recommended by some authors so as to detect the immediacy of venous drainage and the risk of venous embolization of cement (Fig. 10.2). Needle repositioning may be necessary if the needle tip is in the basi-vertebral vein. However, not all authors have found this step to be helpful or necessary, pointing out that the flow characteristics of contrast and cement are very different. Many no longer recommend performing a venogram as it often yields no useful information. The vertebral bodies are extremely vascular under any circumstances, and it is difficult to

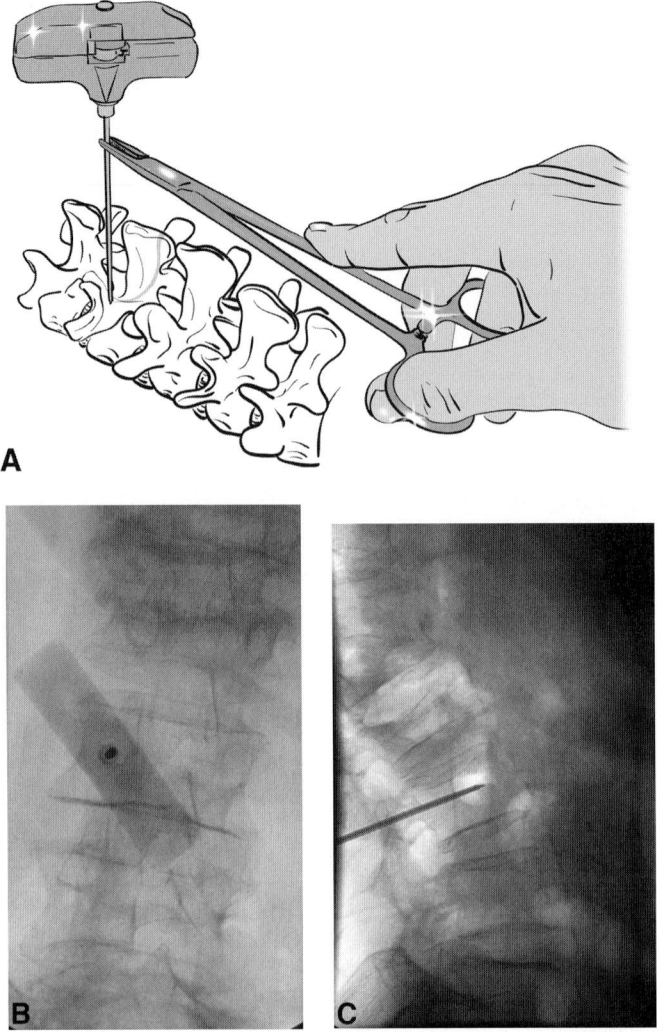

FIGURE 10.1 • *Needle Approach for Vertebroplasty.*
It is important to start the needle off on the correct path. Once an incorrect transpedicular path is established, it is very difficult to correct. A long-handled forceps can be used to straighten the needle under the fluoroscope (A). Some operators give the needle a tap of a hammer to embed it into the cortex over the pedicle and thus assure that drifting of the needle tip does not occur.

The AP fluoroscopic image (B) shows the needle shaft superimposed on the pedicle, and ideally one would like to preserve this image through the needle placement process. Particular emphasis should be placed on not transgressing the medial cortex of the pedicle, lest a dural tear occur. To encourage the needle tip to drift toward the center of the vertebral body as it advances (and thus obviate the need for a bilateral needle placement), some operators suggest angling the fluoroscope a little more laterally. While preserving visualization of the pedicular cortex, a more oblique angulation will allow the needle to describe a slightly lateral to medial course as it advances. Thus the spinous process is a little off center in this image.

The lateral view (C) in the same patient shows the position of the needle tip at the junction of the middle and anterior third of the vertebral body, a good position at which to start the injection. This relatively normal-proportioned vertebral body was being treated prophylactically in a patient with multiple fractures, which were also treated at the same session. When vertebroplasty was first introduced, it was thought that treating multiple levels at one treatment session was safe. However, until more reliable data are available on the safety of this procedure, restricting the treatment to one or two levels per treatment session is suggested to the reader as a safety measure.

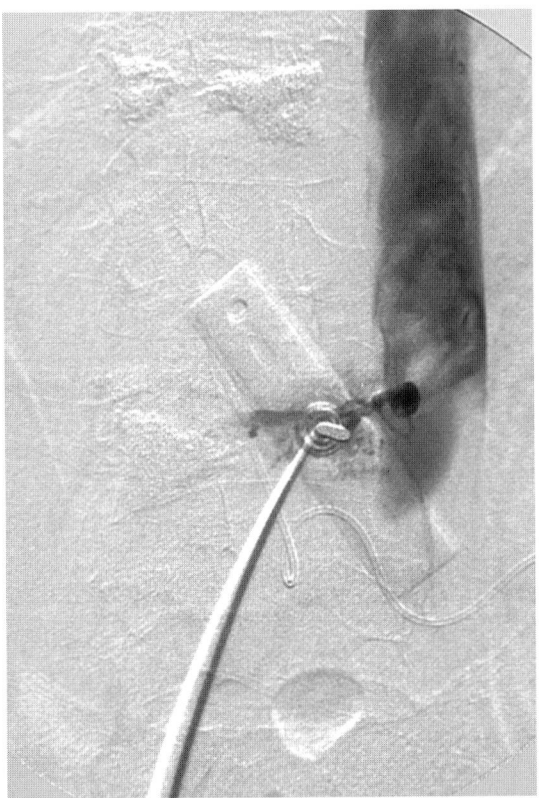

FIGURE 10.2 • *Venogram.*
There are mixed opinions on the value of performing a venogram. Lingering contrast afterwards can be a severe hindrance in visualizing the advancing cement. In this patient, however, the promptness of venous flow to the inferior vena cava reminds one of the ease with which embolization of methylmethacrylate to the lungs could be induced. Very careful monitoring of the cement under high-quality fluoroscopy is imperative during these procedures.

avoid what appears to be immediate venous opacification in most patients. For certain tumors contrast can diffuse into and linger in the tumor tissue and obscure subsequent visualization of cement. Similarly, if contrast leaks into the intervertebral disc space during the venogram, it can linger there for the duration of the case. This can be an extreme hindrance during subsequent cement injections as it can be difficult to know whether the cement is extruding into the disc space or not.

Mixing of the Methylmethacrylate Cement
Methylmethacrylate orthopedic cement is available from a number of vendors and is supplied as a sachet of powder and a glass bottle of liquid monomer. Some suppliers already mix barium with the powder moiety, but the level of barium is not adequate for fluoroscopic visualization. Additional sterile barium is imperative for adequate visualization of the cement. Some authors have used tantalum or tungsten powder for opacification, but most agree that barium in liberal quantities is the best agent.

A problem with barium is the need to mix it with the methylmethacrylate powder thoroughly to achieve an even preparation without clumping. A sterile pestle can be used or improvised from tabletop items.

Recommended Powder Mixture

- Methylmethacrylate powder 30 g (1 sachet)
- 2 bottles of barium sulfate 6 g each
- Tobramycin 1.2 g (optional, less commonly advocated now than when the procedure was still new in the United States)

The mixture of PMMA powder, Tobramycin, and opacifying agent(s) are ground as homogeneously as possible in a sterile bowl. To husband out the supply of powder, the mixture of approximately 55 ml can be divided into 2 or 3 aliquots, so that one begins the mixing with the liquid monomer with more manageable batches. A glass syringe is necessary for decanting and holding the liquid monomer due to the solvent effects of the monomer on plastic syringes. Working with the mixture over a chilling basin of ice, insulated for sterility by a plastic sheet, can prolong the working time (<10 minutes) of the mixed paste.

A commercially available sealed system for mixing the cement components is available (Parallax). This has the advantage of allowing the mixture to be shaken thoroughly without exposing the room to the vapors and greatly reduces the time involved in the procedure. The quantities of powder and liquid are prescribed according to

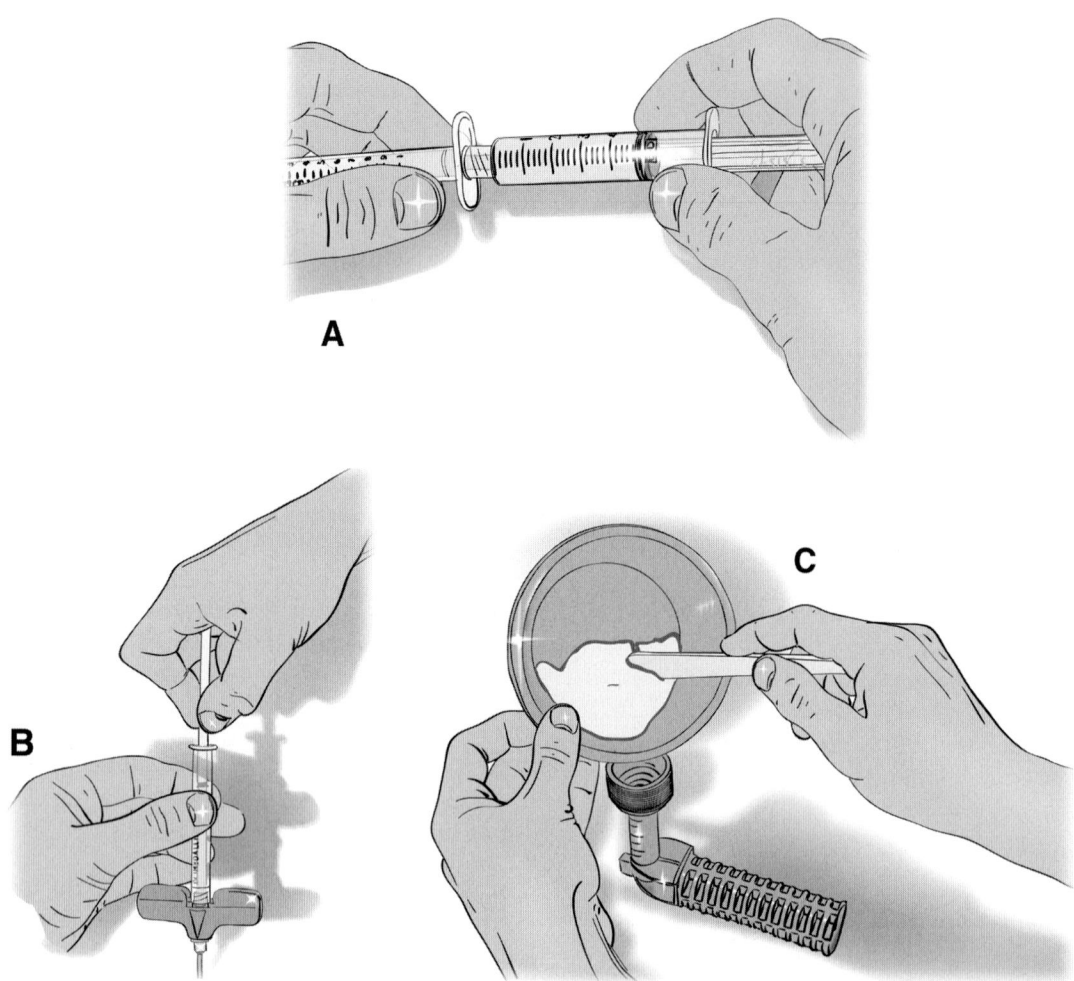

FIGURE 10.3 • *Cement Mixing and Injection.*
Cement can be injected with small syringes or with patent devices available from various vendors. Single-ml syringes can be backloaded from a larger syringe by an assistant as illustrated (A). There might be considerable resistance within the needles at times, and it is important to prevent sudden uncontrolled injections of cement with a drop in resistance. Holding the syringe as illustrated (B) so that one's fingers will act a brake will help. Cement can be mixed openly in a sterile basin and poured into the reservoir of a crank device as illustrated (C). The latter may give longer working time for the cement and reduce vapor exposure. A crank pump (D) also has the advantage of allowing biplane monitoring of the cement injection because the hands are removed from under the fluoroscope.

The closed mixing system from Parallax is highly recommended for ease of cement preparation and for reduction of personnel exposure to the noxious vapors of the mixing solution. A plastic beaker (E) is provided containing approximately 5 ml of barium tracer powder. The powder monomer is added to this for a total of 19 ml. With mixing of the powder and barium some settling to a volume less than 19 ml will be observed. After one has mixed the two dry components together, one adds 7.5–8 ml of liquid monomer. A long needle can be used (F) to assure an even distribution of liquid through the beaker. Note that the syringes must be of glass or other material resistant to the solvent effects of the liquid monomer. Finally, the beaker is shaken thoroughly and allowed to stand for a minute before decanting it into the injector device. The dividends of time and effort saved by using this closed mixing system are enormous.

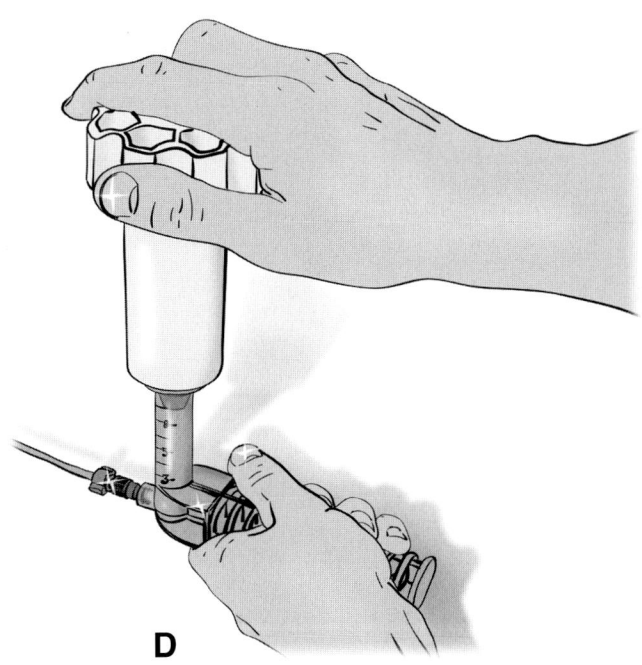

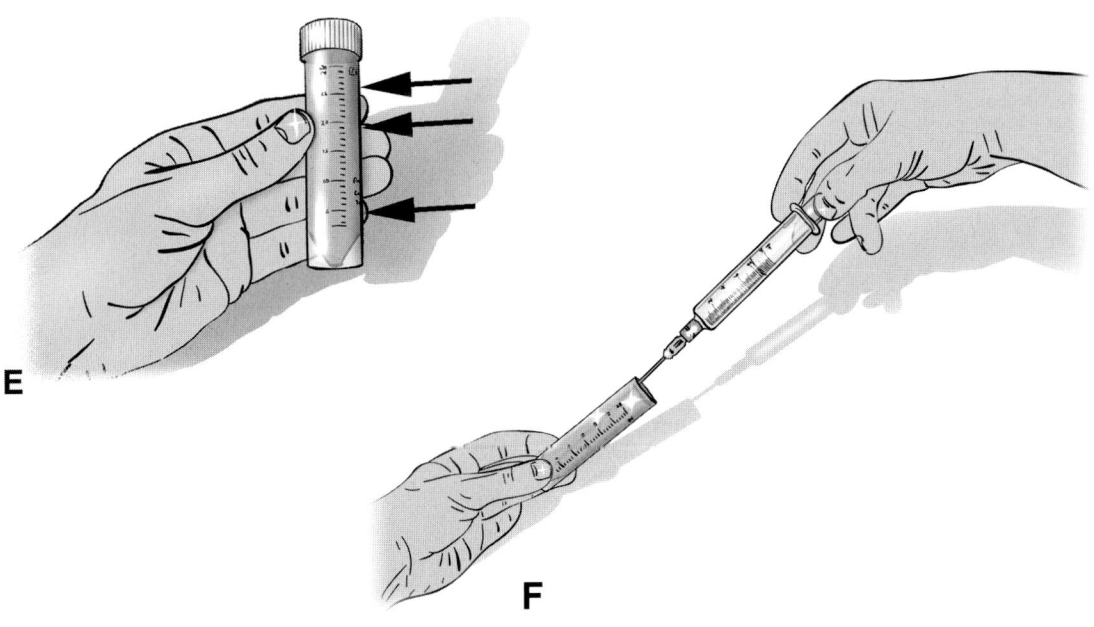

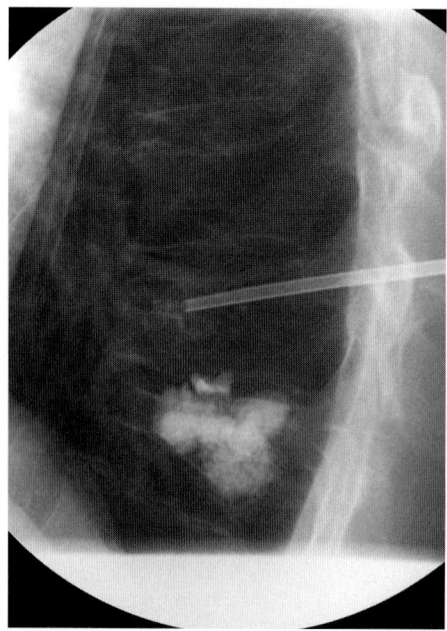

FIGURE 10.4 • *Extrusion of Cement into the Disk Space.*
A lateral view of the needle position in preparation for vertebroplasty shows extrusion of cement into the disk space above the vertebral body previously injected. This should be inconsequential to the patient. The more important considerations are detecting any venous emboli of cement during the injection or extrusion of cement posteriorly into the spinal canal.

formula. It is highly recommended as an alternative to the mixing and measuring protocol described above.

Injecting the Methylmethacrylate Cement
The PMMA cement can be injected with a crank device specifically marketed by a number of vendors for this purpose, or hand injections with 1-ml Luer-Lock syringes can be performed. Exposure to air and initiation of the polymerization process are the countervailing forces at this stage, and therefore isolation of the paste within the crank device may provide an advantage in this respect. In either event, the preparation of the paste from a mixing of the liquid and powder components depends a little on the learning curve of the operator (Fig. 10.3). A smoothly flowing viscous preparation is necessary, and a useful rule of thumb is that if it is too viscous to be suctioned into a 1-ml syringe or to drip freely from a spatula, it will probably be too difficult to inject via a 13 G needle within a short space of time.

Several strategies have been canvassed when using syringes. While the primary operator is injecting the cement, an assistant loads the 1-ml syringes. This is done by backloading the 1-ml syringes from a 3-ml or 5-ml syringe by removing the plunger from the 1 ml syringe and backloading the paste. Alternatively, one could load a number of 1-ml syringes at the beginning and then decant a small droplet of polymerizing cement from the tip of each 1-ml syringe at the time of each syringe interchange.

Clumping of the cement within the needle is a problem as the case progresses. Pushing hard on the syringe runs the risk of a sudden cement injection

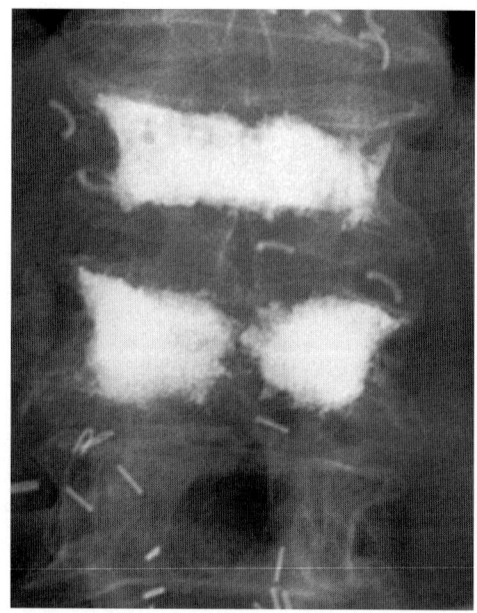

FIGURE 10.5 • *Postvertebroplasty Plain Film.*
A plain film following two-level vertebroplasty shows a satisfactory appearance at each level. The cement spontaneously filled the entire body at the upper level from a single injection. Bilateral needle placement was necessary at the lower level.

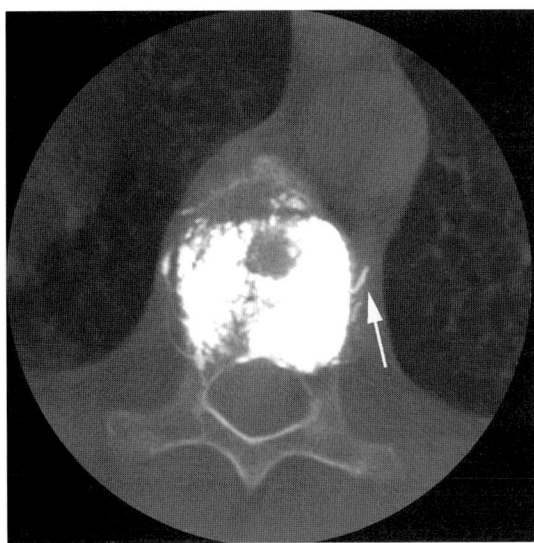

FIGURE 10.6 • *Postvertebroplasty CT I.*
A CT scan following vertebroplasty shows satisfactory filling of the body, with inconsequential migration of cement into a paravertebral vein (arrow).

injected by a unilateral or bilateral approach (Fig. 10.5).

Postprocedure Patient Care
Following the procedure the patient is log-rolled onto a stretcher and maintained on bedrest for at least a few hours until the PMMA is hardened. Most patients are kyphotic or otherwise uncomfortable with simple supine positioning, so commonsense accommodations to body habitus such as towel or pillow positioning are necessary. Adequate postprocedure analgesia with nonsteroidal agents or short-term prescription of narcotic agents is usually necessary. A postprocedure CT scan will also allay any patient or operator concerns about the precise location of any questionable cement extrusions that were unclear under fluoroscopy (Figs. 10.6, 10.7). Generally, patients can go home the night of the procedure.

if the resistance gives way. The blunt trochar of the needle can be used to clear the shaft if this happens. If the obstruction is insurmountable, the needle can be replaced. A guide can be fashioned from the blunt trochar to direct the replacement needle into the vertebral body. However, the hole in the bone when viewed end-on is usually easy to see fluoroscopically, and a replacement needle will usually slide down the same route within the bone without difficulty.

The sealed crank system available from various vendors extends the working time of the cement, reduces personnel exposure to vapors, and reduces the likelihood of exposing the operator's hands in the primary radiation beam. It is highly recommended.

Injection of the cement is monitored carefully on the fluoroscope (Fig. 10.4). Particular attention is given to the epidural space and the posterior margins of the vertebral column. Therefore, positioning the lateral image intensifier to profile the spinal canal is very important. Usually 2–10 ml of cement are used per vertebral body,

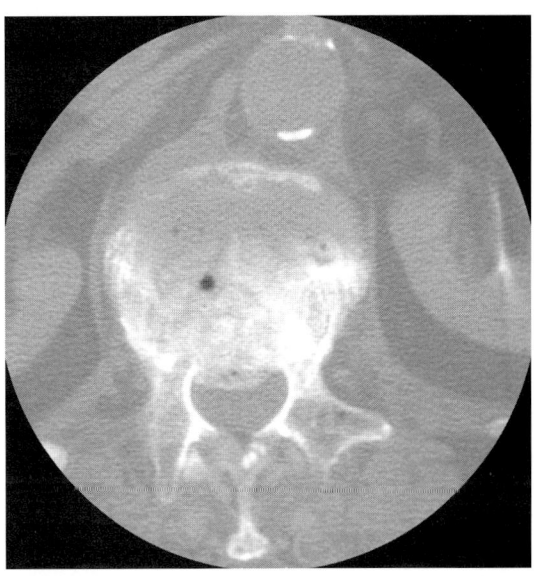

FIGURE 10.7 • *Postvertebroplasty CT II.*
A postvertebroplasty CT at the level of an intervertebral disc shows retropulsion of the cortical margin into the spinal canal. Fortunately, this was stable compared with the preprocedure CT. In the thoracic spine one should be extremely cautious about performing vertebroplasty in situations of compromise of the canal. The risks of spinal compression are quite real.

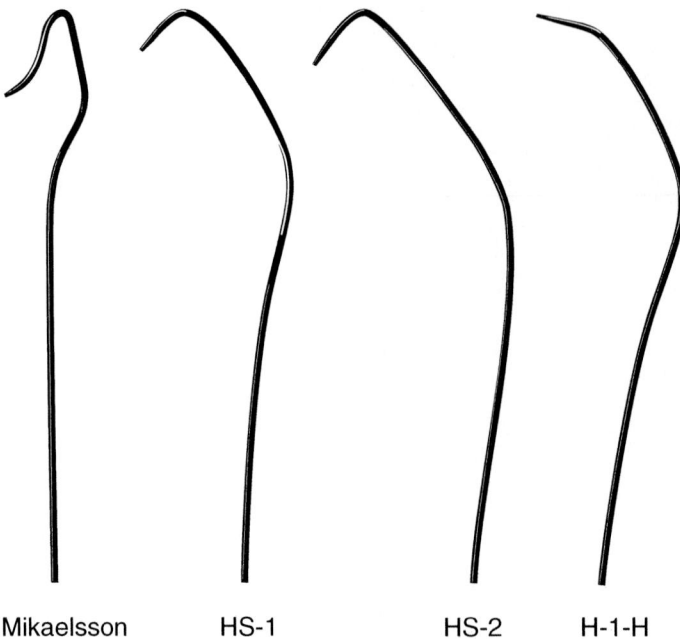

FIGURE 10.8 • Several spinal catheters are available from various vendors. There is a smooth progression from craniad to caudad in the orientation of the segmental arteries. The higher vessels tend to point cephalad and therefore an upward-pointing catheter such as the H-1–H modified Headhunter catheter is often most suitable. The most caudad vessels point inferiorly at their origin; inferiorly directed catheters such as the HS-2 or Simmons catheters tend to perform well in this location. The Mikaelsson catheter is a little more difficult to use than the other catheters, and, as a general rule, one will use more contrast finding a straightforward vessel ostium with it than with other catheter shapes. However, when all others have failed to lodge in a particularly difficult vessel, the Mikaelsson catheter can be relied upon to come through.

Spinal Arteriovenous Malformations

Arteriovenous malformations of the spine are classified by location. Four categories are recognized:

- Paravertebral arteriovenous malformation and fistulas
- Dural arteriovenous fistulas
- Perimedullary arteriovenous fistulas
- Intramedullary arteriovenous malformations/fistulas

Paravertebral Arteriovenous Malformations and Fistulas

Vascular malformations adjacent to the spinal cord can present with myelopathic symptoms and signs, and can mimic in many ways the appearance of a true spinal cord arteriovenous malformation (Figs. 10.8–10.10). These lesions are rare. Spinal cord involvement with a paravertebral AVM can be seen as part of a metameric AVM in Cobb's syndrome involving all three embryonic tissue layers. When paravertebral AVMs drain into the epidural veins, they can generate mass-effect on the cord. They may also present with venous hypertension through transmission of venous pressure into the intradural veins of the spine, and thus can mimic the clinical appearance of a spinal dural AVF or a perimedullary fistula. Isolated cases of epidural and intradural venous hypertension have been reported from pelvic arteriovenous malformations or masses with arteriovenous shunting. Such lesions are rare.

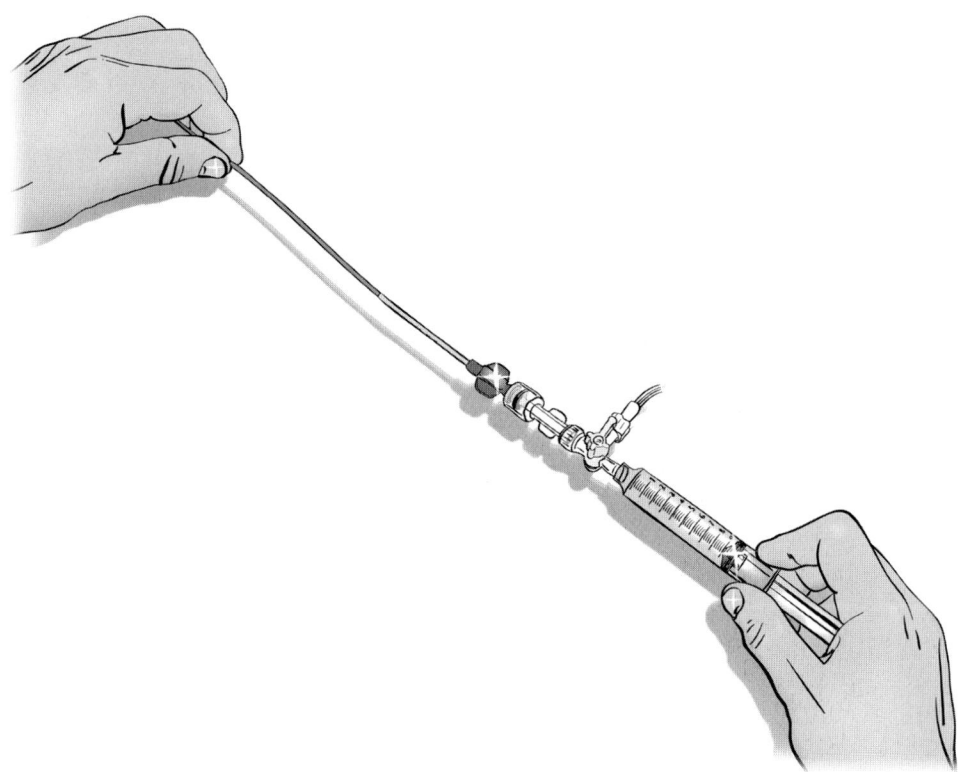

FIGURE 10.9 • *Spinal Angiography Technique.*
Spinal angiography only takes a little practice to eliminate any intimidation of novelty that it may hold. A swivel adapter interposed between the syringe and the catheter will allow independent motion with the left hand. When the catheter tip finds the desired arterial pedicle, a little tension must be added to the catheter to encourage it to stay there for the duration of the run. In a recurved catheter, e.g., Mikaelsson, this means pulling down a little on the catheter. When the catheter is seated well, the stopcock can be switched to the injector for the run, and the process resumed immediately following the run.

Spinal Dural Arteriovenous Fistulas (SdAVF)

Dural AVFs of the spine are the most common type of spinal AVM seen in most series (Figs. 10.11–10.13). They are acquired lesions of late adulthood in which a small fistula or rete appears along the spinal dura, usually in the axilla of a dural sleeve around a nerve root, most often in the lumbar area. A segmental artery, e.g., a branch of the vertebral artery, an intercostal artery, lumbar artery, etc., normally gives a dural branch near the neural foramen. When a SdAVF is established, this dural branch feeds the fistula, draining intradurally. Branches of the skull base can be involved at the cephalad end of the neural axis, while the median or lateral sacral arteries can be involved in the pelvis. Therefore, the entire neural axis needs to be studied in patients suspected of having a SdAVF.

These lesions are most commonly tiny and very slowly flowing. Their significance lies in their effect on the venous field. Normally, the state of venous pressure in the intradural venous plexus is insulated from the surrounding epidural veins. Venous flow along the medullary veins emanating from the cord is normally centrifugal toward the epidural veins. When a SdAVF becomes established, flow is then reversed in one of the draining medullary veins and becomes centripetal. Although the rate of flow in

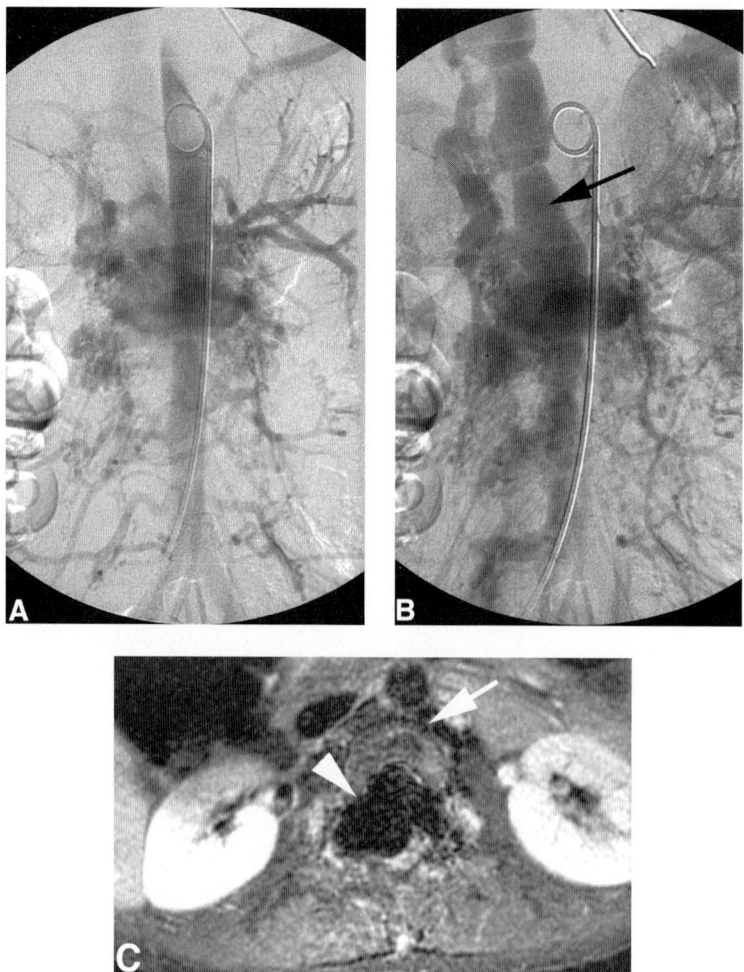

FIGURE 10.10 • *Paravertebral Arteriovenous Malformation.*
An 11-year-old girl presenting with high-output cardiac failure was found to have a large AVM on abdominal aortogram during cardiac catheterization. The aortogram (A, arterial phase; B, venous phase) showed a profusion of retroperitoneal lumbar arteries opacifying a large AVM and draining cephalad via a hugely enlarged intracanalicular vein (arrow in B).

The contrast-enhanced axial MRI examination (C) showed the enlarged intracanalicular vein (arrowhead) and remodeling of the posterior vertebral bodies (arrow), but the question of involvement of the spinal cord was still difficult to answer. The cord itself appeared normal on the sagittal MRI images (D). The spinal angiogram demonstrated that the cord itself was not involved with the AVM. No posterior spinal or anterior spinal arteries could be seen supplying the AVM, implying that the AVM was paravertebral in location. However, the spinal arteries in this patient demonstrate how vigilant one must be in searching for spinal arteries and sites of potential disaster at all times. The left L2 injection (E) via a Mikaelsson catheter shows no evidence of a spinal artery, and there is prominent opacification of the AVM.

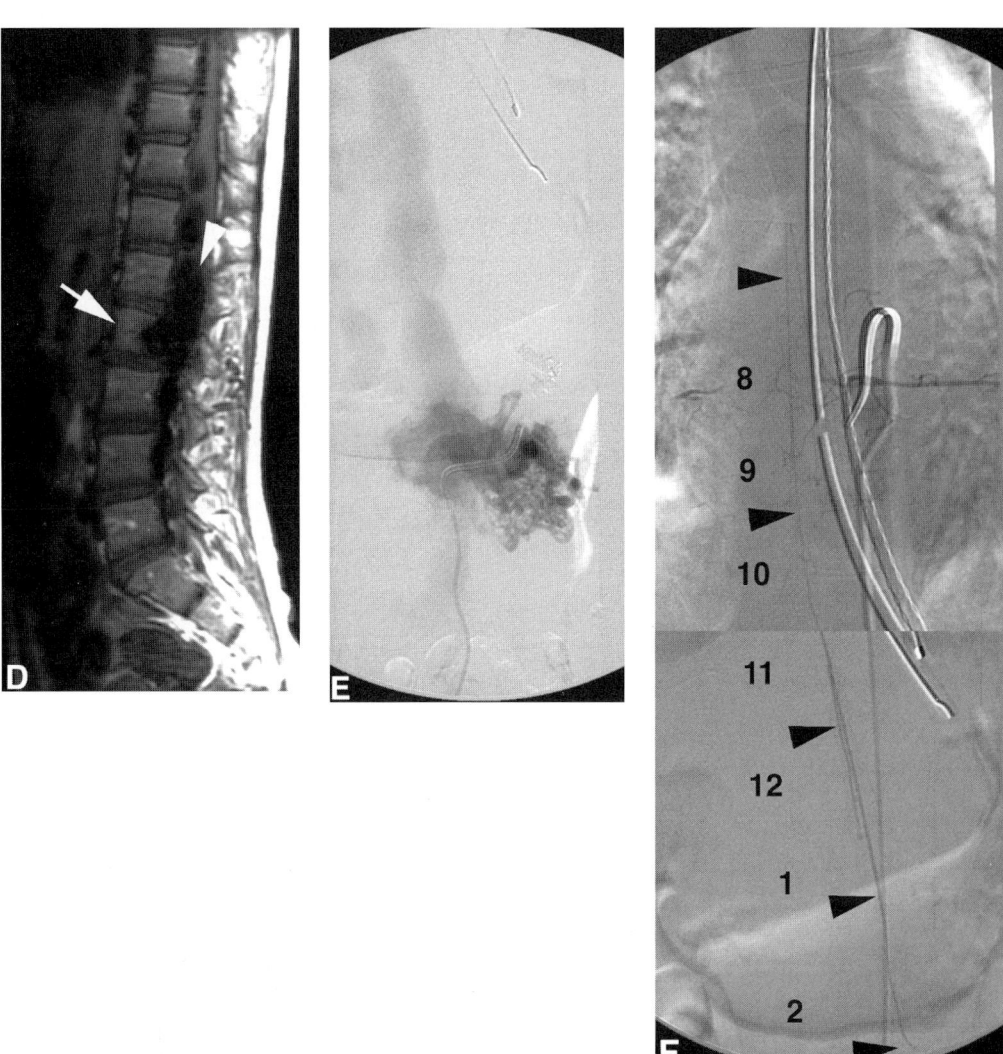

The anterior spinal artery was seen at left T8 and showed no evidence of AVM opacification. However, the anterior spinal artery takes an unusual course and bevels off to the left as it descends, ending abruptly at the neural foramen of L2-L3. A composite image (F) from two runs via the left T8 pedicle shows the course of the anterior spinal artery. The right-sided pedicles are numbered for reference. The anterior spinal artery (arrowheads) is abruptly cut off at the L2-L3 level. Therefore, one deduces that the sump of the AVM is drawing blood down the anterior spinal artery to the L2-L3 level, and the original conclusion that the L2 artery does not have a spinal artery is incorrect. It is present, albeit reversed in flow. This raises the question of inadvertent antegrade embolization of the anterior spinal artery during the course of treatment.

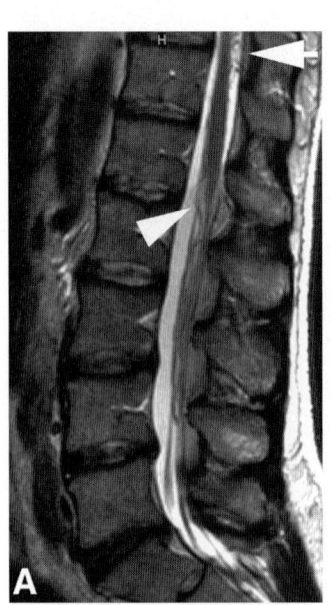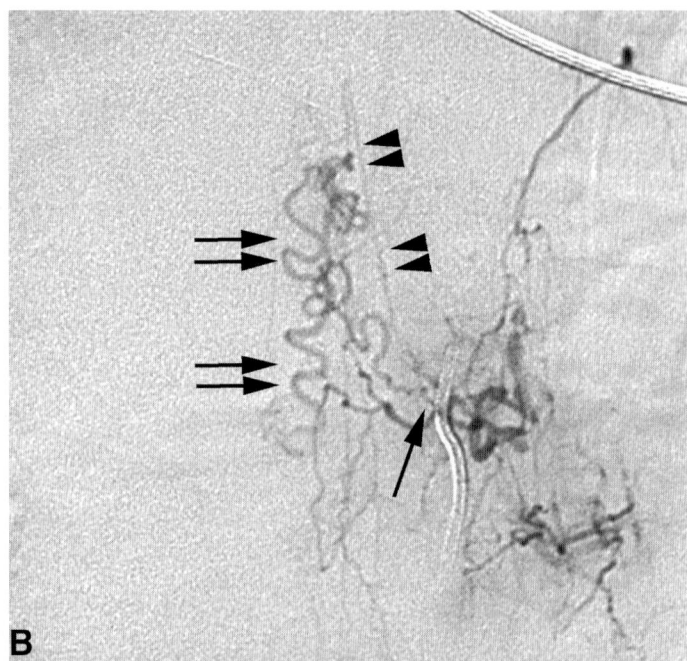

FIGURE 10.11 • *Spinal Dural AVF of Left T12.*
A sagittal T2-weighted MRI image (A) in a middle-age male patient presenting with clinical features typical of spinal venous hypertension shows abnormal flow voids on the dorsal surface of the cord (arrow) and a serpentine singularity among the structures of the cauda equina (arrowhead).

Spinal angiography showed the lesion at left T12 (B) with a later image from this run demonstrating the extensive spinal plexus of distended veins. However, careful examination of the images shows that there is a posterior spinal artery present (double arrowheads), which precludes safe acrylate glue embolization at this level. The fistula is seen in the neural foramen as an irregular segment of vessel (arrow), which changes caliber as it opens into the veins (double arrows). A third unmarked vessel extending medially from the left T12 pedicle represents a superimposed muscular branch.

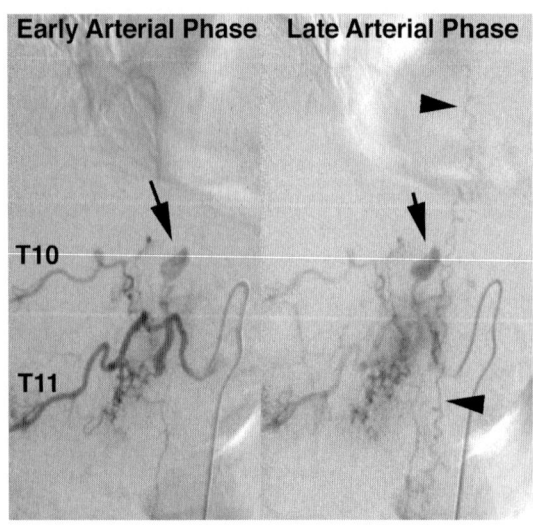

FIGURE 10.12 • *Variant of Spinal Dural AVF.*
A 68-year-old lady progressed from being normal to complete paraparesis and incontinence over a 2-week period. A spinal angiogram was performed on the basis of an abnormal MRI examination and showed opacification of an epidural varix or pouch (arrow) at the right T11 injection. This pouch then drained intradurally with the typical appearance of spinal venous stasis (arrowheads). At surgery the extradural pouch was located and resected with the fistula. The patient made a complete recovery.

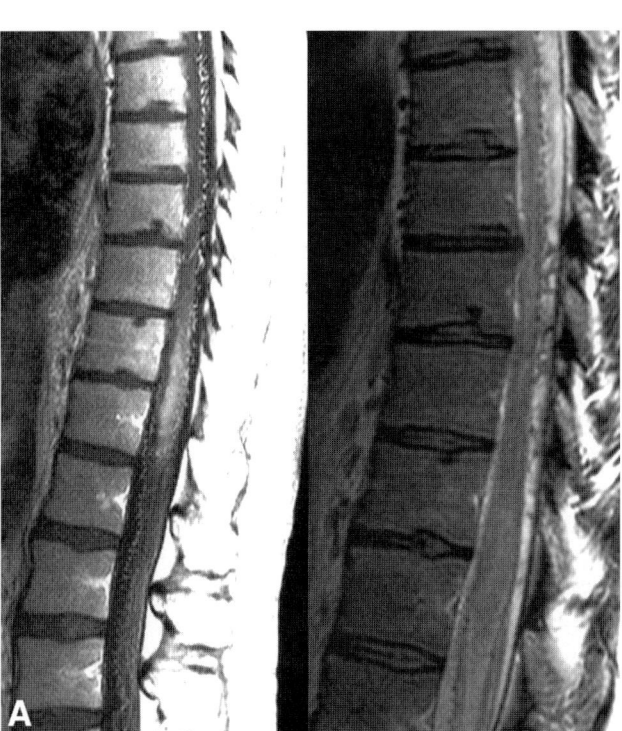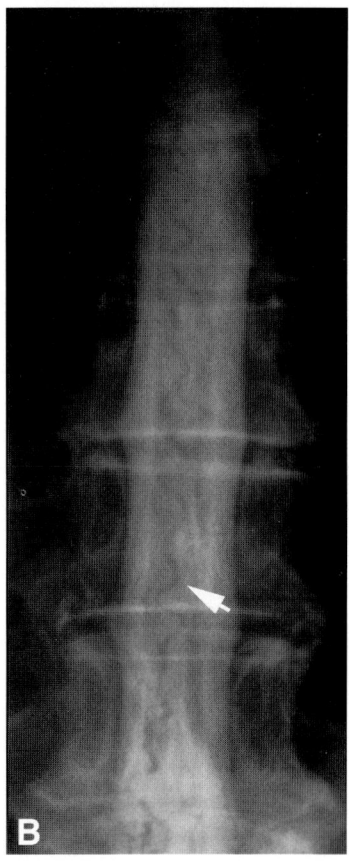

FIGURE 10.13 • *Spinal Dural AVF on MRI and Myelography.*
Because SdAVF is a curable disease in the early stages of physiologic decline, it is important to recognize the disease the first time it comes for imaging. However, not many patients will be as floridly abnormal as in these images chosen for print quality. A sagittal enhanced T1 MRI and T2 MRI (A) show the characteristic features of an expanded, edematous conus with enhancement. Numerous flow voids, which enhance with gadolinium, extend over the dorsal and ventral surfaces of the cord. A myelogram (B) shows the serpentine filling defect of a distended vein (arrow) within the thecal column.

the fistula is very slow, the capacitance of the venous system of the cord (at least in patients who are symptomatic) is limited and quickly overwhelmed. Consequently, the venous plexus of the cord becomes distended and stagnant. Venous hypertension alters the arteriovenous gradient of the spine and flow becomes slow in the distal anterior spinal artery. The cord becomes swollen and edematous with breakdown of the blood-CNS barrier. This was originally described as the syndrome of Foix-Alajouanine, i.e., a venous infarction of the cord.

Spinal function deteriorates in a characteristic fashion. Patients typically present in late middle age or later. Regardless of the site of the SdAVF, the most vulnerable area of the cord is the distal reach of the anterior spinal artery circulation, i.e., the conus. Symptoms typically start with weakness of the lower extremities and sensory disturbances that evolve into an ascending pattern of sensation loss, often with a clearly demarcated level. Patients may not spontaneously volunteer symptoms of autonomic dysfunction, but when asked they commonly have had episodes of sphincter incontinence and sexual dysfunction. The course of events may vary in speed, with some patients becoming wheelchair-bound and incontinent within a matter of weeks. Others may have a history extending over a year or more.

When the disease is detected early in the course, these patients generally respond excellently to treatment either by surgery or embolization. When the extreme effects of the disease are long-established, complete reversal of clinical symptoms is less likely after treatment. Even when treatment by embolization or surgery is delayed for months or years after onset of symptoms, however, the majority of patients still show some improvement with treatment.[31] It is common for patients presenting with this disease to have had MRI and other examinations previously in which the diagnosis was overlooked or misinterpreted. Some patients will be diagnosed as having spinal tumors and may undergo biopsy in the course of evaluation. The longer the delay before correct diagnosis, the less chance there is of a complete recovery from the condition. Therefore, the most important function of an interventional neuroradiologist in this disease is reminding one's diagnostic colleagues from time to time of this entity so that the condition is correctly diagnosed at the first session of imaging. Serpentine filling defects on a myelogram examination, for example, can be very subtle prospectively but should be noticed, as this may represent the patient's only chance for an expeditious diagnosis. Similarly, on MRI examination an expansile mass of the conus with gadolinium enhancement may not necessarily represent a tumor, especially if the pattern of edema extends very high in the cord and the surface of the cord is studded with enhancing vessels. Typically, the MRI examination in this condition shows expansion of the conus, with or without enhancement that can be focal or diffuse. The T2-weighted MRI images show expansion of the cord too, with variable degrees of hyperintense signal within the cord.

Spinal angiography must be performed with meticulous recording of the levels injected and of those not found or yet to be injected (Figs. 10.8, 10.9). A worksheet of the runs performed should be kept by the technologist during the case. If the internal iliac arteries, median sacral artery, and segmental arteries have all been adequately seen, then the examination must be extended to include the vertebral arteries, the internal carotid arteries, the external carotid arteries, and the ascending cervical and thyrocervical trunks, so as to include the dura of the entire spinal axis. The locations of the anterior spinal arteries and posterior spinal arteries are important in defining the risks of attempted embolization in adjacent pedicles. The state of flow in the anterior spinal artery will also help in some patients to confirm the disease state. Commonly there will be slowing of flow in the anterior spinal artery and delayed washout of contrast in the arterial phase. The venous phase of the anterior spinal artery injection will also be abnormal with prominent, delayed congestion.[32] Each run must be continued well into the venous phase of adjacent normal tissue because of the slow filling of these fistulas. Any run that is impaired by bowel motion or shift of the catheter will need to be repeated.

Embolization of SdAVFs can be curative if the lesion can be embolized without risk to the spinal arteries. Coils and particles are not adequate for this purpose, as they have a significant risk of allowing immediate or delayed recanalization. Only acrylate liquid glue injections reaching and filling the adjacent vein are acceptable as a therapeutic alternative to surgery.[33] If successful embolization cannot be accomplished or fails, placing a small platinum coil in the feeding artery as close as possible to the fistula can be very useful as a fluoroscopic and visual guide to the surgeon during subsequent surgery.

Perimedullary Arteriovenous Fistulas

Perimedullary fistulas are intradural lesions situated on the surface of the spinal cord (Fig. 10.14). A feeder from an anterior or posterior spinal artery connects directly with a spinal vein without a definable nidus. While rupture from a vein or an aneurysm of a feeding pedicle can present with subarachnoid hemorrhage, it is more common for these patients to present with symptoms and MRI findings very similar to those seen with the state of

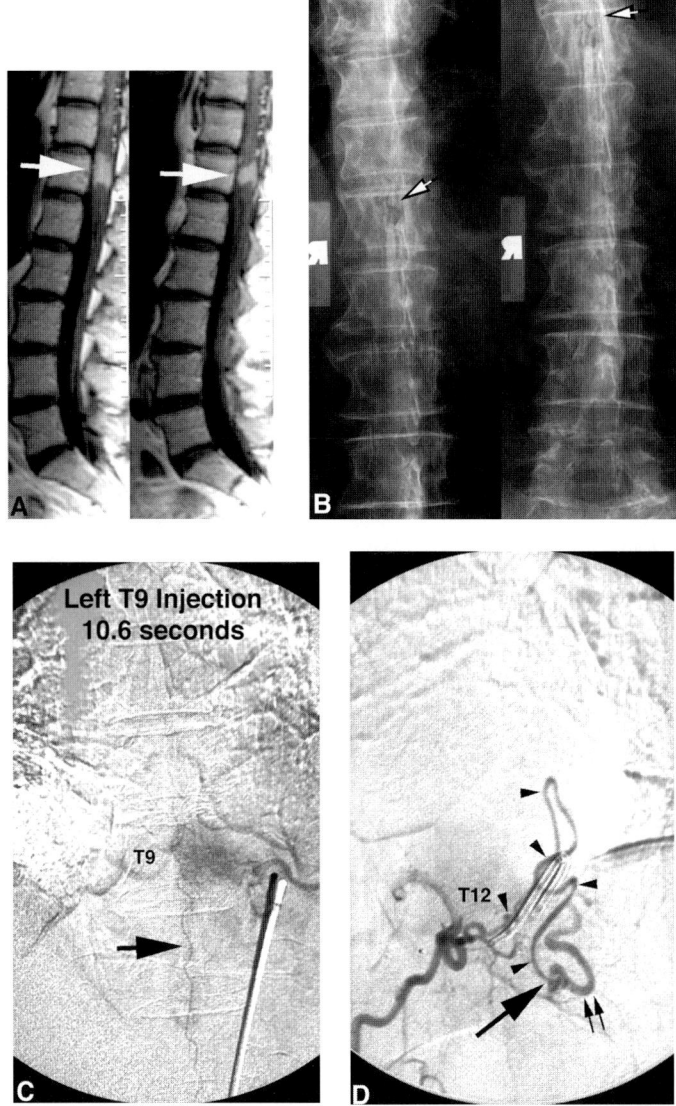

FIGURE 10.14 • *Perimedullary Spinal AVM.*
A middle-age female presenting with myelopathic signs after treatment for breast carcinoma some years previously was at first thought to have metastatic disease to the conus (A, MRI with gadolinium). However, a single metastasis to the conus in the absence of disease elsewhere would be unusual, and a second MRI (shown) demonstrated enhancing vessels on the dorsum of the conus. Marked expansion and enhancement of the conus is present (arrow).

A myelogram examination (B) showed subtle intrathecal serpentine filling defects (arrows). A spinal angiogram was undertaken. The anterior spinal artery was seen at left T9 (C) and showed no evidence of direct supply to an AVM. However, the injection is abnormal in that at 10.6 seconds into the run after a 2-second injection, the anterior spinal artery is still opacified throughout its course. This indicates a slowing of arterial flow due to the alteration of the arterio-venous gradient of the spinal circulation.

The abnormality at right T12 (D) is most likely categorized as a perimedullary fistula. The right T12 injection opacifies a characteristic hairpin posterior spinal artery (arrowheads), which descending behind the cord abruptly changes caliber at the fistula (arrow) causing subsequent opacification of the veins (double arrow).

venous hypertension found in SdAVFs. However, patients with perimedullary AVFs are more likely to present in early adulthood to early middle age, in contrast to the later presentation of SdAVFs. The onset and progress of clinical symptoms can be rapid. Perimedullary fistulas are classified according to the state of flow in the fistula by Merland,[34] but some perimedullary fistulas do not fit easily into a clear schema.

Type 1 Perimedullary Fistula

This is a simple fistula from the anterior spinal or posterior spinal artery to the venous plexus with slow flow. The feeding artery is not particularly dilated in appearance, and the veins are small or minimally dilated. Catheterization of the distal feeding artery is therefore usually not possible, and thus embolization is usually not an option. Embolization from a relatively distal location of a posterior spinal artery fistula with particles is sometimes advocated as possible. However, because one cannot be sure that recanalization will not occur and because the posterior surface of the spinal cord is relatively easy to visualize surgically, many neurosurgeons prefer to treat these lesions surgically.[33]

Type 2 Perimedullary Fistula

This lesion has more flow than the Type 1 perimedullary fistula and has dilatation of the feeding artery and draining veins. More distal catheterization of the feeding artery with a microcatheter is therefore an option for some of these patients with a view toward embolization. However, this should be undertaken with extreme caution, if at all. Somatosensory evoked potential (SEP) and motor evoked potential (MEP) monitoring during the embolization is a prudent precaution. Provocative testing in association with SEP and MEP monitoring can be used as a guide for embolization by injecting sodium amytal 50–75 mg and lidocaine 20–40 mg via the microcatheter prior to attempting embolization.[35] This monitoring is usually performed by staff from the neuroanesthesia or neurophysiology departments experienced in this technique. A 10% change in the latency period of the signal after a challenge, or a 60% drop in amplitude is taken as a positive (i.e., dangerous) result. Surgical technique for closing Type 2 perimedullary fistulas is well established and successful.

Type 3 Perimedullary Fistula

This variant is described as having giant vessels on the arterial and venous side. Because of the size and tension of the vessels, surgical exploration of these lesions is more problematic. Embolization with balloons, coils, or acrylate glue may represent the safest option.

Mourier et al.[36] reported on a series of 35 patients with fistulas of types 1, 2, and 3 treated by embolization or surgery. Half of the patients with types 1 and 2 improved with treatment and the other half remained stable. Type 3 patients who could be successfully embolized did exceptionally well. The failure of successfully embolized patients with types 1 and 2 disease to improve consistently was thought by the authors to represent the effects of prolonged venous ischemia prior to treatment.

Intramedullary Spinal Arteriovenous Malformations

Intramedullary spinal AVMs typically present with either a spinal or subarachnoid hemorrhage and thus with a catastrophic neurologic event. Sometimes patients may have a superimposed gradual pattern of progressive decline (Fig. 10.15). Mass-effect, venous hypertension from the venous effects of the AVM, or local ischemic "steal" are possible modes of pathophysiology, but are predominant only in the minority of patients. Patients typically are seen in childhood or early adulthood. Multiple spinal AVMs can be seen in systemic nonmetameric syndromes such as Osler-Rendu-Weber and Klippel-Trenaunay syndromes, and in the metameric Cobb syndrome.[37] Flow tends to be fast in the majority of intramedullary AVMs (80%), and related arterial or venous aneurysms were seen in 20% to 44% of the arterial or venous components in various large series.[31,38] The angiographic presence of a nidal aneurysm correlates strongly with the patient's risk of subarachnoid hemorrhage. Af-

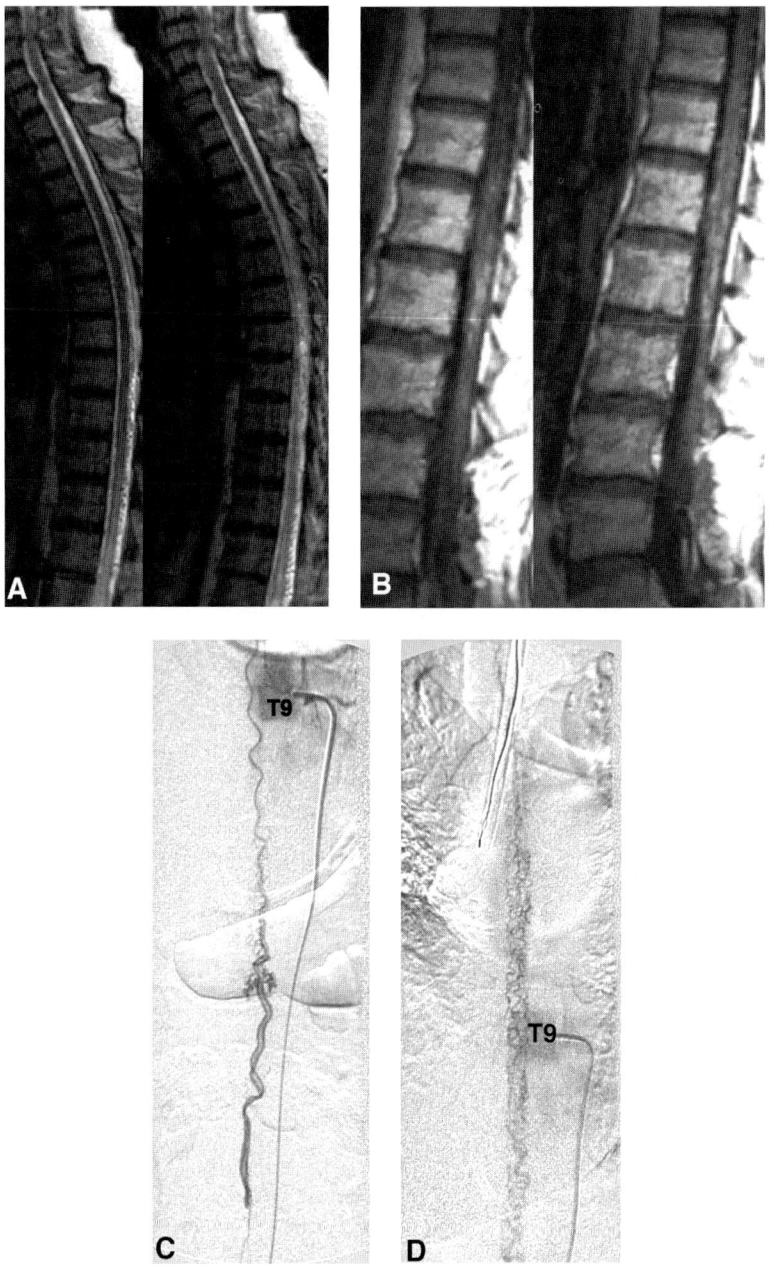

FIGURE 10.15 • *Intraparenchymal Spinal AVM.*
A late middle-age female with a remote history of surgical release of a tethered cord presented with rapidly progressive myelopathic symptoms. An MRI examination showed conus hyperintensity and abnormal flow voids on the surface of the cord on the T2-weighted images (A). The T1 contrast-enhanced images (B) showed tethering of the cord and expansion of the enhancing conus.

Spinal angiography shows an AVM filling from the anterior spinal artery from left T9. The arterial phase (C) demonstrates how the anterior spinal artery doubles back up the posterior aspect of the cord to supply the well-circumscribed nidus of the AVM. The venous phase (D) of a left T9 run centered higher shows the extensive venous congestion of the cord.

ter endovascular treatment of the spinal AVM, flow-related aneurysms may regress or disappear.[39]

Although the possibility of recanalization of intramedullary AVMs after particle embolization is acknowledged by all authors, most still recommend particles (150–500 μm) as safer than cyanoacrylate for intramedullary embolization.[31,40] Particle size, however, is a critical factor. Particles smaller than 50 μm have the ability to penetrate the sulcocommisural branches of the anterior spinal artery and cause infarctions, which may not be seen angiographically.[41] Electrophysiological monitoring is potentially very important during such high-risk spinal embolizations. Although high rates of angiographic recanalization were seen following particle embolization of spinal AVMs in a series of 35 patients by Biondi et al., 80% showed sustained clinical improvement at long-term follow-up following one or more embolization sessions.[42]

Two types of intramedullary spinal AVM are recognized:

- A discrete, compact nidus surrounded by normal cord tissue is usually termed a Glomus type AVM. They respond better than Juvenile Type lesions to treatment. Surgical excision in collaboration with preoperative particle embolization is the most favored approach. Embolization with particles is recommended by most authors as palliative or as a preoperative treatment, provided that microcatheter access can be gained close to the AVM so as to minimize the risks of collateral cord damage.[40] Favorable results were reported in most patients by Bao and Ling[41] in one of the largest modern series using combined treatment.
- A more diffuse AVM infiltrating into surrounding tissue, often with some expansion of the cord and demonstrating larger vessels, is termed a Juvenile Type Spinal AVM. These lesions are rare and are difficult to treat. Most authorities advocate palliative rather than definitive treatment because the risks of mortality and morbidity are so high.[41] Some juvenile spinal AVMs can extend over many segments of the spine and can extend through the subarachnoid space to involve the dural and paradural structures.[33]

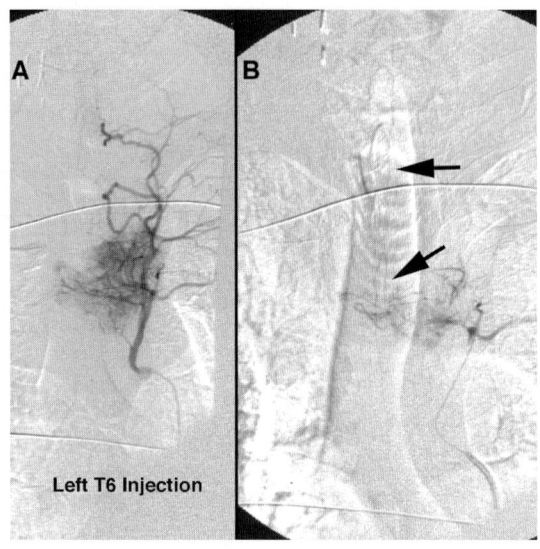

FIGURE 10.16 • *Metastatic Thyroid Carcinoma.*
A left T6 injection (A) in an elderly male patient with metastatic follicular cell carcinoma of the thyroid shows a prominent tumor blush. This tumor was so vascular that surgery to stabilize the spine had to be abandoned due to torrential blood loss. In preparation for embolization, it is important always to perform a microcatheter injection at the point of planned embolization. This run (B) more selectively from the same level shows the presence of an anterior spinal artery (arrows), indicating the degree of risk involved in this procedure. Fibered coils were used instead of particles as a result of this finding.

SPINAL TUMOR EMBOLIZATION

Extramedullary tumors of the vertebral bodies can be extraordinarily vascular to a degree that impairs surgical resection or fixation attempts. Metastatic renal cell carcinoma, thyroid carcinoma (Fig. 10.16), paraganglioma (Fig. 10.17), melanoma, giant cell tumors, or aggressive hemangiomas can frequently induce such severe bleeding during fixation or stabilization procedures that surgery has to be abandoned. Preoperative embolization and devascularization of such tumors can make the tumor bed more manageable from a surgical point of view and can significantly reduce the degree of intraoperative bleeding by a factor of 2 to 3.[43–49] Embolization can

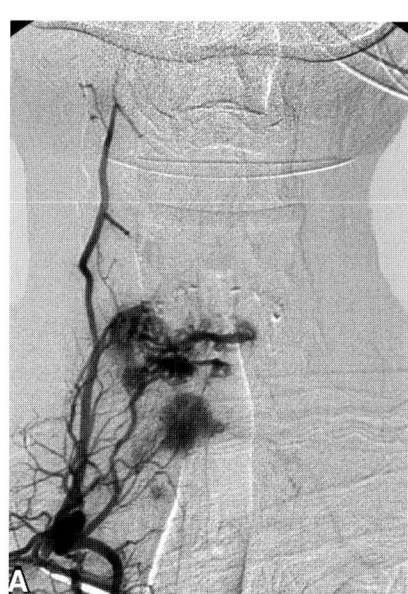
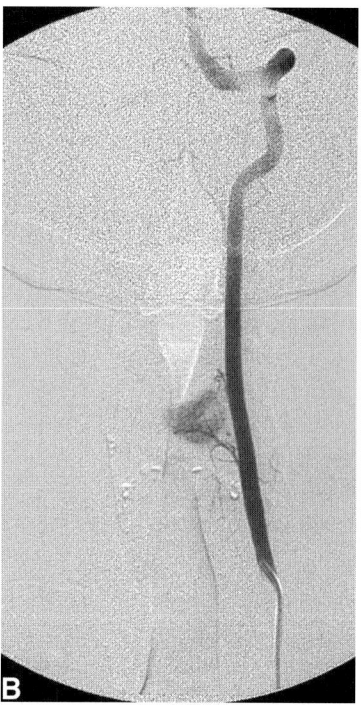
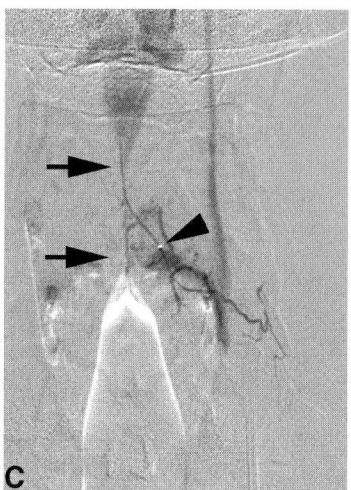

FIGURE 10.17 • *Metastatic Paraganglioma.*
Metastatic paraganglioma can be extremely vascular, as was the case in this 24-year-old male patient requiring multiple procedures in preparation for orthopedic stabilization (A, right thyrocervical trunk injection). The left vertebral artery injection (B) shows more tumor opacifying in the mid-cervical level. Illustrating the point made in case 10.16, a superselective injection (C) made via a microcatheter (arrowhead) at this level shows the anterior spinal artery (arrows), which could not be seen on the previous injection.

be performed via a transarterial approach using coaxial microcatheters or by direct needle puncture of the tumor.

Transarterial embolization of vascular extramedullary spinal tumors is most commonly performed using PVA (150–250 μm) particles, Gelfoam, coils, or less commonly alcohol or acrylate glue. In a study comparing the effects of various embolic agents in hypervascular spinal metastases, Berkefeld et al.[49] found that PVA particles (150–250 μm) were significantly more effective at reducing perioperative blood loss by more than a factor of 2 compared with coil embolization. Direct-puncture techniques can allow devascularization and debulking of tumor with acrylate glue and alcohol, or stabilization with methylmethacrylate as described for vertebroplasty. In all instances a primary source of concern is inadvertent embolization of the anterior and posterior spinal arteries. Before such a procedure it is prudent to extend the spinal angiogram until the normal anterior spinal artery is visualized in full. Transarterial or direct-puncture embolization should be performed very carefully, especially when the anterior spinal artery is not well seen. When it is well seen remote from the tumor, there is still potential for the arterial pedicle at the level of tumor involvement to connect unseen with the anterior spinal axis through branches not seen initially due to hemodynamic effects.

An anterior spinal artery arising from the same pedicle as the intended embolization is generally seen as a contraindication to embolization.[43,47] In extreme circumstances, coil embolization can be performed in the pedicle in question if one is confident of being distal to the origin of the anterior spinal artery. When the spinal artery is from the pedicle immediately adjacent to the site of planned embolization, the potential for anastomoses from one level to the next should prompt extreme caution and use of larger size PVA particles. As a general rule, as the embolization progresses in this and other circumstances, repeat DSA runs should be performed to monitor any change in hemodynamics, allowing emergence of a critical vessel or of a dangerous collateral vessel. Proximal embolization of a pedicle feeding the posterior spinal artery with coils is unlikely to cause a clinically significant injury. However, caustic agents such as acrylate glue or alcohol, if they penetrate the posterior spinal artery, are likely to produce clinically evident injuries.[50] Physiologic monitoring of sensory and motor evoked potentials during spinal embolizations can be helpful when challenge infusions of lidocaine or amytal are given intraarterially beforehand.

In the high thoracic region multiple arterial sources of flow to hypervascular tumors are commonly seen. In addition to the immediately contiguous arterial segmental levels, the costocervical, thyrocervical, and vertebral arteries represent sites of significant flow to such tumors and will need to be evaluated accordingly.

Intramedullary hypervascular tumors are rare and consist almost exclusively of spinal hemangioblastomas. Preoperative embolization of spinal hemangioblastomas has been reported by some authors with favorable surgical opinions on the ease of subsequent surgery and degree of intraoperative blood loss.[43,51] Particle embolization to the tumor can be performed if distal access is sufficient. Proximal coil occlusion of feeding arteries may also be sufficiently helpful for surgical purposes.

References

1. GALIBERT P, DERAMOND H, ROSAT P, LE GARS D (1987) Preliminary note on the treatment of vertebral angioma by percutaneous acrylic vertebroplasty. *Neuro-Chirurgie* 33:166–168.
2. MARTIN JB, JEAN B, SUGIU K, SAN MILLAN RUIZ D, PIOTIN M, MURPHY K, RUFENACHT B, MUSTER M, RUFENACHT DA (1999) Vertebroplasty: clinical experience and follow-up results. *Bone* 25:11S–15S.
3. BOSTROM MP, LANE JM (1997) Future directions. Augmentation of osteoporotic vertebral bodies. *Spine* 22:38S–42S.
4. TOHMEH AG, MATHIS JM, FENTON DC, LEVINE AM, BELKOFF SM (1999) Biomechanical efficacy of unipedicular versus bipedicular vertebroplasty for the management of osteoporotic compression fractures. *Spine* 24:1772–1776.
5. BELKOFF SM, MARONEY M, FENTON DC, MATHIS JM (1999) An in vitro biomechanical evaluation of bone cements used in percutaneous vertebroplasty. *Bone* 25:23S–26S.
6. MELTON LJ (1997) Epidemiology of spinal osteoporosis. *Spine* 22:2S–11S.

7. COOK DJ, GUYATT GH, ADACHI JD, THE MULTICENTER VERTEBRAL FRACTURE STUDY GROUP (1993) Quality of life issues in women with vertebral fractures due to osteoporosis. *Arthritis Rheum* 36:750–756.
8. GOLD DT (1996) The clinical impact of vertebral fractures: Quality of life in women with osteoporosis. *Bone* 18:185S–189S.
9. JENSEN ME, EVANS AJ, MATHIS JM, KALLMES DF, CLOFT HJ, DION JE (1997) Percutaneous polymethylmethacrylate vertebroplasty in the treatment of osteoporotic vertebral body compression fractures: technical aspects. *AJNR* 18:1897–1904.
10. MATHIS JM, PETRI M, NAFF N (1998) Percutaneous vertebroplasty treatment of steroid-induced osteoporotic compression fractures. *Arthritis Rheum* 41:171–175.
11. CORTET B, COTTEN A, BOUTRY N, FLIPO RM, DUQUESNOY B, CHASTANET P, DELCAMBRE B (1999) Percutaneous vertebroplasty in the treatment of osteoporotic vertebral compression fractures: an open prospective study. *J Rheumatol* 26:2222–2228.
12. DERAMOND H, DEPRIESTER C, GALIBERT P, LE GARS D (1998) Percutaneous vertebroplasty with polymethylmethacrylate. Technique, indications, and results. *Radiol Clin N A* 36:533–546.
13. IDE C, GANGI A, RIMMELIN A, BEAUJEUX R, MAITROT D, BUCHHEIT F, SELLAL F, DIETEMANN JL (1996) Vertebral haemangiomas with spinal cord compression: the place of preoperative percutaneous vertebroplasty with methyl methacrylate. *Neuroradiology* 38:585–589.
14. WEILL A, CHIRAS J, SIMON JM, ROSE M, SOLA-MARTINEZ T, ENKAOUA E (1996) Spinal metastases: indications for and results of percutaneous injection of acrylic surgical cement. *Radiology* 199:241–247.
15. GARMATIS CJ, CHU FC (1978) The effectiveness of radiation therapy in the treatment of bone metastases from breast cancer. *Radiology* 126:235–237.
16. SALAZAR OM, RUBIN P, HENDRICKSON FR, KOMAKI R, POULTER C, NEWALL J, ASBELL SO, MOHIUDDIN M, VAN ESS J (1986) Single-dose half-body irradiation for palliation of multiple bone metastases from solid tumors. Final Radiation Therapy Oncology Group report. *Cancer* 58:29–36.
17. CONVERY FR, GUNN DR, HUGHES JD, MARTIN WE (1975) The relative safety of polymethylmethacrylate. A controlled clinical study of randomly selected patients treated with Charnley and ring total hip replacements. *J Bone Joint Surg Am* 57:57–64.
18. CASTEL E, LAZENNEC JY, CHIRAS J, ENKAOUA E, SAILLANT G (1999) Acute spinal cord compression due to intraspinal bleeding from a vertebral hemangioma: two case-reports. *Europ Spine J* 8:244–248.
19. DERAMOND H, WRIGHT NT, BELKOFF SM (1999) Temperature elevation caused by bone cement polymerization during vertebroplasty. *Bone* 25:17S–21S.
20. PADOVANI B, KASRIEL O, BRUNNER P, PERETTI-VITON P (1999) Pulmonary embolism caused by acrylic cement: a rare complication of percutaneous vertebroplasty. *AJNR* 20:375–377.
21. PINTO PW (1993) Cardiovascular collapse associated with the use of methylmethacrylate. *AANA Journal* 61:613–616.
22. SCHEMITSCH EH, JAIN R, TURCHIN DC, MULLEN JB, BYRICK RJ, ANDERSON GI, RICHARDS RR (1997) Pulmonary effects of fixation of a fracture with a plate compared with intramedullary nailing. A canine model of fat embolism and fracture fixation. *J Bone Joint Surg Am* 79:984–996.
23. ELMARAGHY AW, HUMENIUK B, ANDERSON GI, SCHEMITSCH EH, RICHARDS RR (1998) The role of methylmethacrylate monomer in the formation and haemodynamic outcome of pulmonary fat emboli. *J Bone Joint Surg Br* 80:156–161.
24. JENSEN ME, KALLMES DF, SHORT JG, SCHWEIKERT PJ, MARX WF (2000) Percutaneous vertebroplasty does not increase the risk of adjacent vertebral fracture—a retrospective study. Proceedings of the 38th annual meeting of the American Society of Neuroradiology, Atlanta, pp. 4–5.
25. CHIRAS J, DEPRIESTER C, WEILL A, SOLA-MARTINEZ MT, DERAMOND H (1997) Percutaneous vertebral surgery. Techniques and indications. *J Neuroradiol* 24:45–59.
26. COTTEN A, DERAMOND H, CORTET B, LEJEUNE JP, LECLERC X, CHASTANET P, CLARISSE J (1996) Preoperative percutaneous injection of methyl methacrylate and N-butyl cyanoacrylate in vertebral hemangiomas. *AJNR* 17:137–142.
27. CLOFT HJ, EASTON DN, JENSEN ME, KALLMES DF, DION JE (1999) Exposure of medical personnel to methylmethacrylate vapor during percutaneous vertebroplasty. *AJNR* 20:352–353.
28. MCLAUGHLIN RE, BARKALOW JA, ALLEN MS (1979) Pulmonary toxicity of methyl methacrylate vapors: an environmental study. *Arch Environ Health* 34:336–338.
29. MCLAUGHLIN RE, REGER SI, BARKALOW JA, ALLEN MS, DAFAZIO CA (1978) Methylmethacrylate: a study of teratogenicity and fetal toxicity of the vapor in the mouse. *J Bone Joint Surg Am* 60:355–358.
30. GANGI A, KASTLER BA, DIETEMANN JL (1994) Percutaneous vertebroplasty guided by a combination of CT and fluoroscopy. *AJNR* 15:83–86.
31. ROSENBLUM B, OLDFIELD EH, DOPPMAN JL, DI CHIRO G (1987) Spinal arteriovenous malformations: a comparison of dural arteriovenous fistulas and intradural AVMs in 81 patients. *J Neurosurg* 67:795–802.
32. WILLINSKY R, LASJAUNIAS P, TERBRUGGE K, HURTH M (1990) Angiography in the investigation of spinal dural arteriovenous fistula. *Neuroradiology* 32:114–116.
33. MERLAND JJ, REIZINE D (1987) Treatment of arteriovenous spinal-cord malformations. *Sem Intervent Radiol* 4:281–290.
34. MERLAND JJ, RICHÉ MC, CHIRAS J (1980) Les fistules artérioveineuses intracanalaires extramédullaires drainage veineuses médullaire. *Journal de Neuroradiologie* 7:271–320.
35. NIIMI Y, BERENSTEIN A (1999) Endovascular treatment of spinal vascular malformations. *Neurosurg Clin North Am* 10:47–71.
36. MOURIER KL, GOBIN YP, GEORGE B, LOT G, MERLAND JJ (1993) Intradural perimedullary arteriovenous fistulae: results of

surgical and endovascular treatment in a series of 35 cases. *Neurosurgery* 32:885–891.

37. Miyatake SI, Kikuchi H, Koide T, Yamagata S, Nagata I, Minami SS, Asato R (1990) Cobb's syndrome and its treatment with embolization. *J Neurosurg* 72:497–499.

38. Biondi A, Merland JJ, Hodes JE, Pruvo JP, Reizine D (1992) Aneurysms of spinal arteries associated with intramedullary arteriovenous malformations. I. Angiographic and clinical aspects. *AJNR* 13:913–922.

39. Biondi A, Merland JJ, Hodes JE, Aymard A, Reizine D (1992) Aneurysms of spinal arteries associated with intramedullary arteriovenous malformations. II. Results of AVM endovascular treatment and hemodynamic considerations. *AJNR* 13:923–931.

40. Riché MC, Melki JP, Merland JJ (1983) Embolization of spinal cord vascular malformations via the anterior spinal artery. *AJNR* 4:378–381.

41. Bao YH, Ling F (1997) Classification and therapeutic modalities of spinal vascular malformations in 80 patients. *Neurosurgery* 40:75–81.

42. Biondi A, Merland JJ, Reizine D, Aymard A, Hodes JE, Lecoz P, Rey A (1990) Embolization with particles in thoracic intramedullary arteriovenous malformations: long-term angiographic and clinical results. *Radiology* 177:651–658.

43. Shi HB, Suh DC, Lee HK, Lim SM, Kim DH, Choi CG, Lee CS, Rhim SC (1999) Preoperative transarterial embolization of spinal tumor: embolization techniques and results. *AJNR* 20:2009–2015.

44. Hess T, Kramann B, Schmidt E, Rupp S (1997) Use of preoperative vascular embolisation in spinal metastasis resection. *Arch Orthop Trauma Surg* 116:279–282.

45. Sundaresan N, Choi IS, Hughes JE, Sachdev VP, Berenstein A (1990) Treatment of spinal metastases from kidney cancer by presurgical embolization and resection. *J Neurosurg* 73:548–554.

46. Gellad FE, Sadato N, Numaguchi Y, Levine AM (1990) Vascular metastatic lesions of the spine: preoperative embolization. *Radiology* 176:683–686.

47. Smith TP, Gray L, Weinstein JN, Richardson WJ, Payne CS (1995) Preoperative transarterial embolization of spinal column neoplasms. *J Vasc Intervent Radiol* 6:863–869.

48. Olerud C, Jonsson H Jr, Lofberg AM, Lorelius LE, Sjostrom L (1993) Embolization of spinal metastases reduces preoperative blood loss. 21 patients operated on for renal cell carcinoma. *Acta Orthopaedica Scandinavica* 64: 9–12.

49. Berkefeld J, Scale D, Kirchner J, Heinrich T, Kollath J (1999) Hypervascular spinal tumors: influence of the embolization technique on perioperative hemorrhage. *AJNR* 20:757–763.

50. Mascalchi M, Cosottini M, Ferrito G, Salvi F, Nencini P, Quilici N (1998) Posterior spinal artery infarct. *AJNR* 19: 361–363.

51. Eskridge JM, McAuliffe W, Harris B, Kim DK, Scott J, Winn HR (1996) Preoperative endovascular embolization of craniospinal hemangioblastomas. *AJNR* 17:525–531.

Chapter 11

Tumor Embolization

Preoperative Devascularization of Tumors

The techniques and principles of embolization of preoperative meningiomas can be generalized to all vascular tumors of the skull base. Although the techniques of preoperative devascularization of vascular tumors of the head and neck have been established for many years, the role of interventional neuroradiology in this arena is still limited to a relatively small number of patients. While it is known that presurgical embolization of meningiomas brings greater ease of surgery in a cost-effective manner, reduced perioperative blood loss, and possibly diminished likelihood of tumor recurrence,[1] the proportion of head and neck tumors suitable for this type of procedure is still the minority. However, a greater role for interventional neuroradiology may evolve in the future with treatment protocols using highly selective infusions of high-dose chemotherapy for squamous carcinoma and other tumors of head and neck.

During angiography of a meningioma the most important information that can be gathered is that which might assist the subsequent surgical resection. Specifically, the state and location of the adjacent veins and venous sinuses, and, if relevant, the possibility of arterial encasement by tumor should not be overlooked during the angiographic examination. Surgical excision of convexity meningiomas is usually a straightforward procedure, and most neurosurgeons do not believe that preoperative embolization is necessary for such situations. Therefore preoperative embolization of meningiomas tends to involve complicated tumors of the floor of the skull, clivus, foramen magnum, or regions of the sphenoid wing adjacent to the orbit. Concerns about arterial anastomoses involving dangerous collaterals to the internal carotid artery, ophthalmic artery, or vertebral artery (Figs. 11.1–11.5) are frequent during such cases. In the region of the orbit or cavernous sinus, the possibility of blindness resulting from particle or alcohol embolization of the central retinal artery of the ophthalmic artery is a risk that should be taken seriously.[2,3] High-quality biplane imaging of the arterial network around the eye and a thorough knowledge of the anatomic possibilities are imperative before proceeding with any embolization.[4] Moreover, the anastomotic pattern of vessels around the eye might change during the course of an embolization, meaning that dangerous collater-

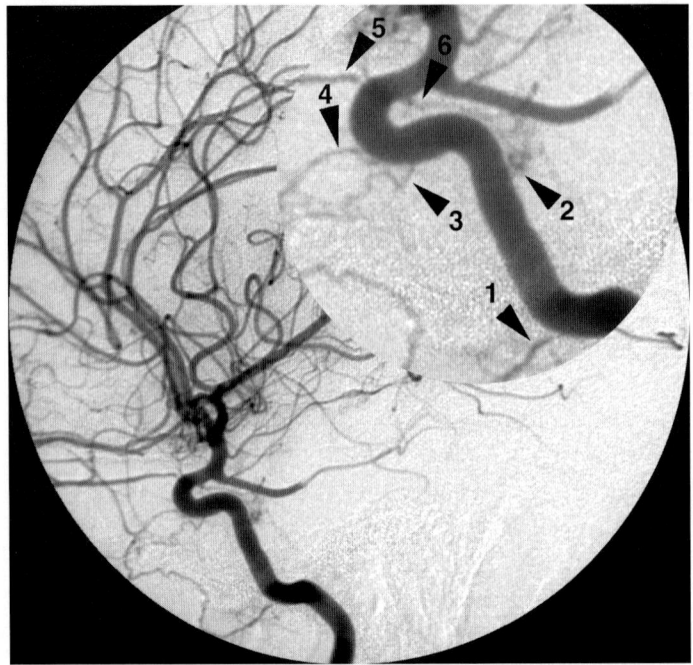

FIGURE 11.1 • *Anatomy of the Internal Carotid Artery Branches.*
A diagnostic image from a routine angiogram (with magnified insert) shows the major nonpathologic branches of the internal carotid artery proximal to the posterior communicating artery in ascending order: (**1**) Mandibulo-vidian branch, (**2**) Meningohypophyseal branches, (**3**) Inferolateral trunk, (**4**) Dorsal ophthalmic artery (?), (**5**) Ventral ophthalmic artery, (**6**) Superior hypophyseal artery.

Any of these arteries can form the basis for dangerous anastomoses to the internal carotid artery from the external carotid artery. (See also Figs. 7.13D, 7.13E.)

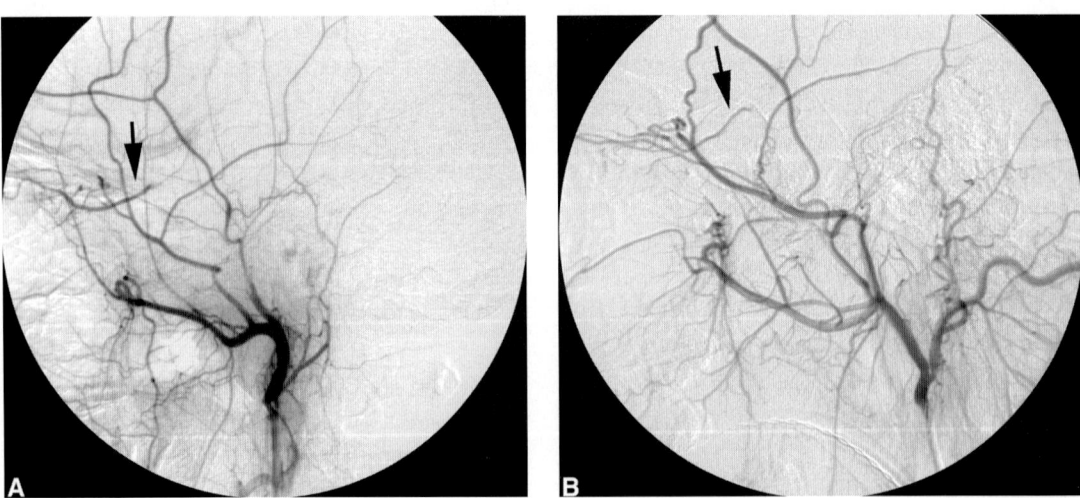

FIGURE 11.2 • *Dangerous Anastomosis to the Ophthalmic Artery.*
External carotid artery injections during the course of evaluation of juvenile angiofibromas in two young males show how readily the ophthalmic artery (arrows) can be opacified from such an injection. This finding does not preclude embolization, but it does require the utmost diligence of technique. (Fortunately, in these cases the tumors did not opacify from the side in question.) Larger particles would be prudent, and they should only be injected gently in a state of free distal flow.

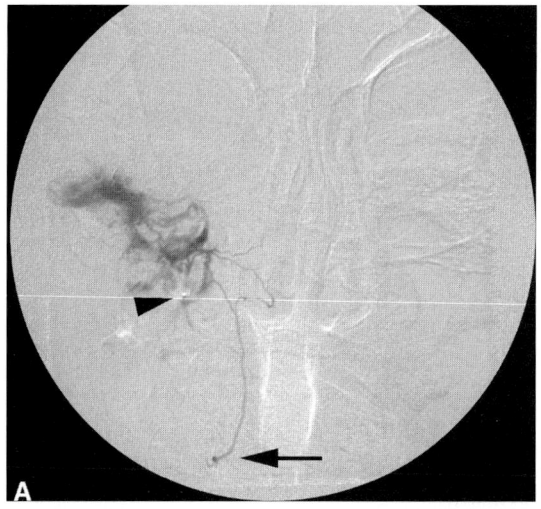 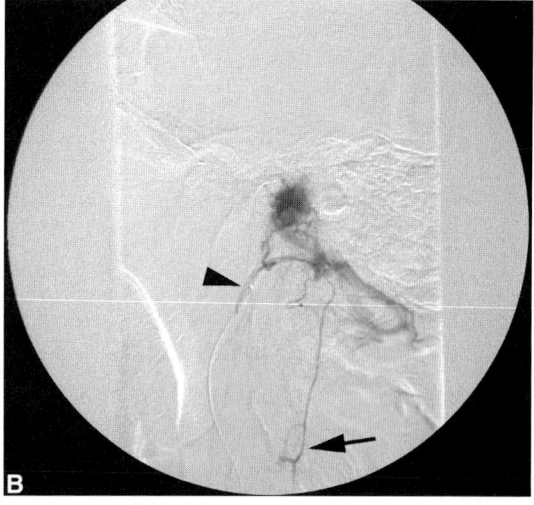

FIGURE 11.3 • *Dangerous Anastomosis to the Vertebral Artery I.*
An elderly patient with an advanced glomus jugulo-tympanicum was referred for embolization. The right ascending pharyngeal artery injection (arrowhead indicates the microcatheter tip) opacifies a sizeable mass of tumor on the AP (A) and lateral views (B). The artery extending inferiorly behind the odontoid process close to the midline is the C3 anastomosis (arrow), the odontoid arcade, connecting the hypoglossal branch of the neuromeningeal trunk to the vertebral artery. This is a very important and common pathway. It is a potential route of inadvertent embolization of the vertebral artery. Aggressive embolization in this location risks collateral embolization to the vertebral artery. It also risks injury to the vasa nervorum of the hypoglossal nerve. Keep the modest importance of embolization in a case such as this in perspective, and avoid unnecessarily aggressive embolization.

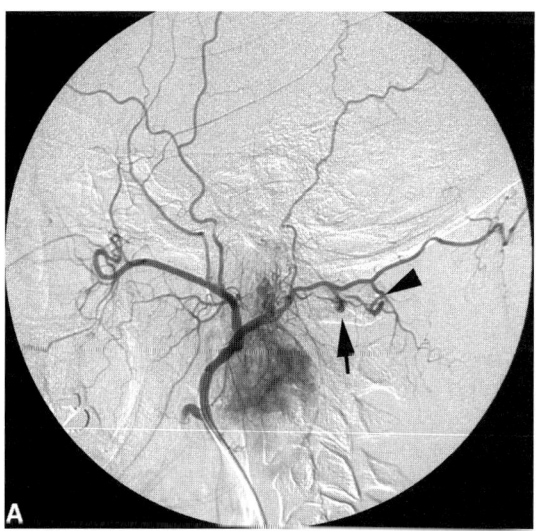 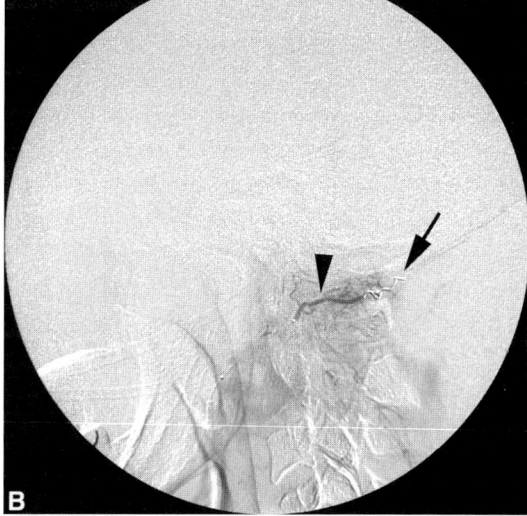

FIGURE 11.4 • *Dangerous Anastomosis to the Vertebral Artery II.*
An occipital artery injection (A, lateral view) in the course of embolization of a glomus tumor demonstrates prominent tumor blush below the jugular foramen. One's attention must be prioritized to the sites of potential danger in all such cases. The C1 branch of the occipital artery (arrowhead) anastomoses with the vertebral artery (arrow) fleetingly. This carries a serious risk of vertebro-basilar embolization of particles.

This can be prevented by depositing a coil (B, arrow) in the occipital artery distal to the tumor, which will prevent particles from accessing the vertebral artery but will allow embolization to proceed proximally more safely (B, taken after coil deposition and particle embolization of the tumor).

als might open up as the embolization progresses.[5] In the region of the cavernous sinus one must be always careful about the possibility of anastomoses to the inferolateral trunk and the meningohypophyseal trunk allowing potential communication between the point of embolization in the external carotid artery and the internal carotid artery. More inferiorly along the clivus, dural branches of the vertebral artery allowing communication between the external carotid artery and the vertebro-basilar system are of most concern. A thorough knowledge of these vessels is required for any skull-base embolization.[6]

Materials and Methods

For long procedures, simple intravenous sedation may be inadequate for patient comfort and safety. Monitored anesthesia care or general anesthesia will often be necessary. Advanced placement of a Foley catheter is rarely an excessive precaution, because the inevitable alternative is placing a urinal bottle or pan under the patient during the case with a catheter in the neck. Some authors recommend prior application of a strip of nitropaste or sublingual calcium antagonists to help diminish the risk of external carotid artery vasospasm during the case. However, transdermal absorption of nitroglycerin may be unpredictable, depending on skin conditions of the patient, and more precise drug delivery can be assured by intraarterial administration of papaverine (30–60 mg) or nitroglycerin (100–300 μg) through the catheter. Intraprocedural heparin to maintain an ACT >200 s is generally prudent to prevent thromboembolic complications. In patients with meningiomas or other intracranial tumors, high-dose steroids during and following the procedure may have a benefit in reducing swelling and edema, especially following aggressive embolization using smaller particles (60–150 μm).[7]

Most external carotid artery embolizations can be accomplished via a 5Fr catheter system, although some 4Fr catheters are available with an 0.038-in inner lumen that will accept a 0.016-in series microcatheter. For ease of flush and contrast injection

FIGURE 11.5 • *Potentially Dangerous Anastomoses in a Young Patient with Juvenile Angiofibroma.*
An MRI examination (A, T1-weighted image with gadolinium) demonstrates the typical expansile appearance of a JNA centered to the right of midline. Flow-voids and some areas of nonvascular necrosis are evident. The right external carotid artery injection (B, AP projection; C, lateral projection) shows the extensive tumor blush transgressing the midline, deriving supply from markedly enlarged long and short sphenopalatine arteries. No dangerous collateral branches can be seen.

The right internal carotid artery injection (D, lateral view), however, shows that there is still potential for danger. As is commonly the case in such young patients, the mandibulo-vidian artery persists and is enlarged (double arrows), supplying the tumor. The inferolateral trunk (arrow) is also enlarged. Both of these vessels represent sites of potential intratumoral anastomoses from external carotid artery to internal carotid artery. Reflux back to the internal carotid artery via intratumoral anastomoses of embolic material could occur if a forceful injection were made in a distal intratumoral branch. This has also been reported with percutaneous direct puncture of vascular masses.

Following embolization with PVA particles 150–250 μm a right external carotid artery injection (E) shows satisfactory devascularization of the tumor. The artery running over the face superficially is the transverse facial artery (arrows).

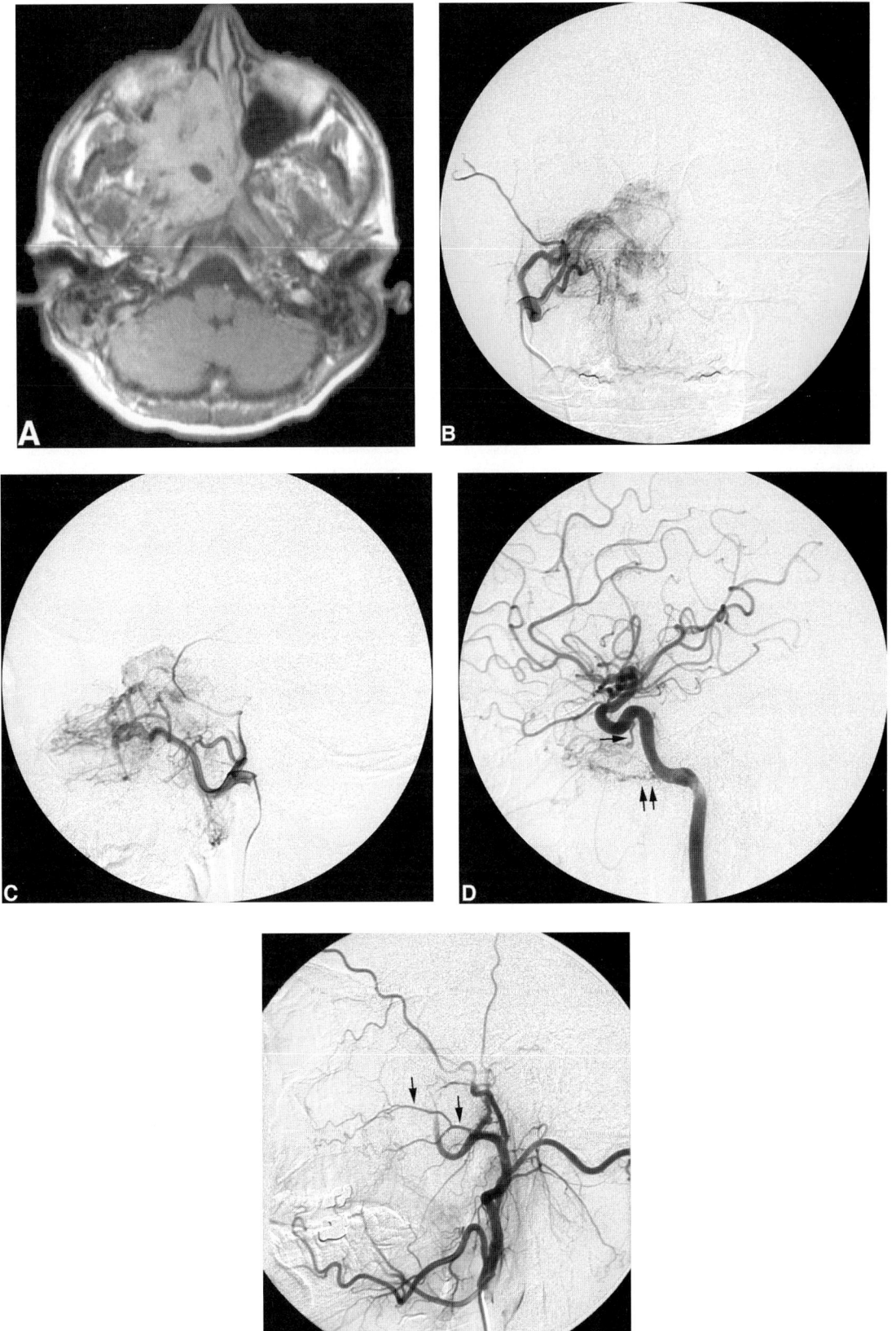

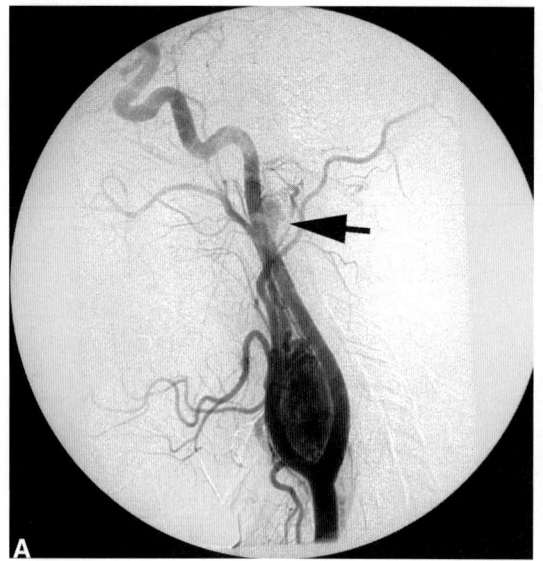 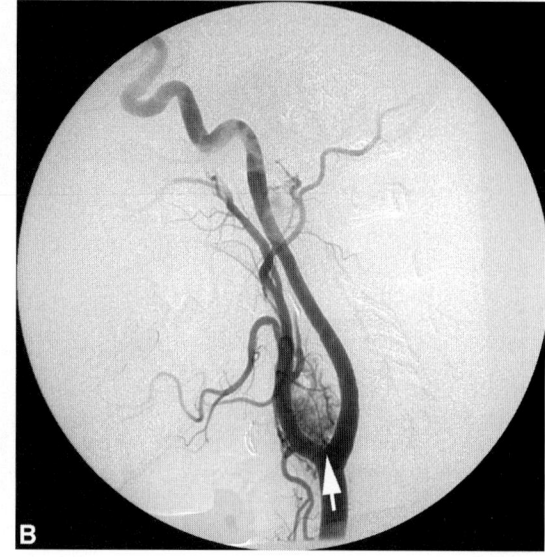

FIGURE 11.6 • *Preoperative Devascularization of a Carotid Body Tumor.*
A preoperative angiogram of the right common carotid artery (A, lateral view) shows splaying of the carotid bifurcation characteristic of a carotid body tumor. There is rapid shunting of blood through the tumor with early venous opacification. A second tumor along the vagus nerve is identified (arrow); it was hitherto unsuspected. It is common during angiography of such patients to identify small tumors that have previously escaped attention. The contralateral side should always be studied on this account.

The lateral view postembolization (B) with PVA 150–250 μm shows adequate devascularization of the tumor. A perfect result would require catheterization of the artery of the carotid body (arrow). However, this would involve unreasonable risk of emboli refluxing into the internal carotid artery. One could place a balloon in the internal carotid artery to prevent antegrade flow of particles during embolization, but to do so would involve loss of perspective on the ancillary importance of this procedure for this patient's welfare.

around the catheter during the case, a 6F or 7F catheter system might be preferred. Any of the currently available hydrophilic microcatheters of 0.016-in inner diameter and corresponding 0.014-in microwires will allow access to the distal branches of the external carotid artery. In unusual circumstances a 0.010-in series microcatheter might be useful to gain more distal access, but this will limit the size of particles and coils that can be embolized. Care should always be exercised to avoid rupturing a microcatheter either with the wire or while injecting Gelfoam pledgets. Proximal rupture of a microcatheter will allow subsequent particles to embolize into incorrect vessels with potentially disastrous results.

Particle Size

The choice of particle size is a balance between risk and efficacy. Smaller particles like Gelfoam powder (Upjohn) 40–60 μm or polyvinyl alcohol (PVA) 50–150 μm penetrate a tumor better than do larger particles and achieve a more lasting and thorough devascularization (Figs. 11.5–11.7). This often involves central necrosis of the tumor and can be demonstrated by postembolization contrast-enhanced MRI or MR spectroscopy.[7,8] However, particles at the smaller end of the size range may carry a higher risk of intraprocedural complications, ophthalmic artery injury, tissue necrosis, or injury to the vasa nervorum of the adjacent cranial

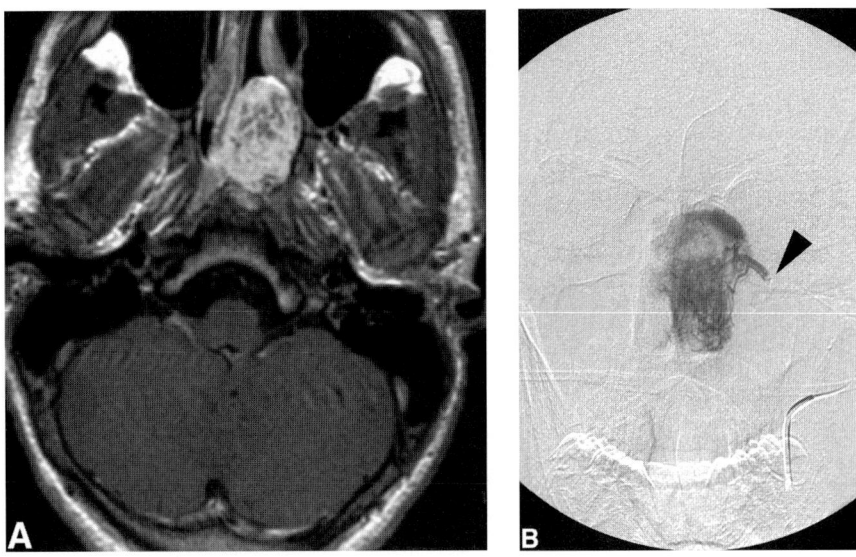
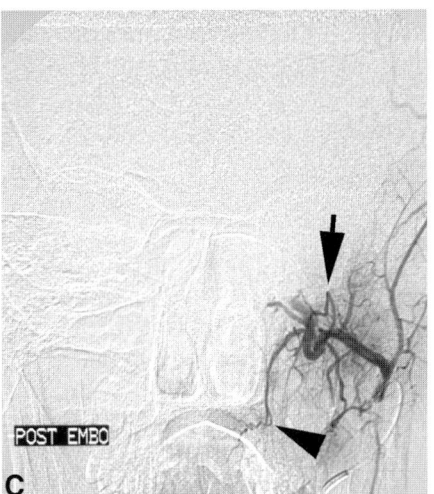

FIGURE 11.7 • *Juvenile Angiofibroma.*
An MRI examination (A, T1-weighted sequence with gadolinium) on a young male with change in voice, nasal stuffiness, and nosebleeds demonstrates an enhancing nasopharyngeal tumor to the left of midline. A preembolization run (B, left external carotid artery AP projection) shows the characteristic hypervascular blush of this tumor. The position of the microcatheter (arrowhead) is distal to the infraorbital artery. There are no dangerous anastomoses present, and this is a good location from which to embolize with PVA 150–250 μm followed by Gelfoam pledgets.

Following embolization (C, left external carotid artery postembolization AP projection) the tumor is adequately devascularized. The infraorbital artery (arrows) is preserved, as is the greater descending palatine artery (arrowhead). Embolizing these vessels inadvertently or through a nonspecific technique might not have any particular consequences, but generally the risk of endangering a critical anastomosis goes up with a more proximal embolization. Furthermore, some patients can experience a deal of facial pain and discomfort when a nonspecific general embolization is conducted. Therefore, unless vessel access is extraordinarily difficult, it is better to be quite targeted in one's embolization technique.

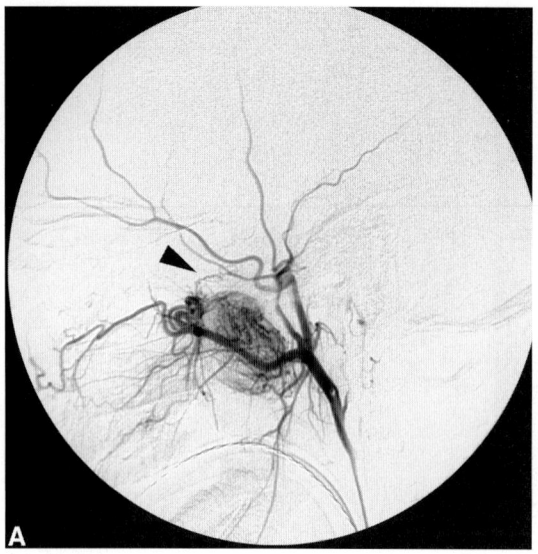 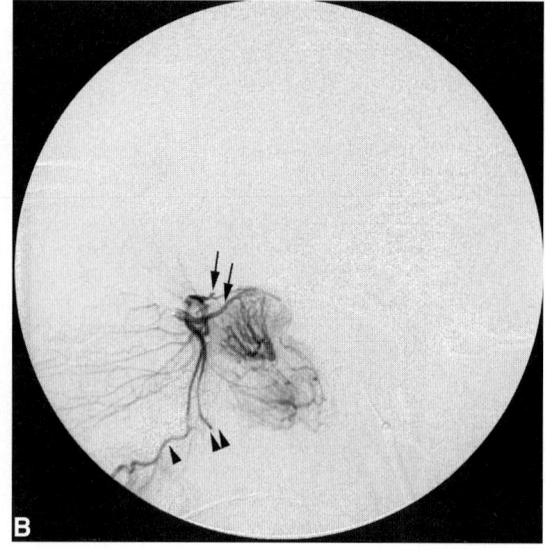

FIGURE 11.8 • *Juvenile Angiofibroma.*
A lateral view of the right external carotid artery (A) shows a characteristic nasopharyngeal blush from a juvenile angiofibroma. The arrowhead indicates the artery of the foramen rotundum, an important dangerous anastomosis between the distal external carotid artery and the inferolateral trunk of the internal carotid artery. This does not preclude embolization in this patient, but indicates the need in all patients for extreme care.

A more selective injection (B) through the microcatheter in the distal left internal maxillary artery allows embolization of the tumor through two posteriorly directed branches (arrows), one of which probably represents the artery of the pterygo-vaginal canal. This is a common anastomosis between the internal maxillary artery and the pharyngeal branches of the accessory meningeal artery. The accessory meningeal artery will sometimes be involved with tumors of this region. The greater (single arrowhead) and lesser descending (double arrowhead) palatine arteries are clearly seen with a characteristic appearance.

nerves.[9–14] For similar reasons, embolization with liquid alcohol or cyanoacrylate glue in the external carotid artery carries a risk of tissue necrosis or cranial nerve necrosis if the vasa nervorum are embolized. On the other hand, with PVA particles over 150 μm in size a lesser degree of tumor penetration is achieved, but the risk of tissue necrosis or cranial nerve injury is extremely small. Generally particles 150–500 μm are used for tumor devascularization with satisfactory results. Caution should be exercised if there is arteriovenous shunting in a tumor. Larger particles ($>$500 μm) are preferred in that situation lest embolic particles should travel unimpeded to the venous field and cause pulmonary symptoms.

Direct Percutaneous Puncture

A variety of hypervascular tumors of the head and neck can respond favorably in terms of presurgical devascularization to direct percutaneous or transnasal puncture by 18–20 gauge needles.[15] A sheath needle can be used at the initial introduction for guiding subsequent coaxial needles when trauma to neurovascular structures is feared. Liquid agents, principally NBCA (n-butyl-cyanoacrylate) and alcohol, are most suited to this technique. Complications involving neurovascular structures or embolic complications from intratumoral anastomoses to critical vessels can be seen with this technique, similar to those of transarterial embolization.[16]

Juvenile Nasal Angiofibroma, Glomus Tumors, and Other Vascular Head and Neck Tumors

The goal of treatment for Juvenile Nasal Angiofibroma (JNA), glomus tumors, and other vascular tumors of the head and neck is total resection and prevention of recurrence (Figs. 11.8–11.10). Embolization has been shown to make a significant contribution to the surgical outcome of these patients. Siniluoto et al.[17] compared a group of JNA patients embolized prior to surgery with a group without preoperative embolization. Embolization reduced perioperative blood loss from an average of 1,510 ml to 510 ml and eliminated the need for blood transfusion. Patients without preoperative embolization also demonstrated disease recurrence in significant numbers compared with those embolized prior to surgery. However, at least one paper[18] suggests an association between preoperative embolization and likelihood of recurrence, but this adverse experience is not generally thought to be commonplace and may have represented a referral bias. Juvenile angiofibromas tend to involve the distal branches of the internal maxillary artery, and concerns about anastomotic branches to the internal carotid artery and ophthalmic artery are similar to those described for embolization of epistaxis in that area. As the tumor enlarges inferiorly and posteriorly, it is common to see involvement of the accessory meningeal artery through its pharyngeal branches. Because these patients are all young males, typically in their early teens, there is a very high prevalence of enlargement of the mandibular artery from the petrous internal carotid artery supplying the tumor directly or indirectly. This represents a potential site of intratumoral or peritumoral anastomoses to the internal carotid artery, underscoring the need for extreme caution during particle embolization. When tumors have enlarged still further to a degree where skull-base invasion or intracranial invasion is evident on the MRI examination, supply from the inferolateral trunk to the tumor as well as from the middle meningeal artery and ophthalmic artery can be seen. As with glomus tumors, the possibility of arteriovenous shunting within a JNA should be considered when flow of blood and particles in contrast is very fast.[19] One might consider the safety of moving to larger particles in such circumstances to avoid pulmonary embolization with particles.

Preoperative embolization of glomus tumors of the head and neck has also been demonstrated to reduce perioperative blood loss, to shrink the tumor in preparation for surgery, and to improve the ease of surgical dissection.[20–22] Preoperative embolization reduces operative blood loss by a factor of 2 to 3, and the beneficial effects are most pronounced in patients with larger tumors where the need for perioperative transfusion is reduced by over 50%.[23] Procedural complications of a slightly different nature prevail during glomus tumor embolization compared with JNA embolization:

- Risk of reflux of particles into the internal carotid artery is a prominent concern when embolizing a carotid body tumor close to the bifurcation. One should be careful not to overestimate the importance or value of the embolization procedure in such instances. The benefits of blood loss at surgery, improved ease of dissection, etc., mentioned above do not warrant taking a risk involving passage of particles to the cerebral circulation. One should be satisfied with an imperfect angiographic appearance rather than risking the patient's welfare in an imprudent manner (Fig. 11.6).
- When embolizing glomus or other tumors at the skull base, anastomoses to the vertebral artery via the C1, C2, or C3 collaterals should be considered vigilantly at all times. Anastomoses from the ascending pharyngeal artery to the internal carotid artery along the back of the clivus or to the vertebral artery via the hypoglossal artery-to-C3 anastomosis must be monitored by superselective microcatheter digital runs before every embolization. Digital runs should be employed liberally as the embolization progresses to detect hemodynamic change in the vascular field. Anastomoses may emerge and grow to hemodynamic significance as the embolization progresses.

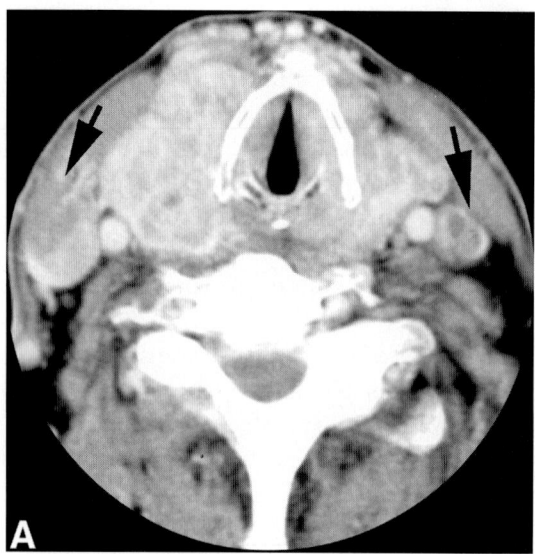
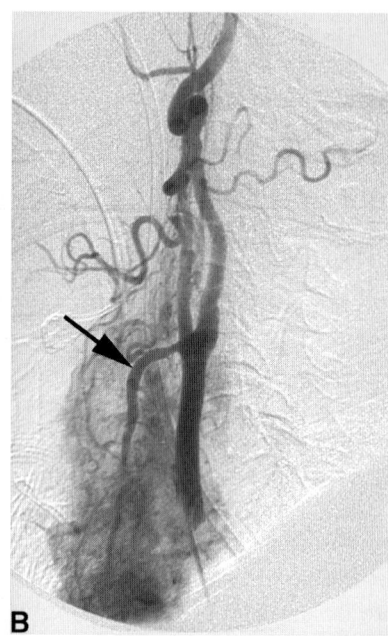

FIGURE 11.9 • *Metastatic Renal Cell Carcinoma.*
An 81-year-old patient with known metastatic renal cell carcinoma to the neck was referred for embolization prior to tracheotomy. A contrast-enhanced CT examination (A) shows tumor investing the thyroid gland and invading both internal jugular veins (arrows). The right common carotid artery injection (B, lateral view) shows the extraordinary extent of disease with marked enlargement of the superior thyroidal artery (arrow). The size of the tumor would probably mean that at least early in the embolization, there is little risk to the procedure. However, things are rarely so simple. Some specific considerations apply:
- Is there prominent shunting to the veins? If so, a long embolization session could amount to a significant embolic load to the lungs, and therefore larger particles might be considered from the outset.
- If the tumor swells from the effects of embolization, what provision has been made to protect the airway? This patient was already intubated for the procedure and was later extubated under direct visualization in the operating room.
- Other prominent routes of supply to this tumor, e.g., thyrocervical trunk, will need to be examined. The cervical contribution to the anterior spinal artery can sometimes arise from this trunk, prompting the need for caution.

- At the skull base, injury to the vasa nervorum of the facial nerve or other lower cranial nerves is a significant concern. This is a risk while embolizing the artery of the stylo-mastoid foramen (usually from the occipital artery or ascending pharyngeal artery). The hypoglossal nerve can be at risk while embolizing the hypoglossal branch of the neuromeningeal trunk (usually from the ascending pharyngeal artery).[24,25] This risk can be reduced by avoiding aggressive embolization with small particles ($<150 \mu m$) and by avoiding alcohol or cyanoacrylate embolic material in these locations.
- When arteriovenous flow seems particularly fast, always beware of the possibility of arteriovenous shunting within the tumor. Using smaller-range particles in such a circumstance could result in pulmonary complications.
- A minority of glomus tumors will demonstrate clinical evidence of catecholaminergic activity,

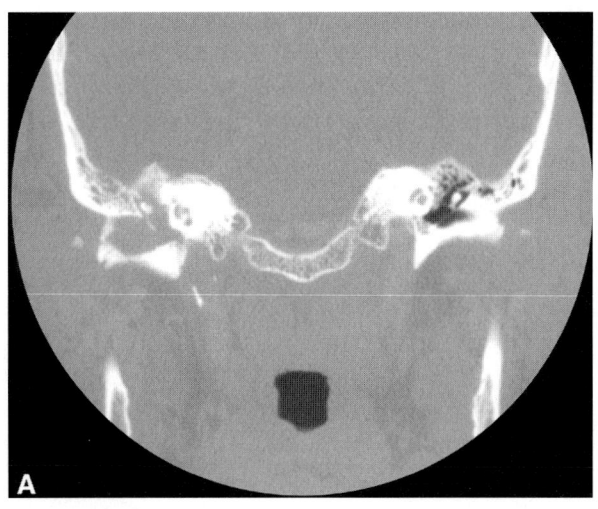 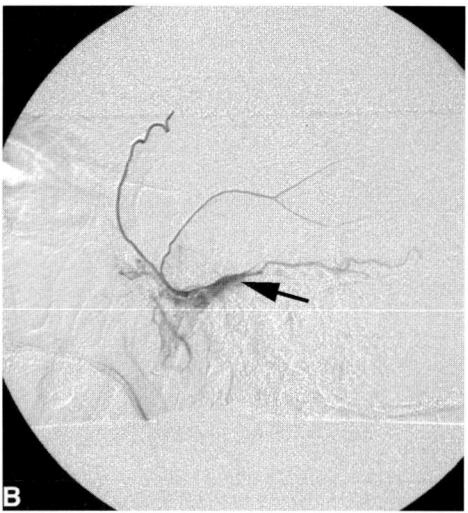

FIGURE 11.10 • *Glomus Tympanicum.*
A coronal CT scan (A) shows the characteristic appearance of expansion and bone permeation of a glomus tumor in the right ear. Among the branches involved with this tumor is the ipsilateral middle meningeal artery (B, lateral view). A proximal branch of the middle meningeal artery (arrow) supplies the tumor. This is probably the petrosal branch, which also supplies the vasa nervorum of the facial nerve. One should be careful, therefore, not to embolize this branch too aggressively.

and this may not be discovered until exacerbated by the embolization procedure.[26,27] This complication requires α-blocking agents and is a contraindication to more commonly used β-blocking agents.
- The appearance of a typical glomus tumor on MRI or angiography can be mimicked by the more aggressive adenocarcinoma of the endolymphatic sac or metastatic paraganglioma (Fig. 11.11, 10.17). Patients with these tumors also benefit from preoperative embolization using similar techniques.[28]

CHEMOTHERAPY

Developing chemotherapy protocols for treatment of brain tumors and of head and neck carcinomas suggest that interventional neuroradiology services may have a larger role to play in the future in these disease states.

Brain Tumors, the Blood-Brain Barrier, and Intraarterial Chemotherapy

The blood-brain barrier (BBB) represents a significant obstacle to effective chemotherapy for primary and metastatic tumors of the brain. When it was first described,[29] the BBB was conceptualized as an anatomic barrier of tight junctions at points of intercellular attachment in the endothelium.[30] More recent understanding of the BBB emphasizes the additional physiologic role of the basal lamina. The BBB is frequently abnormal within brain tumors, hence the enhancement of tumors seen on CT or MRI, but it remains sufficiently intact particularly at the proliferating edges of the tumor to prevent diffusion of chemotherapeutic agents in effective concentrations into the tumor. Factors influencing drug permeability of the BBB include:

- lipid solubility (expressed as the octanol/water partition coefficient)

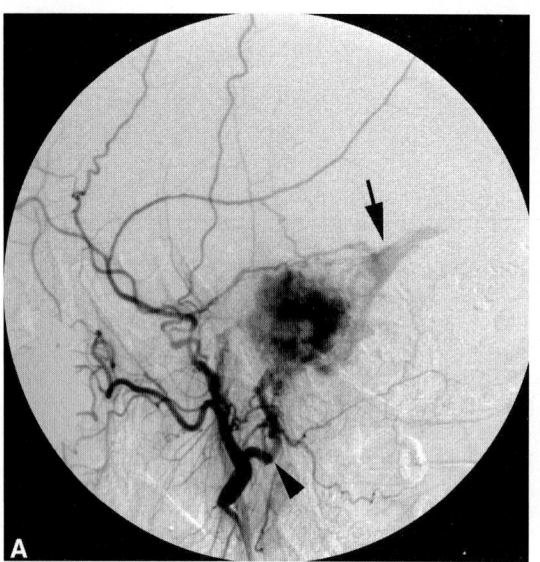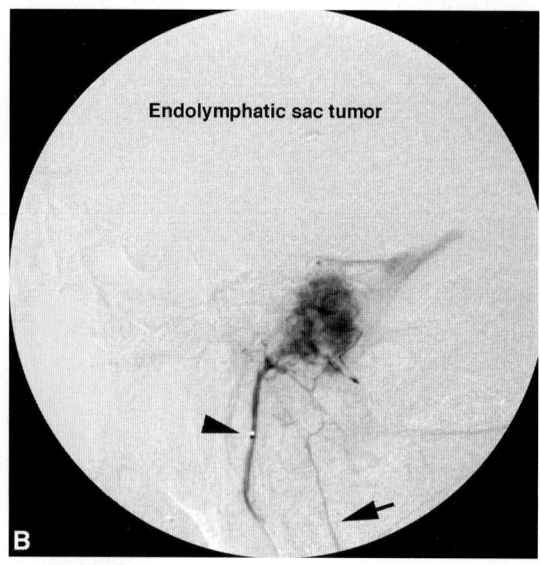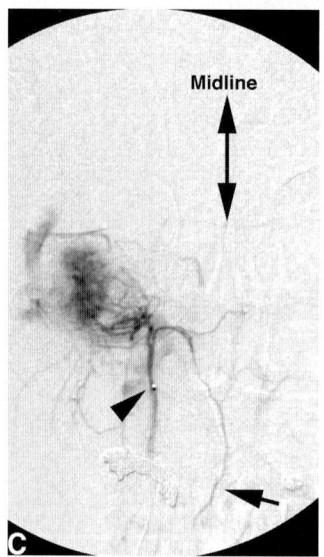

FIGURE 11.11 • *Endolymphatic Sac Tumor of the Petrous Bone.*
Among the many vascular tumors that can mimic the angiographic appearance of a glomus tumor is an endolymphatic sac tumor. This patient's tumor has invaded the sigmoid sinus (A, left external carotid artery, lateral view) with retrograde opacification of the transverse sinus (arrow). The posterior auricular artery is prominently involved (arrowhead). An injection in the hypoglossal branch of the right ascending pharyngeal artery (B, lateral view; C, AP view) shows the tumor again. The microcatheter tip is indicated by the arrowhead. The arrow indicates the dangerous C3 anastomosis to the ipsilateral vertebral artery, as described in Fig. 11.3.

- molecular mass,
- electric charge

Water-soluble agents with a molecular weight of 180 or more are effectively excluded by the BBB, while most chemotherapeutic agents have a mass between 120 and 1,200.[31] Stratagems to circumvent the impermeability of the BBB have attempted to harness the physiologic processes of transcytosis, endocytosis, or cell transport mechanisms mediated by specific receptors. For example, monoclonal antibodies attached to chemotherapeutic agents can be designed to bind to specific receptors on the BBB. An alternative stratagem is to induce a transient injury of the BBB and allow a window of opportunity during which chemotherapy agents can be delivered effectively. Osmotic disruption of the BBB with intraarterial infusions of mannitol, saline, urea, lithium chloride, ethylene glycol, or hyperosmolar contrast have had some in vitro and clinical success with treatment of CNS lymphoma, germ cell tumors, and primary neuroectodermal tumors.[32–35] The understanding of the "cell-shrinking" effect of the hyperosmolar challenge involved with these agents has given way to a realization that the disruption of the BBB may be related to triggering of protein kinase mediated intracellular ion fluxes and activation of nitric oxide production within the endothelium.

Osmotic disruption of the BBB is a nonfocal phenomenon and, in fact, has a more pronounced effect in normal areas of brain than in the area of tumor. A more focused insult to the BBB in the region of brain tumors has been made possible through the recognition that the BBB of tumors is deficient in γ-glutamyltranspeptidase. This enzyme is responsible for the inactivation of leukotrienes, an important mediator of the inflammatory response. Leukotriene C_4, adenosine, histamine, and particularly bradykinin are among the endogenous agents that have been recognized to induce transient permeability of the BBB of tumors.[36–39] Bradykinin and its synthetic analog, RMP-7, are currently the focus of research with emphasis on delivery of chemotherapeutic agents such as carboplatin and methotrexate to brain tumors.[40] Carboplatin is a second-generation cisplatin analogue with an improved safety profile for renal, gastrointestinal, and CNS toxicity. With a molecular mass of 371 daltons it is effectively excluded from tumor by an otherwise intact BBB.[41] RMP-7 is a synthetic derivative of bradykinin with a longer half-life and greater specificity for the bradykinin B_2 receptor. Bradykinin receptors are found on the endothelium of brain capillaries, and their activation is coupled to secondary intracellular messenger systems involving G-proteins, phosphoinositol turnover, and calcium fluxes. These messenger systems in turn induce nitric oxide-related cytoskeletal structural changes responsible for alterations in cellular junctional zones.[42] This results in a greater permeability of the BBB to chemotherapy agents.[43] The permeability effects of B_2 receptor activation are inhibited by administration of nitric oxide synthase inhibitors and corticosteroids.[44] On the other hand, the permeability effects of bradykinin and RMP-7 are enhanced in brain tissue that has been previously irradiated.[31,45] It is possible that a tachyphylaxis or receptor down-regulation occurs within 20–30 minutes of administration of RMP-7, resulting in attenuation of the permeability effect and restoration of a functionally intact BBB. This implies that the window of opportunity for delivery of chemotherapy may be very short and could limit the efficacy of this delivery stratagem.

Systemic administration of bradykinin or RMP-7 is limited by significant cardiovascular side effects. This limitation can be circumvented by intracarotid infusion of a lower dose of RMP-7 while achieving an adequate disruption of the BBB,[31,46] typically in conjunction with an intracarotid infusion of a chemotherapy agent. Intracarotid infusion of RMP-7 in animal studies has been shown with autoradiographic techniques to improve intratumoral delivery of smaller drug agents (100–300 daltons) by a factor of 2 to 4, while delivery of larger agents (up to 70,000 daltons) is improved by a factor of 10 to 12.[46,47] The relative specificity of the RMP-7 effect on tumor tissue makes this agent the focus of ongoing research into a clinical role in the treatment of brain tumors. Questions of safety and efficacy are not yet answered.

From the point of view of the interventional neuroradiologist, while clinically relevant doses of intracarotid RMP-7 seem safe so far, concerns about the safety of the invasive procedure and side effects of the chemotherapeutic agents deserve specific consideration. The global cognitive effect of such high-dose intraarterial chemotherapy is a major area of concern. Procedure-related technical concerns also apply. In the anterior circulation, positioning of the microcatheter for delivery of high doses of chemotherapy is important. It is necessary to avoid selective infusion of the drug into the ophthalmic artery, anterior choroidal artery, or posterior communicating artery, and therefore surveillance of the stability of the microcatheter during the case is important. Selective streaming of the chemotherapy agent into even the inferolateral trunk is potentially hazardous. In the limited experience gained already with these techniques, injuries to the retina[48,49] and paracavernous cranial nerves[50] have already been reported. A pulsatile pattern of drug delivery to avoid streaming effects may be necessary.[51,52]

In the posterior circulation selective infusions of cisplatin and carboplatin carry a significant risk of ototoxicity side effects with an incidence of high-frequency hearing loss of over 75%.[53–55] The ototoxic effects of these drugs are more severe with advancing age and with the concurrent use of furosemide as part of the aggressive hydration stratagem used in many such protocols. To diminish the ototoxic effects, microcatheter infusions of chemotherapeutic agents are made with the tip located above the level of the anterior inferior cerebellar arteries.[52] Additional potential for diminishing the toxic effects of cisplatin and carboplatin may lie with systemic administration of a neutralizing rescue agent. Sodium thiosulfate inactivates cisplatin and carboplatin with its thiol group that binds with the electrophilic platinum, forming an easily excreted inactive complex.[41,56,57]

Head and Neck Carcinoma

For advanced carcinoma of the head and neck intraarterial chemotherapy protocols offer the promise of greater therapeutic potential in the near future. While the BBB is not a concern in this location, stratagems similar to those described above for intraarterial chemotherapy for brain tumors are used. Local intraarterial delivery of high-dose chemotherapy to head and neck carcinomas with systemic administration of rescue agents in conjunction with radiotherapy can achieve complete tumor regression in otherwise inoperable cases.[58–60] The RADPLAT study, RTOG 96-15, involves a local intraarterial infusion of cisplatin 150 mg/m^2 in the external carotid artery in conjunction with an intravenous infusion of sodium thiosulfate 9 g/m^2 once per week for 4 weeks. Patients receive daily radiotherapy throughout. Renal and bone marrow toxicity effects are substantially reduced in this manner. Ototoxicity effects are still seen in approximately 25% of patients but are mostly confined to higher frequencies.[61] Patients with advanced local disease in this protocol have so far demonstrated a greater than 90% rate of complete regression of disease.[60,62] Procedural questions for the interventional neuroradiologist will relate to division of dose in the case of bilateral disease, which may require insertion of bilateral catheters. Additional caution may be necessary in the case of severe common carotid bifurcation atherosclerotic disease, which is common in this population of patients. A coaxial microcatheter for delivery of the drug can be used in this instance. Although there is evidence that delayed delivery of sodium thiosulfate can be effective for neutralizing cisplatin, the RTOG 96-15 protocol requires that the intravenous infusion of the rescue agent be commenced 3 minutes before the intraarterial infusion of cisplatin. As it is not rare to have intravenous lines malfunction unnoticed under the drapes of the angiography suite for considerable periods of time, an additional precaution that will bring peace of mind is placing an intravenous line in the femoral vein at the time of catheterization of the femoral artery. This line can be used for administration of the rescue agent and gives the neuroradiologist complete supervision of the drug protocol. Eye protection and skin protection for the angiography suite personnel are important when treating patients with highly concentrated chemotherapy agents of this nature. Specific handling protocols for spillage or disposal of exposed equipment are necessary.

References

1. DEAN BL, FLOM RA, WALLACE RC, KHAYATA MH, OBUCHOWSKI NA, HODAK JA, ZABRAMSKI JM, SPETZLER RF (1994) Efficacy of endovascular treatment of meningiomas: evaluation with matched samples. *AJNR* 15:1675–1680.
2. AHUJA A, GIBBONS KJ (1994) Endovascular therapy of central nervous system tumors. Review, 68 refs. *Neurosurg Clin North Am* 5:541–554.
3. TERADA T, KINOSHITA Y, YOKOTE H, TSUURA M, ITAKURA T, KOMAI N, NAKAMURA Y, TANAKA S, KURIYAMA T (1996) Preoperative embolization of meningiomas fed by ophthalmic branch arteries. *Surg Neurol* 45:161–166.
4. NELSON PK, SETTON A, CHOI IS, RANSOHOFF J, BERENSTEIN A (1994) Current status of interventional neuroradiology in the management of meningiomas. *Neurosurg Clin North Am* 5:235–259.
5. MORRIS PP (1999) Interventional neuroradiology in the treatment of brain tumors. *Neuroimag Clin N A* 9:767–778.
6. LASJAUNIAS P, BERENSTEIN A (1987) in *Surgical Neuroangiography*. Vol.2. Berlin-Heidelberg-New York: Springer-Verlag.
7. WAKHLOO AK, JUENGLING FD, VAN VELTHOVEN V, SCHUMACHER M, HENNIG J, SCHWECHHEIMER K (1993) Extended preoperative polyvinyl alcohol microembolization of intracranial meningiomas: assessment of two embolization techniques. *AJNR* 14:571–582.
8. GRAND C, BANK WO, BALERIAUX D, MATOS C, DEWITTE O, BROTCHI J, DELCOUR C (1993) Gadolinium-enhanced MR in the evaluation of preoperative meningioma embolization. *AJNR* 14:563–569.
9. BERETTA L, DELL'ACQUA A, GIORGI E, NAPOLITANO L, TOMMASINO C, RIGHI C, FERRARI DA PASSANO C, MOTTI E (1992) Complications during preoperative embolization in intracranial meningioma. *Minerva Anestesiologica* 58:111–114.
10. KALLMES DF, EVANS AJ, KAPTAIN GJ, MATHIS JM, JENSEN ME, JANE JA, DION JE (1997) Hemorrhagic complications in embolization of a meningioma: case report and review of the literature. *Neuroradiology* 39:877–880.
11. HAYASHI T, SHOJIMA K, UTSUNOMIYA H, MORITAKA K, HONDA E (1987) Subarachnoid hemorrhage after preoperative embolization of a cystic meningioma. *Surg Neurol* 27:295–300.
12. SUYAMA T, TAMAKI N, FUJIWARA K, HAMANO S, KIMURA M, MATSUMOTO S (1987) Peritumoral and intratumoral hemorrhage after gelatin sponge embolization of malignant meningioma: case report. *Neurosurgery* 21:944–946.
13. TERADA T, KINOSHITA Y, YOKOTE H, TSUURA M, ITAKURA T, KOMAI N, NAKAMURA Y, TANAKA S, KURIYAMA T (1996) Preoperative embolization of meningiomas fed by ophthalmic branch arteries. *Surg Neurol* 45:161–166.
14. TERADA T, NAKAI E, TSUMOTO T, ITAKURA T (1997) Iatrogenic arteriovenous fistula of the middle meningeal artery caused during embolization for meningioma—case report. *Neurologia Medico-Chirurgica* 37:677–680.
15. CASASCO A, HERBRETEAU D, HOUDART E, GEORGE B, HUY TB, DEFFRESNE D, MERLAND JJ (1994) Devascularization of craniofacial tumors by percutaneous tumor puncture. *AJNR* 15:1233–1239.
16. CASASCO A, HOUDART E, BIONDI A, JHAVERI HS, HERBRETEAU D, AYMARD A, MERLAND JJ (1999) Major complications of percutaneous embolization of skull-base tumors. *AJNR* 20:179–181.
17. SINILUOTO TM, LUOTONEN JP, TIKKAKOSKI TA, LEINONEN AS, JOKINEN KE (1993) Value of preoperative embolization in surgery for nasopharyngeal angiofibroma. *J Laryngol Otol* 107:514–521.
18. MCCOMBE A, LUND VJ, HOWARD DJ (1990) Recurrence in juvenile angiofibroma. *Rhinology* 28:97–102.
19. SCHROTH G, HALDEMANN AR, MARIANI L, REMONDA L, RAVEH J (1996) Preoperative embolization of paragangliomas and angiofibromas. Measurement of intratumoral arteriovenous shunts. *Arch Otolaryngol Head Neck Surg* 122:1320–1325.
20. YOUNG NM, WIET RJ, RUSSELL EJ, MONSELL EM (1988) Superselective embolization of glomus jugulare tumors. *Ann Otol Rhinol Laryngol* 97:613–620.
21. TRAN BA HUY P, DEFFRENNES D, BRETTE MD, GEORGE B, THUREL C, GELBERT F, MERLAND JJ, WASSEF M (1987) Tympanic and jugular paragangliomas. II. Angiographic, surgical and irradiation treatment. Results. Indications. Apropos of 25 cases. *Annales de Oto-Laryngologie et de Chirurgie Cervico-Faciale* 104:489–499.
22. FRUHWIRTH J, KOCH G, KLEIN GE (1996) Preoperative angiographic embolization of carotid glomus tumors. A method for improving operability. *HNO* 44:510–513.
23. MURPHY TP, BRACKMANN DE (1989) Effects of preoperative embolization on glomus jugulare tumors. *Laryngoscope* 99:1244–1247.
24. HERDMAN RC, GILLESPIE JE, RAMSDEN RT (1993) Facial palsy after glomus tumour embolization. *J Laryngol Otol* 107:963–966.
25. MARANGOS N, SCHUMACHER M (1999) Facial palsy after glomus jugulare tumour embolization. *J Laryngol Otol* 113:268–270.
26. MATISHAK MZ, SYMON L, CHEESEMAN A, PAMPHLETT R (1987) Catecholamine-secreting paragangliomas of the base of the skull. Report of two cases. *J Neurosurg* 66:604–608.
27. KREMER R, MICHEL RP, POSNER B, WANG NS, LAFOND GP, CRAWHALL JC (1989) Catecholamine-secreting paraganglioma of glomus jugulare region. *Am J Med Sci* 297:46–48.
28. MUKHERJI SK, CASTILLO M (1996) Adenocarcinoma of the endolymphatic sac: imaging features and preoperative embolization. *Neuroradiology* 38:179–180.
29. EHRLICH P (1906) *Collected Studies in Immunity*. New York: John Wiley, 567–595.
30. RAPOPORT SI, ROBINSON PJ (1986) Tight-junctional modifi-

cation as the basis of osmotic opening of the blood-brain barrier. *Ann N Y Acad Sci* 481:250–267.
31. Kroll RA, Neuwelt EA (1998) Outwitting the blood-brain barrier for therapeutic purposes: osmotic opening and other means. *Neurosurgery* 42:1083–1099.
32. McAllister LD, Doolittle ND, Guastadisegni PE, Kraemer DF, Lacy CA, Crossen JR, Neuwelt EA (2000) Cognitive outcomes and longterm followup results after enhanced chemotherapy delivery for primary central nervous system lymphoma. *Neurosurgery* 46:51–61.
33. Elliott PJ, Hayward NJ, Huff MR, Nagle TL, Black KL, Bartus RT (1996) Unlocking the blood-brain barrier: a role for RMP-7 in brain tumor therapy. *Experimental Neurol* 141:214–224.
34. Dahlborg SA, Henner WD, Crossen JR, Tableman M, Petrillo A, Braziel R, Neuwelt EA (1996) Non-AIDS primary CNS lymphoma: first example of a durable response in a primary brain tumor using enhanced chemotherapy delivery without cognitive loss and without radiotherapy. *Cancer J Sci Am* 2:166–174.
35. Dahlborg SA, Petrillo A, Crossen JR, Roman-Goldstein S, Doolittle ND, Fuller KH, Neuwelt EA (1998) The potential for complete and durable response in non-glial primary brain tumors in children and young adults with enhanced chemotherapy delivery. *Cancer J Sci Am* 4:110–124.
36. Black KL, Baba T, Pardridge WM (1994) Enzymatic barrier protects brain capillaries from leukotriene C4. *J Neurosurg* 81:745–751.
37. Black KL, King WA, Ikezake K (1990) Selective opening of the blood-brain barrier by intracarotid infusion of leukotriene C4. *J Neurosurg* 72:912–916.
38. Inamura T, Black KL (1994) Bradykinin selectively opens blood-tumor barrier in experimental brain tumors. *J Cereb Blood Flow Metabol* 14:862–870.
39. Inamura T, Nomura T, Ikezaki K, Fukui M, Pollinger G, Black KL (1994) Intracarotid histamine infusion increases blood tumor permeability in RG2 glioma. *Neurol Res* 16:125–128.
40. Inamura T, Nomura T, Bartus RT, Black KL (1994) Intracarotid infusion of RMP-7, a bradykinin analog: a method for selective drug delivery to brain tumors. *J Neurosurg* 81:752–758.
41. Elferink F, van der Vijgh WJ, Klein I, Pinedo HM (1986) Interaction of cisplatin and carboplatin with sodium thiosulfate: reaction rates and protein binding. *Clin Chem* 32:641–645.
42. Nakano S, Matsukado K, Black KL (1996) Increased brain tumor microvessel permeability after intracarotid bradykinin infusion is mediated by nitric oxide. *Cancer Res* 56:4027–4031.
43. Matsukado K, Inamura T, Nakano S, Fukui M, Bartus RT, Black KL (1996) Enhanced tumor uptake of carboplatin and survival in glioma-bearing rats by intracarotid infusion of bradykinin analog, RMP-7. *Neurosurgery* 39:125–133.

44. Matsukado K, Nakano S, Bartus RT, Black KL (1997) Steroids decrease uptake of carboplatin in rat gliomas—uptake improved by intracarotid infusion of bradykinin analog, RMP-7. *J Neuro-Oncol* 34:131–138.
45. Fike JR, Gobbel GT, Mesiwala AH, Shin HJ, Nakagawa M, Lamborn KR, Seihan TM, Elliott PJ (1998) Cerebrovascular effect of the bradykinin analog RMP-7 in normal and irradiated dog brain. *J Neuro-Oncol* 37:199–215.
46. Riley MG, Kim NN, Watson V, Gobin YP, LeBel CP, Black KL, Bartus RT (1998) Intra-arterial administration of carboplatin and the blood brain barrier permeabilizing agent, RMP-7: a toxicologic evaluation in swine. *J Neuro-Oncol* 36:167–178.
47. Koga H, Inamura T, Ikezaki K, Nomura T, Samoto K, Fujui M (1996) Increased delivery of a new cisplatin analogue (254-S) in a rat brain tumor by intracarotid infusion of bradykinin. *Neurol Res* 18:244–247.
48. Wu HM, Lee AG, Lehane DE, Chi TL, Lewis RA (1997) Ocular and orbital complications of intraarterial cisplatin. A case report. *J Neuro-Ophthalmol* 17:195–198.
49. Millay RH, Klein ML, Shults WT, Dahlborg SA, Neuwelt EA (1986) Maculopathy associated with combination chemotherapy and osmotic opening of the blood-brain barrier. *Am J Ophthalmol* 102:626–632.
50. Alderson LM, Noonan PT, Choi IS, Henson JW (1996) Regional subacute cranial neuropathies following internal carotid cisplatin infusion. *Neurology* 47:1088–1090.
51. Cloughesy TF, Black KL, Gobin YP, Farahani K, Nelson G, Villablanca P, Kabbinavar F, Vineula F, Wortel CH (1999) Intra-arterial Cereport (RMP-7) and carboplatin: a dose escalation study for recurrent malignant gliomas. *Neurosurgery* 44:270–278.
52. Cloughesy TF, Gobin YP, Black KL, Vinuela F, Taft F, Kadkhoda B, Kanninavar F (1997) Intra-arterial carboplatin chemotherapy for brain tumors: a dose escalation study based on cerebral blood flow. *J Neuro-Oncol* 35:121–131.
53. Assietti R, Olson JJ (1996) Intra-arterial cisplatin in malignant brain tumors: incidence and severity of otic toxicity. *J Neuro-Oncol* 27:251–258.
54. Williams PC, Henner WD, Roman-Goldstein S, Dahlborg SA, Brummett RE, Tableman M, Dana BW, Neuwelt EA (1995) Toxicity and efficacy of carboplatin and etoposide in conjunction with disruption of the blood-brain tumor barrier in the treatment of intracranial neoplasms. *Neurosurgery* 37:17–27.
55. Wetmore SJ, Koike KJ, Bloomfield SM (1997) Profound hearing loss from intravertebral artery cisplatin. *Otolaryngol Head Neck Surg* 116:234–237.
56. Neuwelt EA, Brummett RE, Remsen LG, Kroll RA, Pagel MA, McCormick CI, Guitjens S, Muldoon LL (1996) In vitro and animal studies of sodium thiosulfate as a potential chemoprotectant against carboplatin-induced ototoxicity. *Cancer Res* 56:706–709.
57. Pfeifle CE, Howell SB, Felthouse RD, Woliver TB, Andrews

PA, MARKMAN M, MURPHY MP (1985) High-dose cisplatin with sodium thiosulfate protection. *J Clin Oncol* 3:237–244.

58. ROBBINS KT, STORNIOLO AM, KERBER C, SEAGREN S, BERSON A, HOWELL SB (1992) Rapid superselective high-dose cisplatin infusion for advanced head and neck malignancies. *Head Neck* 14:364–371.

59. LOS G, BLOMMAERT FA, BARTON R, HEATH DD, DEN ENGELSE L, HANCHETT C, VICARIO D, WEISMAN R, ROBBINS KT, HOWELL SB (1995) Selective intra-arterial infusion of high-dose cisplatin in patients with advanced head and neck cancer results in high tumor platinum concentrations and cisplatin-DNA adduct formation. *Cancer Chemother Pharmacol* 37:150–154.

60. KERBER CW, WONG WH, HOWELL SB, HANCHETT K, ROBBINS KT (1998) An organ-preserving selective arterial chemotherapy strategy for head and neck cancer. *AJNR* 19:935–941.

61. MADASU R, RUCKENSTEIN MJ, LEAKE F, STEERE E, ROBBINS KT (1997) Ototoxic effects of supradose cisplatin with sodium thiosulfate neutralization in patients with head and neck cancer. *Arch Otolaryngol Head Neck Surg* 123:978–981.

62. WEISMAN RA, CHRISTEN RD, JONES VE, KERBER CW, SEAGREN SL, ORLOFF LA, GLASSMEYER SL, HOWELL SB, ROBBINS KT (1998) Observations on control of N2 and N3 neck disease in squamous cell carcinoma of the head and neck by intraarterial chemoradiation. *Laryngoscope* 108:800–805.

Chapter 12

Trauma and Hemorrhage

THE TECHNIQUES of interventional neuroradiology can be used to control a variety of vascular injuries in the head and neck that are difficult to control through other means.

Triage

When called about a patient in whom control of hemorrhage or potential hemorrhage is the principal concern, there are four initial points of concern to ask about the patient in triage of the procedure:

1. *What is the hemodynamic state of the patient?* How stable are the patient's vital signs, and what is the hematocrit? Has the patient been cross-matched at the blood-bank and are units of blood available for transfusion if further bleeding occurs? Most specifically, is this an absolute emergency situation for which a room must be cleared at once, or can the procedure be worked into the schedule of the day in a more orderly fashion?
2. *Does the site of bleeding or potential bleeding affect the airway?* If so, intubation of the patient by an anesthesia team for protection of the airway is of paramount importance. A supine, sedated patient bleeding even a small amount into the nasopharynx or oropharynx is at high risk for aspiration (Fig. 12.1).
3. *What precisely is known clinically about the side and exact site of hemorrhage?* Frequently, patients who are actively bleeding from the head and neck will be brought to the angiography suite with packing or other tamponading material in place. This will hinder the ease with which sites of hemorrhage can be seen angiographically. It will help enormously in expediting the identification of the site of hemorrhage if communication is established with the clinical team who first saw the hemorrhage. Metallic markers or other markers can be placed externally on the patient over the relevant site of hemorrhage to focus the angiographic search.
4. *Who is available for consent for the procedure?*

General Principles

The techniques and devices used for control of bleeding are the same as for other procedures described in other chapters, but with reference to the procedure itself in this instance the following general principles apply:

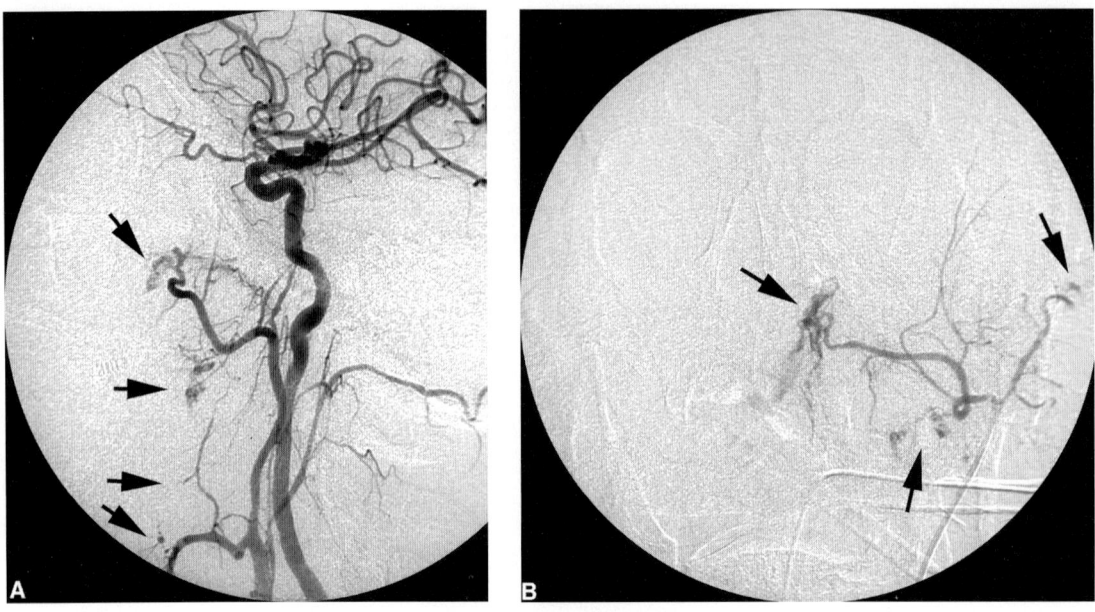

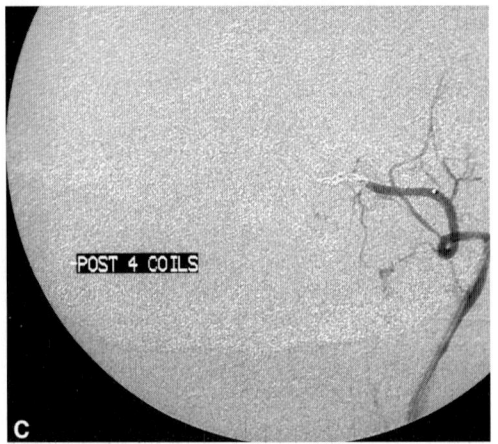

FIGURE 12.1 • *Severe External Carotid Artery Bleeding.*
The appearance of angiographic extravasation of contrast is often understated compared with the clinical state of the patient. This 82-year-old male patient involved in an automobile accident was intubated at the scene, and his facial bleeding was extensively packed and tamponaded by external and oral application of bandaging. Despite these measures his bleeding continued to be fulminant. In such a case as this, all haste is necessary to prepare the room, table, etc., while the patient is en route from the emergency room. The left external carotid angiogram (A, lateral view) shows multiple sites of extravasation from the distal and proximal internal maxillary artery, the ascending palatine artery, and the facial artery. The internal carotid artery is not injured.

The internal maxillary artery was catheterized with a microcatheter (B, AP view) but PVA particles of 500–750 μm continued to extravasate freely from the distal site of hemorrhage. The internal maxillary artery was therefore occluded with four small fibered coils advanced through the microcatheter with a coil-pusher (C, AP view), and the remainder of the external carotid bleeders were occluded with Gelfoam and PVA. The patient had visceral injuries and the trauma team was waiting to take the patient to the operating room for an emergency laparotomy. While speed and some cutting of corners are necessary in such circumstances, one should be very careful when working close to the common carotid bifurcation. Gelfoam pledgets, in particular, can become lodged in the microcatheter, requiring additional force to dislodge them. The possibility of reflux to the internal carotid artery is ever present in such circumstances.

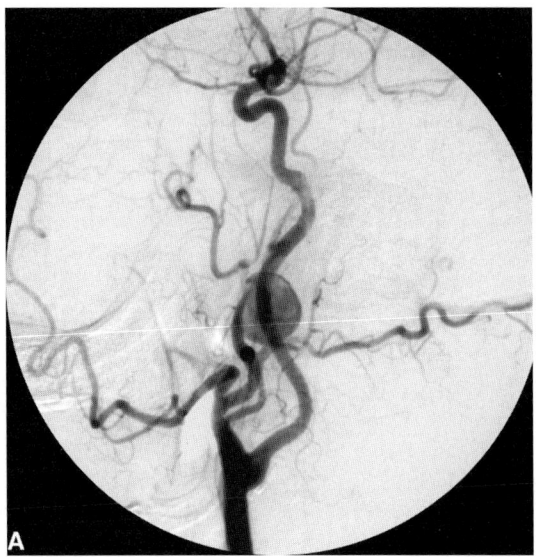
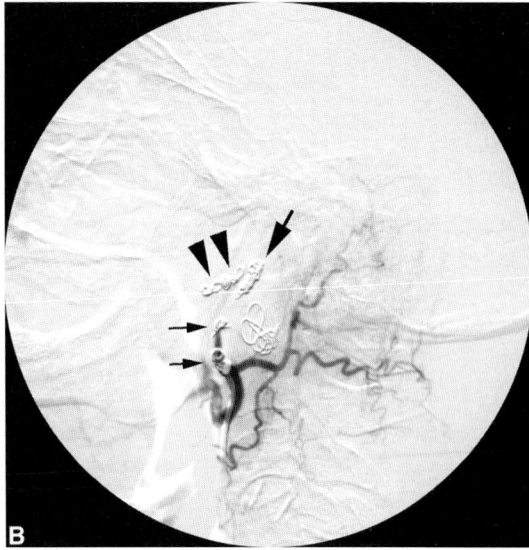

FIGURE 12.2 • *External Carotid Artery Pseudoaneurysm.*
Blunt injury to the right side of the face was followed by severe swelling in this 45-year-old patient. A CT (not shown) demonstrated an enhancing pseudoaneurysm confirmed by angiography (A, lateral view). The primary concern on the first angiogram is the state of the internal carotid artery. In this patient the injury is confined to the distal external carotid artery below the origin of the superficial temporal artery.

A pseudoaneurysm such as this is best treated by trapping with coils. Fortunately a wire could be steered past the pseudoaneurysm and subsequently used to guide a microcatheter. However, there was not sufficient intact artery distal to the pseudoaneurysm below the superficial temporal artery to hold a coil, and the first coil placed prolapsed into the pseudoaneurysm (B, lateral view). Therefore, the superficial temporal artery (large arrow) and internal maxillary artery (double arrowheads) were each selected in turn and occluded proximally with coils. Then the external carotid artery proximal to the pseudoaneurysm was occluded with fibered coils (small arrows), leaving the origin of the posterior auricular artery intact. No path of reconstitution of the pseudoaneurysm remains.

- Patients who have had multiple transfusions for hemorrhage may be coagulopathic. This can thwart one's efforts to achieve hemostasis in the external carotid artery circulation as described below and can also be the source of problems with groin closure. A single-wall needle technique may be worth considering at the outset of the procedure with the anticipation of using an arteriotomy closure device.
- For patients who are potentially or actually hemodynamically unstable, a femoral vein 5Fr or 6Fr sheath can be placed easily and quickly at the beginning of the case and can be used for emergency resuscitation should the occasion arise.

- Of foremost importance is expeditious identification of the site of hemorrhage. In a hemodynamically at-risk patient, immediate focus should be placed on stopping the bleeding. Techniques such as wedging the introducer catheter proximally in the damaged vessel or external tamponade of the bleeding site with a forceps and tightly rolled gauze should not be overlooked while endovascular devices are in preparation. In extreme circumstances, one should not hesitate to subordinate concern for thromboembolic complications to the more imminent risk of exsanguination. Therefore, control of hemorrhage with a balloon catheter inflated within the vessel may

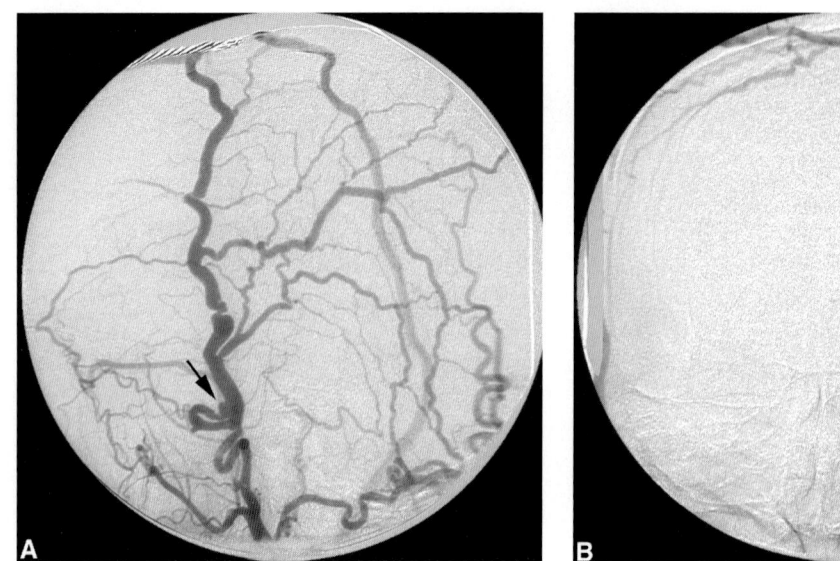

FIGURE 12.3 • *Blunt Injury to the Head with Arteriovenous Fistula. Venous Thrombosis Following Closure of a Fistula.*
A young adult experienced mild swelling of the left temple and experienced a loud bruit following a blow to the head from a baseball. Angiography (A, lateral view, left external carotid artery) demonstrates a laceration of the left superficial temporal artery with a fistula to the adjacent scalp veins (arrow). The AP view (B) also demonstrates the extraordinary distension of the scalp veins distal to the fistula extending cephalad.

The fistula was closed in a standard fashion. A microcatheter was steered through the fistula and fibered coils were laid densely on the venous side of the fistula until the packing process backed into the arterial side (C, lateral view). Because the flow was so great, more coils were necessary then might appear intuitively obvious (arrows).

A minor complication in this patient illustrates the potential for serious postocclusion problems when a high-flow fistula or AVM is closed abruptly, leaving a patulous venous field behind. The patient was discharged home the evening of the procedure, but was seen 2 days later complaining of severe, painless swelling over the left side of his head. The left temple was alarmingly distended, but soft to the touch. The edema extended over his brow closing the left eye. No clinical evidence of infection or recurrence of the fistula was present. A CT examination (D) demonstrated the probable cause of his condition to be thrombosis of an extensive field of scalp veins (arrowhead), which had presumably thrombosed spontaneously following the sudden therapeutic occlusion. His condition resolved uneventfully over some days with antiinflammatory agents and application of warm compresses.

The same phenomenon has been described with a less innocuous impact in similar conditions in the intracranial circulation. Sudden therapeutic closure of carotid cavernous fistulas or brain arteriovenous malformations leaves open the possibility of acute thrombosis of the distended venous field. This can result in venous infarctions of the brain or visual loss due to thrombosis of the superior ophthalmic vein. Additionally, back-thrombosis of a distended arterial feeder can threaten a proximal arterial branch. Prophylactic anticoagulation of patients with sudden closure of a high-flow fistula is probably a precaution best used liberally to prevent this occasional complication.

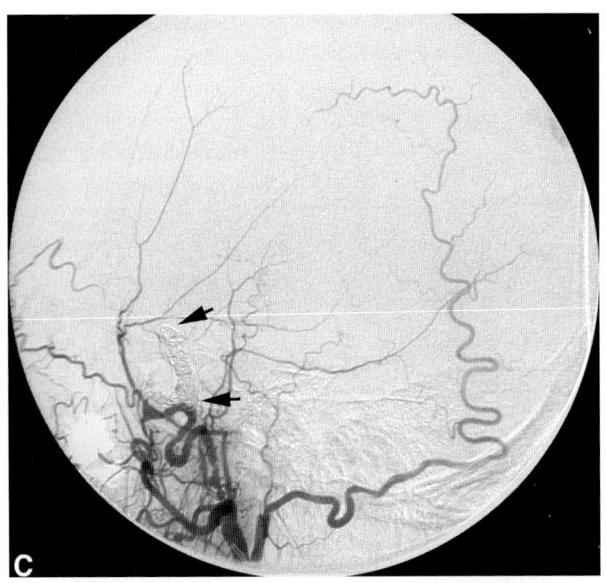

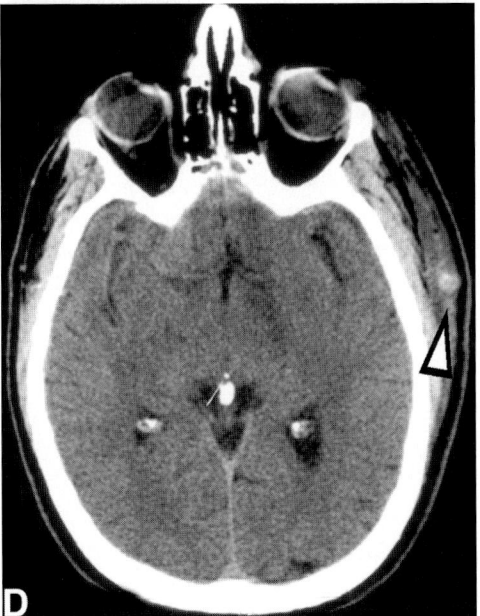

- be necessary in dire circumstances, while other devices are being prepared or while the patient is being transferred to the operating room for surgical control.
- When the site of hemorrhage is unknown, an early focus of concern during the procedure is identifying whether or not the cerebral vessels, internal carotid artery and vertebral artery, are involved, or if the hemorrhage is coming from an external carotid artery source. If the bleeding is from the internal carotid artery or vertebral artery, all therapeutic alternatives and risks should be at least considered before attempting an endovascular sacrifice of the vessel. Under emergency conditions, an angiographic evaluation of the state of collateral flow to the distal ter-

ritory must be made as quickly as possible and the vessel then occluded with coils or balloons.

- It is ironic how surprisingly difficult it is to stop blood flow when one needs to do so. The external carotid artery has a remarkable capacity for providing distal collateral flow through innumerable small vessels. Therefore, for any proximal or mid-external carotid artery laceration or site of bleeding, proximal and distal control of the bleeding site is almost always necessary (Fig. 12.2). This may mean catheterizing the vessel distal to the trauma site and starting the occlusion procedure distally, or it may mean controlling the collateral routes of flow by subsequent catheterization of other branches.
- Furthermore, while a single micro-coil in the wrong location during an intracranial aneurysm embolization can cause no end of trouble, a single microcoil in a bleeding external carotid branch can be surprisingly ineffective at achieving vessel closure (Fig. 12.3). In other words, it usually requires many more 0.018-in fibered micro-coils than one might initially anticipate to close a medium size external carotid artery branch. If the patient is hemodynamically unstable, one should have a low threshold for resorting to 0.035-in or 0.038-in coils placed via the main catheter to achieve immediate vessel closure.

External Carotid Artery Injuries

A variety of postsurgical or posttraumatic external carotid artery injuries may come to the attention of the interventional neuroradiology service. As described above, advance communication about the precise site of hemorrhage can focus one's search for the injured vessel. Serious injuries are frequently very small and innocuous appearing on the angiogram unless active extravasation is present (Fig. 12.4). Even if a bleeding site is not identified for sure, with advance clinical information an educated guess can be made, and prophylactic embolization of the most likely sites conducted.

FIGURE 12.4 • *Delayed Rebleeding from an Arterial Laceration.*

Delayed or secondary bleeding is a common phenomenon presenting within 2 weeks of the original trauma or surgery. It may be related to secondary infection, breakdown of granulation tissue, or use of nonsteroidal pain medications. In this patient presenting with severe facial bleeding following an assault, the right common carotid artery injection (A, lateral view) shows some spasm of the internal carotid artery (arrowheads) and complete occlusion of the external carotid artery distal to the linguo-facial trunk and ascending pharyngeal artery. A suspicious irregularity of the proximal facial artery (arrow) was seen and an offer made to embolize the vessel with coils. The bleeding was controlled clinically by that time, and the managing surgical team declined treatment of the injured facial artery.

Two weeks later, the patient presented anew with a pulsatile mass of the right oropharynx, shown by CT (B, arrowhead) to be a partially enhancing pseudoaneurysm. A right common carotid angiogram (C, lateral view) shows the pseudoaneurysm that has arisen at the previously identified irregularity of the facial artery (arrow). The external carotid artery continues to be occluded, and the distal internal maxillary artery is reconstituted via the buccal artery (labeled b). The previously seen irregularity of the internal carotid artery has resolved.

After coil embolization with trapping of the facial artery pseudoaneurysm and preservation of the lingual artery (D, lateral view, right external carotid artery), the pattern of reconstitution of the internal maxillary artery is changed due to elimination of the buccal artery as an effective route of reconstitution. The ascending pharyngeal artery (labeled asc.ph.) through the superior branch of the pharyngeal trunk reconstitutes the internal maxillary artery via the pterygovaginal artery (labeled pt.vag.).

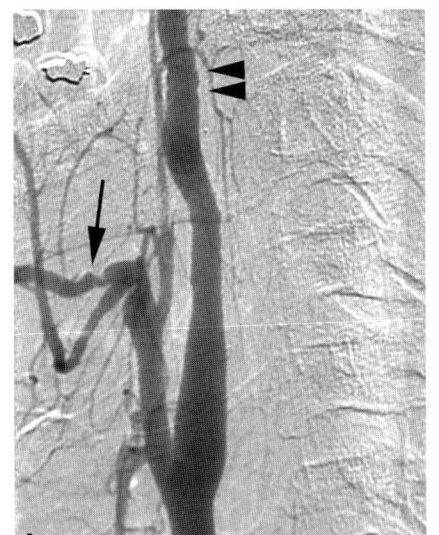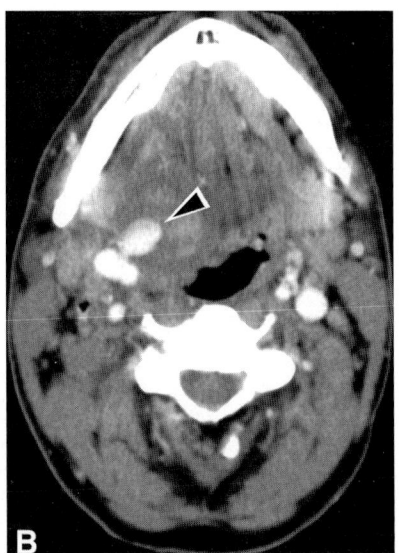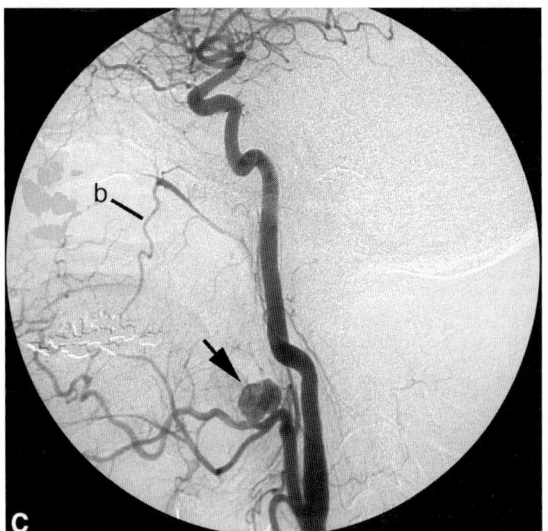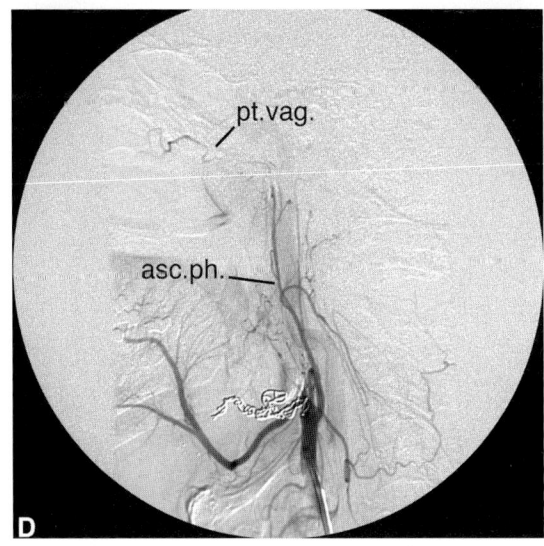

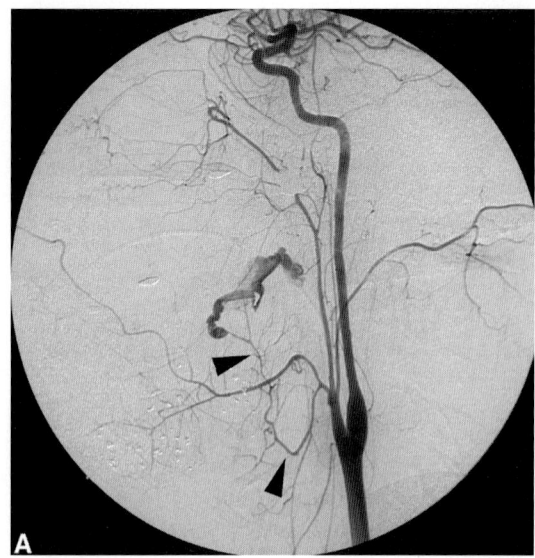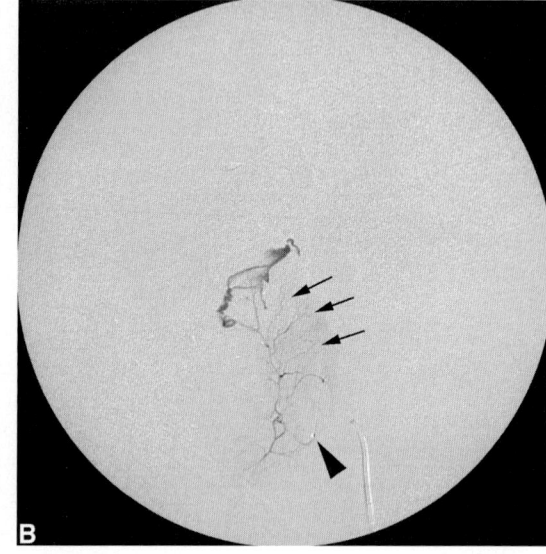

FIGURE 12.5 • *Gunshot Wound to the Lingual Artery.*
This intubated patient demonstrates the importance of protecting the airway in patients with bleeding into the mouth, nose, or pharynx. A gunshot wound traverses the tongue (A, lateral view, left common carotid artery) with bullet fragments creating subtraction artifact in the floor of the mouth and over the internal maxillary artery. The internal carotid artery is stretched and mildly spastic, but shows no injury. Free extravasation into the oropharynx from the lingual artery (arrowheads) is seen.

The lingual and facial arteries can be very difficult to catheterize distally, but success can often be achieved by selecting them proximally with a microwire, and then using the microcatheter-wire combination to lodge the introducer catheter into the artery ostium. Wedging the catheter initially with a standard guide-wire will often induce spasm and prevent the microcatheter from exiting the catheter. In this case the bleeding site (B, microcatheter injection into lingual artery lateral view) could not be reached and the bleeder was embolized from a point a little beyond the arrowhead. PVA particles of 350–500 μm in dilute suspension were used successfully followed by a pledget of Gelfoam. One must be careful in the lingual artery due to the terminal nature of the ranine branches (arrows), where aggressive embolization with small particles could induce mucosal necrosis.

For extreme distal small-vessel injuries, particle embolization with PVA or Gelfoam sponge is conducted using a microcatheter (Fig. 12.5). For more proximal injuries, fibered coils are preferable with a view toward gaining proximal and distal control. Close to the carotid bifurcation there is a risk of reflux of particulate materials into the internal carotid artery. Therefore coils are always preferred when reflux is a risk. Acrylate materials can be used in the external carotid artery for endovascular control of bleeding or percutaneous closure of pseudoaneurysms. However, because of the risk of end-tissue necrosis, these applications are uncommon.

POST-TONSILLECTOMY BLEEDING

Removal of the adenoids and tonsils is one of the most commonly performed childhood surgeries, with an estimated 286,000 such procedures performed per year in the United States.[1] One of the most serious complications following tonsillectomy and adenoidectomy is recurrent hemorrhage with an incidence of approximately 2% to 3%.[2–4] Post-tonsillectomy hemorrhage accounts for the majority of fatalities following tonsillectomy and accounts for most causes of protracted post-tonsillectomy hospitalizations (Figs. 12.6, 12.7). Primary

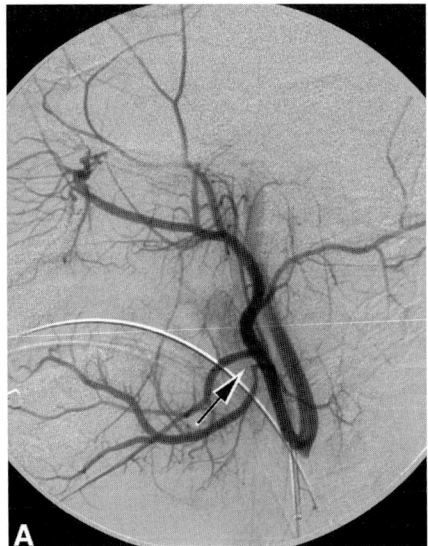 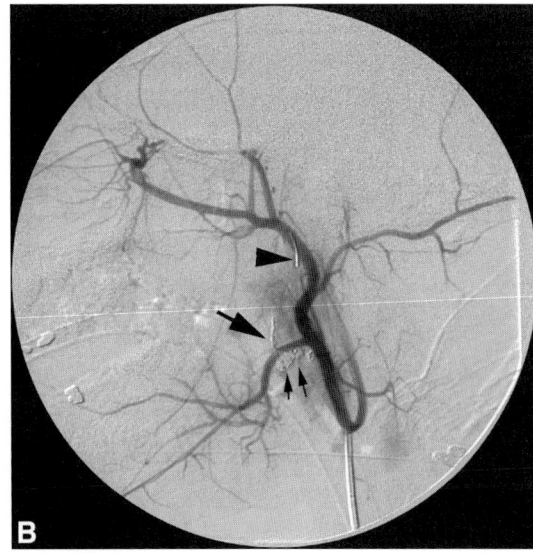

FIGURE 12.6 • *Post-Tonsillectomy Bleeding in a Child I.*
An 8-year-old girl suffered recurrent heavy bleeding over a 3-day period following tonsillectomy and adenoidectomy. Despite repeated transfusions, her hematocrit at the time of transfer was 25%. After intubation an external carotid angiogram (A, lateral view) shows an irregularity of the proximal lingual artery, but no evidence of pseudoaneurysm or extravasation.

Because the identified irregularity was very close to the external carotid artery trunk, it was thought possible that a coil occlusion of that segment might spill back into the external carotid artery trunk, blocking access to more distal sites of bleeding. A suspiciously truncated branch of the ascending pharyngeal artery was therefore embolized first with straight coils (arrowhead in B, external carotid artery angiogram postembolization), as was the ascending palatine branch of the facial artery (arrow). However, upon selecting the lingual artery, the force of a microcatheter injection was sufficient to induce free extravasation of contrast, confirming this as the certain site of bleeding. The microcatheter tip was seen to be in an extravascular site, but was not retracted. Curved coils were deposited outside the artery and packed back into the arterial lumen to eliminate the bleeding. Using 3-mm curved coils (B, postembolization, small arrows), it was possible to preserve the external carotid artery trunk. Reconstitution of the lingual artery from the contralateral side is commonly seen, although in this patient robust reconstitution distal to the coils is present by virtue of prompt anastomoses from the proximal facial artery.

bleeding occurring within 24 hours of surgery is thought to be related to surgical technique, vessel injury, or other reasons for difficulties with hemostasis such as coagulopathy or von Willebrand's disease.[5] Secondary bleeding occurring after 24 hours is thought most likely related to breakdown of the surgical field from factors such as infection, old age, chronic tonsillitis, or use of nonsteroidal anti-inflammatory drugs.[4,6] It typically presents 5–10 days following surgery, and the degree of bleeding can be quite serious.

Surgical measures to control the bleeding include clot removal and direct ligation of the arterial bleeders, electrocautery, application of silver nitrate, infiltration with vasoconstrictive drugs, or ligation of the external carotid artery or its branches.[7,8] Endovascular treatment is also an option for control of post-tonsillectomy bleeding or pseudoaneurysms,[9,10] particularly when primary measures have failed.

After excluding an injury of the internal carotid artery as the foremost angiographic priority, there are a typical few important branches of the exter-

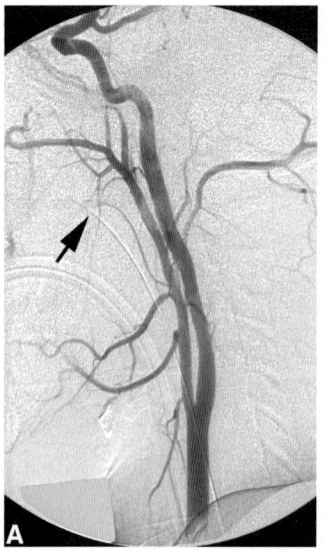
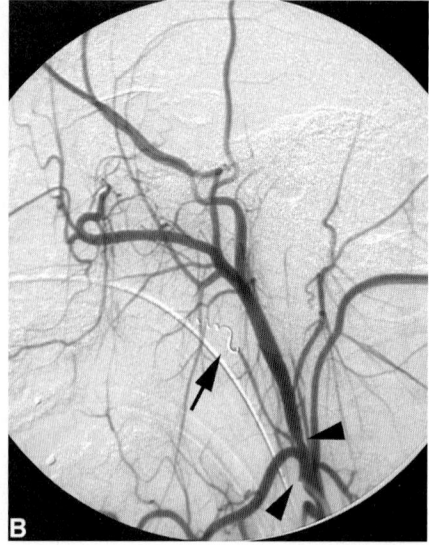

FIGURE 12.7 • *Post-Tonsillectomy Bleeding in a Child II.*
In this child presenting following tonsillectomy with a similar clinical sequence of events described for Fig. 12.6, the bleeding site was identified as the ascending palatine artery. A common carotid injection (A, lateral view) shows the internal carotid artery to be intact. A truncation of the ascending palatine artery (arrow) arising from the external carotid artery is noted. Extravasation was seen on a microcatheter injection, and the vessel was embolized with two curved coils (arrows in B, external carotid artery injection, lateral view). Notice how the minimal catheter-related spasm (arrowheads in B) does not appear significantly different from the evidence of hemorrhage sites illustrated in Figs. 12.4A or 12.6A, underscoring the need for a common carotid angiogram before selecting the external carotid branches.

nal carotid artery that can be involved with post-tonsillectomy hemorrhage (Fig. 12.8).

- The ascending palatine artery from the facial artery or directly from the external carotid artery trunk is frequently involved along the inferior aspect of the surgical bed.
- Along the superior aspect of the bed the lesser descending palatine artery from the internal maxillary artery is sometimes involved, too.
- The ascending pharyngeal artery must also be evaluated. The pharyngeal trunk from the ascending pharyngeal artery can give a superior pharyngeal branch to the nasopharynx, anastomosing there with the accessory meningeal artery. It can also send a collateral laceral branch intracranially toward the inferolateral trunk of the internal carotid artery, raising the risk of embolization of the intracranial vessels. The middle and inferior pharyngeal branches may send branches to the faucial pillars and be involved with post-tonsillectomy bleeding.
- Larger proximal branches such as the lingual artery or the external carotid artery itself may be injured.[11,12]
- The possibility of an injury to the internal carotid artery should always be evaluated at the beginning of the case before proceeding to the external carotid artery.[13] A common carotid injection at the beginning will be helpful for this. Furthermore, an initial common carotid injection will help to avoid the situation of misinterpreting wire-related spasm in the proximal external carotid artery as posttraumatic change. Vasospasm induced by wire manipulation can confound one's interpretation of the angiographic

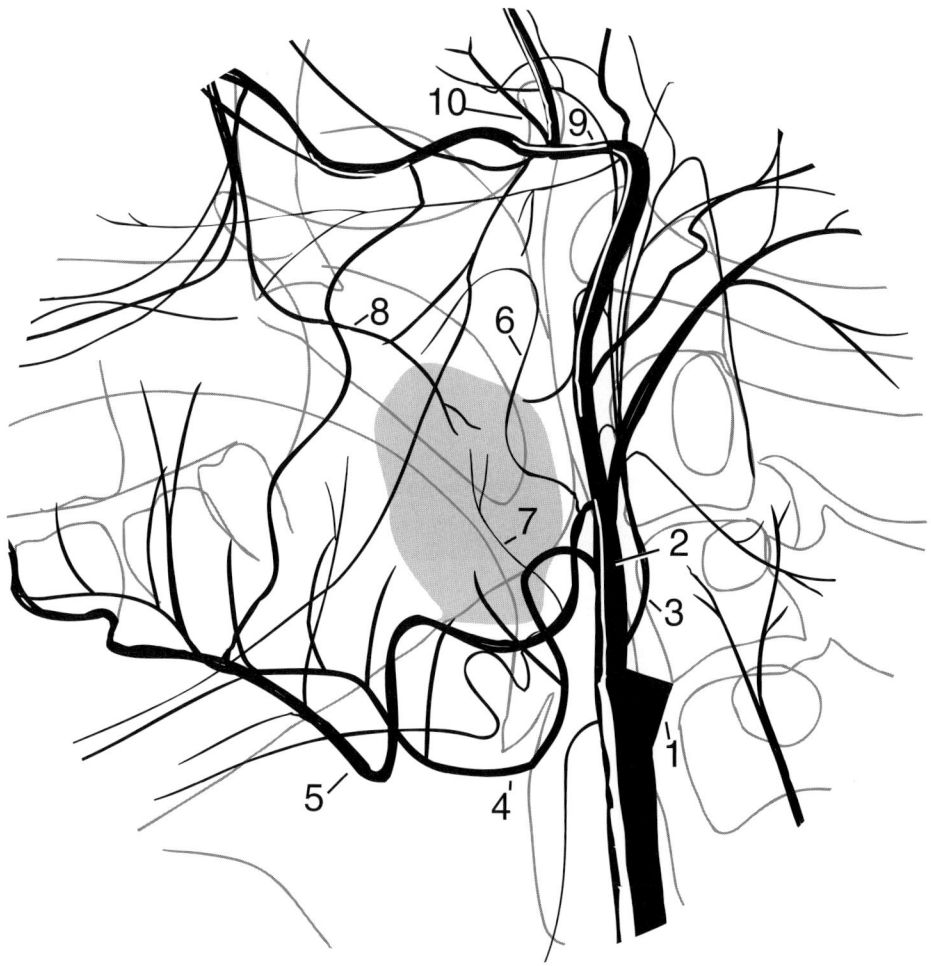

FIGURE 12.8 • *Sites of Post-Tonsillectomy Bleeding.*
Sometimes the site of hemorrhage in a child with post-tonsillectomy hemorrhage can be difficult or impossible to identify angiographically. Clinical knowledge of the site and side of hemorrhage is imperative. The commonly involved branches are illustrated, and in a patient in whom no definite bleeder is seen, empirical embolization is justifiable in circumstances of repeated transfusions and falling hematocrit.

The first priority is to assure that the internal carotid artery (1) is not involved. Sites of inadvertent arterial injury or postincision bleeding will be sometimes seen in:
- the external carotid trunk (2) *(common)*,
- ascending pharyngeal artery (3),
- proximal lingual artery (4) *(common)*,
- proximal facial artery (5),
- the ascending palatine artery (6) arising either from the facial artery or the external carotid artery *(common)*,
- tonsillar branches from the proximal linguo-facial trunk (7),
- the lesser descending palatine artery (8) from the distal internal maxillary artery (9),
- the accessory meningeal artery (10) following adenoidectomy.

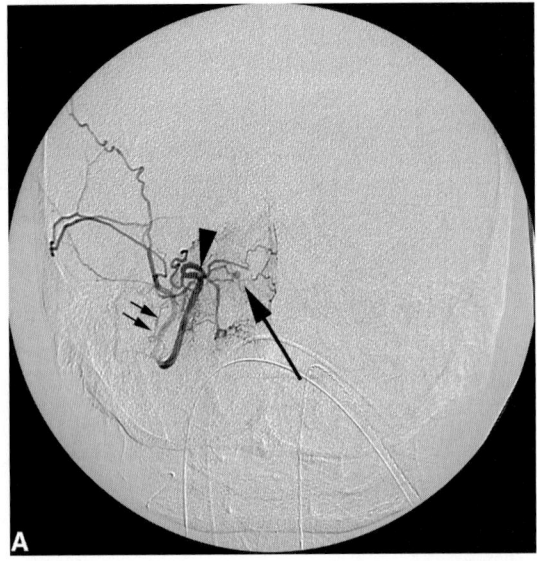 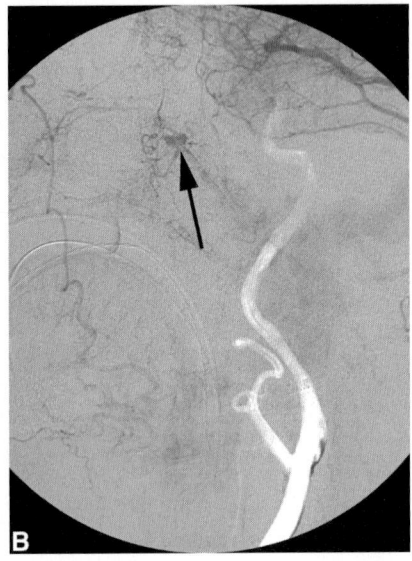

FIGURE 12.9 • *Severe Posterior Epistaxis in an 80-Year-Old Patient.*
• An AP (A, microcatheter injection into the right internal maxillary artery, AP view, arterial phase) and lateral view (B, right common carotid artery, lateral view of venous phase) in an elderly patient with recurrent severe epistaxis over the course of a month demonstrates an unusual finding of a pseudoaneurysm (arrow). This is most likely due to free extravasation enclosed by surrounding clot and nasal packing. Usually patients with posterior epistaxis just demonstrate prominence and beading of the sphenopalatine arteries. The AP view (A) performed via a microcatheter (tip marked with arrowhead) shows how easily reflux within the internal maxillary artery can extend back to potentially dangerous vessels such as the middle meningeal artery (double arrow). Orbital anastomoses from the latter could jeopardize the ophthalmic artery during particle embolization. Most commonly epistaxis embolization is performed from a location similar to that demonstrated using dilute PVA particles 150–250 μm suspended in contrast followed by Gelfoam pledgets. The facial artery on the side ipsilateral to the bleeding is also embolized distally with a small volume of dilute particles to suppress reconstitution of the nasal mucosa from the angular branch.

images, leading to uncertainty whether the findings were present before the case started. Therefore, an initial nonselective injection of the cervical carotid system is often very useful as an initial screen of the internal carotid artery and as a reference for subsequent findings in the external carotid artery.

Postsurgical Vascular Injury

Significant hemorrhage can be seen following a variety of surgical procedures presenting acutely or in a delayed manner. These include:

- Any kind of facial reconstructive surgery involving maneuvers such as a LeFort osteotomy of the maxilla or lateral osteotomy reduction of the mandible.[13,14]
- Transsphenoidal pituitary surgery.[15]
- Endoscopic nasal surgery.
- Middle ear surgery, particularly in the setting of variant anatomy such as an aberrant internal carotid artery or persistent stapedial artery.[16]

As with other causes of trauma, the initial angiographic question is whether the internal carotid artery is involved or injured. When a postsurgical or trauma patient presents with epistaxis, the possibility of an internal carotid artery injury with pseudoaneurysm formation within or adjacent to the sphenoidal sinus should always be considered.

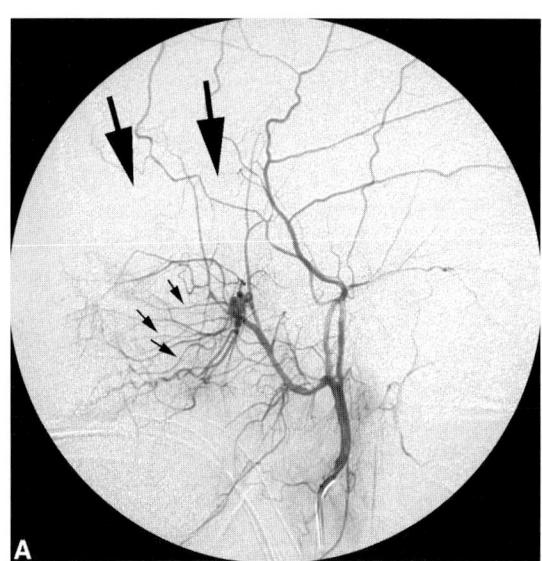 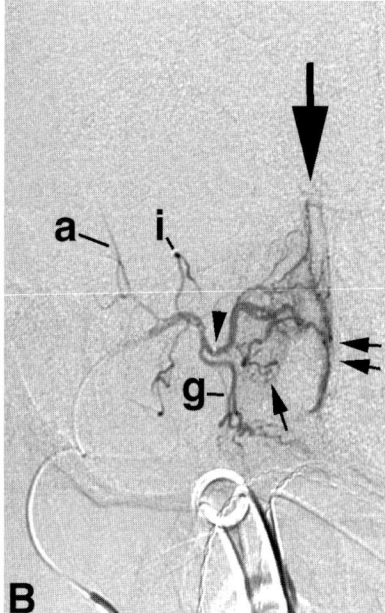

FIGURE 12.10 • *Posterior Epistaxis Angiographic Evaluation.*
Angiographic findings more typical than those seen in Fig. 12.9 are seen in this patient presenting with a falling hematocrit and repeated bleeding. The patient has been intubated for the procedure. The lateral view of the right external carotid artery (A) shows a standard configuration anatomy, with just slightly greater than usual prominence of the sphenopalatine arteries (small arrows). The absence of opacification (large arrows) of the territory or course of the ophthalmic artery is auspicious from the point of view of potentially dangerous anastomoses (see Figs. 11.2A, 11.2B). However, the run must be repeated with a microcatheter before embolization is performed. The internal maxillary artery run (B, AP view) shows the beaded irregular appearance of the long sphenopalatine arteries (double arrows) along the midline (large arrow) and of the short sphenopalatine arteries (single small arrow), typical of this disease state.

In image B, the microcatheter tip (arrowhead) is situated just distal to the origin of the greater descending palatine artery (labeled g), and reflux to the anterior deep temporal artery (labeled a) and infraorbital artery (labeled i) is also present. Some reflux of PVA particles into the greater descending palatine artery during embolization is desirable and will discourage reconstitution of the septal mucosal branches through the incisive canal of the hard palate at the distal reaches of this artery. Reflux of particles into the infraorbital artery or anterior deep temporal artery will serve no therapeutic purpose and could be hazardous.

In such cases angiographic evaluation of the collateral vessels in the Circle of Willis is important because immediate endovascular trapping of the pseudoaneurysm and closure of the lacerated vessel may prove necessary.[17,18]

EPISTAXIS

Spontaneous epistaxis is broadly divided into two groups according to the location of the hemorrhage—anterior and posterior. Epistaxis is a common complaint experienced by a large segment of the general population on at least one occasion. Most of these never reach medical attention.

Anterior epistaxis is a benign, venous bleed from Kiesselbach's plexus or Little's area anteriorly on the nasal septum. It is thought to be related to changes in temperature or humidity, intercurrent infection, physical irritation, or allergies. Hyperemic mucosa along the septum bleeds easily and becomes encrusted, leading to a cycle of irritation, nose-picking, and recurrent bleeding. Anterior epistaxis is usually easily controlled by nose-pinching, or rarely by electrical or chemical cautery of the offending mucosa.

Posterior epistaxis is a much less common problem and is usually related to arterial bleeding behind the inferior turbinate close to the sphenopalatine foramen (Figs. 12.9, 12.10). In contrast to the slow ooze of anterior epistaxis, posterior epistaxis tends therefore to be brisk, often fulminant, and alarming to the patient. It is most commonly seen in older patients with atherosclerotic disease. It can be related to hypertension, coagulopathies, or hereditary teleangiectasia (Osler-Rendu-Weber syndrome). Nonidiopathic causes such as trauma, postsurgical injuries, etc., may need to be considered in some patients.

Embolization therapy for posterior epistaxis is usually invoked when primary control measures such as direct cautery or nasal packing have failed. Traditional surgical therapy for epistaxis has involved direct surgical clipping of the internal maxillary artery and its terminal branches. However, clipping for epistaxis involves a failure rate of 15% to 22% due to incomplete clipping, or emergence of collateral vascular pathways.[19] Since 1974 when Sokoloff et al.[20] described the techniques of embolization for posterior epistaxis, management of intractable epistaxis by endovascular means has grown in acceptance. Particle embolization of the internal maxillary artery and, when necessary, the ipsilateral facial artery achieves a success rate for control of idiopathic epistaxis of 82% to 97%.[21–24] Complications such as end-tissue necrosis, scarring, blindness,[25] or facial nerve paralysis have been seen following epistaxis embolization,[26] but, in general, complications are uncommon, with most reported incidences between 0.1% and 3%.[22,23] The most important procedural factors are avoiding dangerous collateral branches to the internal carotid artery or the ophthalmic artery and avoiding use of particles that are either too small or too large (usually a size range of 150–500 μm is satisfactory). The second greatest procedural risk is aspiration of pooled blood in the nasopharynx.

FIGURE 12.11 • *Carotid-Jugular Fistula.*
A young adult presented with a loud bruit and swelling of the left side of his neck following a stabbing. The left common carotid angiogram (A, AP view; B, lateral view) shows occlusion of the left external carotid artery and absence of intracranial flow from the internal carotid artery distal to the site of a large carotid-jugular fistula. The internal jugular vein is compressed (arrow) by hematoma, and therefore much of the venous flow from the fistula is directed superiorly toward the cavernous sinuses (double arrows) and the pharyngeal venous plexus (arrowheads).

The status of the distal cervical internal carotid artery can be deduced as patent by virtue of retrograde flow down to the fistula site as seen on the lateral view of the right vertebral artery injection (arrow in C). In this case, two therapeutic embolizations were performed (D, left vertebral artery injection postembolization).

1. Latex balloons were navigated on a microcatheter stiffened with a wire past the internal carotid artery pseudoaneurysm up to the cavernous segment (uppermost double arrowhead) and deposited distal and proximal (lower single arrowhead) to the pseudoaneurysm, thus trapping it.
2. To prevent secondary bleeding from the lacerated external carotid artery, coils were deposited into the stump (single arrow). The left vertebral artery injection shows prompt reconstitution of the supraclinoid internal carotid artery via the posterior communicating artery. There is prompt reconstitution of the left external carotid artery via the C1-occipital anastomosis (double arrows).

Alternatives for preserving the internal carotid artery in this patient did not exist and were not necessary in view of his excellent native collateral flow. A covered stent might become a more viable option in the future using vein graft material or synthetic covering. Alternatively, balloon deposition on the venous side of a fistula such as this or transvenous embolization might be considerations in patients with more favorable anatomy at the site of the fistula.

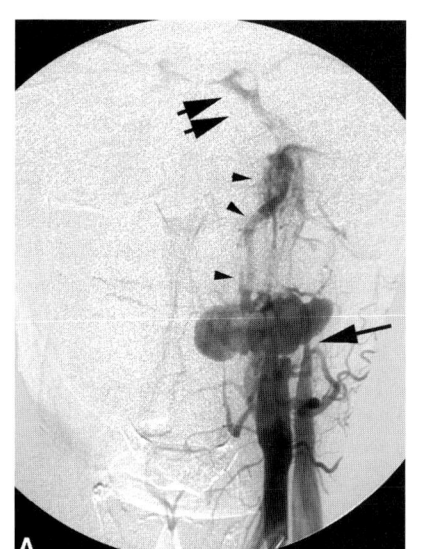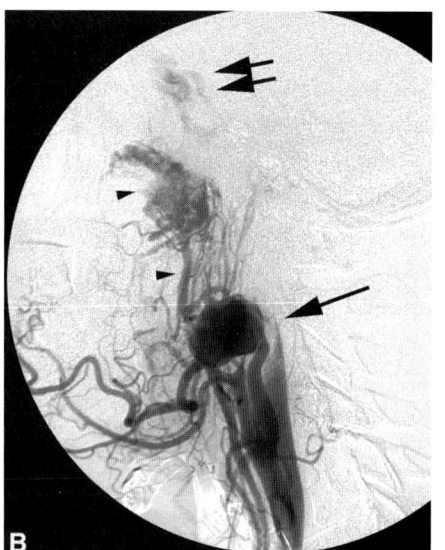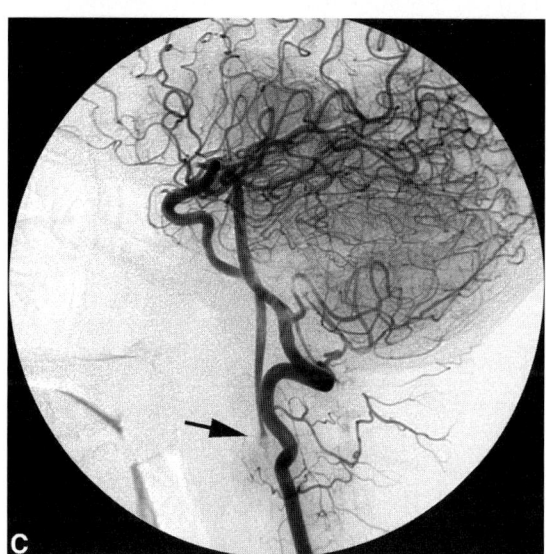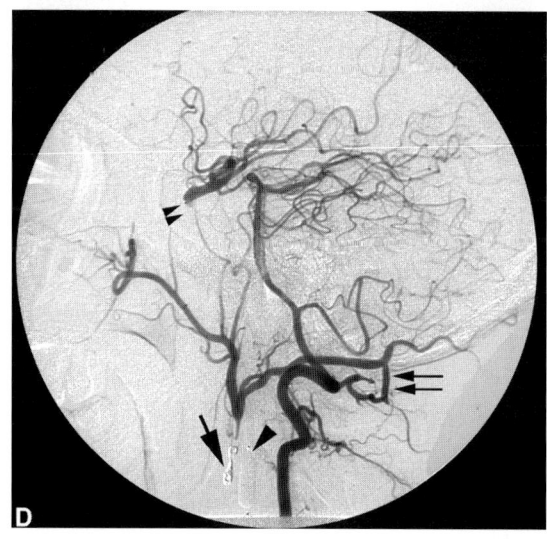

Even with nasal packing in place, slow oozing of blood into the nasopharynx is common, with a risk of aspiration while the patient is supine. Therefore epistaxis embolization is usually more safely performed under general anesthesia with airway protection. The techniques used for idiopathic posterior epistaxis embolization are equally applicable to posttraumatic epistaxis following penetrating injury or gunshot wounds.[27] Usually embolization of the internal maxillary artery is conducted through a microcatheter advanced to the distal point of arborization of the vessel into the *short and long sphenopalatine arteries*. These serve the lateral and septal areas of the narine mucosa, respectively, and will account for most areas of bleeding. It is usually desirable to embolize also the *greater descending palatine artery* in order to eliminate it as an important distal collateral route to the septal mucosa. The greater descending palatine artery usually arises distal to the infraorbital artery, and thus by careful injection of particles the latter can usually be spared. By penetrating the vessels distally with particles in the range of 150 µm or larger, the potential for immediate distal collateralization of the territory is reduced. Smaller particles have a risk of mucosal necrosis and greater ease of reflux into dangerous anastomoses. Larger particles >500 µm may lodge too proximally in the vessel and fail to achieve a satisfactory reduction in the perfusion of the vessel. This failure will encourage collateral branches from the ethmoidal arteries, the facial artery, or the accessory meningeal artery to reconstitute the supply to the nasal mucosa. When embolization of the internal maxillary artery is completed, some anterior septal blush from the distal angular branch of the facial artery is commonly seen. The *facial artery* is usually selected on the side of bleeding and catheterized as far distally as possible before embolizing lightly (3–6 ml of dilutely suspended particles) in this territory to reduce the distal mucosal territory of the facial artery. Excessive embolization in the facial artery can be hazardous, especially if small particles are used, and causes a great deal of patient discomfort, trismus, and facial pain afterwards. Rarely, other branches of the external carotid artery that can reach the nasal septum may need to be con-

FIGURE 12.12 • *Vertebro-Jugular Fistula.*
A middle-age female patient presented with intermittent, pulsatile blood loss from the left side of her neck following a domestic stabbing. The left vertebral artery demonstrates a high-flow fistula from the mid-cervical segment to the ipsilateral jugular vein (A, AP view). The jugular vein is compressed by hematoma with restriction of antegrade flow. In fact, later images showed that the fistula drained through the intracranial sinuses to the contralateral internal jugular vein. The lateral view of the left vertebral artery (B) shows the tract of the fistula well (arrow), and also shows on one image only from the run that a small lick of contrast (arrowhead) extends distal to the fistula before being washed back into the tract. This is an important indicator of the potential for slipping a balloon past the fistula further up into the left vertebral artery.

The right vertebral artery injection (C) also shows prominent filling of the fistula by retrograde opacification of the previously unseen distal left vertebral artery, and confirms the likelihood that a straight balloon microcatheter will pass the fistula. Two silicone balloons mounted on extended-tip microcatheters did bypass the fistula quite easily. The positioning of the upper balloon (D) is probably not high enough. Ideally the C1 and C2 anastomoses of the vertebral artery should be below the uppermost balloon. In that manner, antegrade flow in the vertebral artery above the balloon would be eliminated and with it any risk of carrying thrombus into the intracranial circulation. However, so great was the flow in this artery that the only position in which the balloon would sit securely was at the first curve of the vertebral artery. The second balloon straddles the fistula itself (E, lateral view unsubtracted) and bulges anteriorly into the fistula (arrowhead).

One of the dangers in a case such as this is that the balloons already placed or a third supporting balloon will cover the origin of the anterior spinal artery, causing spinal cord ischemia. This is a particular danger in the C4 to C6 region. Therefore, before detaching the second balloon a 5–10 minute period of observation was conducted with testing of the patient's spinal function before detaching the balloon. A run of the left vertebral artery was then performed (D) to check for the presence of an anterior spinal artery. Similarly, before detaching a third balloon (F), a long period of observation of the patient was conducted.

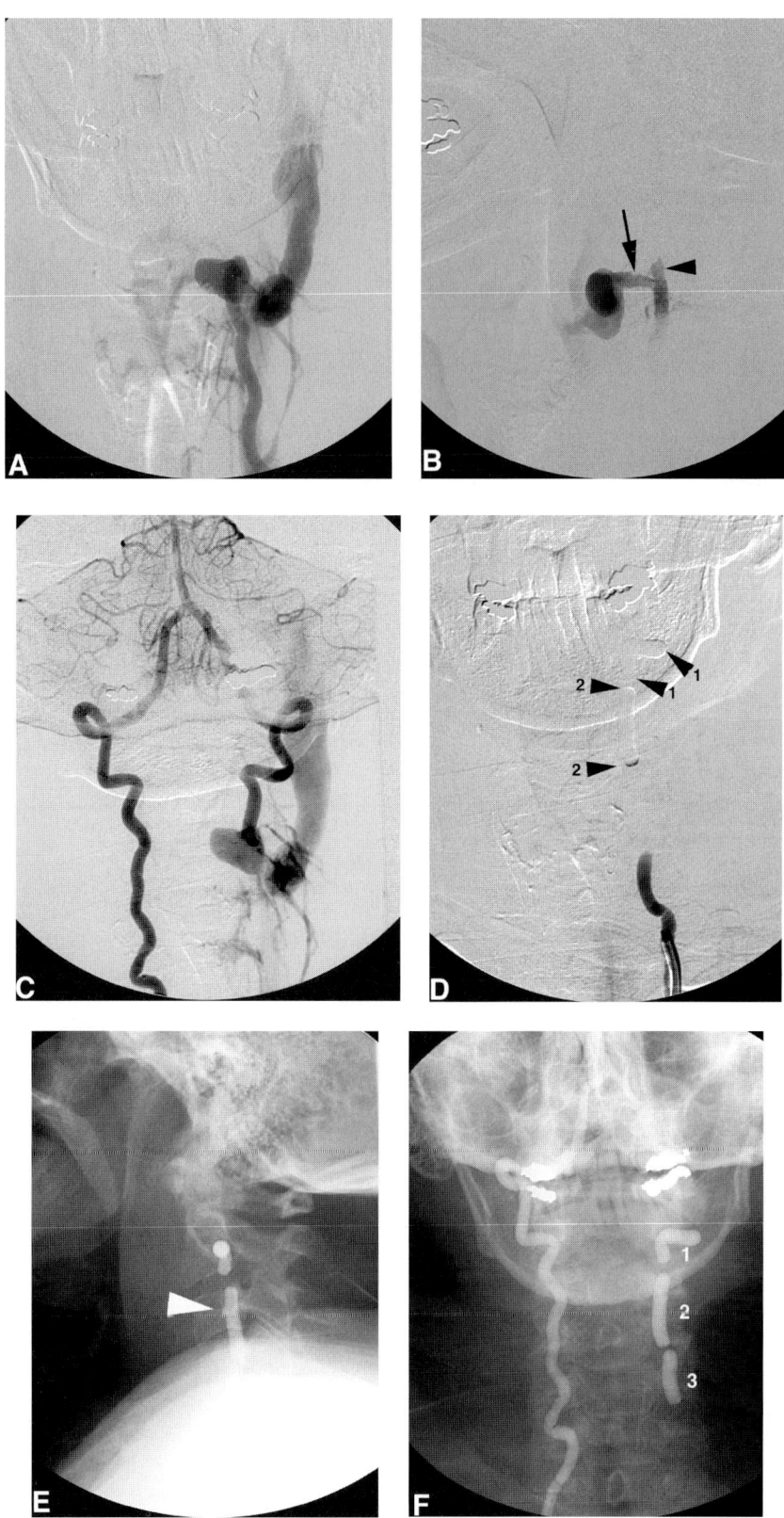

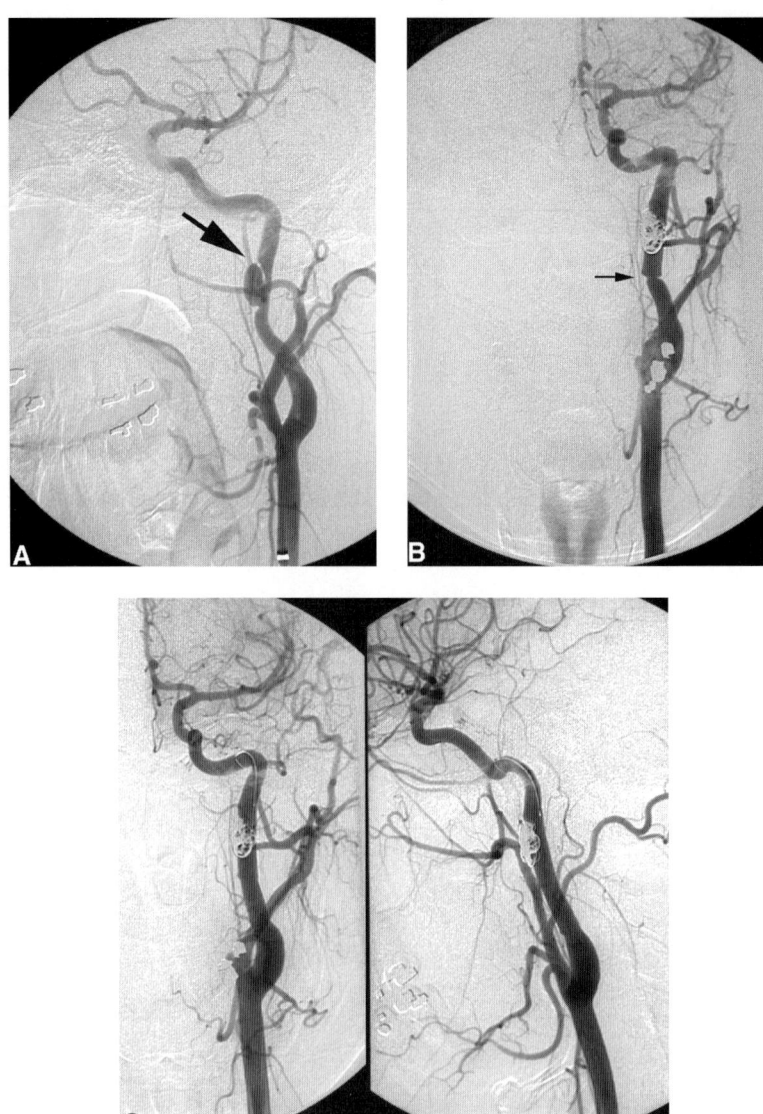

FIGURE 12.13 • *Internal Carotid Artery Pseudoaneurysm Treated by Stenting and Coiling.*
A 32-year-old female patient sustained multiple injuries in an automobile accident in which her neck and thorax were pinned against the road by the wheel of her car. Three months after discharge from hospital, she presented anew with a loud bruit on the left side, found to be related to a pseudoaneurysm of the left internal carotid artery with significant narrowing of the vessel just before the skull base (A, left common carotid artery, oblique view).
After premedication with clopidogrel and aspirin, heparin and eptifibatide were used during the procedure as described in Chapter 4 for placement of a SMART (Cordis) 8 × 20 mm stent across the pseudoaneurysm. The pseudoaneurysm was then catheterized with a microcatheter through the struts of the stent and embolized with GDCs. The posttreatment images (B, left common carotid artery, AP view) looked reasonable, except for a prominent web of spasm (arrow) at the proximal end of the stent. It was assumed that this spasm would disappear over time, but on return 3 months later it appeared worse and resisted a low-pressure balloon angioplasty, suggesting that it had become fibrotic. Consequently, a second stent was placed overlapping the first (C) with a more satisfactory sustained appearance. An asymptomatic contralateral internal carotid artery pseudoaneurysm, more shallow than the left, did not narrow the artery on the right side to the same degree and was treated with antiplatelet agents only.

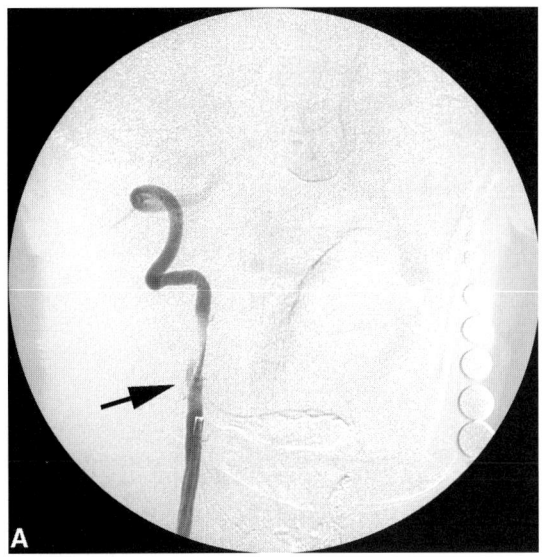
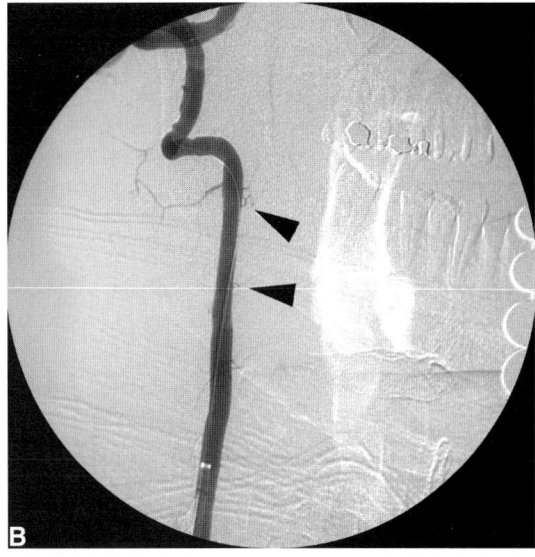

FIGURE 12.14 • *Iatrogenic Dissection of the Right Vertebral Artery.*
A severe dissection of the distal cervical vertebral artery was induced by the guide-wire in a 45-year-old adult described elsewhere (arrow in A, right vertebral artery, AP projection). His intracranial posterior circulation was already severely compromised by intracranial stenoses and thrombosis, making this additional injury more serious. Fortunately, it was possible to cross the dissection with a Choice PT 0.014-in wire (Boston Scientific) and mend the dissection site with a NIR 4 × 30 mm stent (Boston Scientific). Side branches of the vertebral artery continue to opacify through the struts of the stent (arrowheads in B). His intracranial angioplasty and stent placement then proceeded without further incident. Notice the early spasm of the high cervical segments of the vertebral artery induced by the wire. Pretreatment of the vertebral arteries with nitroglycerin and papaverine may be pivotally important in such patients before proceeding to the intracranial circulation.

sidered for embolization. They are usually involved when there has been a previous proximal ligation or clipping, and include the *transverse facial artery*, and the arteries of the nasopharynx including the pharyngeal branches of the *ascending pharyngeal artery* and the *accessory meningeal artery*, or the *ascending palatine artery*.

Embolization of the nasal septum may be ineffective if there are prominent ethmoidal branches from the ophthalmic artery descending through the cribriform plate accounting for the hemorrhage from the nasal mucosa. Although it is technically feasible to embolize branches of the ophthalmic artery, this is rarely done due to the risk of retinal artery occlusion unless the patient is already blind.[28] Patients with bleeding from ethmoidal branches of the ophthalmic artery are usually considered more suitable for clipping.

The most important anastomotic dangers during embolization of the internal maxillary artery for epistaxis are:

- The artery of the foramen rotundum to the inferolateral trunk of the internal carotid artery.
- The Vidian artery, or mandibular artery if present, to the petrous internal carotid artery.
- The ethmoidal arteries of the nasal septum connecting to the ophthalmic artery.
- The deep temporal branches of the internal maxillary artery connecting to the ophthalmic artery.
- Particles inadvertently refluxing into the middle meningeal artery may find access to the oph-

thalmic artery. The possibility of meningeal to ophthalmic anastomoses as a potential site of hazard should not be overlooked.

Internal Carotid and Vertebral Artery Injuries

Injuries to the internal carotid artery and vertebral artery from blunt or penetrating injury are common. In patients with blunt injury and cervical spine injury, arterial injury rates of approximately 10% to 24% are detectable by MRA, Doppler examination, or angiography.[29-30] However, most of these flaps and small dissections remain asymptomatic. With penetrating trauma from projectiles or knives, the types of arterial injuries seen tend to be more serious, involving occlusions, fistulas (Figs. 12.11, 12.12), and pseudoaneurysms (Fig. 12.13). These injuries can sometimes be managed using endovascular techniques for vessel or fistula closure. Stent technology offers the possibility of vessel preservation with repair of lacerations or pseudoaneurysms in conjunction with other devices or stent-coverings.[32] For isolated injuries these devices are quite successful at preserving the vessel lumen and providing a basis for restoration of the vessel wall (Fig. 12.14). However, the question of the dangers of anticoagulation for the procedure and antiplatelet therapy in the acute setting in patients with other visceral or cerebral traumatic injuries is a restriction on the application of these devices.

References

1. Hall MJ, Kozak LJ, Gillum BS (1997) National survey of ambulatory surgery: 1994. *Statistical Bulletin—Metropolitan Insurance Companies* 78:18–27.
2. Chowdhury K, Tewfik TL, Schloss MD (1988) Post-tonsillectomy and adenoidectomy hemorrhage. *J Otolaryngol* 17:46–49.
3. Colclasure JB, Graham SS (1990) Complications of outpatient tonsillectomy and adenoidectomy: a review of 3,340 cases. *Ear Nose Throat J* 69:155–160.
4. Myssiorek D, Alvi A (1996) Post-tonsillectomy hemorrhage: an assessment of risk factors. *Int J Pediatr Otorhinolaryngol* 37:35–43.
5. Allen GC, Armfield DR, Bontempo FA, Kingsley LA, Goldstein NA, Post JC (1999) Adenotonsillectomy in children with von Willebrand disease. *Arch Otolaryngol Head Neck Surg* 125:547–551.
6. Smith I, Wilde A (1999) Secondary tonsillectomy haemorrhage and non-steroidal anti-inflammatory drugs. *J Laryngol Otol* 113:28–30.
7. Steketee KG, Reisdorff EJ (1995) Emergency care for post-tonsillectomy and postadenoidectomy hemorrhage. *Am J Emerg Med* 13:518–523.
8. Franco KL, Wallace RB (1987) Management of postoperative bleeding after tonsillectomy. *Otolaryngolog Clin North Am* 20:391–397.
9. Weber R, Keerl R, Hendus J, Kahle G (1993) The emergency: traumatic aneurysm in the area of the head-neck. *Laryngo-Rhino-Otologie* 72:86–90.
10. Mitchell RB, Pereira KD, Lazar RH, Long TE, Fournier NF (1997) Pseudoaneurysm of the right lingual artery: an unusual cause of severe hemorrhage during tonsillectomy. *Ear Nose Throat J* 76:575–576.
11. Karas DE, Sawin RS, Sie KCY (1997) Pseudoaneurysm of the external carotid artery after tonsillectomy. A rare complication. *Arch Otolaryngol Head Neck Surg* 123:345–347.
12. Mitchell RB, Pereira KD, Lazar RH, Long TE, Fournier NF (1997) Pseudoaneurysm of the right lingual artery: an unusual cause of severe hemorrhage during tonsillectomy. *Ear Nose Throat J* 76:575–576.
13. Bendor-Samuel R, Chen YR, Chen PK (1995) Unusual complications of the LeFort I osteotomy. *Plast Reconstruct Surg* 96:1289–1296.
14. Rogers SN, Patel M, Beirne JC, Nixon TE (1995) Traumatic aneurysm of the maxillary artery: the role of interventional radiology. A report of two cases. *Int J Oral Maxillofacial Surg* 24:336–339.
15. Raymond J, Hardy J, Czepko R, Roy D (1997) Arterial injuries in transsphenoidal surgery for pituitary adenoma; the role of angiography and endovascular treatment. *AJNR* 18:655–665.
16. Glasscock ME, Seshul M, Seshul MB (1993) Bilateral aberrant internal carotid artery case presentation. *Arch Otolaryngol Head Neck Surg* 119:335–339.
17. Han MH, Sung MW, Chang KH, Min YG, Han DH, Han MC (1994) Traumatic pseudoaneurysm of the intracavernous ICA presenting with massive epistaxis: imaging diagnosis and endovascular treatment. *Laryngoscope* 104:370–377.
18. Uzan M, Cantasdemir M, Seckin MS, Hanci M, Kocer N, Sarioglu AC, Islak C (1998) Traumatic intracranial carotid tree aneurysms. *Neurosurgery* 43:1314–1320.
19. Montgomery WW, Reardon EJ (1980) in *Controversies in Otolaryngology*. Philadelphia: J.B.Saunders 315–319.
20. Sokoloff J, Wickbom I, McDonald D, Brahme F, Goergen TC, Goldberger LE (1974) Therapeutic percutaneous embolization in intractable epistaxis. *Radiology* 111:285–287.
21. Parnes LS, Heeneman H, Vinuela F (1987) Percutaneous embolization for control of nasal blood circulation. *Laryngoscope* 97:1312–1315.

22. Vitek JJ (1991) Idiopathic intractable epistaxis: endovascular therapy. *Radiology* 181:113–116.
23. Strutz J, Schumacher M (1990) Uncontrollable epistaxis. Angiographic localization and embolization. *Arch Otolaryngol Head Neck Surg* 116:697–699.
24. Siniluoto TMJ, Leinonen AS, Karttunen AI, Karjalainen HK, Jokinen KE (1993) Embolization for the treatment of posterior epistaxis. An analysis of 31 cases. *Arch Otolaryngol Head Neck Surg* 119:837–841.
25. Moreau S, De Rugy MG, Babin E, Courtheoux P, Valdazo A (1998) Supraselective embolization in intractable epistaxis: review of 45 cases. *Laryngoscope* 108:887–888.
26. Wehrli M, Leiberherr U, Valavanis A (1988) Superselective embolization for intractable epistaxis: experience with 19 patients. *Clin Otolaryngol Allied Sci* 13:415–420.
27. Borsa JJ, Fontaine AB, Eskridge JM, Song JK, Hoffer EK, Aoki AA (1999) Transcatheter arterial embolization for intractable epistaxis secondary to gunshot wounds. *J Vasc Intervent Radiol* 10:297–302.
28. Moser FG, Rosenblatt M, De La Cruz F, Silver C, Burde RM (1992) Embolization of the ophthalmic artery for control of epistaxis. Report of two cases. *Head Neck* 14:308–311.
29. Rommel O, Niedeggen A, Tegenthoff M, Kiwitt P, Botel U, Malin J (1999) Carotid and vertebral artery injury following severe head or cervical spine trauma. *Cerebrovasc Dis* 9:202–209.
30. Friedman D, Flanders A, Thomas C, Millar W (1995) Vertebral artery injuries after acute cervical spine trauma: rate of occurrence as detected by MR angiography and assessment of clinical consequences. *AJR* 164:443–447.
31. Weller SJ, Rossitch E Jr, Malek AM (1999) Detection of vertebral artery injury after cervical spine trauma using magnetic resonance angiography. *J Trauma-Inj Infect Crit Care* 46:660–666.
32. Bejjani GK, Monsein LH, Laird JR, Satler LF, Starnes BW, Aulisi EF (1999) Treatment of symptomatic cervical carotid dissections with endovascular stents. *Neurosurgery* 44:755–760.

Chapter 13

Thrombolysis and Treatment of Acute Stroke

Background

The ideal treatment for ischemic stroke involves removal of vascular obstruction, protection of the injured brain, and restoration of function. Irreversible brain injury probably begins about 5 minutes after onset of complete global ischemia, which does not allow much scope for completely effective therapy.[1] However, degrees of ischemia and vascular occlusion are variable in symptomatic patients, which means that some stroke patients can be helped considerably by aggressive treatment within the first few hours of onset. Measures aimed at improving perfusion pressure within the affected area of brain should be effective at limiting the degree of tissue damage following an ischemic event. The most obviously effective strategy would involve removal of the occlusive lesion (Fig. 13.1). Therefore, the possibility of thrombolytic therapy by intravenous and intraarterial routes has been examined in a number of trials. The earliest trials involved use of intravenous streptokinase administered to patients within periods up to 4 days following stroke. Treated groups of patients demonstrated poorer outcomes and higher rates of hemorrhagic transformation compared with controls.[2]

The preoccupation with avoiding hemorrhagic transformation of stroke has been an overarching concern in the design and execution of subsequent thrombolytic trials. It has also, in the opinion of some, been a significant obstacle in clinical practice to the aggressive implementation of thrombolytic therapy. Intravenous thrombolytic therapy for stroke is safe and effective for most stroke patients when given within 3 hours of onset, possibly even longer. However, implementation of this therapy has been slow to find currency for reasons related to public health awareness, institutional inertia, and perception of risk. The major modern trials of thrombolysis have confined therapy to the first few hours of ischemia. The European Cooperative Acute Stroke Study (ECASS) administered t-PA in doses of 1.1 mg/kg intravenously and later at 0.9 mg/kg intravenously to patients within 6 hours of onset of symptoms.[3] The results showed a statistically nonsignificant trend toward efficacy on the part of the drug. The National Institute of Neurological Disorders and Stroke (NINDS) trial of t-PA was a double-blind, placebo controlled trial of

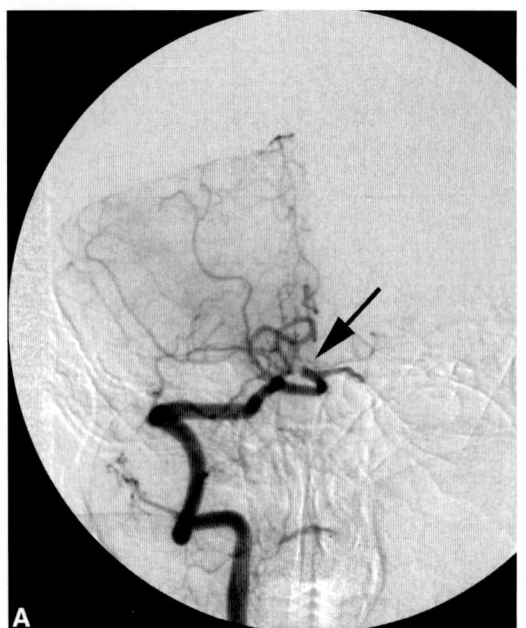 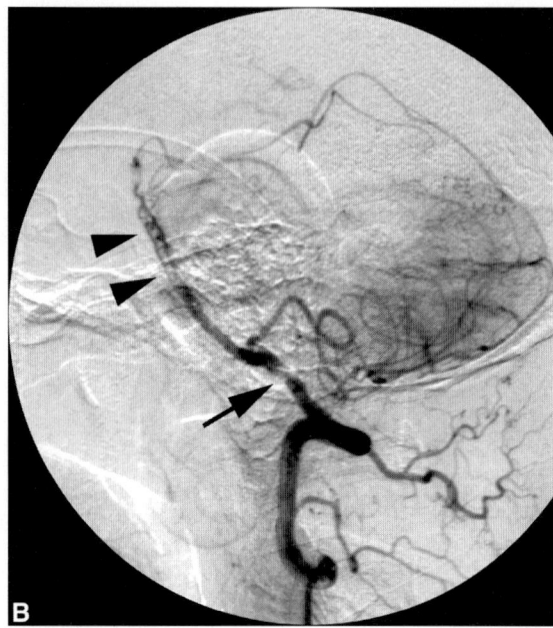

FIGURE 13.1 • *Emergency Thrombolysis for Basilar Artery Thrombosis.*
A 45-year-old male patient presented with cranial nerve deficits, signs of cerebellar infarction, and progressive obtundation. An emergency angiogram demonstrated complete occlusion of the proximal basilar artery (arrow in A, right vertebral artery injection, Towne's projection). An emergency thrombolysis was performed using 650,000 units of urokinase introduced into the right vertebral artery by microcatheter. The patient's neurological status improved, but he began to complain of severe headache. Therefore, although considerable intracranial basilar thrombus persisted (arrowheads in B, right vertebral artery injection postthrombolysis) the procedure was discontinued. A prominent stenosis of the intradural right vertebral artery is present (arrow in B). An angiogram 48 hours later (Fig. 5.6A) showed no evidence of thrombus, and his right vertebral artery stenosis was successfully stented (Fig. 5.6B).

Images courtesy of Dr. J. Mewborne of Greenville NC.

0.9 mg/kg intravenous t-PA (10% as bolus and the remainder over an hour) administered to stroke patients within 3 hours of onset.[4] The results showed a statistically significant difference in long-term outcome in favor of the drug compared with placebo, even taking into account an increased rate of hemorrhage with t-PA. Patients treated with t-PA were at least 30% more likely to have minimal or no disability at 3-month follow-up compared with control patients. However, a double-blind trial similar in design to the NINDS study failed to show a favorable result from treatment of ischemic stroke with r-tPA 0.9 mg/kg intravenously when treatment was given between 3 and 6 hours following onset.[5]

INTRAARTERIAL THROMBOLYSIS

Just as the favorable results of intravenous thrombolytic trials have been slow to take root, the more invasive and specialized limitations on the availability of endovascular treatment of stroke have restricted development of this modality of effective stroke therapy. However, Edwards et al.[6] have demonstrated that establishment of an effective stroke response team is possible in a determined community hospital, with tangible improvement in patient outcome following intraarterial thrombolysis delivered within 6 hours of stroke.

Intraarterial thrombolysis performed within 6

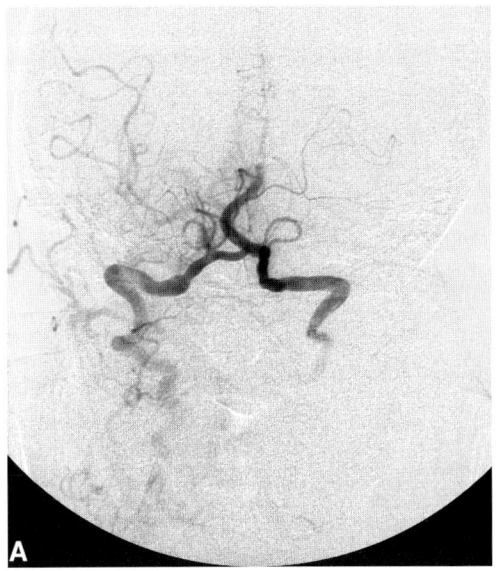 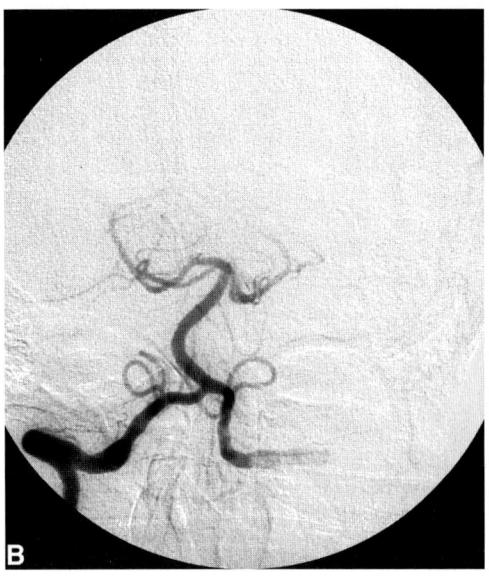

FIGURE 13.2 • *Emergency Thrombolysis Following Embolus during Angiography.*
An 80-year-old female developed an embolus to the distal basilar artery following a maneuver in the aortic arch involving an exchange length wire (A). Many misadventures of this nature have occurred because of adherent platelets and thrombus along the length of an exchange wire during catheter exchanges. Exchange length wires in the aortic arch should probably be used only in a last resort and, at that, only in patients protected by heparin or antiplatelet agents. With immediate heparinization and prompt thrombolysis via a microcatheter with 600,000 units of urokinase, her posterior circulation quickly (<2 hours) resumed a normal appearance (B).

hours of onset of acute ischemic stroke improves patient outcome compared with conservative management (Figs. 13.1–13.3).[7,8] The PROACT II study of acute ischemic stroke in the middle cerebral artery[6] randomized patients to receive 9 mg of intraarterial recombinant prourokinase (r-pro-UK) with low-dose heparin or treatment with heparin only. The middle cerebral artery was catheterized with a microcatheter and wire and 9 mg of r-pro-UK were delivered over a 2-hour infusion into the proximal middle cerebral artery. Mechanical clot disruption was prohibited during the trial to prevent any non–drug-related therapeutic effects. Heparin was administered as a 2,000 u bolus with infusion of 500 u per hour. Recanalization rates were 66% in the r-pro-UK group and 18% in the control group. Despite an increased rate of early symptomatic hemorrhagic transformation of cerebral infarction with r-pro-UK (10.2% versus 2%), ultimate hemorrhage and mortality rates were similar, while neurologic outcome for the r-pro-UK group as measured by a Rankin score of 2 or less was better (40% versus 25%).

A rate of 10.2% for symptomatic hemorrhagic transformation with intraarterial thrombolysis was higher in the PROACT II trial than in trials of intravenous t-PA (6.4% in the NINDS trial,[4] 7.2% in the ATLANTIS r-tPA trial,[5] 8.8% in the ECASS II trial).[3] Other uncontrolled studies of intraarterial thrombolysis have demonstrated rates of symptomatic and nonsymptomatic hemorrhage ranging from 14% to 38% following thrombolysis, but the degree of heparin use in these was higher than would currently be thought optimal.[9,10] In general, better clinical outcomes have been reported with earlier treatment, when thrombolysis is successful

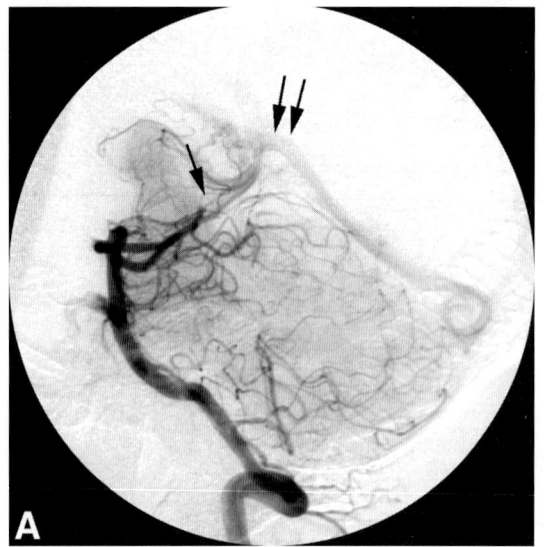 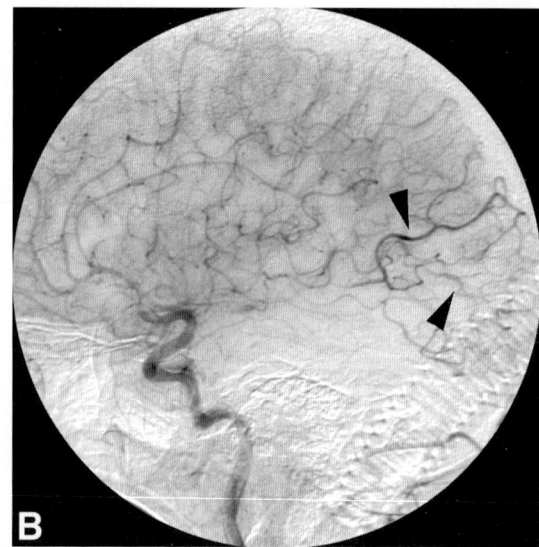

FIGURE 13.3 • *Importance of Collateral Circulation in Assessment of Treatment Decisions.*
An elderly patient presenting with complete basilar artery thrombosis responded fairly well over the course of an hour to intraarterial instillation of 1.2 million units of urokinase. A DSA run following urokinase (A, left vertebral artery, lateral view) shows that the basilar artery is completely cleared, but there is abrupt termination of the posterior cerebral arteries by thrombus (single arrow). The left internal carotid angiogram (B, lateral view) shows prompt reconstitution of the distal cortical branches of the right posterior cerebral artery (arrowheads) suggesting that all major obstacles to cerebral flow have been cleared, and the procedure was terminated. Note the early venous opacification in image A (double arrows) suggesting that at least some infarction has occurred in the posterior circulation. Nevertheless, the patient made a meaningful recovery and returned to independent living.

in achieving early recanalization, and when the patient has a milder clinical deficit at presentation.

The patient populations, severity of middle cerebral artery occlusion, and the time of treatment make comparison between various intraarterial and intravenous thrombolytic trials difficult. For instance, the overall mortality rate in the ECASS II trial was 10.6%, whereas rates of 25% (treated with r-pro-UK) and 27% (control) were seen in the PROACT II study. This suggests that the patient population studied in the PROACT II study had more severe strokes than in some of the intravenous trials. It seems reasonable to assume that risks factors associated with likelihood of hemorrhagic transformation in the intravenous trials might also be pertinent to patients treated with intraarterial drugs. Attention to these factors might improve patient triage for intraarterial treatment. In the NINDS trial of intravenous t-PA independent variables associated with risk of hemorrhage were:

- Mass-effect on CT prior to treatment.
- Brain edema represented by hypodensity on CT prior to treatment.
- Severity of clinical condition prior to treatment.[11]
- The ECASS II study of intravenous t-PA identified pretreatment hypodensity on CT greater than 33% of the MCA territory as a risk factor for subsequent hemorrhage.[12]

There is a consensus that intravenous thrombolytic agents are less effective at achieving middle cerebral artery recanalization when there is a complete occlusion present than in situations of partial occlusion. Tomsick et al.[13] demonstrated that the presence of a dense MCA sign on CT prior to treatment, indicating a complete occlusion, predicted a poor outcome for patients treated with IV t-PA. The results of the ECASS II trial of intravenous alteplase demonstrated only a weak nonstatistically significant effect from 0.9 mg/kg administered intravenously in patients treated within 6 hours of onset of ischemia, perhaps in part for this reason.[3] The potential weakness of the intravenous approach argues for the theoretically better chances of recanalization with an intraarterial direct delivery of drug. Furthermore, the therapeutic efficacy of ancillary techniques and devices during intraarterial thrombolysis was not fully utilized in the PROACT II study. The capacity to perform mechanical clot disruption with a wire or microballoon, clot extraction with a microsnare, or rheolytic clot fragmentation and extraction with rheolytic catheters, in addition to the capacity to perform emergency angioplasty and stenting of critical occlusive lesions mean that the recanalization rates seen with intraarterial r-pro-UK or intraarterial t-PA could represent an underestimation of the efficacy of the intraarterial approach to stroke treatment.

Technical and Procedural Considerations

A decision for or against intraarterial thrombolysis is best made by a team of specialists working together as a stroke team. The major component of leadership in this respect inevitably falls on the team neurologist who is best experienced to evaluate the patient's neurological condition. However, the best efforts are achieved through collaborative teamwork. The interventional neuroradiolgist's principal responsibilities involve:

- Communication with the patient's family concerning consent for the procedure, impressing upon them the need for a speedy decision. As they will have to live with the results of the procedure, an informed realistic consent regarding risks and benefits is ethically necessary.
- Organization of a rapidly responsive team involving technologists, nurses, assistants, and in many instances the department of anesthesia. More people involved with the procedure can often mean more potential for delay. Time is very important in treatment of stroke patients; every 5 minutes lost in mustering the endovascular team equates with long-term functional loss for the patient. Therefore, it is often tempting and sometimes appropriate to forgo procedural delays incurred by such considerations as involvement of an anesthesia team, insertion of a Foley catheter, replacement of marginal intravenous lines, etc. However, protection of the airway in severely obtunded patients or those with posterior circulation ischemia is a vitally important consideration for the safe outcome of the patient.
- Communication with the stroke team before, during, and after the endovascular procedure. It is very unpleasant for the neurology team to take care of a patient with complications or an adverse outcome related to procedural decisions in which they perceive, correctly or incorrectly, that they had no hand.

Dose

Most experience with intraarterial thrombolysis was obtained with urokinase. Typical doses for superselective intracranial administration ranged as high as 1–1.2 million units, occasionally as high as 2 million units, usually delivered over the course of an hour or so. Since the withdrawal of urokinase from the commercial market, recombinant tissue plasminogen activator (r-tPA) is effectively the only agent available in common use for this purpose. Commonly, this agent is formulated to a solution of 1 mg/ml and administered intraarterially at rates of up to 1 mg/minute through a microcatheter. The optimal or maximal dose is not known for certain. Intraarterial dose ranges of up to a total of 20 mg are commonly endorsed,[14] but greater efficacy and reasonable risk have been shown with doses as high as 40 mg.[15]

Arterial Puncture

A double-wall puncture technique might raise concern for posterior-wall bleeding during the case following administration of thrombolytic agents. Fortunately, this is surprisingly uncommon. However, in patients who are already anticoagulated or receiving thrombolytic agents intravenously, caution at the arterial puncture site is warranted. A single-wall arterial puncture technique in such patients is probably safer, and at that probably best done using an 0.018-in micropuncture kit. This will minimize bleeding from inadvertent venous punctures or arterial side-wall punctures.

Size and Length of Arterial Sheath

Stroke patients tend generally to be older, frequently hypertensive, and often have significant peripheral vascular disease involving the great vessels of the aortic arch and the iliac arteries. Longer (30 cm) sheaths may be necessary in such patients to straighten the iliac arteries sufficiently to allow catheter manipulation. Therefore, at the outset if the course of the wire in the iliac system appears tortuous or difficult, a long sheath inserted at the beginning will avoid considerable delays later.

Microcatheters can be inserted coaxially via 5 French introducer catheters. The advantage of a 5 Fr system is ease of control of the arterial puncture site afterwards. However, there are few, if any, other advantages. Disadvantages include:

- Smaller catheters are less stable in the cervical vessels while advancing coaxial microcatheters.
- With a coaxial microcatheter in place, effective diagnostic runs cannot be performed via the 5 Fr outer catheter to monitor for progress or complication.
- Larger mechanical devices such as snares, angioplasty balloons, and stents cannot generally fit through a 5 Fr catheter. One has the option of starting the case with a 5 Fr sheath and deciding later to up-size if necessary. However, this again involves unnecessary delay. Furthermore, since the advent of effective arterial closure devices, the concern of arterial closure in the setting of thrombolytic and anticoagulant agents has become relatively minor. A 7 Fr introducer catheter and some larger lumen 6 Fr catheters (0.067-

FIGURE 13.4 • *Mechanical Clot Disruption Using a Compliant Balloon.*
A 73-year-old female undergoing diagnostic angiography for evaluation of a dural AVM of the left cavernous sinus developed an embolic complication in the left middle cerebral artery. The initial run (A, left internal artery, AP projection) shows complete patency of the left middle cerebral artery and faint opacification of the left superior ophthalmic vein (arrowhead, also seen in C). She became profoundly plegic on the right side and aphasic, with complete occlusion of the left middle cerebral artery (B, arrow).

Heparin and a bolus of saline were administered. An emergency thrombolysis was performed via a microcatheter, but after 14 mg of t-PA had been delivered into the occlusion site no impact on the clot could be discerned and the middle cerebral artery remained completely occluded.

The 5 Fr system was exchanged for a 6 Fr introducer catheter. A Sentry balloon (Target) was passed over a 0.010-in wire to the site of the clot and inflated gently with contrast in multiple locations and dragged through the clot. This, in association with a bolus of abciximab, opened the vessel somewhat (arrow in C), with immediate improvement in her clinical examination. Although her clinical examination did not normalize for some days while in the ICU on heparin, she ultimately made a complete recovery with no clinical sustained evidence of a significant infarction.

CT scans (D) performed immediately after the thrombolysis and later that night show a commonly seen phenomenon of contrast staining (white arrow) following thrombolysis procedures. This is often misinterpreted as hemorrhage. It probably represents areas of blood-brain-barrier breakdown and infarction, in variable measures in different patients. It usually clears completely within 24 hours or less, as was the case in this patient.

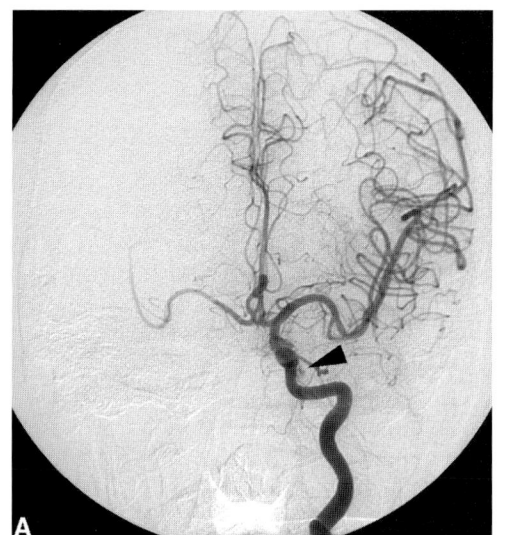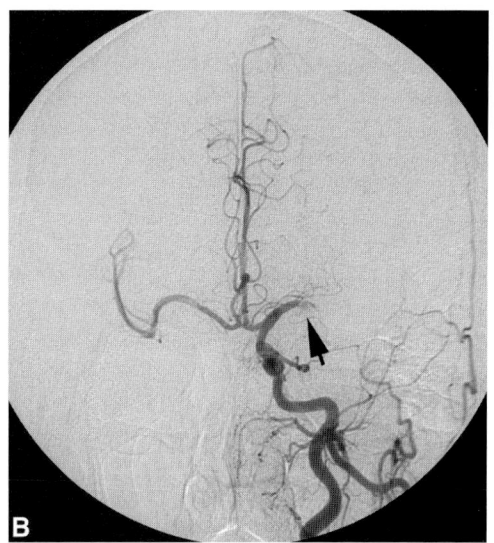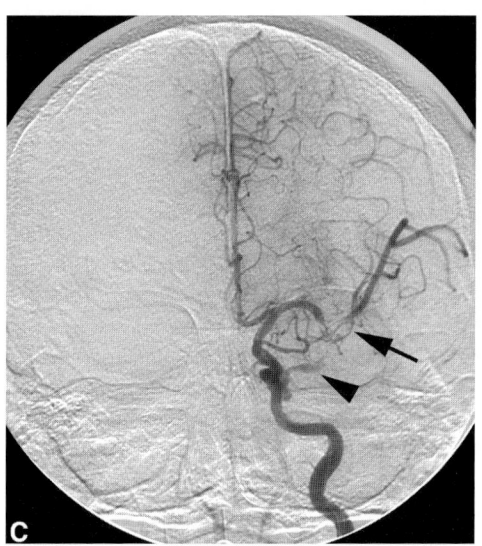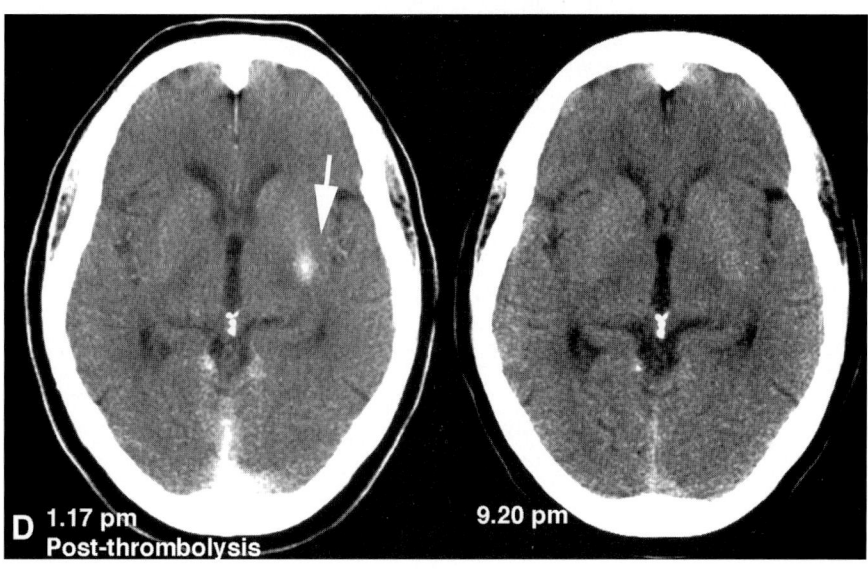

in) will allow one maximal flexibility for insertion of additional necessary devices as a case progresses.

Mechanical Clot Disruption

In a patient with slow or ineffective response to intraarterial thrombolytic agents, or in whom one has a concern for minimizing the dose of thrombolytic agent, clot disruption and fragmentation aimed at increasing the surface area of clot exposed to the thrombolytic agent can be very effective (Fig. 13.4). This can be accomplished with a number of devices.

Balloons

Soft compliant balloons such as the Endeavor balloon (Boston Scientific) or wire-directed balloons such as the Commodore (Cordis), Sentry (Target), or Equinox (MTI) can be inserted via a 6 Fr introducer catheter and used to fragment clot within the internal carotid artery, basilar artery, or even the middle cerebral artery. Coronary angioplasty balloons can be used for a similar purpose but are generally stiffer to use. Occasionally, it has been possible to pull the semi-inflated balloon back into the introducer catheter and extract the debris from the arterial circulation by evacuating the introducer catheter. All of these balloons have the potential to cause arterial dissection through overinflation or arterial rupture in the intradural circulation. Great care is necessary therefore in situations where one is performing this procedure blindly, i.e., where absence of flow prevents acquisition of a roadmap or a digital run to give one an advance knowledge of the arterial anatomy. Blindly inserted devices have a remarkable tendency to find the posterior inferior cerebellar artery, the anterior choroidal artery, or a posterior communicating artery. Even mild inflation of a balloon in these vessels can cause arterial rupture.

Wires

A microwire can be used fairly safely and effectively to probe and fragment intraluminal clot. Again, this

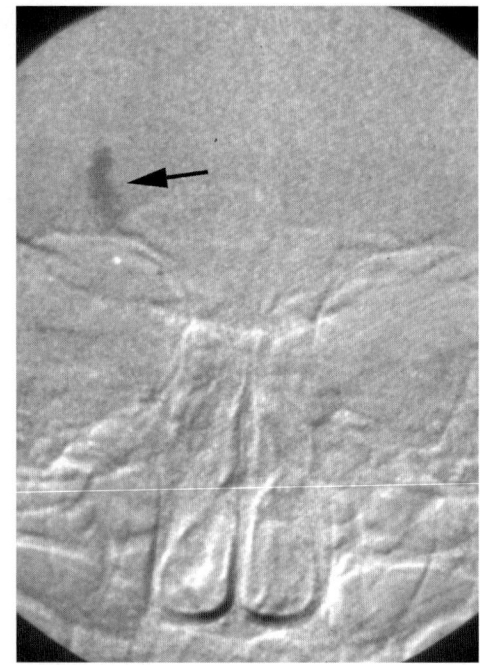

FIGURE 13.5 • *Extravasation of Contrast.*
A roadmap image during middle cerebral artery thrombolysis indicates free extravascular flow of contrast from the tip of the microcatheter into the basal ganglia. It is important to be aware of the potential for intracranial perforation of the delicate cerebral arteries in all cases. When an occlusion prevents roadmap outlining of the vessel to be navigated, a rounded J curve on the wire is the safest way of probing the arterial lumen.

procedure when necessary is performed without having the benefit of being able to perform a roadmap or run of the targeted vessel. Therefore probing the clot with the wire must be gentle to avoid the risk of arterial perforation or dissection (Fig. 13.5). It is probably most safely performed with a generous J curve at the tip. This will prevent inadvertent selection of minor side-branches of the internal carotid artery (typically a blindly inserted microwire will unfailing find the ophthalmic artery, posterior communicating artery, and anterior choroidal artery, in that order). A tortuous basilar artery can also be very difficult to catheterize blindly with a mildly curved microwire. By forming a generous J on the microwire, one has the best chance of staying within the main arterial lumen. By working the J back and forth within the thrombosed segment of vessel, effective fragmentation of the clot can be accomplished. In the event of discovery of an intracranial stenosis, however, crossing the stenosis will be difficult and inadvisable with a J-curve. Reshaping or replacement of the wire will be necessary.

Microcatheter

Passing the microcatheter over the wire on multiple occasions through the area of thrombosis can be effective at clot fragmentation and may help in the formation of channels within the thrombus. An additional technique that may be effective is to inject heparinized saline into the clot at high speed with a 1-ml syringe. As long as the microcatheter is not wedged in a small branch, this maneuver is very unlikely to cause arterial harm and may be effective at lysing clot.

Snares

Snare devices (Microvena, Target) are available which involve a microcatheter shaft and a microwire fashioned into a loop that can be tightened. Occasionally, a snare trawled repeatedly through the clot can be very effective in breaking it up. Some operators have even been able to extract intact emboli of established hard clot in this manner when they identified that the clot was not responding to acute fibrinolysis.

Rheolytic Devices

Several companies are developing catheter systems that involve a high-velocity jet of saline at the tip directed back into the shaft of the catheter. The Venturi effect of the jet generates a suction effect at the tip, which causes thrombus to be drawn toward and macerated by the high-speed saline jet. Such devices are already in use in the coronary field and have potential to be used effectively in the treatment of arterial and venous thrombotic disease.[16,17]

EMERGENCY ANGIOPLASTY AND STENT PLACEMENT

Discovery of a critical extracranial or intracranial stenosis during the course of a thrombolytic ther-

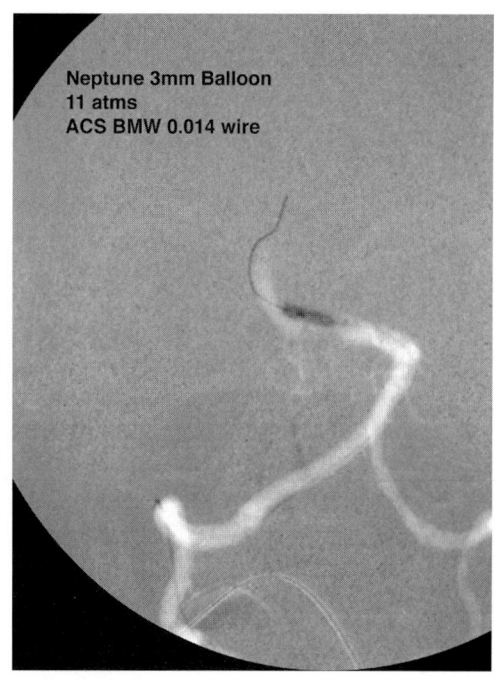

FIGURE 13.6 • *Impromptu Angioplasty during Emergency Thrombolysis I.*
This patient described in Fig. 1.2 presented with complete basilar thrombosis. After failure of sustained improvement following urokinase, he responded finally to administration of abciximab and a balloon angioplasty of the lower basilar artery. A Neptune 3-mm balloon (Bard) was inflated to 11 atm over an ACS Balance Middle Weight 0.014-in wire with excellent results (see Fig. 1.2D).

apy is fairly common (Figs. 13.6, 13.7). In the past, there was a reluctance to treat such lesions acutely, mostly due to inexperience and a perception that such treatment amplified the procedural risks for a particular patient. However, it is likely that refraining from such impromptu definitive revascularization at the time of thrombolysis is a mistake and that angioplasty can be performed with a reasonable risk.[18] Commonly, in the setting of critical occlusive lesions, acute or subacute reaccumulation of thrombus occurs and causes an immediate downturn in the fortunes of a patient who might otherwise do well.

One should therefore not be hesitant to perform an extempore angioplasty or even stent placement

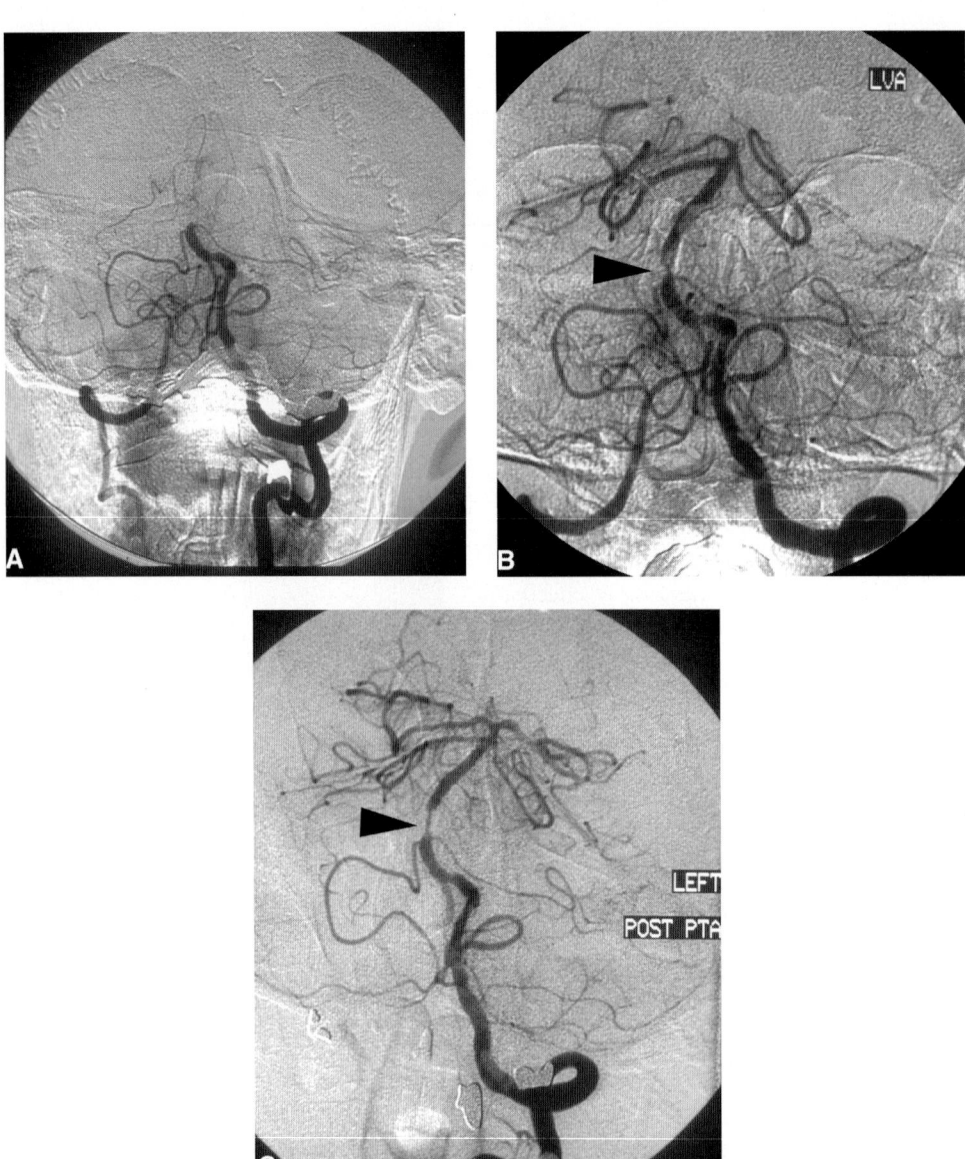

FIGURE 13.7 • *Angioplasty during Emergency Thrombolysis II.*
An elderly patient presenting with basilar thrombosis above the level of the anterior inferior cerebellar arteries (A, left vertebral artery injection, Caldwell projection) was treated with 1 million units of urokinase intraarterially. He demonstrated persistent clot above a severe basilar stenosis (arrowhead in B, post-urokinase). Even a very timid angioplasty using a 2-mm Fastealth balloon (Target) was sufficient to improve flow considerably and contribute to dissolution of the remaining clot (C, post PTA). This case dates from some time ago. Now administration of GPIIb/IIIa inhibitors in association with more robust angioplasty and probable stent placement in the stenosis would constitute a better level of care for this patient.

in acute stroke patients following the guidelines described in Chapters 4 and 5. Specific considerations in the acute emergency setting dwell on the absence of premedication with antiplatelet agents. Intravenous aspirin is available in some countries and can be used at such a juncture. If a stent is necessary to maintain vessel patency, the complication of acute stent thrombosis can be monitored angiographically. Occasionally heparinization can be adequate to prevent acute thrombosis, and the patient can be started on antiplatelet agents after the procedure with a loading dose of 300–450 mg of clopidogrel with aspirin. However, typically one is attempting to avoid simultaneous use of heavy heparinization and thrombolytic agents, and an alternative to consider involves use of the GPIIb/IIIa inhibitor agents (Fig. 1.2). Eptifibatide and tirofiban may be slightly less potent and thus slightly less likely to cause hemorrhagic intracranial complications in the setting of acute stroke than abciximab, although this is conjectural. Experience with abciximab in the setting of acute infarcts has been so far very favorable and free of hemorrhagic complications.[19] An additional advantage of these agents in the setting of acute thrombolysis or acute in-stent thrombosis is that part of the loading bolus can be delivered very effectively via a microcatheter directly into the stent or thrombus.

Contraindications to Intraarterial Thrombolysis

Contraindications to treatment of a devastating illness such as stroke are relative. Before throwing in the towel on a stroke patient because of a contraindication listed on a drug advisory sheet, alternatives might be considered.

- *Established neurological damage.* Clearly, large established areas of infarction, cerebral hemorrhage, or cerebral edema represent contraindications to use of thrombolytic agents, but perhaps mechanical clot disruption or extraction might still be a consideration to reduce the likelihood of further loss of tissue.

- *Recent surgery or trauma.* The risk of bleeding from thrombolytic agents or GPIIb/IIIa inhibitors in the setting of recent surgery or tissue trauma is probably overemphasized by sources concerned with liability and regulatory compliance. For individual patients calculated risks can be taken with fully informed family consent. For such patients a heavy procedural emphasis on clot disruption and minimization of the dose of thrombolytic agent is prudent. Common sense is always a more useful guide than published lists of contraindications or guidelines.

- *Pregnancy and other "absolute" contraindications.* Particularly in the setting of a posterior circulation occlusive lesion where established mortality rates approach 100%, it is difficult to rationalize withholding treatment for a patient who has not yet reached a point of obviously irreversible decline. Short of this, all absolute contraindications become relative, even pregnancy. However, a cautionary note to remember in discussing the procedural consent with family members of all patients with posterior circulation difficulties is the possibility of severely impaired neurologic outcome and a virtual or actual "locked-in" syndrome as an outcome. Probably most if not all patients and families would consider this a worse outcome than death.

References

1. Zivin JA (1998) Factors determining the therapeutic window for stroke. *Neurology* 50:599–603.
2. Zivin JA (1999) Thrombolytic stroke therapy: past, present, and future. *Neurology* 53:14–19.
3. Hacke W, Kaste M, Fieschi C, von Kummer R, Davalos A, Meier D, Larrue V, Bluhmki E, Davis S, Donnan G, Schneider D, Diez-Tejedor E, Trouillas P (1998) Randomised double-blind placebo-controlled trial of thrombolytic therapy with intravenous alteplase in acute ischaemic stroke (ECASS II). Second European-Australasian Acute Stroke Study Investigators. *Lancet* 352:1245–1251.
4. Anonymous (1995) Tissue plasminogen activator for acute ischemic stroke. The National Institute of Neurological Disorders and Stroke rt-PA Stroke Study Group. *N Engl J Med* 333:1581–1587.
5. Clark WM, Albers GW (1999) The Atlantis rt-PA (Alteplase) Acute Stroke Trial: final results. *Stroke* 30:234.

6. EDWARDS MT, MURPHY MM, GERAGHTY JJ, WULF JA, KONZEN JP (1999) Intraarterial cerebral thrombolysis for acute ischemic stroke in a community hospital. *AJNR* 20:1682–1687.
7. FURLAN A, HIGASHIDA R, WECHSLER L, GENT M, ROWLEY H, KASE C, PESSIN M, AHUJA A, CALLAHAN F, CLARK WM, SILVER F, RIVERA F (1999) Intra-arterial prourokinase for acute ischemic stroke. The PROACT II study: a randomized controlled trial. *JAMA* 282:2011.
8. DEL ZOPPO GJ, HIGASHIDA RT, FURLAN AJ, PESSIN MS, ROWLEY HA, GENT M (1998) PROACT: a phase II randomized trial of recombinant pro-urokinase by direct arterial delivery in acute middle cerebral artery stroke. PROACT Investigators. Prolyse in Acute Cerebral Thromboembolism. *Stroke* 29:4–11.
9. GÖNNER F, REMONDA L, MATTLE H, STURZENEGGER M, OZDOBA C, LÖVBLAD KO, BAUMGARTNER R, BASSETTI C, SCHROTH G (1998) Local intra-arterial thrombolysis in acute ischemic stroke. *Stroke* 29:1894–1900.
10. JAHAN R, GOBIN YP, GLENN B, DUCKWILER GR, VINUELA F (1998) Transvenous embolization of a dural arteriovenous fistula of the cavernous sinus through the contralateral pterygoid plexus. *Neuroradiology* 40:189–193.
11. ANONYMOUS (1997) Intracerebral hemorrhage after intravenous t-PA therapy for ischemic stroke. The NINDS t-PA Stroke Study Group. *Stroke* 28:2109–2118.
12. VON KUMMER R, BOZZAO L, BASTIANELLO S, MANELFE C (1997) Extent of ischemic brain edema and the response to plasminogen activators in acute hemispheric stroke. *Stroke* 28:270.
13. TOMSICK T, BROTT T, BARSAN W, BRODERICK J, HALEY EC, SPILKER J, KHOURY J (1996) Prognostic value of the hyperdense middle cerebral artery sign and stroke scale score before ultraearly thrombolytic therapy. *AJNR* 17:79–85.
14. LEWANDOWSKI CA, FRANKEL M, TOMSICK TA, BRODERICK J, FREY J, CLARK W, STARKMAN S, GROTTA J, SPILKER J, KHORY J, BROTT T (1999) Combined intravenous and intraarterial r-TPA versus intraarterial therapy of acute ischemia stroke: Emergency Management of Stroke (EMS) Bridging Trial. *Stroke* 30:2598–2605.
15. QURESHI AI, SURI FK, SHATLA AA, RINGER AJ, FESSLER RD, ALI Z, GUTERMAN LR, HOPKINS LN (2000) Intraarterial recombinant tissue plasminogen activator for ischemic stroke: an accelerating dosing regimen. *Neurosurgery* 47:473–479.
16. OPATOWSKY MJ, MORRIS PP, REGAN JD, MEWBORNE JD, WILSON JA (1999) Rapid thrombectomy of superior sagittal sinus and transverse sinus thrombosis with a rheolytic catheter device. *AJNR* 20:414–417.
17. DOWD CF, MALEK AM, PHATOUROS CC, HEMPHILL JC 3RD (1999) Application of a rheolytic thrombectomy device in the treatment of dural sinus thrombosis: a new technique. *AJNR* 20:568–570.
18. NAKAYAMA T, TANAKA K, KANEKO M, YOKOYAMA T, UEMURA K (1998) Thrombolysis and angioplasty for acute occlusion of intracranial vertebrobasilar arteries. Report of three cases. *J Neurosurg* 88:919–922.
19. THE ABCIXIMAB IN ISCHEMIC STROKE INVESTIGATORS (2000) Abciximab in Acute Ischemic Stroke. A randomized, double-blind, placebo-controlled, dose-escalation study. *Stroke* 31:601–609.

Chapter 14

Venous Thrombotic Disease

CEREBRAL VENOUS THROMBOSIS is associated with a variety of systemic illnesses, sepsis, pregnancy, coagulation defects, and autoimmune states. Deficiencies of antithrombin III, protein C, protein S, and factor V Leiden, or an increase in anticardiolipin A antibodies may be identified in patients with this disorder, but a precise pathogenesis may not be identifiable in 25% to 35% of patients.[1] The disease is frequently overlooked clinically and on CT imaging, in part due to a low clinical suspicion of the disease stemming from its ability to simulate the clinical appearance of benign intracranial hypertension, neoplasms, encephalitis, or cerebrovascular accident.[2] However, MRI with contrast, MR venography, and CT angiography all enhance reader sensitivity to this disease. The prognosis of the disease is unpredictable and variable. Mortality rates up to 33% can be reported depending on the underlying disease state and the presence or absence of hemorrhagic venous infarcts.[3]

Endovascular techniques offer the potential for direct pharmacological and physical dissolution of venous clot in the dural sinuses (Fig. 14.1). Several techniques have been used successfully including:

- Instillation of urokinase or t-PA via a microcatheter in acute doses equivalent to intraarterial cerebral thrombolysis, or in a prolonged infusion with an indwelling microcatheter similar to that used for peripheral arterial thrombolysis.[4–13] Access to the dural sinuses is usually gained from a transfemoral approach, but occasionally a direct retrograde internal jugular stick has been used. Even direct puncture of the anterior cranial fontanelle in infants with a 21G needle for prolonged instillation of urokinase has been performed safely by Higashida et al.[14]
- Clot extraction with a snare.[4,15]
- Clot fragmentation with a rheolytic catheter device.[16–18] Several catheter devices are in development which use the Venturi effect generated by a jet of high-pressure saline to attract and fragment nearby clot. Due to the absence of moving parts the likelihood of tissue damage from these devices should be low, although their safety and efficacy for treatment of cerebral arterial and venous thrombosis are yet to be demonstrated (Fig. 14.2).[19–21]
- Clot fragmentation with coronary angioplasty balloons or other balloons (Fig. 14.3).[22]

The angiographic and clinical success of these techniques in published case series has been generally good, with most patients making a successful recovery and with few reports of hemorrhagic com-

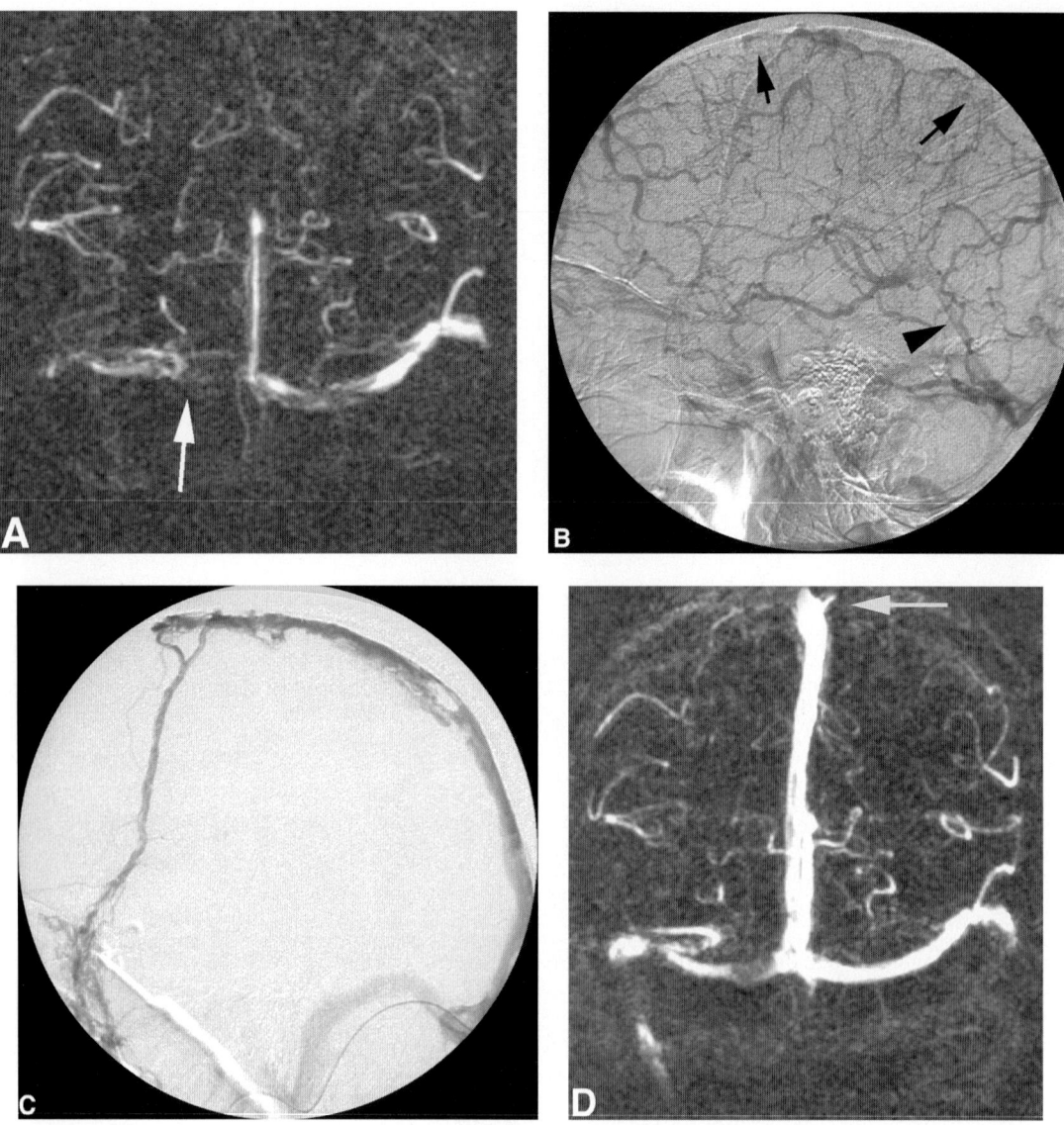

FIGURE 14.1 • *Combined Thrombolytic and Mechanical Clot Disruption of Dural Sinus Thrombosis.* An MRV phase-contrast study of the brain (A) in a 67-year-old female demonstrates absence of detectable flow in the superior sagittal sinus and attenuation of flow in the right transverse sinus (arrow). The venous phase of the right carotid angiogram (B, lateral view) shows absence of opacification of the superior sagittal sinus (arrows) and poor flow in the straight sinus (arrowhead). The venous field throughout the right hemisphere is disordered with late congestion of vessels and generalized poor outflow.

After a combination of thrombolytic therapy with urokinase delivered directly into the sinuses via a microcatheter and clot fragmentation with the Angiojet catheter (Possis) and coronary angioplasty balloons, a venogram (C, lateral view) shows the much improved appearance of the cleared venous sinus. With continued anticoagulation following the endovascular treatment, her clinical condition improved and an MRV done 2 days later (D) shows resumption of flow in the superior sagittal sinus (arrow) and improved flow in the right transverse sinus.

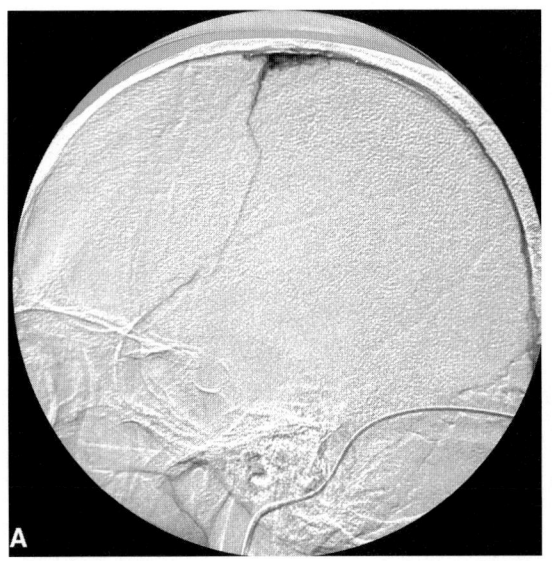 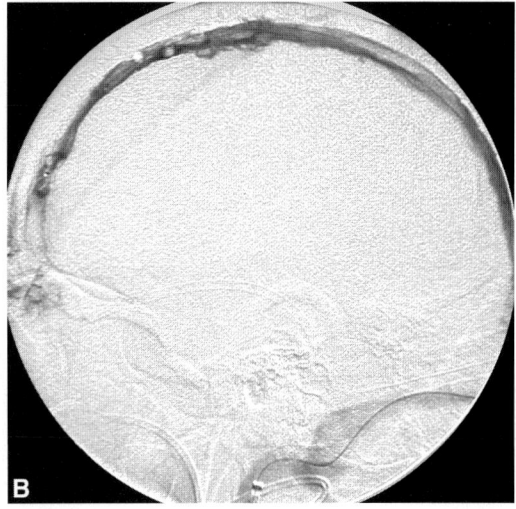

FIGURE 14.2 • *Efficacy of Rheolytic Clot Fragmentation.*
A venogram of a thrombosed superior sagittal sinus (A, lateral view) after infusion of 600,000 units of urokinase shows resumption of antegrade flow down the sinus, but the channel is narrow and slow. Immediately after passage of a rheolytic catheter through the right transverse sinus and superior sagittal sinus, rapid antegrade flow is evident with substantial fragmentation of the clot (B).

plications following thrombolysis. However, these reports are not randomized studies, and selection criteria for patients treated in this manner are variable from one hospital to another and from one occasion to another. Heparinization of patients with dural sinus thrombosis has been reported to have an 80% favorable outcome with very low mortality compared with only a 10% favorable outcome and 30% mortality with placebo therapy,[23] but such favorable results are not consistently seen.[24] The question of endovascular treatment of venous thrombotic disease usually arises when patients on anticoagulant therapy have exacerbation of clinical symptoms or imaging signs of worsening disease or intracranial hemorrhage.

Indications for Endovascular Treatment

Venous infarcts with or without hemorrhagic transformation or neurologic decline with propagation of clot despite heparinization, or development of cerebral venous hypertension and edema are commonly seen in acutely ill patients. In these patients continuing systemic anticoagulation may be manifestly ineffective or contraindicated. Other incidental contraindications to systemic anticoagulation may be present. In such patients it is justifiable to consider endovascular treatment, even in the setting of cerebral hemorrhage.[25] Alternatively, endovascular treatment might be justifiable at the time of initial presentation in a patient who is neurologically intact but who has an overwhelming burden of sinus thrombus or thrombosis of the deep venous system.

The point has been made by Dowd et al.[17] that a potentially critical difference in treatment philosophy may be necessary in the endovascular treatment of venous thrombotic disease compared with arterial thromboembolic disease. The large volume of clot contained within the thrombosed dural sinuses in such patients is several orders of magnitude greater than that encountered during transarterial thrombolytic interventions. Dose limitations on thrombolytic drugs prevent a corresponding magnification of the dose used in arterial

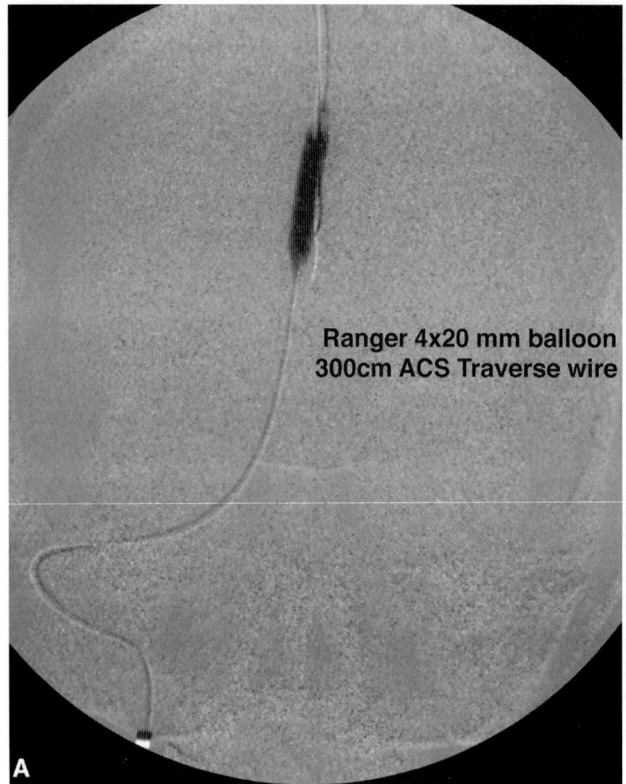
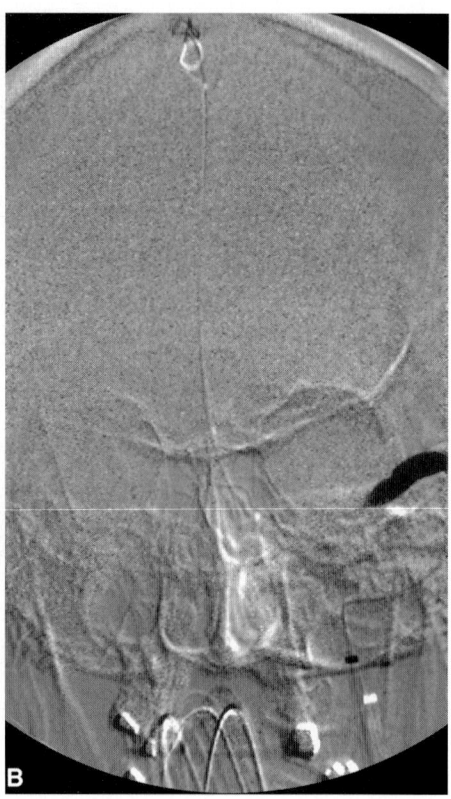

FIGURE 14.3 • *Use of Coronary Wire-Directed Balloons in the Dural Sinuses.*
In a patient with extensive dural sinus thrombosis a 4-mm Ranger balloon catheter was passed easily over a 0.014-in wire to the anterior aspect of the superior sagittal sinus (A) and dragged back through the clot into the right transverse sinus. To relieve the left transverse sinus, the left jugular vein was catheterized (B) and the process repeated on that side.

cases. Therefore the possibility of mechanical fragmentation or extraction of clot from the dural sinuses has attracted some attention using either extraction snares[4,15] or rheolytic catheters.[16,17]

TECHNIQUES

Experience with the endovascular treatment of cerebral venous thrombosis is limited to a small number of case reports and case series. However, the published results of treatment are almost uniformly encouraging for the safety and efficacy of these techniques. Generally, a transarterial angiogram is helpful to confirm the diagnosis and to evaluate the severity of venous hypertension. It may be better, however, to avoid an arterial puncture completely. The diagnosis of venous thrombosis can be made noninvasively with CT or MR imaging, and the need for anticoagulant therapy in this group of patients can mean that an arteriotomy site becomes an otiose undertaking resulting in avoidable complications.

- Transvenous access to the jugular bulb is gained by a transfemoral approach or by a direct jugular stick.[22] The right transverse sinus is larger in most patients and represents a more direct route of intracranial passage, regardless of whether it is involved with the disease or not.
- The intracranial navigation of the microwire is usually most safely and most easily performed by allowing the wire to prolapse into a wide J shape

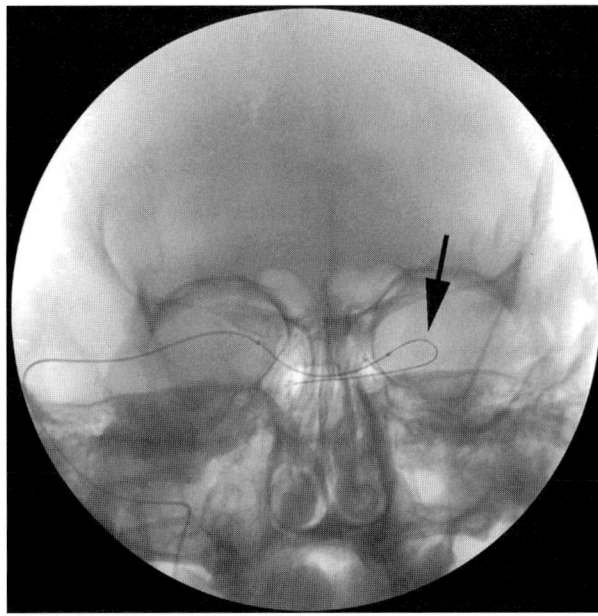

FIGURE 14.4 • An image of the left transverse sinus being catheterized from the right with a microcatheter. The generous curve on the tip of the leading wire is the best assurance of avoiding inadvertent probing and injury of a parenchymal vein. A two-marker microcatheter was inadvertently opened, but this had no impact on the case.

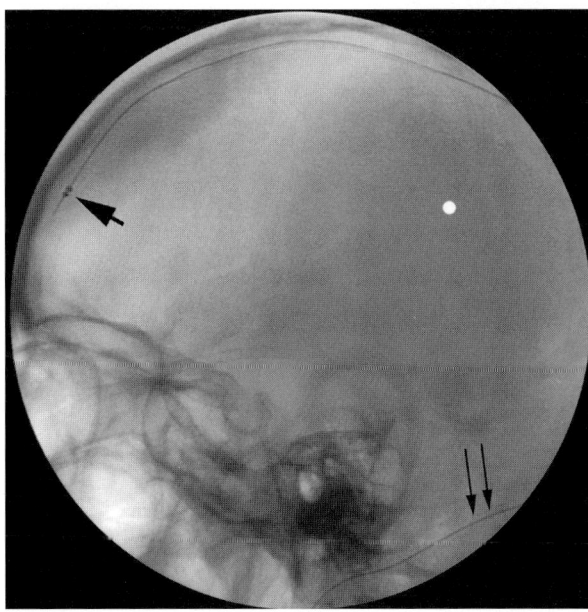

FIGURE 14.5 • An image of the Angiojet 5 Fr rheolytic catheter in the superior sagittal sinus (arrow). The relatively straight course of the right sigmoid sinus (double arrow) in this patient was the main factor that determined the technical feasibility of this procedure.

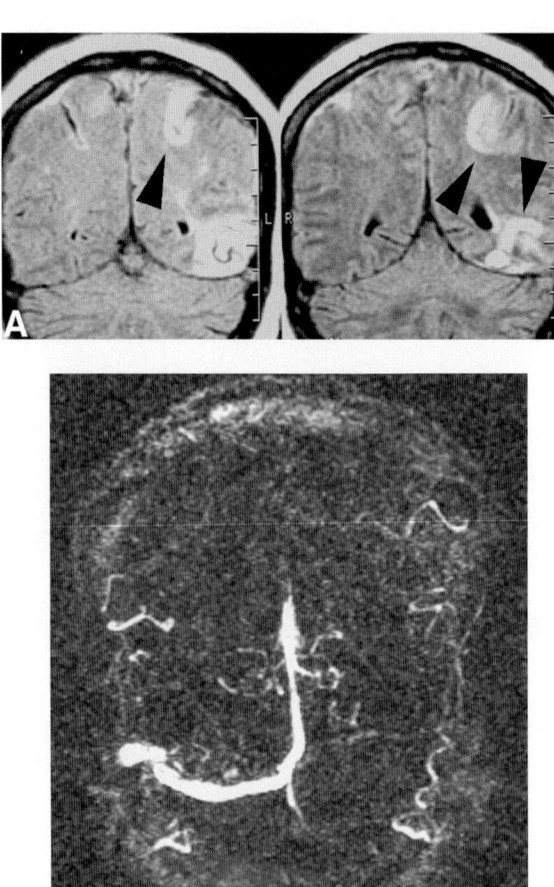

FIGURE 14.6 • *Dural Sinus Thrombosis I.*
A 67-year-old female presenting with extensive dural sinus thrombosis deteriorated clinically despite heparinization. An MRI examination confirmed the diagnosis and demonstrated venous infarctions in multiple locations (arrowheads in A, FLAIR images). A phase contrast MRV (B) showed venous flow in the straight sinus and right transverse sinus only. A lateral view venogram (C) performed via a microcatheter in the superior sagittal sinus shows the absence of normal antegrade drainage of contrast. The patient was treated with a combination of infusion of urokinase into the dural sinuses, balloon angioplasty of the clot, and passage of the Angiojet rheolytic catheter (D, lateral view).

Following treatment, a venogram demonstrates the improved flow in the sinuses (E, lateral view). The patient's clinical course improved immediately with continuation of anticoagulation.

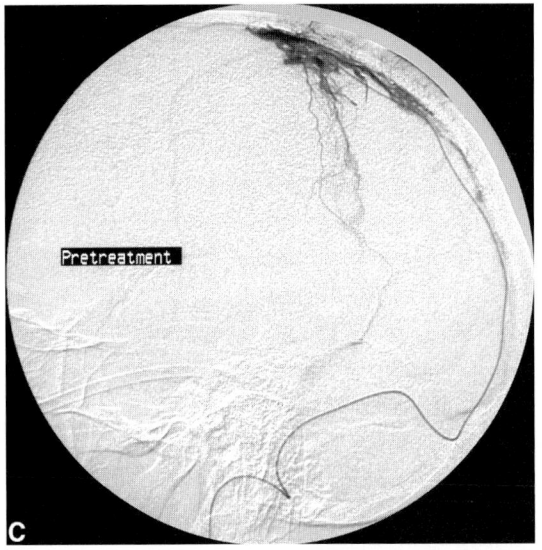
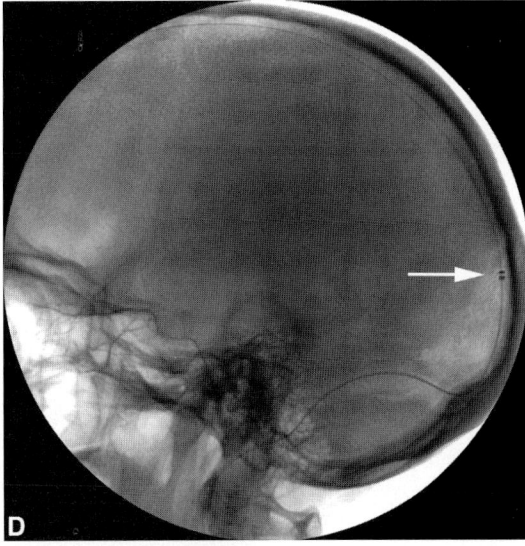
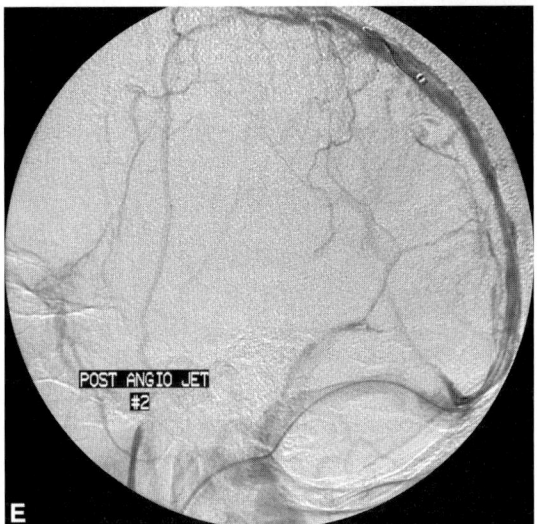

(Fig. 14.4). This will serve to cleave the fresh clot within the sinus while advancing the wire, and will also prevent inadvertent blind selection of a small parenchymal vein ostium opening into the sinus.
- The 5 Fr version of the Angiojet Rheolytic device (Possis) is stiff compared with standard microcatheters. To avoid buckling into the right atrium during advancement, it can be helpful from a transfemoral approach to place a 90-cm 7 Fr sheath with a coaxial 90- to 100-cm 7 Fr catheter (Figs. 14.5–14.7). The combined stiffness of the two coaxial introducer devices gives greater support. Any coronary 300-cm 0.014-in wire at the floppy end of the spectrum can be used to guide the Angiojet catheter.
- Generally, it is straightforward to advance a microwire and microcatheter into the superior sagittal sinus from the region of the torcular. However, when working in the AP plane, it is easy to mistake the progress of the wire as being in the superior sagittal sinus when, in fact, the straight sinus has been catheterized. Therefore, unless one is specifically interested in the deep venous system with its inherent risk of greater vessel fragility

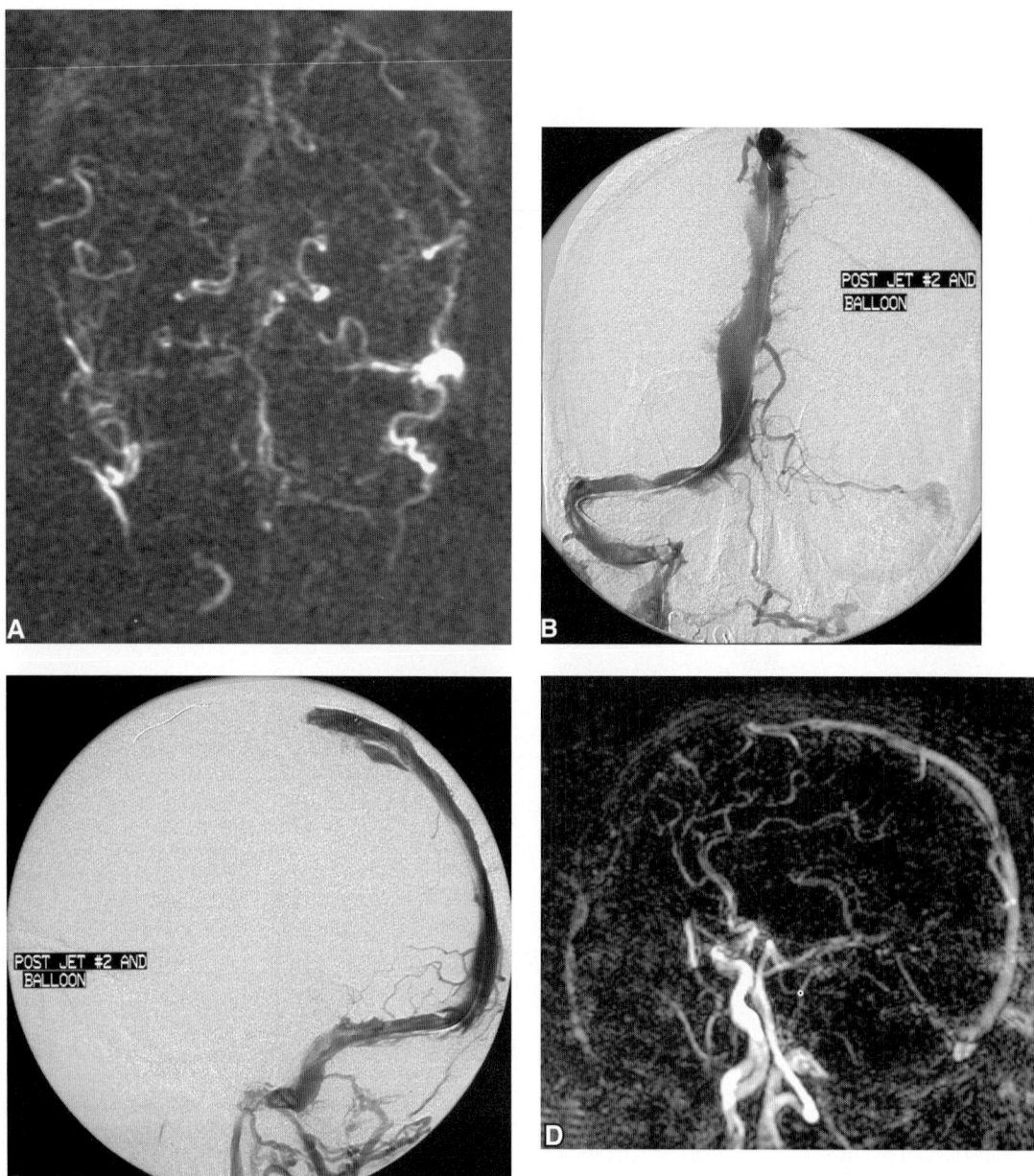

FIGURE 14.7 • *Dural Sinus Thrombosis II.*
A middle-age female patient presenting with extensive dural sinus thrombosis demonstrates almost complete absence of flow-signal in the dural sinuses on phase-contrast MRV (A, coronal projection). Venograms following treatment as in Fig. 14.6 show considerable improvement in antegrade flow in the AP (B) and lateral (C) projections. This improved venous flow is sustained on an MRV on the following day (D, sagittal projection).

compared with the dural sinuses, it is better to avoid this mistake, particularly with larger devices.

- Different infusion protocols of thrombolytic agents have been used involving either an acute high-dose infusion aimed at immediate resolution of thrombosis, or a slower prolonged infusion with a fixed hourly rate given over the course of 1–2 days. Both protocols appear to be effective. An acute infusion of up to a million units of urokinase has been given over 2–3 hours by some authors with resumption of antegrade flow and clinical recovery of the patient.[11] Alternatively, an acute bolus of 10 mg of t-PA was given by Kim et al. to nine patients with dural sinus thrombosis[9] followed by an infusion of 16 mg/hr for 3 hours and then 5 mg/hr until resolution of the thrombus was seen at 8–43 hours.

References

1. Deschiens MA, Conard J, Horellou MH, Ameri A, Preter M, Chedru F, Samama MM, Bousser MG (1996) Coagulation studies, factor V Leiden, and anticardiolipin antibodies in 40 cases of cerebral venous thrombosis. Stroke 27:1724–1730.
2. Ameri A, Bousser MG (1994) Cerebral venous thrombosis: clinical diagnosis. Annales de Radiologie 37:101–107.
3. Cantú C, Barinagarrementaria F (1993) Cerebral venous thrombosis associated with pregnancy and puerperium. Stroke 24:1880–1884.
4. Philips MF, Bagley LJ, Sinson GP, Raps EC, Galetta SL, Zager EL, Hurst RW (1999) Endovascular thrombolysis for symptomatic cerebral venous thrombosis. J Neurosurg 90:65–71.
5. Barnwell SL, Higashida RT, Halbach VV, Dowd CF, Hieshima GB (1991) Direct endovascular thrombolytic therapy for dural sinus thrombosis. Neurosurgery 28:135–142.
6. Barnwell SL, Clark WM, Nguyen TT (1994) Safety and efficacy of delayed intraarterial urokinase therapy with mechanical clot disruption for thromboembolic stroke. AJNR 15:1817–1822.
7. Holder CA, Bell DA, Lundell AL, Ulmer JL, Glazier SS (1997) Isolated straight sinus and deep cerebral venous thrombosis: successful treatment with local infusion of urokinase. Case report. J Neurosurg 86:704–707.
8. Horowitz MB, Purdy P, Unwin H (1997) Treatment of dural sinus thrombosis using selective catheterization and urokinase. Ann Neurol 38:58–67.
9. Kim SY, Suh JH (1997) Direct endovascular thrombolytic therapy for dural sinus thrombosis: infusion of alteplase. AJNR 18:639–645.
10. Smith TP, Higashida RT, Barnwell SL, Halbach VV, Dowd CF, Fraser KW, Teitelbaum GP, Hieshima GB (1994) Treatment of dural sinus thrombosis by urokinase infusion. AJNR 15:801–807.
11. Spearman MP, Jungreis CA, Wehner JJ, Gerszten PC, Welch WC (1997) Endovascular thrombolysis in deep cerebral venous thrombosis. AJNR 18:502–506.
12. Tsai FY, Higashida RT, Matovich V, Alfieri K (1992) Acute thrombosis of the intracranial dural sinus: direct thrombolytic treatment. AJNR 13:1137–1141.
13. Frey JL, Muro GJ, McDougall CG, Dean BL, Jahnke HK (1999) Cerebral venous thrombosis. Combined intrathrombus tPA and intravenous heparin. Stroke 30:489–494.
14. Higashida RT, Helmer E, Halbach VV, Hieshima GB (1989) Direct thrombolytic therapy for superior sagittal sinus thrombosis. AJNR 10:S4–S6.
15. Bagley LJ, Hurst RW, Galetta S, Teener J, Sinson GP (1998) Use of a microsnare to aid direct thrombolytic therapy of dural sinus thrombosis. AJR 170:784–786.
16. Opatowsky MJ, Morris PP, Regan JD, Mewborne JD, Wilson JA (1999) Rapid thrombectomy of superior sagittal sinus and transverse sinus thrombosis with a rheolytic catheter device. AJNR 20:414–417.
17. Dowd CF, Malek AM, Phatouros CC, Hemphill JC 3rd (1999) Application of a rheolytic thrombectomy device in the treatment of dural sinus thrombosis: a new technique. AJNR 20:568–570.
18. Scarrow AM, Williams RL, Jungreis CA, Yonas H, Scarrow MR (1999) Removal of a thrombus from the sigmoid and transverse sinuses with a rheolytic thrombectomy catheter. AJNR 20:1467–1469.
19. Wagner HJ, Stefan MH, Pitton MB, Weiss W, Wess M (1997) Rapid thrombectomy with a hydrodynamic catheter: results from a prospective, multicenter trial. Radiology 205:675–681.
20. Sharafuddian MJA, Hicks ME, Jenson ML, Morris JE, Drasler WJ, Wison GJ (1997) Rheolytic thrombectomy with use of the Angiojet-F105 catheter: preclinical evaluation of safety. J Vasc Intervent Radiol 8:939–945.
21. Sharafuddin MJA, Hicks ME (1997) Current status of percutaneous mechanical thrombectomy, I. General Principles. J Vasc Intervent Radiol 8:911–921.
22. Novak Z, Coldwell DM, Brega KE (2000) Selective infusion of urokinase and thrombectomy in the treatment of acute cerebral sinus thrombosis. AJNR 21:143–145.
23. Einhäupl KM, Villringer A, Meister W (1991) Heparin treatment in sinus venous thrombosis. Lancet 338:597–600.
24. Preter M, Tzourio C, Ameri A (1996) Long-term prognosis in cerebral venous thrombosis. Follow up of 77 patients. Stroke 27:243–246.
25. Rael JR, Orrison WW Jr, Baldwin N, Sell J (1997) Direct thrombolysis of superior sagittal sinus thrombosis with coexisting intracranial hemorrhage. AJNR 18:1238–1242.

Chapter 15

Arteriovenous Malformations of the Brain

ARTERIOVENOUS MALFORMATIONS of the brain are uncommon disorders with a prevalence of <1%.[1,2] The incidence of asymptomatic AVMs in autopsy series is very small, and therefore it can be assumed that most or virtually all AVMs become symptomatic during a lifetime. An increased prevalence of AVMs is seen in certain conditions such as hereditary hemorrhagic teleangiectasia.[3] The morbidity and mortality associated with AVMs are primarily related to the propensity of these lesions to bleed spontaneously into the brain parenchyma or into the subarachnoid space. Other epiphenomena related to AVMs such as deep or cortical venous hypertension, arterial steal, or hydrocephalus are usually of lesser importance. Approximately half of AVMs present with intracranial hemorrhage,[4] with an initial mortality rate of approximately 10% and morbidity of 25% to 58%.[5,6] However, the prospects for meaningful recovery following intracranial hemorrhage from an AVM seem better than those following intracranial hemorrhage from other causes such as aneurysmal rupture or hypertension.[7]

The principal question posed by a newly diagnosed AVM is how best to treat it and how to advise the patient accordingly of his/her best interests.

The natural history of AVMs is thought to be that of an annual risk of hemorrhage of 2% to 4% per year[5,8,9] and an annual risk of mortality of 1% per year.[5] To calculate the remaining lifetime accumulated risk of hemorrhage from an AVM, the multiplicative law of probability can be invoked, assuming an annual rate of bleeding of 3%:

$$\text{Risk} = 1 - 0.97^{\text{expected years of remaining life}}$$

For instance, a 50-year-old with 25 years of remaining life expectancy does not have a 3% × 25 = 75% risk of bleeding at least once, but rather a calculated risk of 53%.[10] This method of calculation assumes that the risk of hemorrhage is uniform from year to year and not influenced by intercurrent symptomatology or a history of a recent bleed at the time of initial presentation. Some studies have suggested that in the first year following a spontaneous AVM hemorrhage, the risk of rebleeding may be as high as 6% to 17.9% initially, subsequently declining to baseline.[4,6,8,9] Similarly, patients presenting initially with seizure may be at a higher risk of subsequent hemorrhage compared with nonseizure and nonhemorrhagic patients.[9] However, other natural history studies have not observed a period of risk elevated above baseline following initial presentation with hemorrhage or otherwise.[5]

Risk Factors Predictive of Hemorrhage

Not all AVMs are the same, and it may be erroneous to apply the same rules of risk to all patients at any given point in their life. A prospective study by Mast et al.[4] of 281 symptomatic AVM patients presenting with and without hemorrhage observed an initial annual rate of hemorrhage of 2% in the nonhemorrhagic group following presentation. The symptomatic group who presented with hemorrhage, on the other hand, had an annual rate of hemorrhage of 17.8% following initial presentation.

The angiographic appearance of AVMs and other clinical features have been found in a number of studies to correlate with a higher risk of hemorrhage. Although inconsistent and contradictory observations are commonplace in the body of literature dealing with AVMs, the following risk factors of hemorrhage are frequently cited:

- Posterior fossa location with greater risk of mortality with hemorrhage.[9]
- Previous hemorrhage.[11]
- Deep venous drainage.[12–14]
- Intraventricular or periventricular locations.[13]
- High feeding artery pressure.[12,13,15]
- A single draining vein[11] or evidence of occlusive changes in the venous channel(s).[16,17]
- Small AVM size.[6,12] Spetzler et al.[15] demonstrated that small AVMs tend to have a higher perfusion pressure than nonhemorrhagic AVMs, providing a physiologic explanation for this observation. Follow-up studies suggest that small AVMs may have a 52% to 86% risk of hemorrhage compared with risks of 10% to 30% for larger AVMs.[6,18] However, in a 10-year follow-up study of 217 patients Crawford et al.,[8] on the other hand, thought that while small AVMs present most commonly with hemorrhage, the subsequent risk of hemorrhage for those patients was probably no greater than the rest of the AVM population.
- Intranidal or other aneurysms found in up to 58% of AVM patients.[13,14,19,20]
- Location in the basal ganglia.[13,14] Deep perforator locations may be exposed to a higher feeding mean arterial pressure, explaining this association.
- Diffuse morphology.[11] However, a different study showed that prominent angiomatous changes around an AVM nidus indicated a lower risk of hemorrhage.[13]
- Feeding by deep perforators.[14]
- Delay in time to peak arterial contrast opacification at angiography.[21]
- Male gender.[4]

Physiological Steal in the Vicinity of AVMs

Since the introduction of "cerebral steal" as a term to describe the effects of an AVM on the perfusion of surrounding brain parenchyma,[22] the concept has grown in scope to a broad understanding that surrounding brain may suffer from chronic hypoperfusion and anoxia due to the presence of the shunt through the AVM. The argument then goes that progressive neurologic injury occurs to the surrounding territories due to chronic hypoxia. However, this understanding has been challenged in recent work, at least as a common source of symptoms and deficits prior to treatment.[23,24] Mast et al.[24] found that progressive neurological deficits unrelated to hemorrhagic events were uncommon (<2%) in a prospective group of 152 AVM patients followed over a mean period of 17 months. Nonprogressive focal neurological deficits (7.2%) did not appear to correlate with any detectable alterations in physiologic flow parameters such as transcranial Doppler indices, intraarterial pressure of the feeding pedicles, or pulsatility indices. There is evidence that complete elimination of circulatory autoregulation in the vicinity of an AVM is probably rare or extremely rare. The state of physiology around an AVM is perhaps best characterized as having an autoregulatory shift to the left, so to maintain perfusion. Oxygen extraction fractions on positron emission tomography (PET)[25] and CO_2 responsiveness[26] remain normal in the vicinity of virtually all AVMs, even though the perfusion pressure (CPP) of the feeding arterial pedicles is reduced.[27] This suggests an adaptation on the part of local brain tissue to the reduced perfusion pressure with preservation of a capacity for autoregulation, and preservation of normal levels of cerebral blood flow (CBF) in most patients. Arterioles adjacent to AVMs retain a vasodilatory response to agents such as verapamil and papaverine but not to vasodilating agents that work via pathways mediated by nitric oxide such as nitroglycerin or sodium nitroprusside.[28]

Normal Perfusion Pressure Breakthrough

A corollary of the contentious paralysis of autoregulatory vasomotor tone in the region of AVMs is the hypothesis that sudden local increases in cerebral perfusion pressure following excision of an AVM account for brain swelling and hemorrhage seen in 2.3% to 15% of patients.[29,30] Large AVMs (>6 cm diameter) may have a postoperative incidence of this phenomenon of up to 50%, particularly in large AVMs centered on watershed or border zones.[30] This phenomenon is termed normal perfusion pressure breakthrough.[31]

Recent research suggests that the causes of this postoperative phenomenon are more complicated that a straightforward hyperperfusion of tissue lacking in autoregulatory capacity. The likelihood of a postoperative hyperemic complication is most closely correlated with global hemispheric changes in cerebral blood flow (CBF) rather than with changes in local perfusion pressure.[29,32] Meyer et al.[23] have hypothesized that patients with postoperative hyperperfusion complications may represent situations in which the compensation mechanisms in surrounding tissues have reached their limits, and being "exhausted" or extinguished are unable to cope with the postoperative changes in CPP. However, evidence suggests that the autoregulation in response to CO_2 around AVMs is intact prior and subsequent to AVM removal.

Global hemispheric cerebral blood flow parameters tend to be increased following resection of a moderate-sized or large AVM, but a simple pressure-passive response in CBF does not seem to be the case in these patients.[33] Therefore, rather than a simple state of vasomotor paralysis, a "shift to the left" of the cerebral autoregulatory curve plotting cerebral blood flow versus cerebral perfusion pressure may be the case with larger AVMs.[34] Other more subtle mechanisms through which increased cerebral perfusion pressures following treatment can cause hyperperfusion complications may include the effects of an excessive state of capillary recruitment or abnormal changes in pH causing tissue edema.[35] Alterations in the pulsatility index of AVM feeding vessels could have an influence on the postoperative physiology of blood flow not reflected in measurements of CPP or CBF.[33]

Microsurgical Treatment of Arteriovenous Malformations

Despite advances in embolization materials and radiosurgery techniques, complete microsurgical excision of an AVM remains the preferred standard of treatment for these lesions. The Spetzler-Martin Grading system[36] scores AVMs (I–VI) on the basis of:

- Size (<3cm = 1 point, 3–6 cm = 2 points, >6 cm = 3 points)
- Eloquence of surrounding brain (noneloquent = 0, eloquent = 1)
- Pattern of venous drainage (superficial = 0, deep = 1)

This simple scoring system has been applied retrospectively and prospectively and has been found to correlate with the risks of postoperative deficits in surgical resection of brain AVMs, either with or without preoperative embolization.[37] On the basis of this scoring system a postoperative death or deficit risk of <1% can be predicted for Grades I and II, <3% for Grade III, 31.2% (21.9% permanent) for Grade IV, and 50% (16.7% permanent) for Grade V. Advocates of this system suggest therefore that surgical treatment of AVMs for Grade IV and V patients is offered only when the patient is experiencing progressive neurological deficits or repeated hemorrhages. Grade VI AVMs are considered inoperable.

Large AVMs (>6 cm) represent a group of higher risk for postoperative edema and normal perfusion pressure hemorrhage, particularly when there are large shunts in the AVM with poor angiographic depiction of surrounding vessels, prominent feeders from the external carotid artery, and a history of progressive or fluctuating neurologic deficits.[38] Staged embolization of the AVM before surgery and careful monitoring of blood pressure after the embolization sessions and following surgery may help to reduce the risk of this complication. Using combined techniques of staged embolization and intraoperative angiographic control, Spetzler et al. were able to treat a series of 24 patients in this category with 92% success and <5% serious complication rates.[38]

In the case of AVMs in children, complete resection of the AVM seems to be the course most likely to restore the child to a normal life. There is evidence that the prognosis for AVMs that become symptomatic in childhood is worse than the case for adults, with higher rates of mortality and rebleeding. Posterior fossa AVMs in children have a mortality of 57%. An overall mortality of 25% was reported for childhood AVMs in all locations in a large Canadian series collected over 40 years.[39] Children in whom complete AVM resection was possible had a 67% rate of normal neurological outcome, and 73% were able to discontinue antiseizure medication. Partial resection of the AVM did not protect against the risk of subsequent rehemorrhage.

Radiotherapy for Arteriovenous Malformations of the Brain

The use of Cartesian coordinates in three dimensions for stereotactic intracranial surgery was described in 1908[40] and subsequently applied to use for intracranial targets.[41,42] Radiosurgery for brain AVMs is an important treatment alternative for some patients. It has specific risks, complications, and benefits, which need to be considered in advising patients on treatment decisions. In general the success rate with radiosurgery of AVMs is a balance between the need for an effective dose on one hand, and the risks of brain injury from higher doses on the other. In round figures a 100% obliteration rate can be expected for AVMs <1 cm diameter, an 88% or greater cure rate can be expected within 2 years of treatment for AVMs measuring less than 4 cm^3, and 58% for AVMs of 4–10 cm^3.[43,44]

A perfect realization of radiation therapy[45] would involve:

- Absolute congruence between the imaging abnormality and the pathologic abnormality (in this case the nidus of the AVM).
- An ability to delineate with absolute precision the targeted volume on the diagnostic images.
- Correspondence between the pathologic abnormality and the intended dose of radiation.
- Accuracy of delivery of the intended dose to the intended target.

The histologic effects of radiation therapy for AVMs are dose-related, and include endothelial proliferation, deposition of calcium and hyalinization in the vascular wall, and variable degrees of thrombosis, demyelination, gliosis, and necrosis. These changes progress over the course of up to 3 years following therapy.[46] The perfect treatment should have:

- No effects on normal tissue related to entrance dose.
- Conformity between the treated volume and the pathologic lesion.
- Rapid fall-off of dose to prevent collateral damage to normal tissues at the margin of the lesion.

The reality of radiation therapy for brain AVMs falls somewhat short of the ideal, and injury to surrounding tissue can be seen on CT or MRI in >27% of patients.[47] Clinically detectable side effects of radiation are seen in a smaller percentage of patients and can be seen 5 years or later following treatment. They are more likely to resolve in patients presenting with seizure, headache, or without hemorrhage.[48]

There are three modalities of stereotactic radiation therapy in use for brain AVMs:

- Proton and Helium Ion Beam Therapy
- Linear Accelerator Radiosurgery (LINAC)
- Gamma Knife Radiosurgery

Proton and Helium Ion Beam Therapy

Accelerated particles generated in a cyclotron are directed linearly in collimated beams from multiple directions toward the targeted lesion. The rate of energy loss from the beam to traversed tissue is initially very small, being inversely proportional to the square of the proton's velocity. With gradual energy loss over the trajectory of the particle, a critical diminution of velocity occurs to a point where the residual energy of the particle is suddenly lost in a small volume of surrounding tissue. This phenomenon is termed the *Bragg peak*. By estimating the attenuating characteristics of the interposed normal tissue and the depth of the targeted lesion, a calculation can be made of the beam characteristics necessary to superimpose the Bragg peak of the beam on the lesion. The size of the territory covered by the Bragg peak of a beam of monoenergetic particles is very small. Therefore, for lesions other than the smallest targets, a modulated beam is necessary to spread out the Bragg peak effects. The advantages of proton beam therapy over other forms of radiation therapy are the negligible size of the exit dose distal to the Bragg peak and the relatively low entrance dose for a single beam. A major disadvantage of this mode of treatment is cost and availability.

Radiation doses from proton beam therapy are usually quoted in terms of biologic effectiveness compared with a reference value of 1 for gamma irradiation from a Cobalt 60 source. The relative biologic effectiveness (RBE) of proton beam therapy compared with Cobalt 60 is usually taken between 1.1 and 1.25, and doses for proton beam therapy are reported in units of *Cobalt Gray Equivalent (CGE)*.

Much of the early data on the efficacy of proton beam therapy is based on the work of Kjellberg, who treated a large variety of intracranial tumors and AVMs between 1961 and 1993 using single-fraction proton radiosurgery. The results from this work were variable with overall 2-year AVM obliteration rates of 20%. Lesions <3 cm in size showed a 2-year complete obliteration rate of 42%. Lesions >3 cm had a complete 2-year obliteration rate of <6%.[49] Using helium ion Bragg peak therapy for patients with AVMs of poor surgical risk, Steinberg et al.[50] had a 2-year obliteration rate of 94% for lesions <4 cm^3, 75% for lesions measuring 4–25 cm^3, and 39% for lesions >25 cm^3. Doses used were scaled down over time from 35 Gy initially to 7.7–19.2 Gy because of dose-related complications (50% complication rates in patients treated with >18 Gy). The current protocol for AVM treatment using proton beam therapy at the Massachusetts General Hospital uses a dose of approximately 15 CGE to the 90% isodose line for AVMs <15 cm^3. Larger AVMs are treated with a lower-dose fractionated protocol over a period of some weeks.[45]

As is the case for other modalities of radiation therapy for brain AVMs, a major disadvantage of this form of therapy is the lack of protection from AVM hemorrhage during the 2-year period following treatment before complete obliteration may occur. There is even some disputed evidence that the risk of hemorrhage may be increased above baseline during this time, 7% to 14%, possibly due to changes in outflow resistance during obliteration.[50,51] Even though recent studies of radiosurgery for AVMs indicate an unchanged risk or an early protective effect from hemorrhage,[52,53] the consideration of hemorrhage during the period of waiting, the potential for radiation-related damage to normal tissue, and overall expense mean that for the present radiation therapy is generally recommended only for AVMs of high surgical risk.[54]

Linear Accelerator Radiosurgery (LINAC) for Brain AVMs

In LINAC radiosurgery multiple arcs of collimated X-ray beams are described sequentially through the patient's head. The patient's head is moved after each gantry rotation, so that multiple non-coplanar arcs of radiation deliver a high dose of energy to the target volume with minimal exposure of the surrounding tissue.[55] LINAC therapy for AVMs has been reported to have a 2-year obliteration rate between 55% and 94% depending on the dose (ranges 10–50 Gy) and size of the AVM.[56–59] Complication rates between 2% and 10% with a dose-related effect have been reported.[60]

Gamma Knife Radiosurgery

The first human neurosurgical use of stereotactically targeted gamma irradiation was in 1968.[42] Using Cobalt 60 as a source of gamma irradiation, modern units use up to 201 sources mounted in a pseudohemispherical array so that all sources can be focused on a single isocenter at 55 cm from the sources.[60] Experience using the gamma knife for treatment of small AVMs has been favorable, with obliteration rates of >74% reported by Pollock et al.[61–63] Modern use of the gamma knife for AVM radiosurgery involves a treatment-planning angiogram performed while the patient wears a radiolucent headframe bearing localization markers, which then allow for accurate targeting.[64] Because of a linear distortion image-intensifier artifact inherent in digital-subtraction angiography, a correction algorithm is necessary to filter the images before targeting is performed.

EMBOLIZATION THERAPY FOR BRAIN ARTERIOVENOUS MALFORMATIONS

The purpose of treatment of an AVM is the prevention of future hemorrhage. Generally, the understanding of AVMs is that complete obliteration of the AVM is necessary to achieve this. The role of embolization of a brain AVM includes:

- Preoperative reduction of flow within the AVM to enhance the safety and feasibility of subsequent microsurgical resection.
- Reduction in size of the nidus to improve the safety of radiotherapy.
- Occlusion of an obvious site of recent bleeding such as an intranidal or feeding pedicle aneurysm. When there is clinical or angiographic evidence that an aneurysm is the site of bleeding, this should be the primary focus of the embolization. This may mean coil embolization of a proximal aneurysm near the Circle of Willis, coil occlusion of the parent artery at or near the site of the aneurysm, or obliteration of the entire pedicle with NBCA, including filling of the aneurysm with glue.
- Occasionally, embolization of a small AVM can be completely therapeutic, e.g., a 14% complete cure rate from embolization alone was reported in a series of 49 patients treated over 4 years by Fournier et al. in Toronto.[65]
- Palliative therapy for an inoperable AVM to reduce shunting and improve neurological deficits related to high intracranial pressure or vascular steal.

Choice of Embolic Material

The earliest embolizations of brain AVMs used 2.5–4.5 mm steel spheres covered with methylmethacrylate.[66] Later 1–6 mm barium-impregnated Silastic spheres were injected directly into the internal carotid artery.[67,68] The choice of an embolic agent for embolization of a brain AVM requires a consideration of the known safety of the agents available, the histologic effects of the agents, and the durability of the response. For preoperative AVM embolization temporary agents might be sufficient, because ultimate revascularization of the nidus is not a concern in such patients. However, there are very few data comparing the safety and efficacy of the various available agents (Figs. 2.20, 15.1–15.5). The principal agents currently used for brain AVM embolization are described in the following sections.

Cyanoacrylate Adhesive

Use of iso-butyl 2-cyanoacrylate (IBCA) has given way to N-butyl cyanoacrylate (NBCA) because the latter has more predictable rheologic qualities and ease of resection in the surgical bed afterwards. NBCA has a higher viscosity, higher surface tension, and lower bonding strength than IBCA, implying that it will form a more uniform intravascular col-

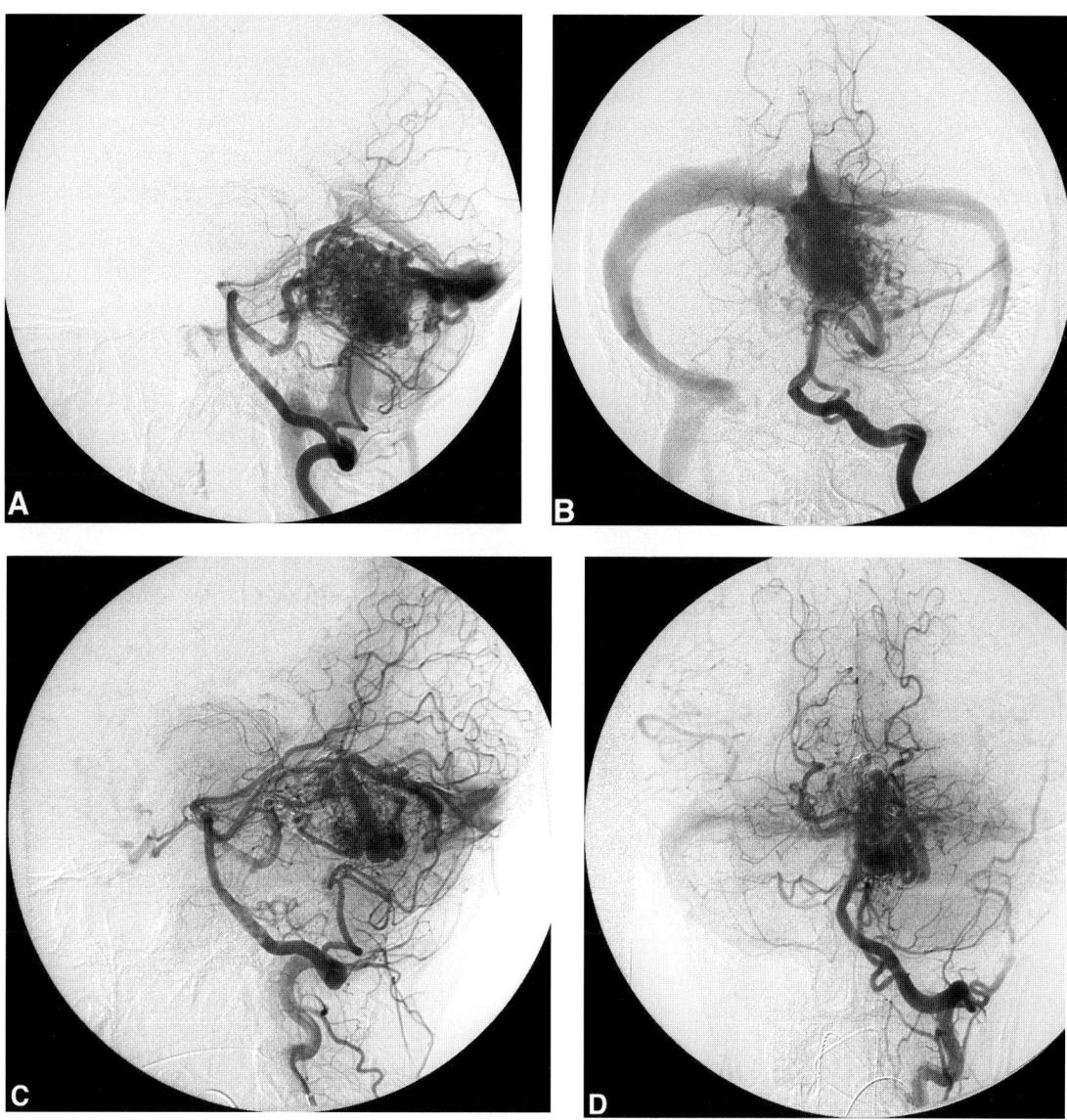

FIGURE 15.1 • *Preoperative Embolization of a Cerebellar AVM.*
A 9-year-old female presented with cerebellar hemorrhage related to an AVM of the cerebellar vermis (A, lateral view; B, AP view). Two months after making a good recovery from her hemorrhage, transarterial preoperative embolization was conducted using flow-guided microcatheters. The AVM was embolized using liquid coils and acrylate with satisfactory reduction in size and volume of flow on the final postembolization DSA run (C, lateral; D, AP). Although the images show that considerable AVM nidus persists, the importance of adjunctive embolization must be kept in perspective. This AVM was subsequently resected with manageable difficulties for the surgeon and an excellent clinical recovery for the patient. Embolization of AVMs with acrylate or any agent involves risks that must be considered carefully. In this patient, embolization beyond that demonstrated would have involved greater risk to cerebellar hemispheric branches than was acceptable and was therefore not performed.

umn of glue with less risk of gluing the microcatheter tip in the vessel.[69] Cyanoacrylate glue is prepared as a tissue adhesive and is commonly used in emergency rooms or in plastic surgery for seamless apposition of lacerated tissues. Its use in brain AVMs is predicated on its liquid character, which allows it to mold to the wall of the nidal vessels where it gels to a solid state causing occlusion of flow. The process of polymerization is fairly immediate when cyanoacrylate glue comes into contact with the ionic milieu of blood. In fact, adhesion of microcatheter tips within the AVM used to be a frequent problem when IBCA was in use and even with NBCA prior to the advent of hydrophilic coating.[70]

Cyanoacrylate is not radiodense and therefore must be opacified with tungsten, tantalum, Ethiodol, or Lipiodol in order to monitor its flow angiographically or fluoroscopically. Generally, the polymerization process is too fast for most AVM injections, and the process is slowed by mixing the cyanoacrylate with a retardant agent such as Ethiodol (occasionally glacial acetic acid is used) in concentrations of 25% glue and higher. Concentrations below 25% usually polymerize too slowly or in a fragmented fashion. Concentrations of 100% are typically used only in high-flow fistulas. The calculations for glue/Ethiodol concentrations during injection are usually based on inexact parameters arising from operator experience. Some have advocated use of formulas based on the time from injection of contrast until opacification of the venous side of the nidus. However, due to convection and mixing within the vessel it is difficult to predict the behavior of a viscous glue preparation based on a water-soluble contrast injection. High-speed filming at 15 frames per second of microdroplet (20 μl) injections of Ethiodol into AVM pedicles demonstrates velocities of flow within AVMs between 6 and 26 cm/s. These velocities indicate that conventional filming rates of 2–4 frames per second with water-soluble contrast are probably very fallible for calculating the behavior of glue.[71] Using this microdroplet technique, Wakhloo et al.[72] estimated that water-soluble contrast injections underestimate the transit time through the

FIGURE 15.2 • A 14-year-old male patient presenting with seizures was referred for preoperative embolization of a left frontal AVM. Although this lies somewhat anterior to the precentral strip, the size of the AVM in relationship to association fibers of the central strip and of Broca's area make it one of considerable risk. Because of the patient's age and anxiety, the procedure could be performed only under general anesthesia (A, left internal carotid artery, AP projection; B, left internal carotid artery, lateral projection).

Electrophysiologic monitoring was performed during the procedure to facilitate selective amytal testing before embolization. This is not an absolutely reliable technique because false negatives can occur. However, a positive result from an injection would certainly discourage embolization.

An AP image from the first DSA run performed in the nidus of the AVM through a flow-directed microcatheter (C) illustrates evidence of one of the many dangers that can be encountered in AVM embolization. A small intranidal vessel adjacent to the microcatheter tip changes caliber immediately into a much bigger draining vein. The contrast density changes from one location to the next, indicating that there are probably multiple sources of fistulous input into this vein, quite close to the microcatheter tip. Therefore the danger here is that embolic material, especially liquid acrylate, could be shorn from the nidus and carried quickly more distally into the veins. This has the potential to cause venous obstruction and acute venous hypertension. The phenomenon of inadvertent venous compromise of an AVM during embolization is one of the most dangerous complications which can occur.

This first fistula was embolized with 80% acrylate (arrowhead on image D, post first day of embolization) while two subsequent fistulas were embolized with liquid coils (small arrows).

After two embolization sessions (E, lateral view) the AVM has been reduced in size and flow sufficiently to render it more manageable at surgery. The patient had slow recovery of speech following surgery, but ultimately over a 6-month period made a complete recovery and resumed normal schooling.

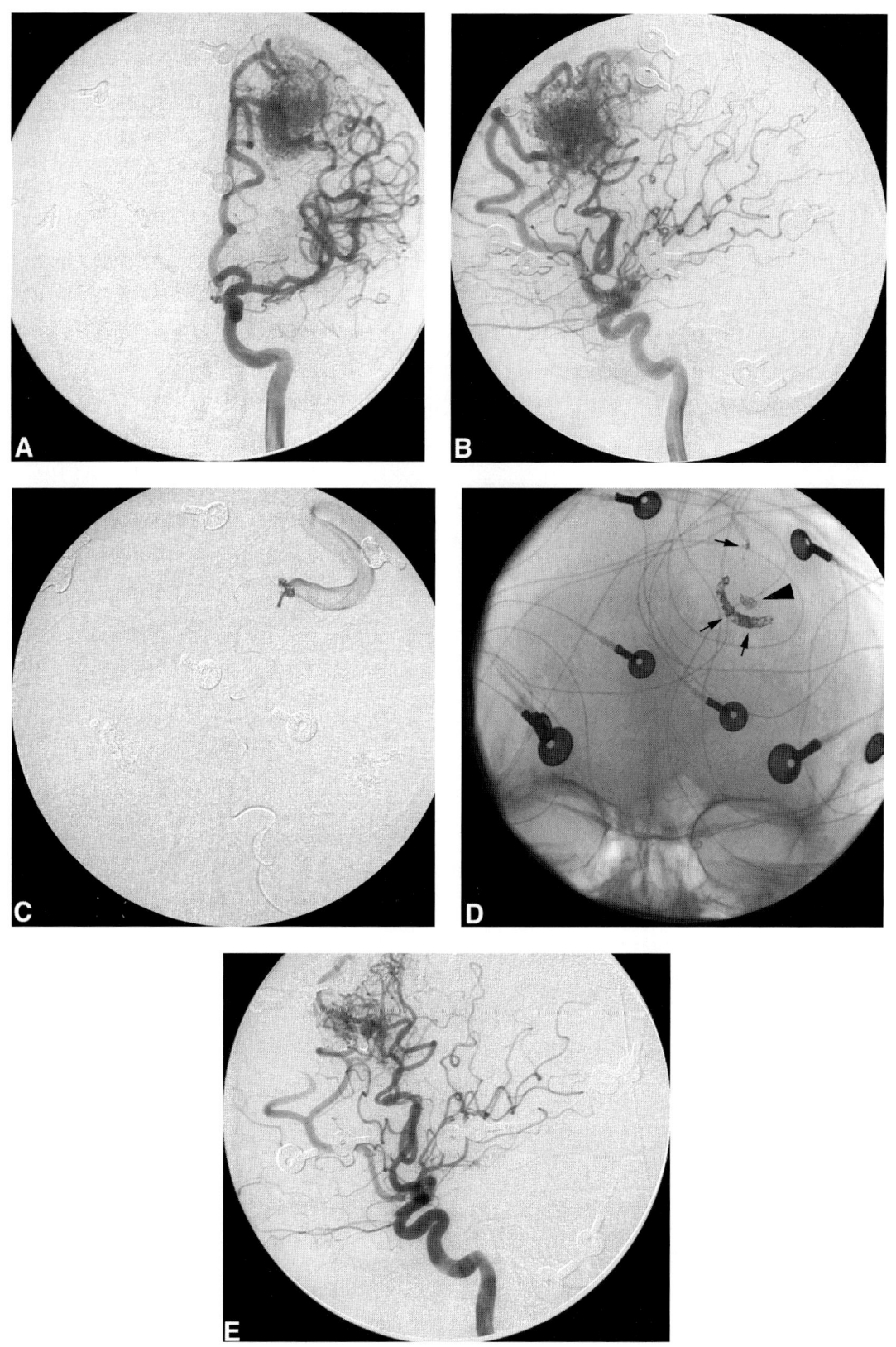

Arteriovenous Malformations of the Brain 299

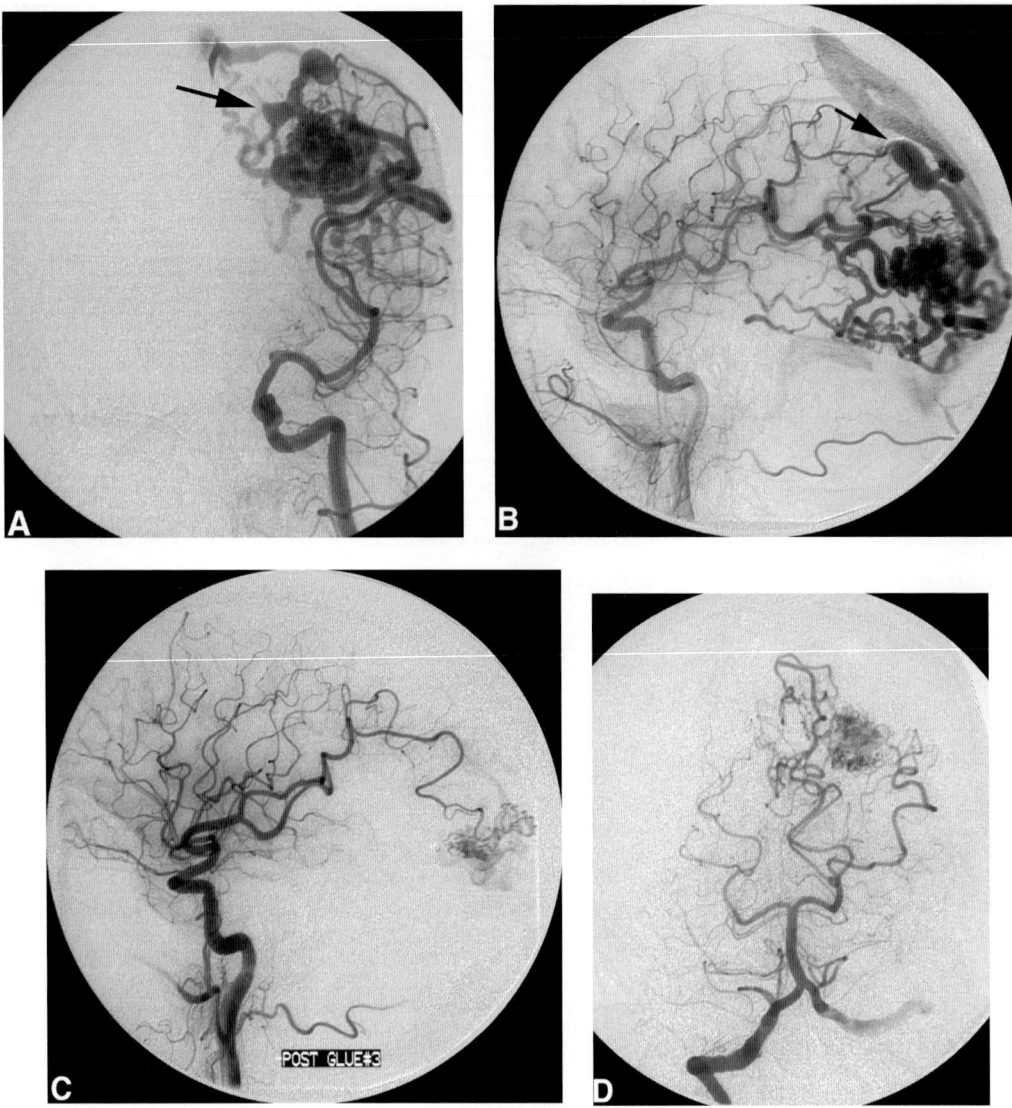

FIGURE 15.3 • For effective reduction of AVM nidal size, penetration of the nidus itself is imperative. Proximal occlusions of feeding vessels will give an illusory reduction in size acutely, but prompt collateral flow to the nidus will be established through other channels.

In this patient a left temporal-occipital AVM derives supply from multiple branches of a duplicated left middle cerebral artery (A, left internal carotid artery, AP view; B, left internal carotid artery, lateral view). A venous varix (arrow) was thought most likely to represent the site of presenting hemorrhage.

Following three uneventful depositions of acrylate in the nidus of the AVM, the lateral view (C, left internal carotid artery injection) and the posterior circulation injection (D) show that the nidus of the AVM continues to opacify partially, through multiple inaccessible channels. The dominant middle cerebral artery feeders to the AVM seen on the lateral view in B are not filling on the early arterial image (C) postembolization. This is a situation that some authors have described as concerning for back-thrombosis due to stagnation. Thrombus forming in a stagnant artery could extend proximally to the next bifurcation, where it could be shorn off and driven into normal brain, causing infarction. Anticoagulation in patients such as this is routinely used following embolization in some centers for this reason.

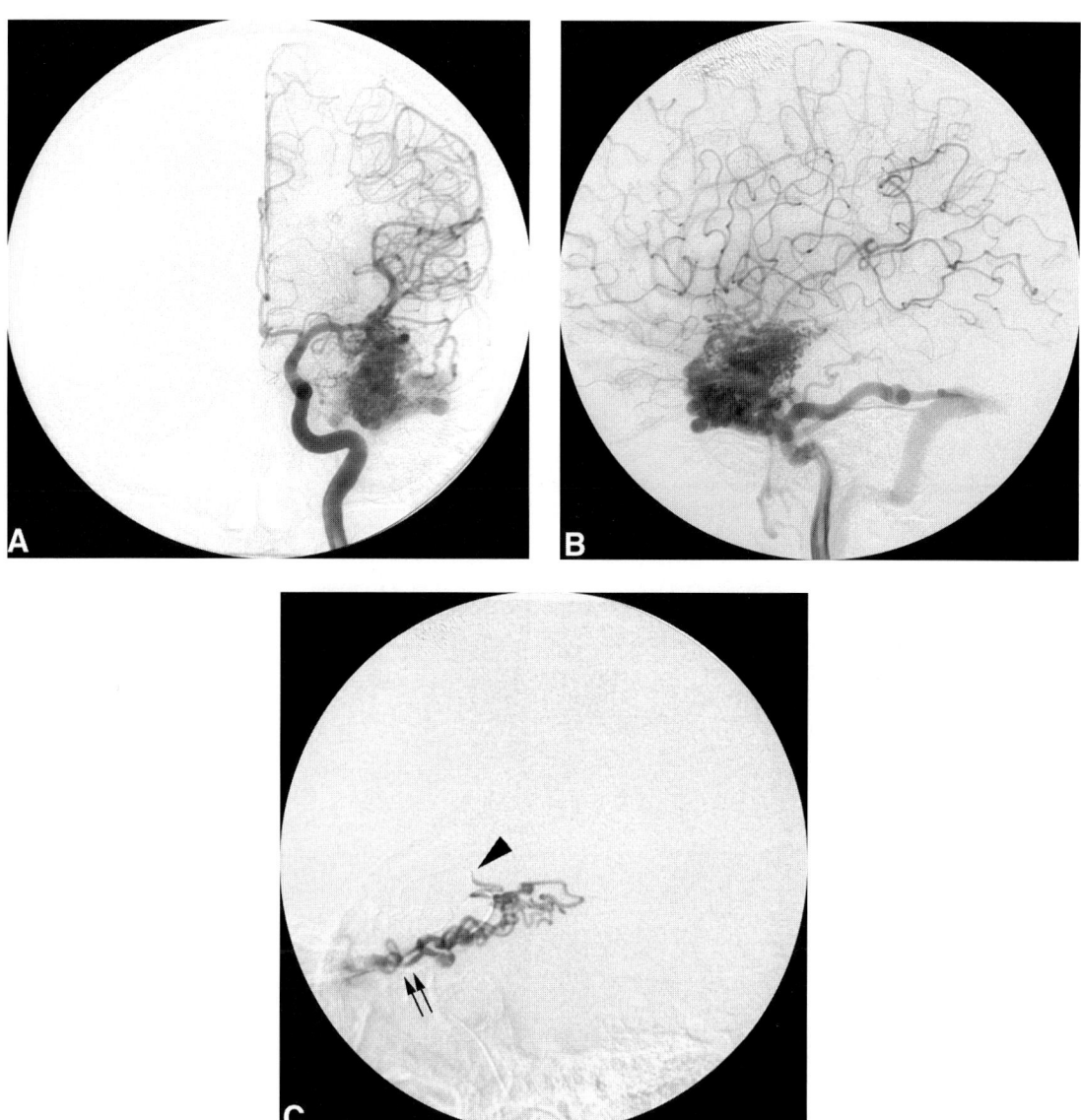

FIGURE 15.4 • *Intranidal Glue Injection with Flow Arrest I.*
The safest and most effective circumstances under which glue can be injected in an AVM prevail when the microcatheter wedges in the nidal channel causing arrest of flow. In these circumstances, a long injection of dilute glue can be made slowly to fill the entire nidal compartment ahead of the microcatheter without the usual risks of losing glue to the venous channels.

A 37-year-old female presenting with a left temporal lobe hemorrhage was referred after recovery for preoperative embolization of a left temporal lobe AVM (A, left internal carotid artery, AP view; B, left internal carotid artery, lateral view, late arterial phase). The AVM is relatively well defined but drains predominantly through a single large vein to the left sigmoid sinus.

The first microcatheter wedged in the nidus of the AVM in flow arrest (C, lateral view). The microcatheter tip is indicated by the arrowhead. Ahead of the microcatheter several nidal channels are opacified over a prolonged course before evidence of washout by other channels can be seen (double arrows). This represents a very favorable set of circumstances for effective and safe injection of dilute acrylate (20% to 30%).

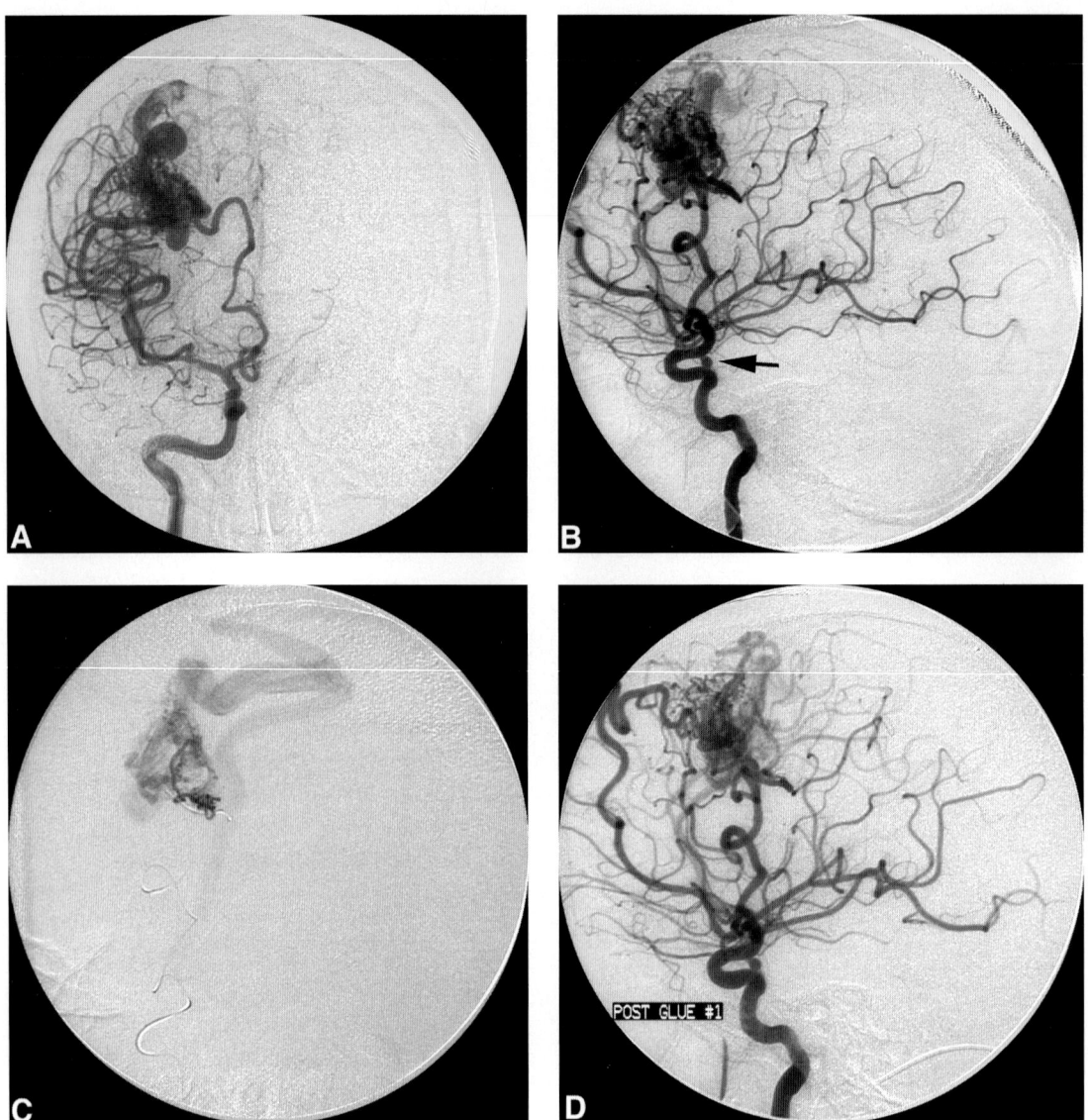

FIGURE 15.5 • *Intranidal Glue Injection with Flow Arrest II.*
A second example of the efficacy of intranidal flow arrest with glue injection is demonstrated. A middle-age female patient presented with seizures and was found to have a right frontal AVM. The pretreatment images (A, right internal carotid artery, AP view; B, right internal carotid artery, lateral view) show a typical wedge-shaped AVM with feeders from the right middle cerebral artery and anterior cerebral artery. An unruptured aneurysm of the posterior communicating artery (arrow) is present. The latter is a significant finding because almost every flow-directed catheter used in this case, regardless of whether it was shaped or not, tried to enter this aneurysm while ascending the carotid artery. One must be very careful not to traumatize any aneurysm en route to an AVM.

   An intranidal microcatheter position, accessed via the right middle cerebral artery, achieved flow arrest (C, lateral view). This allowed an accurate prolonged injection of glue into the nidus. After the first injection of glue, the change in the AVM is already discernible (D, right internal carotid artery, lateral view).

nidus by as much as a factor of 2. It is possible that an ineffable process of calculation deriving from the experience of the operator is likely to guide the choice of concentration of glue rather than a simple calculation based on angiographic estimates of velocities. The effects of cumulative experience with NBCA have been demonstrated with reduction of complications rates with embolization from 52% to 22% in a 6-year period for one group of operators.[73]

Cyanoacrylate embolization causes an effectively permanent occlusion of the injected vessel. Clinical reports of recanalization or dissolution of the glue do occur, but they are uncommon.[74,75] Histologic evidence of recanalization or at least partial capillary permeation of intravascular casts of NBCA was seen in all patients 3 months beyond embolization in a series by Gruber et al.,[76] but the clinical or angiographic significance of this, if any, was not prominently obvious to the authors. The histologic effects of IBCA were examined at different times following brain AVM embolization by Vinters et al.[77] Cyanoacrylate causes an intense inflammatory mural reaction of foreign-body giant cells and perivascular cuffing with mononuclear cells surrounding the embolized vessel in the acute phase.[78] Mural necrosis with extramural or intramural acrylate was commonly seen, and necrosis of surrounding parenchyma was seen up to 3.5 months following the procedure. The ischemia induced by NBCA embolization is thought to represent a powerful stimulus to the release of angiogenic cytokines such as vasoactive endothelial growth factor, fibroblast growth factor, and other factors aimed at promoting revascularization and capillary regrowth. Although there is histologic evidence, therefore, of time-related dissolution and capillary repermeation of NBCA embolic material, the occlusion of AVM vessels induced by acrylate is thought to be effectively permanent from a clinical point of view.

A comparison of the histologic effects of IBCA and PVA was conducted in the celiac circulation of pigs by White et al.[79] The histologic effects of IBCA were intense, with total vessel thrombosis associated with foreign-body giant cell reactions, and chronic inflammatory changes represented by lymphocytes and plasma cells. In some cases the internal elastic lamina of the embolized vessel was disrupted. Collateral damage to surrounding tissues was prominent with hepatic, splenic, and mucosal infarctions being common. The particulate agent, Ivalon (PVA), by comparison caused a much less intense inflammatory reaction with few giant cells and only mild intimal proliferation.

It should be emphasized that preoperative embolization of AVMs with NBCA has been shown to have a clinically detectable effect on patient outcome. In a nonrandomized study by Jafar et al.[80] embolization with NBCA was found to be effective in preoperative preparation of large AVMs in terms of reducing postsurgical complications, hemorrhage, and death to the equivalent of those seen in smaller nonembolized AVMs. This study also found that AVMs containing NBCA were easily manipulated and cut with a microscissors. A study of embolization-with-surgery versus surgery alone from Columbia-Presbyterian Medical Center also demonstrated that despite the bias that the surgery-only patients had smaller AVMs and lower Spetzler-Martin Grades, nevertheless the embolization-with-surgery patients had a better short-term and long-term outcome.[81]

Polyvinyl Alcohol Particles (PVA)
Polyvinyl alcohol particles are favored by some authors as the safest and most manageable embolic agent when the purpose of embolization is preparation for surgery.[82] This may have been particularly true when IBCA was the alternative which caused a hard intranidal cast that was difficult to cut during surgery. NBCA has a more favorable surgical character in this respect. A single-institution review comparing experience with PVA and NBCA ultimately favored the latter agent[83] as being at least as effective as PVA and having fewer overall complications, in part due to a lower risk of postsurgical complications in the acrylate group. Furthermore, AVMs in eloquent areas had a greater chance of being reduced permanently with NBCA compared with PVA to a size that then allowed use of radiosurgery.

PVA particles are manufactured in size ranges from 150 μ to 2,000 μm and are injected in dilute suspension through a microcatheter. Larger particle sizes require a more dilute suspension to avoid clumping of particles in the microcatheter and occlusion of the shaft. One of the principal dangers associated with use of PVA for AVM embolization is that it is difficult to know whether the particles are flowing through the AVM and thence to the pulmonary circulation. Deaths have occurred from this phenomenon, particularly if there is any variability in the quality control of the particle sizes.[84]

Recanalization of an AVM following particulate embolization with PVA occurs with higher frequency than is the case for NBCA. Mathis et al.[85] found that PVA was a satisfactory embolization agent for large AVMs (>3 cm diameter) in preparation for radiosurgery. Recanalized AVM nidus, however, was seen in 12% of patients where embolized AVM was excluded from the treatment field. In a study of embolization of brain AVMs by Sorimachi et al. using predominantly PVA with adjunctive use of other materials, a regrowth or recanalization rate of 43% was seen at 1 month or later following the embolization.[86] Even among those cases with initially complete nidus obliteration, a recurrence rate of up to 80% was seen.

Coils

The coils used in AVMs are usually small, fibered or unfibered, short coils injected through a 0.016-in or 0.010-in microcatheter. A newer alternative is the Liquid Coil of ultrathin platinum wire. These coils have the advantage of being capable of flowing more distally in a tortuous vessel with less likelihood of snagging on a deformed or kinked microcatheter tip, compared with standard-fibered microcoils.[87] They can be inserted with a saline push via a standard microcatheter or a flow-directed microcatheter, and a coil-pusher is not necessary. Larger coils extruded by a pusher or GDC coils may be particularly helpful in occluding large high-flow fistulas, which are hazardous to embolize with liquid adhesive and which are likely to be less responsive to radiosurgery.

Dehydrated Alcohol

Alcohol is in use at a few centers for AVM embolization. It is a caustic agent that scleroses the endothelium of the vessel, causing thrombosis and occlusion. Doses used are limited to <0.5–1 ml/kg body weight.[88] Particular risks with intravascular use of alcohol include elevated pulmonary pressure and cardiovascular collapse. Advocates of alcohol as an embolic agent advise insertion of a Swan-Ganz catheter in the pulmonary artery prior to treatment to allow infusion of vasodilators if signs of elevated pressure begin.

Other Agents

Numerous alternative embolic agents for AVMs have been used in the past, including spherules of different material, polymer thread, 6-0 silk thread, gelatin particles, Avitene (denatured collagen), autologous clot, etc., but none is in common use today for a variety of reasons. A mixture of PVA, 30% alcohol, and Avitene, for instance, was abandoned due to a high recanalization rate of 40%.[89] Silk has been associated with a fulminant vasculitic histologic response and a high rate of clinical hemorrhage and death following embolization.[90] Although several authors[91,92] found silk to be satisfactory as an embolic agent without histologic evidence of fulminant angionecrosis, nevertheless its progress cannot be evaluated fluoroscopically. This potentially increases the risk of inadvertent embolization through reflux, compounded by the high pressures that may be necessary to inject it.

It is likely that the near future will bring a number of agents to market based on alternative adhesive and nonadhesive liquid materials. Agents requiring use of the solvent dimethyl sulfoxide (DMSO) will require dedicated microcatheters to prevent material incompatibility between the solvent and hub plastics.[93]

Complications of AVM Embolization

Any step in the embolization process from insertion of the arterial sheath to hemostasis after the case, and later postprocedure care in the intensive care unit can involve risks to the patient affecting ultimate outcome. Transient exacerbation of symptoms including minor events such as headache can occur in up to 50% of patients following an AVM embolization.[65] Permanent morbidity related to aneurysmal rupture, delayed bleeding, or intraprocedural ischemia occurs with a risk of between 5.1% and 8% with an embolization-related mortality of 0% to 2%.[65,69,80]

Arterial perforation of an aneurysm or wall of the artery by the microwire or microcatheter is usually seen in 1% or less of cases. Intraprocedural and postprocedure hemorrhage can be seen also and is usually thought to be related to inadvertently early compromise of the outflow veins with elevation of intranidal pressure. The same phenomenon can happen during AVM surgery, too. Therefore, during embolization with liquid adhesive—particularly early in the process—embolization of glue to the veins should be thoroughly avoided as it represents one of the most serious sources of procedure-related hemorrhage. Delayed venous hemorrhage may also occur when dilated stagnant veins remain after a partial or complete embolization. Progressive thrombosis of the veins can occur and cause nidal hemorrhage or venous infarction of normal parenchyma.[94] Progressive back-thrombosis of dilated stagnant formerly feeding arteries may also occur and be a cause of thrombotic infarction of adjacent or remote territories, depending on the degree of retrograde thrombosis that occurs (Fig. 15.3). This phenomenon may be more likely in older patients, and low-level heparinization or antiplatelet medication may be a prudent prophylactic therapy to reduce the likelihood of this phenomenon.[95]

Superselective Functional Testing

In general, it is necessary to have the patient absolutely still (i.e., asleep) during injection of cyanoacrylate so as to avoid any collateral damage through unseen reflux to normal vessels. The risk of patient motion or agitation is usually more common and more troublesome than the risk of not being able to discern normal from abnormal territories during an AVM embolization. Therefore, many authors favor use of general anesthesia more and more during AVM embolization, but the use of superselective functional testing on an awake patient may have application in particularly delicate or uncertain situations.

A short-acting barbiturate agent can be injected via the microcatheter and the patient can then be tested clinically for deficits before proceeding to embolization. Han et al.[96] used sodium thiopental (30–50 mg) in 38 patients and found the test helpful in being able to predict deficits related to the embolization. Other deficits were also seen but were related to reflux of embolic material or to spasm, and the authors thought that false-negative results were not seen with this technique in their series of patients. Rauch et al.[97] used sodium amytal 30 mg for superselective Wada testing in conjunction with EEG monitoring. Out of 109 vessels 23 were positive, but only half of these positive tests were evident clinically. The authors recommended reconstituting the amytal in saline at a concentration of 12.5 mg/ml rendering an osmotic concentration of 413 mOs/L. This is because of some evidence that amytal may have a noxious effect on the endothelium of intracranial arteries at high concentration.[98] Rauch et al.[97,99] concluded that embolization following a positive superselective amytal test correlated with a 67% risk of a resultant neurologic complication. They also pointed out that the alterations in the hemodynamics of an AVM during progressive embolization mean that the results of a selective amytal test can change from initially negative to positive in the course of a procedure, as can the risk change from initially low to high, due to opening of collateral pathways and side-branches with reduction of the nidal sump-effect.

Microcatheter Choice during AVM Embolization

The catheters available for AVM embolization can be categorized as either flow-directed (floppy-tip, small inner lumen) or wire-guided (stiffer construction, larger inner lumen). Wire-directed microcatheters with hydrophilic coating and braided construction are capable of very distal access without kinking at tight turns. The advantage of wire-guided catheters is that they allow embolization of a larger variety of materials, e.g., different types of coils, liquids, threads, a wide range of PVA particles, etc. Flow-guided microcatheters are a little more difficult to use, but they can now be steered or supported proximally with newer small-bore wires so as to gain more distal access than standard microcatheters could achieve.

When embolizing with NBCA, the use of microwires and microcatheters with hydrophilic coating has had a significant impact on the ease of distal access right into the AVM nidus. Use of hydrophilic coating on microwires improves the ability to achieve an intranidal catheterization even with nonhydrophilic microcatheters, according to Aletich et al.[100] Hydrophilic coating on the microcatheter also has a significant impact on lessening the risk of gluing the microcatheter tip to the glue cast. In vitro testing by Mathis et al. demonstrated a reduction of intravascular friction by 30% to 35% with hydrophilic coating and a significantly reduced force necessary to extract a microcatheter from a cast of NBCA.[101]

Technique of Glue Injection

Cyanoacrylate is usually injected into brain AVMs under conditions of systemic hypotension and/or bradycardia to reduce the likelihood of excessive venous permeation of the glue cast.[102]

After verifying the position of the microcatheter tip as satisfactory, the first step is to withdraw all slack from the microcatheter before preparing for the injection. The microcatheter is withdrawn slowly until the loop nearest the tip begins to unfurl. This step is important because slack will impact deleteriously on the immediacy of the response of the microcatheter tip to a sudden pull from outside the patient. This delay could make the difference between gluing the tip in the patient or not.

Next, the view that one will use during the injection is set up and angiograms through the microcatheter obtained, which will act as a guide for monitoring the progress of the subsequent glue injection. Note is made of any proximal normal branches that might be vulnerable to refluxing glue and of the appearance of wash-in from the side of nonopacified feeders that one might particularly wish to avoid. An intuitive or other calculation of the velocity of flow and desired depth of penetration of the glue is made to formulate a concentration for injection. The ideal situation for injection of glue is where the tip occludes the flow in the vessel. This allows a slow, controlled injection of dilute (25%) glue into the nidus over a period of several minutes.[103]

Suspensions of NBCA with opacifying agents and Ethiodol or Lipiodol can be injected slowly as a continuous column over periods of up to several minutes or as a discrete bolus "sandwiched" between columns of 5% dextrose. With both techniques the microcatheter hub must be cleansed thoroughly and flushed with 5% dextrose because blood or saline will initiate the polymerization process. The injections are usually made under conditions of systemic hypotension with mean arterial pressures of 80–90 mm Hg. At the end of the injection, the microcatheter and introducer catheter are usually pulled together sharply of a piece, this being done to avoid any inadvertent embolization of glue to the arterial tree during removal of the microcatheter by an adherent droplet being shorn off at the tip of the main catheter. The risk of this happening and of adhering the microcatheter in the body is much reduced since the introduction of hydrophilic coating.

Postembolization Patient Management

Patients are routinely monitored in a neurointensive care unit for at least 24 hours following an embolization procedure.[104] In addition to general neurologic and medical welfare of the patient, the principal concerns are:

- *Headache.* Postembolization headache is a common phenomenon occurring in up to 50% of AVM patients. Generally the headache is manageable with low doses of narcotic agents, and it generally improves quickly. A persistent or severe headache is unusual, however, and may indicate some other complication.

- *Normal perfusion pressure breakthrough edema or hemorrhage.* To prevent this, routine steroid medication and careful monitoring of blood pressure is very important. With reference to large AVMs, some authors recommend confining each embolization session to only 2–4 pedicles and allowing at least 7–10 days between embolizations. It is hypothesized that staging the embolization over several weeks will allow an acclimatization of local hemodynamics to the effects of the procedure. Normal perfusion pressure breakthrough and elevation of ICP >25 mm Hg following surgical resection of AVMs is additionally treated actively with loop diuretic agents, intravenous mannitol, hyperventilation (for PCO_2 <30 mm Hg), and pentobarbital suppression (10 mg/kg loading dose and 2–5 mg/kg per hour) with EEG monitoring.[30] Similar aggressive measures will occasionally be necessary following embolization-related complications.
- *Ischemia due to back-thrombosis of arterial feeders.* When a patulous arterial feeder is left stagnant and slowly draining after an embolization, prolongation of heparinization for 24 hours or longer after the procedure is generally advised (Fig. 15.3).
- *Venous thrombosis.* Again, prolongation of heparinization may be considered prudent for patients thought to be at risk for imminent fulminant venous thrombosis (Fig. 12.3).
- *CT scanning for clinical evidence of complications.* If focal hematoma with mass-effect develops for any reason, surgical evacuation may become necessary.

References

1. McCormick WF (1984) Pathology of Vascular Malformations of the Brain. In: Wilson CB, Stein BM, eds. *Intracranial Arteriovenous Malformations.* Baltimore: Williams and Wilkins; 44–63.
2. Berman MF, Sciacca PR, Pile-Spellman J, Stapf C, Sander Connolly E, Mohr JP, Young WL (2000) The epidemiology of brain arteriovenous malformations. *Neurosurgery* 47:389–397.
3. Kikuchi K, Kowada M, Sasajima H (1994) Vascular malformations of the brain in hereditary hemorrhagic teleangiectasia (Rendu-Osler-Weber disease). *Surg Neurol* 41:374–380.
4. Mast H, Young WL, Koennecke HC, Sciacca RR, Osipov A, Pile-Spellman J, Hacein-Bey L, Duong H, Stein BM, Mohr JP (1997) Risk of spontaneous haemorrhage after diagnosis of cerebral arteriovenous malformation. *Lancet* 350:1065–1068.
5. Ondra SL, Troupp H, George ED, Schwab K (1990) The natural history of symptomatic arteriovenous malformations of the brain: a 24-year follow-up assessment. *J Neurosurg* 73:387–391.
6. Graf CJ, Perret GE, Torner JC (1983) Bleeding from cerebral arteriovenous malformations as part of their natural history. *J Neurosurg* 58:331–337.
7. Hartmann A, Mast H, Mohr JP, Koennecke HC, Osipov A, Pile-Spellman J, Duong DH, Young WL (1998) Morbidity of intracranial hemorrhage in patients with cerebral arteriovenous malformation. *Stroke* 29:931–934.
8. Crawford PM, West CR, Chadwick DW, Shaw MDM (1986) Arteriovenous malformations of the brain. Natural history in unoperated patients. *J Neurol Neurosurg Psychiatry* 49:1–10.
9. Fults D, Kelly DL Jr (1984) Natural history of arteriovenous malformations of the brain: a clinical study. *Neurosurgery* 15:658–662.
10. Kondziolka D, McLaughlin MR, Kestle JR (1995) Simple risk predictions for arteriovenous malformation hemorrhage. *Neurosurgery* 37:851–855.
11. Pollock BE, Flickinger JE, Lundsford LD, Bissonette DJ, Kondziolka D (1996) Factors that predict the bleeding risk of cerebral arteriovenous malformations. *Stroke* 27:1–6.
12. Kader A, Young WL, Pile-Spellman J, Mast H, Sciacca RR, Mohr JP, Stein BM (1994) The influence of hemodynamic and anatomic factors on hemorrhage from cerebral arteriovenous malformations. *Neurosurgery* 34:801–807.
13. Marks MP, Lane B, Steinberg GK, Chang PJ (1990) Hemorrhage in intracerebral arteriovenous malformations: Angiographic determinants. *Radiology* 176:807–813.
14. Turjiman F, Massoud TF, Vinuela F, Sayre JW, Guglielmi G, Duckwiler G (1995) Correlation of the angioarchitectural features of cerebral arteriovenous malformations with clinical presentation of hemorrhage. *Neurosurgery* 37:856–862.
15. Spetzler RF, Hargraves RW, McCormick PW, Zabramski JM, Flom RA, Zimmerman RS (1992) Relationship of perfusion pressure and size to risk of hemorrhage from arteriovenous malformations. *J Neurosurg* 76:918–923.
16. Vinuela F, Nombela L, Roach MR, Fox AJ, Pelz DM (1985) Stenotic and occlusive disease of the venous drainage system of deep brain AVMs. *J Neurosurg* 63:180–184.
17. Mansmann U, Meisel J, Brock M, Rodesch G, Alvarez H, Lasjaunias P (2000) Factors associated with intracranial

hemorrhage in cases of cerebral arteriovenous malformation. *Neurosurgery* 46:272–281.
18. Itoyama Y, Uemura S, Ushio Y, Kuratsu J, Nonaka N, Wada H, Sano Y, Fukumura A, Yoshida K, Yano T (1989) Natural course of unoperated intracranial arteriovenous malformations: study of 50 cases. *J Neurosurg* 71:805–809.
19. Turjiman F, Massoud TF, Vinuela F, Sayre JW, Guglielmi G, Duckwiler G (1994) Aneurysms related to cerebral arteriovenous malformations: superselective angiographic assessment in 58 patients. *AJNR* 15:1601–1605.
20. Perata HJ, Tomsick TA, Tew JM Jr (1994) Feeding artery pedicle aneurysms: association with parenchymal hemorrhage and arteriovenous malformation in the brain. *J Neurosurg* 80:631–634.
21. Norris JS, Valiante TA, Wallace MC, Willinsky RA, Montanera WJ, terBrugge KG, Tymianski M (1999) A simple relationship between radiological arteriovenous malformation hemodynamics and clinical presentation: a prospective, blinded analysis of 31 cases. *J Neurosurg* 90:673–679.
22. Feindel W, Yamamoto YL, Hodge CP (1971) Red cerebral veins and the cerebral steal syndrome. Evidence from fluorescein angiography and microregional blood flow by radioisotopes during excision of an angioma. *J Neurosurg* 35:167–179.
23. Meyer B, Schaller C, Frenkel C, Schramm J (1998) Physiological steal around AVMs of the brain is not equivalent to cortical ischemia. *Neurolog Res* 20(suppl 1):S13–S17.
24. Mast H, Mohr JP, Osipov A, Pile-Spellman J, Marshall RS, Lazar RM, Stein BM, Young WL (1995) "Steal" is an unestablished mechanism for the clinical presentation of cerebral arteriovenous malformations. *Stroke* 26:1215–1220.
25. Fink GR (1992) Effects of cerebral angiomas on perifocal and remote tissue: a multivariate positron emission tomography study. *Stroke* 23:1099–1105.
26. Young WL, Pile-Spellman J, Prohovnik I, Kader A, Stein BM (1994) Evidence for adaptive autoregulatory displacement in hypotensive cortical territories adjacent to arteriovenous malformations. *Neurosurgery* 34:601–610.
27. Fogarty-Mack P, Pile-Spellman J, Hacein-Bey L, Osipov A, DeMeritt J, Jackson EC, Young WL (1996) The effect of arteriovenous malformations on the distribution of intracerebral arterial pressures. *AJNR* 17:1443–1449.
28. Joshi S, Young WL, Pile-Spellman J, Fogarty-Mack P, Sciacca RR, Hacein-Bey L, Duong H, Vulliemoz Y, Ostapkovich N, Jackson T (1997) Intra-arterial nitrovasodilators do not increase cerebral blood flow in angiographically normal territories of arteriovenous malformation patients. *Stroke* 28:1115–1122.
29. Young WL, Kader A, Ornstein E, Baker KZ, Ostapkovich N, Pile-Spellman J, Fogarty-Mack P, Stein BM (1996) Cerebral hyperemia after arteriovenous malformation resection is related to "breakthrough" complications but not to feeding artery pressure. The Columbia University Arteriovenous Malformation Study Project. *Neurosurgery* 38:1085–1093.
30. Awad IA, Magdinec M, Schubert A (1994) Intracranial hypertension after resection of cerebral arteriovenous malformations. Predisposing factors and management strategy. *Stroke* 25:611–620.
31. Spetzler RF, Wilson CB, Weinstein P, Mehdorn M, Townsend J, Telles D (1978) Normal perfusion pressure breakthrough theory. *Clin Neurosurg* 25:651–672.
32. Kato Y, Sano H, Nonomura K, Kanno T, Katada K, Takeshita G, Toyama H (1997) Normal perfusion pressure breakthrough syndrome in giant arteriovenous malformations. *Neurolog Res* 19:117–123.
33. Young WL, Kader A, Prohovnik I, Ornstein E, Fleischer LH, Ostapkovich N, Jackson LD, Stein BM (1993) Pressure autoregulation is intact after arteriovenous malformation resection. *Neurosurgery* 32:491–496.
34. Spetzler RF, Hamilton MG (1993) Pressure autoregulation is intact after arteriovenous malformation resection. *Neurosurgery* 33:772–774.
35. Hoffman WE, Charbel FT, Edelman G, Abood C (1996) Brain tissue response to CO_2 in patients with arteriovenous malformation. *J Cerebral Blood Flow Metabol* 16:1383–1386.
36. Spetzler RF, Martin NA (1986) A proposed grading system for arteriovenous malformations. *J Neurosurg* 65:476–483.
37. Hamilton MG, Spetzler RF (1994) The prospective application of a grading system for arteriovenous malformations. *Neurosurgery* 34:2–6.
38. Spetzler RF, Zabramski JM (1998) Surgical management of large AVMs. *Acta Neurochirurgica—Supplementum* 42:93–97.
39. Kondziolka D, Humphreys RP, Hoffman HJ, Hendrick EB, Drake JM (1992) Arteriovenous malformations of the brain in children: a forty year experience. *Can J Neurol Sci* 19:40–45.
40. Horsley V, Clarke RH (1908) The structure and functions of the cerebellum examined by a new method. *Brain* 31:45–124.
41. Leksell L (1951) The stereotaxic method and radiosurgery of the brain. *Acta Chirurgica Scandinavica* 102:316–319.
42. Leksel L (1968) Cerebral radiosurgery I. Gammathalamotomy in two cases of intractable pain. *Acta Chirurgica Scandinavica* 134:585–595.
43. Lunsford LD, Kondziolka D, Flickinger JC, Bissonette DJ, Jungreis CA, Maitz AH, Horton JA, Coffey RJ (1991) Stereotactic radiosurgery for arteriovenous malformations of the brain. *J Neurosurg* 75:512–524.
44. Karlsson B, Lindquist C, Steiner L (1997) Prediction of obliteration after gamma knife surgery for cerebral arteriovenous malformations. *Neurosurgery* 40:425–430.
45. Harsh G, Loeffler JS, Thornton A, Smith A, Bussiere M,

CHAPMAN PH (1999) Stereotactic proton radiosurgery. *Neurosurg Clin North Am* 10:243–256.
46. CHANG SD, SHUSTER DL, STEINBERG GK, LEVY RP, FRANKEL K (1997) Stereotactic radiosurgery of arteriovenous malformations: pathologic changes in resected tissue. *Clin Neuropathol* 16:111–116.
47. VOGES J, TREUER H, LEHRKE R, KOCHER M, STAAR S, MULLER RP, STURM V (1997) Risk analysis of LINAC radiosurgery in patients with arteriovenous malformation (AVM). *Acta Neurochirurgica—Supplementum* 68:118–123.
48. FLICKINGER JC, KONDZIOLKA D, LUNSFORD LD, POLLOCK BE, YAMAMOTO M, GORMAN DA, SCHOMBERG PJ, SNEED P, LARSON D, SMITH V, MCDERMOTT MW, MIYAWAKI L, CHILTON J, MORANTZ RA, YOUNG B, JOKURA H, LISCAK R (1999) A multi-institutional analysis of complication outcomes after arteriovenous malformation radiosurgery. *International J Radiation Oncol Biol Physics* 44:67–74.
49. KJELLBERG RN, HANAMURA T, DAVIS KR, LYONS SL, ADAMS RD (1983) Bragg-Peak proton-beam therapy for arteriovenous malformations of the brain. *N Engl J Med* 309:269–274.
50. STEINBERG GK, FABRIKANT JI, MARKS MP, LEVY RP, FRANKEL KA, PHILLIPS MH, SHUER LM, SILVERBERG GD (1991) Stereotactic Helium ion Bragg peak radiosurgery for intracranial arteriovenous malformations. *Stereotactic Functional Neurosurg* 57:36–49.
51. COLOMBO F, POZZA F, CHIEREGO G, FRANCESCON P, CASENTINI L, DE LUCA G (1994) Linear accelerator radiosurgery of cerebral arteriovenous malformations: current status. *Acta Neurochirurgica Supplementum* 62:5–9.
52. POLLOCK BE, FLICKINGER JC, LUNSFORD LD, BISSONETTE DJ, KONDZIOLKA D (1996) Hemorrhage risk after stereotactic radiosurgery of cerebral arteriovenous malformations. *Neurosurgery* 38:652–659.
53. KARLSSON B, LINDQUIST C, STEINER L (1996) The effect of gamma knife surgery on the risk of rupture prior to AVM obliteration. *Minimally Invasive Neurosurg* 39:21–27.
54. PORTER PJ, SHIN AY, DETSKY AS, LEFAIVE L, WALLACE MC (1997) Surgery versus stereotactic radiosurgery for small, operable cerebral arteriovenous malformations: a clinical and cost comparison. *Neurosurgery* 41:757–766.
55. FOOTE KD, FRIEDMAN WA, BUATTI JM, BOVA FJ, MEEKS SA (1999) Linear accelerator radiosurgery in brain tumor management. *Neurosurg Clin North Am* 10:203–242.
56. FRIEDMAN WA, BOVA FJ, MENDENHALL WM (1995) Linear accelerator radiosurgery for arteriovenous malformations: the relationship of size to outcome. *J Neurosurg* 82:180–189.
57. LOEFFLER JS, ALEXANDER EI, SIDDON RL (1989) Stereotactic radiosurgery for intracranial arteriovenous malformations using a standard linear accelerator. *International J Radiation Oncol Biol Physics* 17:673–677.
58. BETTI O, MUNARI C, ROSIER R (1992) Traitement radiochirugical avec accelerateur lineaire des 'petites' malformations arterio-veineuses intracranienne. *Neurochirurgie* 38:27–134.
59. ENGENHART R, WOWRA B, DEBUS J (1994) The role of high-dose single-fraction irradiation in small and larger intracranial arteriovenous malformations. *International J Radiation Oncol Biol Physics* 30:521–529.
60. MEHTA MP (1995) The physical, biologic, and clinical basis of radiosurgery. *Curr Probl Cancer* 19:265–329.
61. POLLOCK BE, GORMAN DA, SCHOMBERG PJ, KLINE RW (1999) The Mayo Clinic gamma knife experience: indications and initial results. *Mayo Clin Proc* 74:5–13.
62. POLLOCK BE, LUNSFORD LD, KONDZIOLKA D (1994) Patient outcomes after stereotactic radiosurgery for "operable" arteriovenous malformations. *Neurosurgery* 35:1–8.
63. POLLOCK BE (1999) Stereotactic radiosurgery for arteriovenous malformations. *Neurosurg Clin North Am* 10:281–290.
64. GUO WY, LINDQVIST M, LINDQUIST C, ERICSON K, NORDELL B, KARLSSON B, KIHLSTROM L (1992) Stereotaxic angiography in gamma knife radiosurgery of intracranial arteriovenous malformations. *AJNR* 13:1107–1114.
65. FOURNIER D, TERBRUGGE KG, WILLINSKY R, LASJAUNIAS P, MONTANERA W (1991) Endovascular treatment of intracerebral arteriovenous malformations: experience in 49 cases. *J Neurosurg* 75:228–233.
66. LUESSENHOP AJ, SPENCE WT (1960) Artificial embolization of cerebral arteries. Report of use in a case of arterionous malformation. *JAMA* 172:1153–1155.
67. LUESSENHOP AJ, KACHMANN R, SHEVLIN W, FERRERO AA (1965) Clinical evaluation of artificial embolization in the management of large cerebral arteriovenous malformations. *J Neurosurg* 23:400–417.
68. LUESSENHOP AJ, VELASQUEZ AC (1964) Observations on the tolerance of the intracranial arteries to catheterization. *J Neurosurg* 21:85–91.
69. VALAVANIS A, YASARGIL MG. (1998) The endovascular treatment of brain arteriovenous malformations. *Adv Tech Stand Neurosurg* 24:131–214, 1998
70. ZOARSKI GH, LILLY MP, SPERLING JS, MATHIS JM (1999) Surgically confirmed incorporation of a chronically retained neurointerventional microcatheter in the carotid artery. *AJNR* 20:177–178.
71. RUDIN S, WAKHLOO AK, LIEBER BB, GRANGER W, DIVANI AA, BEDNAREK DR, HOPKINS LN (1999) Microdroplet tracking using biplane digital subtraction angiography for cerebral arteriovenous malformation blood flow path and velocity determinations. *AJNR* 20:1110–1114.
72. WAKHLOO AK, LIEBER BB, RUDIN S, FRONCKOWIAK MD, MERICLE RA, HOPKINS LN (1998) A novel approach to flow quantification in brain arteriovenous malformations prior to enbucrilate embolization: use of insoluble contrast (Ethiodol droplet) angiography. *J Neurosurg* 89:395–404.
73. WIKHOLM G, LUNDQVIST C, SVENDSEN P (1995) Transarterial embolization of cerebral arteriovenous malformations:

improvement of results with experience. *AJNR* 16:1811–1817.
74. Klara PM, George ED, McDonnell DE (1985) Morphological studies of human arteriovenous malformations. Effects of isobutyl 2-cyanoacrylate embolization. *J Neurosurg* 63:421–425.
75. Rao VR, Mandalam KR, Gupta AK (1989) Dissolution of isobutyl 2-cyanoacrylate on long-term follow-up. *AJNR* 10:135–141.
76. Gruber A, Mazal PR, Bavinzski G, Killer M, Budka H, Richling B (1996) Repermeation of partially embolized cerebral arteriovenous malformations: a clinical, radiologic, and histologic study. *AJNR* 17:1323–1331.
77. Vinters HV, Lundie MJ, Kaufmann JCE (1986) Long-term pathological follow-up of cerebral arteriovenous malformations treated by embolization with bucrylate. *N Engl J Med* 314:477–483.
78. Schweitzer JS, Chang BS, Madsen P, Vinuela F, Martin NA, Marroquin CE, Vinters HV (1993) The pathology of arteriovenous malformations of the brain treated by embolotherapy. II. Results of embolization with multiple agents. *Neuroradiology* 35:468–474.
79. White RI, Strandberg JV, Gross GS, Barth KH (1977) Therapeutic embolization with long-term occluding agents and their effects on embolized tissues. *Radiology* 125:677–687.
80. Jafar JJ, Davis AJ, Berenstein A, Choi IS, Kupersmith MJ (1993) The effect of embolization with N-butyl cyanoacrylate prior to surgical resection of cerebral arteriovenous malformations. *J Neurosurg* 78:60–69.
81. DeMeritt JS, Pile-Spellman J, Mast H, Moohan N, Lu DC, Young WL, Hacein-Bey L, Mohr JP, Stein BM (1995) Outcome analysis of preoperative embolization with N-butyl cyanoacrylate in cerebral arteriovenous malformations. *AJNR* 16:1801–1807.
82. Purdy PD, Batjer HH, Risser RC, Samson D (1992) Arteriovenous malformations of the brain: choosing embolic materials to enhance safety and ease of excision. *J Neurosurg* 77:217–222.
83. Wallace RC, Flom RA, Khayata MH, Dean BL, McKenzie J, Rand JC, Obuchowski NA, Zepp RC, Zabramski JM, Spetzler RF (1995) The safety and effectiveness of brain arteriovenous malformation embolization using acrylic and particles: the experiences of a single institution. *Neurosurgery* 37:606–615.
84. Repa I, Moradian GP, Denher LP (1989) Mortalities associated with the use of a commercial suspension of polyvinyl alcohol. *Radiology* 170:395–399.
85. Mathis JA, Barr JD, Horton JA, Jungreis CA, Lunsford LD, Kondziolka DS, Vincent D, Pentheny S (1995) The efficacy of particulate embolization combined with stereotactic radiosurgery for treatment of large arteriovenous malformations of the brain. *AJNR* 16:299–306.
86. Sorimachi T, Koike T, Takeuchi S, Minakawa T, Abe H, Nishimaki K, Ito Y, Tanaka R (2000) Embolization of cerebral arteriovenous malformations achieved with polyvinyl alcohol particles: angiographic reappearance and complications. *AJNR* 20:1323–1328.
87. Ha-Kawa SK, Kariya H, Murata T, Tanaka Y (1998) Successful transcatheter embolotherapy with a new platinum microcoil: the Berenstein Liquid Coil. *Cardiovasc Intervent Radiol* 21:297–299.
88. Yakes WF, Rossi P, Odink H (1996) How I do it. Arteriovenous malformation management. *Cardiovasc Intervent Radiol* 19:65–71.
89. Vinuela F (1995) The safety and effectiveness of brain arteriovenous malformation embolization using acrylic and particles (Comment). *Neurosurgery* 37:615–616.
90. Deveikis JP, Manz HJ, Luessenhop AJ, Caputy AJ, Kobrine AI, Schellinger D, Patronas N (1994) A clinical and neuropathologic study of silk suture as an embolic agent for brain arteriovenous malformations. *AJNR* 15:263–271.
91. Song JK, Eskridge JM, Chung EC, Blake LC, Elliott JP, Finch L, Niakan C, Maravilla KR, Winn HR (2000) Preoperative embolization of cerebral arteriovenous malformations with silk sutures: analysis and clinical correlation of complications revealed on computerized tomography scanning. *J Neurosurg* 92:955–960.
92. Schmutz F, McAuliffe W, Anderson DM, Elliott JP, Eskridge JM, Winn HR (1997) Embolization of cerebral arteriovenous malformations with silk: histopathologic changes and hemorrhagic complications. *AJNR* 18:1233–1237.
93. Murayama Y, Vinuela F, Ulhoa A, Akiba Y, Duckwiler GR, Gobin YP, Vinters HV, Greff RJ (1998) Nonadhesive liquid embolic agent for cerebral arteriovenous malformations: preliminary histopathological studies in swine rete mirabile. *Neurosurgery* 43:1164–1175.
94. Duckwiler GR, Dion JE, Vinuela F, Reichmann A (1992) Delayed venous occlusion following embolotherapy of vascular malformations in the brain. *AJNR* 13:1571–1579.
95. Miyasaka Y, Kurata A, Tanaka R, Irikura K, Yamada M, Fujii K (1998) The significance of retrograde thrombosis following removal of arteriovenous malformations in elderly patients. *Surg Neurol* 49:399–405.
96. Han MH, Chang KH, Han DH, Yeon KM, Han MC (1994) Preembolization functional evaluation in supratentorial cerebral arteriovenous malformations with superselective intraarterial injection of thiopental sodium solution. *Acta Radiologica* 35:212–216.
97. Rauch RA, Vinuela F, Dion J, Duckwiler G, Amos EC, Jordan SE, Martin N, Jensen ME, Bentson J (1992) Preembolization functional evaluation in brain arteriovenous malformations: the ability of superselective amytal test to predict neurologic dysfunction before embolization. *AJNR* 13:309–314.
98. Chaloupka JC, Vinuela F, Sakai N, Vinters HV, Robert J, Duckwiler GR (1994) Potential toxic effects of superselective injection of amobarbital sodium on microvasculature: a study in an animal model. *AJNR* 15:1529–1536.

99. Rauch RA, Vinuela F, Dion J, Duckwiler G, Amos EC, Jordan SE, Martin N, Jensen ME, Bentson J, Thibault L (1992) Preembolization functional evaluation in brain arteriovenous malformations: the superselective amytal test. *AJNR* 13:303–308.
100. Aletich VA, Debrun GM, Koenigsberg R, Ausman JI, Charbel F, Dujovny M (1997) Arteriovenous malformation nidus catheterization with hydrophilic wire and flow-directed catheter. *AJNR* 18:929–935.
101. Mathis JM, Evans AJ, DeNardo AJ, Kennett K, Crandall JR, Jensen ME, Dion JE (1997) Hydrophilic coatings diminish adhesion of glue to catheter: an in vitro simulation of NBCA embolization. *AJNR* 18:1087–1091.
102. Pile-Spellman J, Young WL, Joshi S, Duong H, Vang MC, Hartmann A, Kahn RA, Rubin DA, Prestigiacomo CJ, Ostapkovich ND (1999) Adenosine-induced cardiac pause for endovascular embolization of cerebral arteriovenous malformations: technical case report. *Neurosurgery* 44:881–886.
103. Debrun GM, Aletich V, Ausman JI, Charbel F, Dujovny M (1997) Embolization of the nidus of brain arteriovenous malformations with n-butyl cyanoacrylate. *Neurosurgery* 40:112–120.
104. Dion JE, Mathis JM (1994) Cranial arteriovenous malformations. The role of embolization and stereotactic surgery. *Neurosurg Clin North Am* 5:459–474.

Index

Page numbers in *italic type* refer to illustrations.

Abciximab, 5, 8, 10–11, *10*
Accessory meningeal artery, 265
ACT. *See* Activated clotting time
Activated clotting time (ACT), 8, 12
Aggrastat. *See* Tirofiban hydrochloride
Air-bag injury, *188*
Aneurysm(s), 55–91
   arterial sacrifice, 81, 83, 85, *87*, 88, *89–90*, 91
   basilar artery, *24*, 74–75
   basilar-tip embolization, 63–64
   carotid-ophthalmic, 61, 65–66
   cavernous carotid, *62*, 85, *87*
   coil embolization of intracranial, 55–57, *56–59*, 60, 61–66, *65*, *67*
   complications of therapy, 76, *77–78*, 79
   double microcatheter for wide-necked, *71*
   intracranial, 24, *24*, *25*, 65, 88, *88–90*, 91
   large ruptured posterior communicating, *61*
   left posterior communicating, *56*, *58*
   occlusion with preservation of parent artery, *56*
   occlusion with sacrifice of parent artery, *57*
   packing and first coils, *67*, *69*
   reconstruction with balloons or stents, 67, *68–69*, 70–71, *70–75*, 76
   rupture during coil embolization, 76, *77*, 77, *78*, 79
   subarachnoid, 88, *89–90*, 91
   3D coils for initial framing, *70*
   thromboembolic complications during embolization, 79–80, *81–86*
   vertebrobasilar junction, *26*, *59*
Angiography
   flush system, 25, 27, *27*, 28
   rotational 3D, 23–24, *25*, *26*
   spinal, *215*, *218*
   thrombolysis following embolus during, *271*
Angioplasty
   balloon, 40, 42–43, *100*, *112*, 123, 125–27, *126–27*, *142–53*, 152–54
   brachiocephalic artery, *100*
   carotid, 95–116
   distal vessel, *150–51*
   intracranial, 121–37, *122*, *152*
   microembolic events during, 106–7
   protection during carotid, 107, *108–9*
   proximal-to-distal vasospasm, *145*
   restenosis, *126–27*
   subclavian artery, *102*, *112*, *115*
   in thrombolytic therapy, 277, *277–78*, 279
   vertebral artery, 107, 109, 111, *111*, *112*, 113–14, *122–23*
Angiojet rheolytic catheter, 281, *282*, *283*
Angioseal device, *52*
Antiplatelet therapy, 1–12, *2–5*

Arterial laceration, *253*
Arterial puncture, 273–74
Arterial sheath, 274
Arterial thrombosis, 1, *3*
Arteriotomy, 47, *50*, *51*, *52*, 53
Arteriovenous malformations
    intramedullary spinal, 222, *223*, 224
    intraparenchymal spinal, *223*
    paravertebral, 214, *216–17*
    See also Arteriovenous malformations of brain; Dural arteriovenous malformations
Arteriovenous malformations of brain, 291–307
    coils, 304
    complications, 304–5
    cyanoacrylate adhesive, 296, 299, 303
    embolization therapy, 296, *297–302*, 299, 303–7
    glue injection, *301–2*, 306
    microcatheter choice, 305–6
    microsurgical treatment, 293–94
    normal perfusion pressure breakthrough, 293
    physiological steal in vicinity of, 292–93
    polyvinyl alcohol particles, 303–4
    postembolization management, 306–7
    radiotherapy for, 294–96
    risk factors predictive of hemorrhage, 292
    superselective functional testing, 305
Ascending palatine artery, 265
Ascending pharyngeal artery, 265
Aspirin, 4, 5–6
Atherosclerotic disease, 7, *56*, 121, 134–35
ATLANTIS r-tPA trial, 271

Balloon(s)
    for aneurysm, 61, *63–64*, 67, 70–71, *71–73*
    angioplasty, *40*, 42–43, *100*, 112, 123, 125–27, *127*, *142–53*
    for carotid cavernous fistulas, *179–87*, 184, 187
    clot disruption, *274–75*, 276–77
    coil embolization, *63–64*, 66, *71–73*
    Commodore, 148
    detachable, 31, *31*, *32*, 33, *33*, 34, *180–83*,184
    Endeavor, 34, *58*, *64*, *145*, *150*, *152*, 276
    Fastealth, *150*
    latex, 31, *32*, *33*, 184
    nondetachable, 34, *182–83*, 187,
    papaverine versus angioplasty, *142–53*, 152–54
    as protection, *108–10*
    Ranger, *122–23*, *128–31*
    reconstructive technique, 67, 70–71
    Sentry, *149*, *274–75*
    silicone, 31, *33*, 184
    stents mounted by, *38*, 39, *39*, *40*, *41*
    test occlusion, 193–200, *194–200*
    wire-directed, *153*, 276–77, *284*
Basilar artery
    aneurysm, 24, *74–75*
    coil embolization of aneurysm, 74–75
    flow to, *122–23*
    focal lesion in proximal, *124*
    stenting, *133*
    thrombosis, 9, *270*, *272*
Bleeding. See Hemorrhage
Blood-brain barrier, 239, 241–42
Blunt injury, *250–51*
Brachiocephalic artery, *100–101*
Bradykinin, 241
Bragg peak, 295
Brain
    arteriovenous malformations, 291–307
    tumors, 239, 241–42

CAPTURE trial, 7, 10
Carotid angioplasty, 95–116
    in high-risk patients, 96, *97–103*, 98, 101
Carotid artery
    anatomy of internal branches, *230*
    aneurysm, *62*, 65
    catheterization, 47, *48*, *49*, 65
    devascularization of tumor, 232, *232–34*, 234
    external injuries, 252, 254
    external pseudoaneurysm, *249*
    injection, *232–33*
    internal injuries, 260–65, *266*
    right internal, *24*, *128–29*, *160*, *232–33*
    severe bleeding of external, *248*
    stenting, *96*, *98*, *99*, *101*, *103*, *104*
    test occlusion of internal, 193–95, *196*, 197
    vasospasm, *150*
    See also Carotid cavernous fistulas
Carotid cavernous fistulas, 177–90
    coil embolization, 187
    combination techniques in treatment, *186–87*
    early treatment, 177–78
    embolic complications following treatment, *185*
    endovascular treatment, 178
    indications for treatment, 178, 180–81
    materials and methods for occluding, *179–90*, 181, 184, 187, 190
    transorbital approach, 187, *189–90*, 190
Carotid-jugular compression protocol, 165–66, *166*

Carotid-jugular fistula, *260–61*
Catheters and catheterization, 27–28
    of carotid arteries, 47, *48*, *49*
    of cavernous sinus, 173, *174–75*, 176
    coaxial, 25
    rheolytic devices, 277, *283*, *284*, *285*
    spinal, *214*
    transorbital venous for carotid cavernous fistulas, *189–90*
    See also Microcatheter(s)
Cavernous carotid aneurysms, 62, 85, 87
Cavernous sinuses, *169*, *170*, *172–73*, *174–75*, 176
Cerebral hyperperfusion syndrome, 101
Cerebral steal, 292
Cerebral vasospasm. *See* Vasospasm
Cerebral venous thrombosis. *See* Venous thrombosis
Cervical arterial dissection, 113–14
Chemotherapy, 239, 241–43
Clopidogrel, 6–7
Clot disruption, *274–75*, *276–77*, 282
Coagulation
    antiplatelet therapy, 1–12, *3*
    cascade, *5*
    heparin sodium, 12–14
    hirudin/lepirudin, 14
    protamine sulfate, 14–15
    thrombolytic agents, 15
Cobalt Gray equivalent, 295
Coil embolization, 55–57, *56–66*
    balloon-assisted, *63–64*, 66, *71–73*
    of carotid cavernous fistulas, 187
    disadvantages, 62, 65, 67
    rupture, 76, *77-78*, 79
    stent-assisted, *73–75*
    thromboembolic complications, 79, *81–86*
Coils
    Guglielmi detachable, 34, *34*, 35, *36*, *36*, 37, 55, *57*
    push and liquid, 37, *37*
Commodore balloon, *148*
Coronary artery stenting, 104–6
Cribriform plate, *167*
Cyanoacrylate adhesive, 296, 298, 303

Dehydrated alcohol, 304
Dipyridamole, *4*
Dragging loop method, *30*
Dural arteriovenous malformations, 159–76
    carotid-jugular compression protocol, 165–66, *166*
    of cavernous sinuses, *169*, *170*, *172–73*, *174–75*, 176
    clinical presentation, 164–65, *165*

of cribriform plate, *167*
endovascular treatment, 167, *168–71*, 172–73, *172–75*, 176
of foramen magnum, *165*
indications for treatment, 166–67
of left transverse sinus with antegrade venous flow, *171*
radiotherapy, 176
of right sigmoid sinus with antegrade parenchymal venous drainage, *172*
risks related to venous sysem, 159, *160–64*
transarterial embolization, 172
transorbital embolization of cavernous sinus, 172–73
transvenous catheterization of cavernous sinus in absence of inferior petrosal sinus, 173, *174–75*, 176
transvenous embolization, 167, *168–71*, 172, *172*, 173
transverse sinus, *173*
See also Carotid cavernous fistulas
Dural sinus thrombosis, *282*, *284*, *286–88*

ECASS. *See* European Cooperative Acute Stroke Study
Electrophysiologic intraprocedural monitoring, 224, 305
Embolization
    of arteriovenous malformations of brain, 296, *297*, *298*, *299–302*, 303-7
    transarterial of dural arteriovenous malformations, 172
    transorbital of dural arteriovenous malformations, 172–73
    transvenous of dural arteriovenous malformations, 167, *168–69*, 172, *173*
    See also Coil embolization
Endarterectomy, 106–7
Endeavor balloon, 34, *58*, *64*, 145, *150*, *152*, 276
Endolymphatic sac tumor, *240*
EPIC trial, 7, 8, 10
EPILOG trial, 7, 8, 10
Epistaxis, 258–60, *258–59*, 262, 265–66
EPISTENT trial, 7
Eptifibatide, *5*, 11
European Cooperative Acute Stroke Study (ECASS), 269, 271-7

Facial artery, *252–54*, 262
Fastealth balloon, *150*
Flush system, 25, 27, *27*, 28

Gamma knife radiosurgery, 296
Gelfoam, 44, *44*
GFX stent, *113*, *114*, *130–31*, 133-7

Glanzmann's thrombasthenia, 4
Glomus tumors, 235, 237–39, *239–40*
Glycoprotein Ib/IX, 1
Glycoprotein IIb/IIIa, 3, *3*, 4, *4*, 5, 7–8
Glycoprotein receptors, 1, *2*, 4
Glycopyrrolate, 114, 116
Greater descending palatine artery, 262
Guglielmi detachable coil, 34, *34*, 35, 36, *36*, 37, 55, *57*
Gunshot wound, *254*

Head and neck tumors, 237, *239–40*, 242–43
Head injury, *250–51*
Helium ion beam therapy, 295
Hemorrhage
    carotid artery, *248*
    delayed rebleeding from arterial laceration, *253*
    epistaxis, 258–60, *258–59*, 262, 265–66
    general principles for control of, 247, 249, 251–52
    intraparenchymal, *162*
    left temporal lobe, *163*
    post-tonsillectomy, 254–56, *255–57*, 258
    risk in arteriovenous malformations of brain, 292
    subarachnoid, *26*, 56, *57*, *61*, *63–64*, 148
    triage, 247
Heparinoids, 13
Heparin sodium, *5*, 12–14
Hirudin, *5*, 14

IMPACT-II trial, 7, 11
Inferior petrosal sinus, 173
Integrilin. *See* Eptifibatide
Integrin α2β1, 2, 4
Intraarterial chemotherapy, 239, 241–42
Intraarterial thrombolysis, 270–73, 279
Intracranial stenotic lesions, 125
Intracranial venous hypertension, *160–61*
Intramedullary spinal arteriovenous malformations, 222, *223*, 224
Intraparenchymal hemorrhage, *162*
Intraparenchymal spinal arteriovenous malformations, *223*
Intravenous cannula, *22*
Introducer sheaths, 27–28

Juvenile nasal angiofibroma, *230–31*, 233, *235–36*, 237–39

Kiesselbach's plexus, 259

Latex balloon, 31, *32*, 33, 184
Lepirudin, 14

LINAC. *See* Linear accelerator radiosurgery
Lindegaard carotid index, 141
Linear accelerator radiosurgery (LINAC), 295–96
Lingual artery, *252–54*
Liquid coils, 37, *37*
Liquid embolic agents, 43
Little's area, 259
Low-molecular weight heparin, 13–14
Luer-lock syringe, *23*

Manometer, *39*
Meningeal artery, *163*, *164*, 265
Meningiomas, 229
Metastatic paraganglioma, *225*
Metastatic renal cell carcinoma, *238*
Methylmethacrylate, 206, 209, 212–13
Microcatheter(s)
    advancing, 47
    for aneurysm, *58*, 70–71, *73*
    for arteriovenous malformation embolization, 305–6
    for clot disruption, 276
    and detachable balloons, *32*, *180–81*, 184
    dragging loop method, *30*
    flow-directed, 28
    hubs, *22*
    wire-directed, 28, 31
Microembolic events, 106–7
Microwires, 28
Middle cerebral artery, *136*, *152–53*, 300
Myocardial infarction, 5–6

NASCET. *See* North American Symptomatic Carotid Endarterectomy Trial
National Institute of Neurological Disorders and Stroke (NINDS), 269–70
Neck tumors. *See* Head and neck tumors
Neutropenia, 6
Nidus, *300–302*
NINDS. *See* National Institute of Neurological Disorders and Stroke
NINDS trial of tPA, 269
North American Symptomatic Carotid Endarterectomy Trial (NASCET), 96–104
Nycomed system, *32*

Ophthalmic artery, *25*, *230*
Osteoporotic compression fractures, 203–4

Palmaz stent, 38, *100, 102*
Papaverine, 154
    side effects and risks, 154–55
    versus balloon angioplasty, *142–53, 152–54*
Paraganglioma, *225*
Paravertebral arteriovenous malformations/fistulas, 214, *216–17*
Perclose arteriotomy closure device, *50*
Perimedullary arteriovenous fistulas, 220, *221,* 222
Petrous bone, *240*
Physiologic steal in vicinity of AVM, 292–93
Platelets
    adhesion, activation, and aggravation, 1, *2, 3, 3,* 4
    antiplatelet therapy, 1–12
Plavix. *See* Clopidogrel
Polyvinyl alcohol, 43–44, *44,* 303–4
Posterior communicating artery, *61,* 146
Posterior inferior cerebellar artery, *130–31*
Postsurgical vascular injury, 258–59
PROACT II study, 271–72
Protamine sulfate, 14–15
Proton beam therapy, 295
Pseudoaneurysm, 88, *249, 253, 264*
PURSUIT study, 11
Push coils, 37

Radiation, 44–47, *45*
Radiotherapy, 176, 294–96
Radius self-expanding stent, *42*
Ranger balloon, *122–23, 128–31*
Refludan. *See* Hirudin
Renal cell carcinoma, *238*
ReoPro. *See* Abciximab
Restenosis, *124, 126–27*
RESTORE trial, 7
Rheolytic devices, 277, *283, 284, 285*
RMP-7, 241–42
Rotational 3D angiography, 23–24, *25, 26*

Safety balloon technique for CCF treatment, *180–84,* 187
Selverstone clamp, 65
Sentry balloon, *149,* 274–75
Sheath, 27–28, 274
Silicone detachable balloon, 31, *33,* 184
SMART stent, *41, 96–97, 110, 264*
Snake venom, 2, 5
Snare, 277
Sphenopalatine arteries, 262
Spine, 203–26
    angiography, *215, 218*

    arteriovenous malformations, 214–15, *216–219,* 219–220, *221, 222, 223,* 224
    catheters, *214*
    dural arteriovenous fistulas, 214–15, *218–19,* 219–20
    paravertebral arteriovenous malformations/fistulas, 214, *216–17*
    perimedullary arteriovenous fistulas, 220, *221,* 222
    tumor embolization, 224, *224–25,* 226
    vertebroplasty, 203–13
Stent(s), 38–42
    for aneurysm, 71, *73–74, 75, 75*
    balloon-mounted, *38, 39, 39, 40*
    basilar artery, *133*
    brachiocephalic artery, *100*
    carotid artery, *96, 98, 99,* 101, *103,* 104, *264*
    coil embolization, *73–75*
    coronary artery, 104–6
    coverage of posterior inferior cerebellar artery, *130–31*
    extracranial use of coronary, 40–41
    GFX, *113, 114, 130–31, 133–37*
    in high-risk patients, 96, *97–103, 98,* 101
    intracranial, 41–42, 121–37
    of intradural right vertebral artery, *132*
    medication protocol for extracranial, 114, 116
    medication protocol for intracranial, 135–36
    middle cerebral artery, *136–37*
    Palmaz, 38, *100–102*
    Radius, *103*
    restenosis, *124*
    self-expanding, 38, *41, 42*
    sizing, *99*
    "slotted tube," *111*
    SMART, *41, 96–97, 110, 264*
    subclavian artery, *102, 112, 115*
    for symptomatic cervical arterial dissection, 113–14
    in thrombolytic therapy, 277, *279*
    vertebral artery, 107, 109, 111, *111–14,* 113–14, *134–35*
    Wall, *41, 98, 99*
Stroke, 6, 10, 269–70
    See also Thrombolysis
Subarachnoid aneurysm, 88, *89–90,* 91
Subarachnoid hemorrhage, *26, 56, 57, 61, 63–64,* 148
Subclavian artery, *102,* 109, 111, *112, 115*
Superselective amytal testing, 305
Supraclinoid right internal carotid artery, *24*
Surgical clipping, 55–57, 62
Surpass balloon, *128–29*
Syringe, *23*

TCD. *See* Transcranial Doppler imaging
Thienopyridines, *4*, 6–7
Thrombocytopenia, 11, 13
Thromboembolic complications, 79–80, *81–86*
Thrombolysis, 269–79
    for basilar artery thrombosis, *270*
    contraindications, 279
    following embolus during angiography, *272*
    intraarterial, 270–73, 279
    technical and procedural considerations, 273–74, 276–77
Thrombolytic agents, *5*, 15
Thrombotic thrombocytopenic purpura, 6
Thyroid carcinoma, *224*, *238*
Ticlid. *See* Ticlopidine hydrochloride
Ticlopidine hydrochloride, 6
Tirofiban hydrochloride, *5*, 11–12
Tissue-type plasminogen activator, 15
Tonsillectomy, 254–56, *255–57*, 258
t-PA. *See* Tissue-type plasminogen activator
Transcranial Doppler imaging (TCD), 106–7, *110*
Transvenous embolization, 167, *168–69*, 172, *173*
Transverse facial artery, 265
Tumor(s)
    brain, 239, 241–42
    chemotherapy, 239, 241–43
    direct percutaneous puncture, 236
    embolization of spinal, 224, *224–25*, 226
    endolymphatic sac, *240*
    glomus, 235, 237–39, *239–40*
    head and neck, 237, *239–40*, 242–43
    juvenile nasal angiofibroma, *230–31*, 233, *235–36*, 237–39
    metastatic renal cell, *238*
    preoperative devascularization, 229, *230–35*, 234, 236
    spinal, 204–5
    thyroid, *224*, *238*

Urokinase, *5*, 15, 273, 283

Vascular injury, postsurgical, 258–59
Vasoseal device, *51*
Vasospasm
    diagnosis, 141
    early intervention, 146–47, 149, 152
    endovascular treatment, 139–55
    of intracranial left internal carotid artery, *150*
    long-term histologic effects, 141, 146
    papaverine versus balloon angioplasty, *142–53*, 152–54
    proximal-to-distal angioplasty, *145*
    risk factors for, 140
Venogram, 207, 209, *209*, 283
Venous hypertension, *160*
Venous thrombosis, *250–51*, 281–89
    dural sinus, *282*, *284*, *286–88*
    indications for endovascular treatment, 283–84
    techniques for endovascular treatment, 284, *285–88*, 287, 289
Vertebral artery
    angioplasty, 107, 109, 111, *112*, 113–14, *122–23*
    dangerous anastomosis to, *231*
    iatrogenic dissection of right, *265*
    injection, 24
    stenting, 107, 109, 111, *111–13*, *132*, *134–35*
    test occlusion, 193
    transbrachial approach to stenosis, *114*
Vertebral hemangioma, 204
Vertebrobasilar junction, *26*, *59*
Vertebro-jugular fistula, *262–63*
Vertebroplasty, 203–13
    for aggressive/malignant spinal tumors, 204–5
    exposure to methylmethacrylate vapors, 206
    injecting methylmethacrylate cement, *210–12*, 212–13
    mixing methylmethacrylate cement, 209, *210–11*, *212*
    needle approach, 207, *208*, 209
    for osteoporotic compression fractures, 203–4
    patient selection and screening, 207
    postprocedure patient care, 213
    postprocedure plain film and CTs, *213*
    recommended powder mixture, 209, 212
    risks and complications, 205–6
    techniques, 207
    venogram, 207, 209, *209*
    for vertebral hemangioma, 204
Virchow's triad, 1
von Willebrand factor, 1, 2, *2*, 5

Wall stent, *41*, *98*, *99*
Wires, 28, *29*, 39, 276
    See also Balloon(s), wire-directed